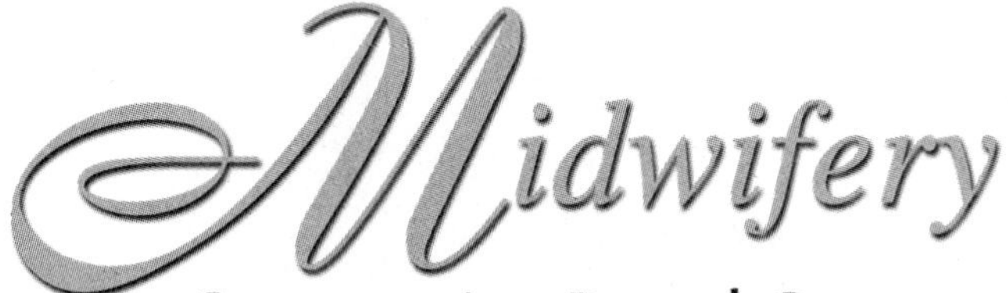

Community-Based Care
During the Childbearing Year

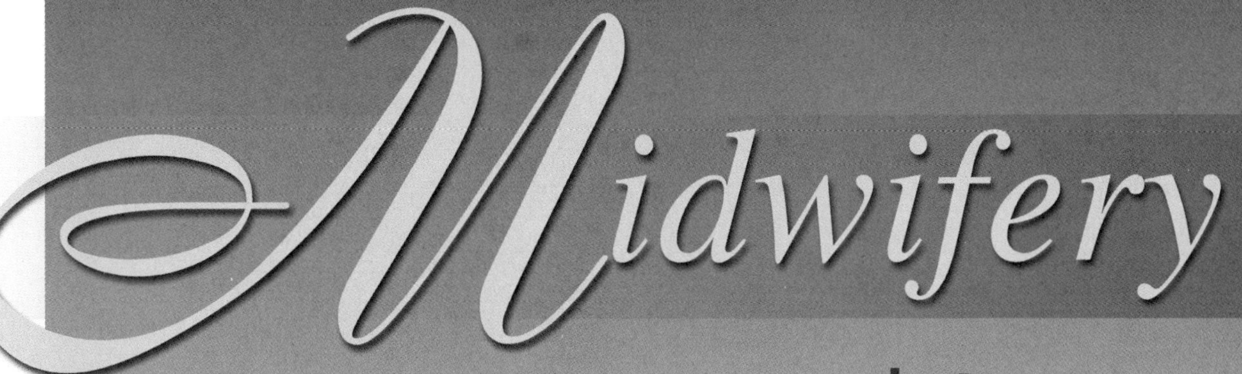

Midwifery

Community-Based Care During the Childbearing Year

Linda V. Walsh, CNM, MPH, PhD
Director, Midwifery Service at Stanford
Associate Professor
University of San Francisco
School of Nursing
San Francisco, California

with 185 *illustrations*

W.B. SAUNDERS COMPANY
A Harcourt Health Sciences Company
Philadelphia London New York St. Louis Sydney Toronto

W.B. SAUNDERS COMPANY
A Harcourt Health Sciences Company

The Curtis Center
Independence Square West
Philadelphia, Pennsylvania 19106

Library of Congress Cataloging-in-Publication Data

Walsh, Linda V.
Midwifery / Linda V. Walsh

p. cm.

Includes bibliographical references and index.

ISBN 0-7216-4716-2

1. Midwifery. 2. Community health services 3. Maternal health services. I. Title

RG950..W35 2001

618.2—dc21 2001020138

Vice President and Publishing Director, Nursing: Sally Schrefer
Senior Editor: Michael S. Ledbetter
Senior Developmental Editor: Lisa P. Newton
Project Manager: Deborah L. Vogel
Production Editor: Mary E. Drone
Design and Layout: Julia Ramirez
Cover photo courtesy of: Peggy S. Matteson

MIDWIFERY
Community-Based Care During the Childbearing Year
ISBN 0-7216-4716-2

Printed in the United States of America

Last digit is the print number: 9 8 7 6 5 4 3 2 1 TG/KPT

Contributors

Catherine Carr, CNM, DrPH
Assistant Professor
Department of Family and Child Nursing
University of Washington
Seattle, Washington

Linda Chapman, RN, DNSc
Professor
Samuel Merritt College
Oakland, California

Jeanne F. DeJoseph, CNM, PhD, FAAN
Assistant Professor (Retired)
University of California, San Francisco
San Francisco, California

Pam England, CNM, MA
Author, *Birthing From Within: an Extra-ordinary Guide to Childbirth Preparation*
Albuquerque, New Mexico

Rob Horowitz, PhD
Author, *Birthing From Within: an Extra-ordinary Guide to Childbirth Preparation*
Albuquerque, New Mexico

Barbara J. Petree, RN, MA
Director, Maternal Child Health Services
El Camino Hospital
Mountain View, California

Alexandra Schott, CNM, MSN
Faculty, Institute of Midwifery
Philadelphia University
Philadelphia, Pennsylvania

Anne Scupholme, CNM, MPH, FACNM
Director, Patient Care Services
Women's Hospital Center
Jackson Memorial Hospital
Miami, Florida

†**Henry O. Thompson,** M.Div., PhD
Adjunct Professor of Ethics
School of Nursing
University of Pennsylvania
Philadelphia, Pennsylvania

Joyce Thompson, CNM, DrPH
Professor, Associate Dean and Director of Graduate Studies and Professional Development
School of Nursing
University of Pennsylvania
Philadelphia, Pennsylvania

Maureen Wolfe, CNM, MSN
Faculty, Institute of Midwifery
Philadelphia University
Philadelphia, Pennsylvania

†Deceased

For Ed,
who, like a good midwife, expressed belief in my ability to deal with this labor and provided unwavering support throughout the process

Preface

Students in women's health care programs that prepare midwives, advanced nurse practitioners, physician associates, and physicians are faced with a wide selection of texts that address physiology, pathophysiology, and specialty areas of practice. Often a text that is strong in clinical management may not provide depth in pathophysiology. Likewise, many physiology and pathophysiology texts do not link the science with clinical decision-making. This text seeks to meet several distinct and essential needs for the learner and for the practicing midwife who seeks to supplement her or his level of knowledge and skills.

First, a solid understanding of the physiology of pregnancy is necessary to interpret data collected through historical and physical assessment. Chapters addressing physiology of pregnancy and continued presentation of physiologic considerations in clinical management are presented to reinforce the importance of understanding findings to identify and interpret deviations from normal.

Second, it is essential that the practitioner become adept at critiquing the professional literature. We are living in a society in which there is ever-increasing dissemination of new knowledge. Thus it is imperative that we prepare practitioners who are able to rapidly incorporate new knowledge into their practices. Such preparation will enhance practitioners' ability to adapt to a rapidly changing practice environment. This text incorporates research studies and findings to facilitate the practitioner's ability to "read the literature" and apply the findings to clinical decision making in a rational manner. The contributors to this book believe, with me, that developing practitioners who can base their management decisions on sound rationale will ultimately improve the quality of women's health care. Unlike texts that expect the practitioner to learn a "cookbook" approach to care delivery, this volume will challenge the reader to broaden the care options considered in order to meet the individual and community needs of childbearing women.

Third, practitioners must develop their own cultural competence to provide appropriate care in our multicultural communities. True women-centered care requires an understanding of these cultural influences on the decision to seek care and the acceptance or rejection of the care strategies suggested by a professional health care provider. It is expected that the integration of cultural aspects of care throughout the volume will stimulate the learner to consistently consider the impact of the woman's beliefs and values on her decision to seek care and follow through on health care recommendations.

Management of care, as used in this text, is the dynamic process of assessing the individual's health status and developing a plan to best meet the health needs of the woman and her child. The care recipient retains an active role in the care management process through communicating her concerns and needs to the provider and choosing strategies and interventions that are consistent with her beliefs and values. The content of this book is that which is seen to be essential for providers working with essentially healthy women. Through development of a thorough understanding of the wide range of "normal" in pregnancy, the clinician can best identify those situations in which consultation with and/or referral to another professional is necessary.

Linda V. Walsh

Acknowledgments

I have definitely come to appreciate that a book is not just the work of the author. Numerous individuals have contributed directly through writing, reading, and discussing the necessary content for this text. Others have contributed indirectly, guiding and shaping me as a midwife, thereby shaping the underlying philosophy of care represented in this volume. Although it is impossible to list everybody by name, several individuals and groups deserve special credit.

First and foremost, I would like to thank the thousands of women and families who have blessed me with the honor of participating in their care during pregnancy and birth. As I often tell students, I continue to learn from women (even after over 20 years of practice), and it is the "taking in" of women's experiences that has made me the midwife I am today. I would also like to thank the many midwives, physicians, and nursing colleagues who have supported me as I pursued my midwifery practice in a variety of sites. They have instilled in me a deep respect for the positive aspects of a multidisciplinary team in providing care for women who often present with diverse needs during their pregnancies and childbearing.

Several midwife mentors who nurtured my professional growth in order to prepare me for a project of this magnitude stand out. Mary Shean, CNM, MPH, guided me through my midwifery education and provided not only the role modeling for professional practice but also the gentle support for me as a mother pursuing midwifery education in the mid-1970s. Her mothering of me when I was a student provided me with a model that I hope I have carried with me as I teach midwifery and undergraduate nursing students. Joyce Thompson, CNM, DrPH, provided me with guidance as I developed my skills as an educator. Many of the issues addressed in this book reflect the expertise she demonstrated as she developed midwifery education with a community focus. Jeanne DeJoseph, CNM, PhD, continues to influence my research activities, helping me to maintain a feminist orientation to ensure that women themselves remain central in our practices and in our research.

I also would like to thank my midwife colleagues in the Midwifery Service at Stanford for sharing their expertise and wisdom at our weekly midwife meetings. Elizabeth Loftus, CNM, MPH, Christine Ludwick, CNM, MSN, Suzi Saunders, CNM, MSN, and Barri Durning, CNM, MSN—you will probably see many of our discussions reflected in these chapters. I would especially like to thank Elizabeth for her wisdom and sharing in discussions about the philosophic and spiritual aspects of midwifery care. These discussions continue to validate what I see as the soul of midwifery.

Of course, no text can reach the bookstores without the expertise and support of the editorial staff. Michael Ledbetter has provided the leadership in moving this from thousands of pages of chapter manuscripts to its final form. Victoria Legnini provided assistance in obtaining the reviews of the chapters, and Lisa Newton and Mary Drone provided the necessary editing and manuscript preparation. With their quick turnaround of drafts, I have come to believe that they must not sleep. I would also like to thank the contributors—colleagues whom I respect tremendously. They contributed not only their expertise in developing their chapters but also significant time in responding to reviewers' comments, thereby strengthening the content.

Finally, the development of this book would not have been possible without the support of my family. They gave me the time and space to add this project to an already busy professional schedule. In doing so they recognized and supported my belief that this would be a significant contribution to the midwifery profession and ultimately to the women and families we serve. For this I am deeply grateful.

Brief Contents

Contents

Unit I

Maternal-Infant Care in the Community

Chapter 1

Midwifery—A Community-Based Model of Care for Childbearing Women

PHILOSOPHY OF CARE FOR CHILDBEARING WOMEN

Health care providers in the United States and most western societies, as well as health care consumers, have come to equate obstetrics with all aspects of pregnancy. However, obstetrics is only one small part of the health care and social support needed to ensure that women and their families experience an environment and have access to resources that will optimize health status for mothers and infants. The World Health Organization (WHO), in its evaluation of the use of birth technology, identified the "fundamental conflict over the way we conceptualise health care" (Wagner, 1994, p. 6). The WHO Perinatal Study Group notes that the "social model of health care conflicts with the medical model. The conflict is the sharpest in the areas of birth and death, in which the social model seems to offer an important contribution to services based on the orthodox medical model" (Wagner, 1994, p. 6). Their recommendations challenge us to reform health care in a way that shifts the paradigm of care from the current disease identification and treatment model to a health promotion model.

When one examines both the common obstetric texts and journals and the rituals surrounding prenatal care and birth, one sees that the obstetrics specialty of medicine is based on a pathology paradigm rather than a health paradigm. This underlying belief system conflicts with the needs of childbearing women, most of whom experience healthy pregnancies. Since its development in the 1930s, the obstetrics specialty has placed an emphasis on the diseases of pregnancy—certainly necessary for improving the health and pregnancy outcomes of women experiencing medical problems. This approach has had a significant influence on the way providers and the general population view childbearing. The concentration of effort to understand and treat medical problems in pregnancy has led to a de-emphasis on the healthy aspects of pregnancy and a subtle devaluing of the supportive measures that facilitate maintenance of health and prevention of problems. High-tech interventions and equipment provide excitement in the field—excitement shared by providers and women alike. Used appropriately, these discoveries have improved the health status of a small proportion of mothers and infants. But overuse and routine reliance on biotechnology eventually limit our understanding of the normal processes of pregnancy and birth. This volume seeks to reestablish a balance between the management necessary for healthy pregnancy and that necessary when problems arise.

Midwifery is different from obstetrics. This is difficult for many comfortable with the American medical system to understand. Midwifery is not merely a subspecialty of obstetrics—a belief held by many physicians. Midwifery is a discipline with its own unique body of knowledge. This body of knowledge explores and explains the healthy aspects of pregnancy and birth, thereby providing rationale for the less intervening, supportive approach used in caregiving. It further incorporates aspects of management that identify problems or potential problems. This ongoing screening for problems identifies women for whom medical intervention is appropriate.

The management proposed in this text is based on a paradigm of health and preventive care that is consistent with the philosophy expressed internationally by the profession of midwifery. The American College of Nurse-Midwives philosophy notes:

> Certified nurse-midwives believe that every individual has the right to safe, satisfying health care with respect for human dignity and cultural variations . . . [and] believe the normal processes of pregnancy and birth can be enhanced through education, health care and supportive intervention.
>
> Nurse-midwifery care is focused on the needs of the individual and family for physical care, emotional and social support, and active involvement of significant others according to cultural values and personal preferences. The practice of nurse-midwifery encourages continuity of care; emphasizes safe, competent clinical management; advocates nonintervention in normal processes; and promotes health education for women throughout the childbearing cycle (American College of Midwives, 1989).

As used in this volume, midwifery is practiced by any practitioner who bases clinical assessment and decision-making on a paradigm of health promotion in the childbearing cycle. The philosophic belief system of midwifery needs to be seen as separate from the professional licensing of health care providers. Physicians and nurses may practice midwifery; they may demonstrate that practice by incorporating the belief system that includes respect for the normalcy of pregnancy, respect for human dignity and cultural differences, and advocacy for nonintervention in normal biophysical processes in their care. Conversely, providers licensed as midwives do not practice midwifery when they structure their practices on a paradigm based on the pathology of pregnancy and use routine interventions based on a biotechnical model of care. In this volume the terms *clinician* and *provider* are used to encompass the many licensed professionals who provide perinatal care services that demonstrate a midwifery philosophy.

Childbearing women and families are best served in a system of health and medical care that provides access to care appropriate for their specific needs. A multidisciplinary group of providers working collaboratively to ensure risk-appropriate care is the model that will best meet the needs of childbearing families. Collaboration, as used in this text, implies respect for the unique knowledge and skills brought by each care provider. Midwives, nurses, nutritionists, and social workers, as well as physicians, are accepted as experts in their own fields and scopes of practice. Each professional accepts responsibility for the aspect of care that is appropriate to her or his preparation. Thus the perinatologist is the expert in managing perinatal problems, whereas the midwife (or obstetrician or family practice physician practicing in a midwifery model) is the expert in addressing the needs of the healthy pregnant woman.

The collaborative approach to care differs from the traditional medical approach in another important way. The woman receiving pregnancy care becomes central to the caring process. Considering that pregnancy is a healthy experience for most women, women themselves should be seen as central to the decision-making process when determining care practices. Certainly other areas of medical care are also noting the effectiveness of the patient-centered approach. For example, individuals experiencing chronic illness are best served by a paradigm of care that differs from the traditional medical model based on frequent use of high-tech intervention. In non-acute care the individual (patient) becomes the expert in what best meets her or his needs. This is radically different from acute care in which the physician or other professional provider is the expert in the particular intervention believed to have a positive effect on the health outcome of the ill individual.

COMMUNITY AS BOTH SITE AND CULTURE

Community can be described both as the physical location of one's home and as the social milieu of a particular area. Most individuals live in community with others. Through community relationships individuals develop and support belief systems about family, health, and illness. These personal beliefs, along with family attitudes and group beliefs, provide the basis for decision-making in health maintenance and illness care.

Childbearing women have always sought support during pregnancy and birth from individuals who were respected for knowledge and skills that improved the chances for a healthy infant and mother. Before the relatively recent acceptance of medical men, particularly specialists in obstetrics, as birth attendants, women and their caregivers shared gender, ethnicity, language, and cultural beliefs. The move to providing care from home to institutions has changed the relationship between caregiver and care recipient dramatically. Although there has been a move to prepare a culturally diverse cohort of care providers, childbearing women usually share few cultural attributes with them.

The Golden Age of Public Health in the 1910s and 1920s and the turbulent times of the late 1960s and early 1970s provided increased interest in moving the center of care from the institution to the community. Public health nursing, with its development of community clinics and home-based services, provided a model of preventive health care that contributed to the decrease in infectious disease and infant mortality in the early part of the century. The Maternal-Infant Care (MIC) programs of the 1960s demonstrated the effectiveness of comprehensive services offered in community clinics. Primarily because of fiscal issues, institutions are once again developing community outreach sites. However, unless care systems that respect the community culture are developed, community members will not accept nor will they access these new services.

COMMUNITY HEALTH NEEDS OF CHILDBEARING WOMEN

Numerous studies have attempted to address the barriers that contribute to the poor use of prenatal care by women in the United States. Both financial and sociocultural factors have been noted. Expansion of the Title XIX program (Medical Assistance) has been one attempt to reduce financial and selected social barriers faced by low income women. Numerous programs and projects have attempted to minimize structural barriers to access such as transportation, child care, and location of clinical services. However, even with these programs, a large number of pregnant women still do not obtain early and consistent prenatal care.

Recent studies have attempted to identify reasons women seek or delay obtaining prenatal care. Campbell et al. (1995) found that, although most women sought care because they desired a healthy baby and/or wanted to maintain their own health, many women delayed care for financial reasons or because they thought that prenatal care was not necessary (p. 461). Their data suggest that a woman's attitude toward her health care provider is "a distinct and powerful factor" that correlates with her intent to enroll and continue in prenatal care. This finding was supported by the work of Leppert, Partner, and Thompson (1996, p. 141), who found that women identified "disinterest of the doctor, . . . lack of respect from doctors, . . . and denial of the privilege of seeing the same doctor at each appointment" as factors that prevented them from seeking prenatal care. Focus group participants believed that "providers do not understand the difficulties they have in getting to appointments on time . . . and that patients on public assistance do not receive a great deal of respect from doctors." The authors argue that the "culture of medicine" often outweighs the ethnicity and personal culture of the provider as a factor that dissuades women from seeking care.

If the needs of women during the childbearing year are to be met, it is essential that mechanisms be developed to enhance the compatibility of the "culture of medicine" with its emphasis on provider as expert, reliance on tests and interventions, and rigid structure with the more social and cultural structure of community-based sites. Innovative programs are being implemented to increase providers' understanding of the cultural components of care. Examples include providing medical, midwifery, and nursing students with experience in community clinics and homes, as well as developing different systems for providing care. Physical removal from the sheltered culture of the medical teaching institution provides an opportunity to appreciate the "real world" experienced by women and their families. Altering provider rotations in a way that enhances continuity of care holds promise for enhancing the development of relationships among providers and their patients.

FROM HOME TO HOSPITAL: HISTORY OF CARE OF CHILDBEARING WOMEN IN THE UNITED STATES

Communities have always identified women who possessed skills and wisdom to assist childbearing women. Although it is intuitive that the indigenous people in North America must have had birth assistants, little is known about their practices. Early midwifery in the United States was strongly influenced by the western European development of midwifery. What little we know about early midwifery comes from midwifery texts, oaths of office, church documents addressing concerns about the association between midwifery and witchcraft, and essays by individuals who observed practice (Achterberg, 1991). Formal education for midwives had begun in the sixteenth century when the Roman physician Soranus' teachings were printed in a book for German midwives. Soranus had written in the fifth century BC that the midwife "must have a good memory; be industrious and patient, moral so as to inspire confidence; be endowed with a healthy mind, and have a strong constitution; and finally she must have long delicate fingers with nails cut short." The midwife was expected to "encourage the patient by cheerful talk, to help her sympathetically, and to be unflinching in any danger so as not to lose her head when giving advise" (Towler and Bramall, 1986). He argued that literacy was essential for the midwife and that preparation should include theoretic and practical education. His teachings proved to be so popular that the German work was translated into English and printed as *The Byrth of Mankynde* in 1540. The first midwife to publish a text was Louise Bourgeois Boursier in 1626. Her writings were translated into *The Compleat Midwives Practice Enlarged,* in which she addressed the consideration of induction of labor before term when there is a contracted pelvis, discussed management of difficult deliveries, and warned midwives of the risk of contracting syphilis when caring for infected women.

Evidence suggests that societies have usually developed formal expectations of birth attendants. Early oaths of office promulgated in Europe reveal the responsibilities held by midwives and the relationship between the midwife and government and church authorities. Church records in England document one oath taken in 1567:

> I, Eleanor Pead, admitted to the office and occupation of a midwife, will faithfully and diligently exercise the said office according to such cunning and knowledge as God hath given me, and that I will be ready to heal and aid as well poor as rich women being in labour and travail of child, in exercising and executing of my said office. Also I will not permit or suffer that any woman being in labour or travail shall name any other to be the father of her child, than only he who is the right and true father thereof; and that I will not suffer any other body's child to be set, brought or laid before any woman delivered of child in the place of her natural child, so far forth as I can know and understand. Also I will not use any kind of sorcery or incantation in the time of travail of any woman; and that I will not destroy the child born of any woman, nor cut, nor pull of the head thereof, or otherwise dismember or hurt the same, or suffer it to be hurt or dismembered by any manner of way or means. Also that at the ministration of the sacrament of baptism in the time of necessity, I will use apt and accustomed words of the same sacrament (Towler and Bramall, 1986).

Oaths of office typically identified standard obligations of midwives. First, midwives were expected to provide care to all women, regardless of ability to pay. Many communities used public funds to pay midwives for their services. Midwives were expected to document paternity, both to ensure paternal support of children and to identify heirs to social standing and assets. In societies in which there might be incentives for swapping children at birth (for example, when a male heir was desired), it was expected that the moral character of the midwife would protect the natural bond between mother and infant.

Oaths also reflected the prevailing religious beliefs. The Church's decision that midwives could baptize infants, a sacrament in the domain of the clergy, was the result of two concerns. First, since there was high infant mortality in the sixteenth century, there was concern that the infant would die before a priest could be summoned. Concern for the soul of the innocent infant supported the act of baptism at the time of birth by someone other than the priest. Second, church officials were concerned that if midwives were not given sanction to work within the usual church teachings, the midwives would use pagan rituals. Although officials respected the work of midwives, there were also fears of midwives' supernatural powers. Indeed, many of the women prosecuted and burned during the witch trials were midwives.

State rather than church regulation of midwifery was introduced in England in 1550 when King Henry VIII created a system in which the bishop of the diocese and a doctor of "physicke" examined midwives. Midwives who did not obtain a license could be imprisoned and/or excommunicated. Enforcement was lax, and most midwives continued to practice without taking an oath (Achterberg, 1991). This method of licensing had components that were reproduced in future efforts to regulate midwives in Europe and America. Registration or licensing was usually controlled by a board or committee of male physicians rather than midwives, and midwifery practice was restricted to the attendance at "normal" births, a term that could be subjectively defined by physicians.

Before the seventeenth century, few medical men were interested in providing care during childbearing. Barber surgeons were occasionally summoned when destructive instruments were needed to deliver a dead fetus, or medical men were called when medical problems arose that the midwife could not handle. The eighteenth century work of William Smellie (identification of mechanisms of labor) and William Hunter (study of the pregnant uterus) stimulated interest in medical management of childbirth, and obstetrics was increasingly introduced in medical school lectures. Even with this interest, until the twentieth century most physicians completed medical education without witnessing a birth.

Midwives in America, like physicians, surgeons, and apothecaries, worked in a largely unregulated environment until the mid-1800s. Even during the colonial period, the Church of England did not require midwives to take oaths of office. However, some local jurisdictions did regulate practitioners. In 1716 New York enacted a law that required midwives to take an oath in which they promised to be "diligent and faithful and ready to help every woman labouring with child as well as the poor as the sick" (Walsh, 1991, p. 8). In addition, midwives promised to assign proper paternity to the child, to practice safely, and to send for "expert midwives" when complications were identified.

Although some medical school faculty allowed midwives to attend their lectures, most schools banned women from enrollment. Midwives continued to be prepared through apprenticeships with an experienced midwife or were self-taught through the mid-nineteenth century. Ulrich's analysis of Martha Ballard's diary found that midwives did not restrict their practices to childbearing (Ulrich, 1990). Mrs. Ballard was called to care for the sick, and, when necessary, prepare the dead. She was skilled in the preparation of salves, syrups, pills, teas, and ointments; and her diary entries document her efforts to control bleeding, reduce swelling, dress burns, and treat numerous diseases, including tuberculosis and scarlet fever. The midwife's ability to provide a variety of services put her in competition with the general physicians in communities and most likely was a factor in the move to eliminate midwifery in this country.

Increased immigration from southern and eastern Europe in the latter half of the nineteenth century brought populations who respected and supported midwifery care for childbearing women. Proprietary schools of midwifery were opened by European midwives and physicians interested in promoting formal education similar to that available in their countries of origin. These schools suffered many of the same problems as the proprietary medical schools of the time—financial instability, limited clinical experience, and lack of a sound theoretic base (Walsh, 1991)—and by 1900 essentially all of them had closed.

By 1910 health professionals and politicians were forced to acknowledge that the United States ranked below other industrialized countries in prevention of maternal and infant deaths. From 1903 to 1912 women activists led by Lillian Wald lobbied for a federal bureau to oversee the protection of children. In 1912 the bill establishing the Children's Bureau, a Division of the Department of Commerce and Labor, was signed into law, and one of the first activities was an investigation of the cause of infant deaths. Although collection of birth and death statistics was not uniform throughout the country, the Bureau estimated that the infant death rate was approximately 124 to 158 per 1000 live births (Ladd-Taylor, 1992). This rate was unacceptably high. The factor that was most strongly associated with infant death was poverty. Women who were widowed or abandoned often resorted to employment that involved long hours in unsafe factory conditions. The Bureau's work provided some of the earliest evidence of the link between maternal health and infant survival.

The Bureau's success in lobbying for federal funding to support maternal-child preventive care projects culminated in the passage of the Sheppard-Towner Maternity and Infancy Act in 1921. Although the act did not directly address midwifery care, it indirectly influenced the demise of midwifery as a central component of childbearing care in the United States. First, by addressing the importance of prevention and treatment of medical problems during pregnancy, the funded projects forced physicians to recognize the association between prenatal services and decreased maternal and infant mortality and morbidity. As prenatal screening and education moved into the services offered by obstetric specialists, they became accepted as medical interventions rather than nursing, midwifery, or social interventions. Second, although the midwifery training projects taught by public health nurses were meant to improve standards of care, they further marginalized midwifery as a secondary system for women without access to obstetricians.

Midwives became an easy target as a source of the unacceptably high maternal and infant mortality rates. Physician arguments about the "midwife problem" in the first two decades of the 1900s reveal gender, race, and ethnic prejudices. The midwife was portrayed as a woman who "goes to the scene of the labor in the ordinary dirty clothes that she has been wearing while doing her household work, taking her satchel containing a handful of absorbent cotton . . . with a few strings or soiled tape for tying off the cord" (Kosmak, 1913).

Other physicians portrayed midwifery practice as follows:

> The midwife is called in question today not because of the popular demand for her services, but because investigation into disease and death has revealed her working in filthy surroundings, and has shocked the medical and lay public into action. The midwife is willing to undertake maternity work that no well-trained obstetrical nurse would think of attempting because in the first place she is ignorant of the situation; she has the overconfidence of half-knowledge; she is usually unprincipled, and callous of the feelings and welfare of her patients and anxious only for her fee (Emmons and Huntingdon, 1912, p. 400).

Although it is clear that some midwives were not well prepared to meet the needs of childbearing women, review of data suggests that maternal and infant mortality rates associated with midwifery care were similar to or less than those of physician-attended births (Devitt, 1979a, 1979b). In many areas midwives worked very closely with physicians in relationships that were collegial rather than supervisory (Borst, 1988; Litoff, 1978; Walsh, 1994). However, even in areas in which midwives were well respected and an integral part of the community, pregnant women increasingly sought care from physicians. Reasons for the move from midwifery to obstetric care include (1) the public's acceptance of the belief that birth was dangerous and required medical intervention; (2) the influence of women reformers who campaigned for the *right* to medical care for all women; (3) the effect of "Americanization" of immigrant families; and (4) the decrease in midwives available to accept cases (Walsh, 1991).

It is interesting to note that, even as the numbers of midwife-attended births decreased, maternal and infant vital statistics did not improve. In fact, maternal mortality increased from 1915 to 1930, most likely because of the increase in medical interventions during labor and birth. A report issued by the New York Academy of Medicine following a 2-year study of the causes of maternal mortality found that the maternal mortality of women cared for by midwives at any point during labor was 1.6 per 1000 live births compared to 4.5 per 1000 in physician-attended cases. Even with well-conducted studies suggesting the positive impact that a midwifery model of care would have on the health and well-being of women and infants, the U. S. health system embraced the medical model of care for childbearing women.

It has been argued that the transition of birth from the home to the hospital has had a stronger effect on women's loss of control over their childbirth experiences than the transition of provider from midwife to physician (Leavitt, 1986). Certainly the move to the hospital removed the woman from an environment where she and her female support system controlled the activities surrounding birth. If a woman disagreed with the birth attendant's care, she would dismiss her or him from the house. However, the move to hospital-based childbirth occurred in tandem with the increased use of technology in medical care. The availability of pharmacologic agents and technology coupled with the obstetric paradigm of controlling the birth process altered care practices dramatically. Since 1930 the use of routine episiotomy, analgesia and anesthesia, electronic fetal monitoring, routine administration of intravenous fluids, instrument-assisted vaginal births, and cesarean delivery have become the norm in American hospitals.

RE-EMERGENCE OF THE MIDWIFE

Early in the movement to decrease infant and maternal mortality, there was a call to develop a new category of birth attendant—the nurse-midwife. Physicians and nurses discussed the potential benefit of preparing obstetric nurses to provide prenatal care and attend normal births. Two distinct projects set the stage for the introduction of the nurse-midwife into the American health care system.

The Maternity Center Association (MCA) was established in New York City 1918 by a group of women and physicians who recognized the need for a coordinated system of prenatal care to address the unacceptably high infant and maternal mortality in the city (Kelly, 1980). By 1920 the MCA was instrumental in opening 30 maternity centers staffed with physicians and public health nurses. From its inception, the MCA recognized the value of prenatal education and became a leader in the production of educational materials for use in individual and group teaching. Under the leadership of Ralph Waldo Lobenstine, MD, chairman of the MCA Medical Board since 1918, and Hazel Corbin, RN, the Association for the Promotion and Standardization of Midwifery was formed in 1931 to establish a model nurse-midwifery service and education program. The Association proposed a curriculum for a nurse-midwifery education program based on the British model of midwifery education and modified to fit into the American health care system. Later in 1931 the Lobenstine Midwifery Clinic opened as a facility for providing prenatal and postpartum care and as a site in which public health nurses could gain midwifery skills. Intrapartum services were offered in the patient's home. The incorporation of nurse-midwives into the network of maternity centers drew opposition from physicians and resulted in physician resignations from the Board of Directors. The School of the Association for the Promotion and Standardization of Midwifery opened in 1932 with Hattie Hemschemeyer, RN, appointed director; Rose McNaught, a nurse-midwife in the Frontier Nursing Service, was the first faculty member. During the first year of operation, Hattie Hemschemeyer was both director and student, graduating as a nurse-midwife with the first class of six graduates in 1933. In 1934, facing financial difficulties, the educational program and the clinic were consolidated under the MCA. The MCA School of Nurse-Midwifery claims its roots as the first American nurse-midwifery education program from this merger.

The first nurse-midwifery service was started in 1925 when Mary Breckinridge brought British-prepared nurse-midwives to Kentucky in response to a plan organized by the Kentucky Committee for Mothers and Babies. In 1928 a change in the articles of incorporation changed the name to Frontier Nursing Service (FNS). Breckinridge had prepared for the project by doing a needs assessment in the mountain area around Hyden, Kentucky, identifying that most care of childbearing women was in the hands of older granny midwives. Public health nurses, trained in Britain as midwives, provided services in districts surrounding the small hospital FNS opened in Hyden. FNS had planned to develop an educational program from its inception, but financial constraints precluded the realization of that goal. The impact of the developing war in Europe on the ability of nurse-midwives to travel between England and the United States and the desire of British midwives to return to their homeland led to the establishment of the Frontier Graduate School of Midwifery in 1939.

Both the MCA and FNS projects demonstrated the safety of nurse-midwifery care, even while providing care to low income women at increased risk for poor pregnancy outcomes. A review of over 6000 births attended by MCA nurse-midwives found a maternal mortality rate of 0.9 per 1000 live births, compared to the national average of 10.4 per 1000 live births. The FNS statistics were equally impressive. A study of over 8000 FNS-attended births found a maternal mortality rate of 1.2 per 1000 live births compared to an overall national average of 3.4 per 1000 during the same time frame. Yet, even with these outcomes, nurse-midwifery did not expand significantly from the 1920s through the 1960s. MCA and FNS each had unique factors that prevented their nurse-midwives from achieving a central position in the health system. MCA, with its location in an urban area rich with influential physicians, had medical board members who ensured that all of the MCA educational materials contained the message that women should see an obstetrician during pregnancy. Nurse-midwives were accepted as appropriate educators of immigrant or granny midwives, administrators of maternal-child health agencies, and educators in schools of nursing. They were *not* promoted as autonomous care providers since they could ultimately become competition for the obstetricians. Those graduates of the MCA educational program who did practice as clinical nurse-midwives usually did so in international health projects, often in mission service.

Conversely, FNS did not have to deal with direct competition from physicians since eastern Kentucky was a medically underserved area. Physicians who served on the FNS medical board knew that their colleagues were not likely to practice in the poor remote area around Hyden and believed that nurse-midwives were the next best alternative to medical care (Ettinger, 1999). But, rather than recognizing FNS as a model that could benefit all childbearing women, health care professionals and the general public saw the project as a romantic and exotic model of care that was not in concert with modern American medicine.

CONSUMER PRESSURE TO CHANGE OBSTETRICS

Opportunities for American women to receive professional midwifery care remained limited until the late 1960s. As late as 1967 only 23% of nurse-midwives were in clinical practice, and almost one-quarter of those were in foreign service (American College of Nurse-Midwifery, 1968). Factors that increased the visibility of midwifery as an alternative to obstetric care included the women's movement and its campaign to give women more power over their health care, the childbirth education movement that empowered women to take back control in the birthing room, and the inclusion of nurse-midwives in federally funded and state-funded multidisciplinary projects to decrease the infant mortality rate and low-birth-weight rate. Midwifery also became visible through the resurgence of lay midwives and home birth, fueled by consumers who rejected the hospital-based obstetric model of care. Groups such as the National Association of Parents and Professionals for Safe Alternatives in Childbirth (NAPSAC), Association for Childbirth at Home International (ACHI), and Home-Oriented Maternity Experience (HOME) joined the La Leche League and International Childbirth Education Association (ICEA) in supporting parents' rights to unmedicated birth without intervention. It was pressure from consumers that led to many of the changes witnessed in maternity units in the 1970s and 1980s. Fathers demanded their right to be with their partners through labor and delivery; parents demanded relaxation of hospital restriction of support people during labor; and women increasingly questioned obstetric routines, including shaving the pubic hair, enemas in early labor, and routine episiotomy. Even with consumer demands for change, midwives continued to face significant barriers to practice. These barriers included restrictive state regulations that required formal contractual agreements with obstetricians, physician refusal to enter into agreements that would facilitate consultation with and referral of patients from midwives, lack of affordable professional liability insurance for midwives (particularly for out-of-hospital birth), lack of direct reimbursement for midwifery services, and continuing consumer confusion about the role and preparation of professional midwives.

THE DEVELOPMENT OF PROFESSIONAL ORGANIZATIONS

Professional organizations serve to define a profession's activities, identify requirements for entry into the profession, determine requirements for continuing competency assessment, promote the search for new knowledge, and communicate knowledge about the profession and its activities to others. The American College of Nurse-Midwives was created when a series of organizational changes left nurse-midwives without a professional body that would represent them. The nurse-midwives who were prepared in the 1930s and early 1940s were able to establish a section within the National Organization of Public Health Nurses (NOPHN). This section developed and implemented the first survey of nurse-midwives in the United States in 1949. When the NOPHN was reorganized and absorbed into the American Nurses Association (ANA) and the National League for Nursing (NLN), neither the ANA nor the NLN would establish a section or council specifically for nurse-midwives. Nurse-midwives were assigned to the Maternal and Child Health–National League for Nursing Interdivisional Council, a body that represented a broad maternity and pediatric constituency. Under the leadership of Sr. M. Theophane Shoemaker, nurse-midwives agreed to form The Committee on Organization in 1954. Within 2 months the group had surveyed nurse-midwives to identify beliefs about organizing, proposed functions for the new organization, developed a definition of the nurse-midwife, proposed educational standards, and circulated two organizational bulletins. In December 1954 46 nurse-midwives met and approved the definition of the nurse-midwife and a statement of the purposes of the organization.

There was much discussion regarding the possible mechanisms for organization. Letters requesting a conference group or council were approved for communication with ANA and NLN, respectively. Neither organization would provide a mechanism for nurse-midwives to be recognized as a specialty group. The Committee explored the potential for the American Association of Nurse-Midwives (AANM), essentially an alumnae association for FNS, to become a national organization. When AANM members did not show interest in the national move, the Committee on Organization proposed the creation of the American College of Nurse-Midwifery. Members of the Committee unanimously approved the proposal in May 1955. After exploration into the process for incorporation, the American College of Nurse-Midwifery was incorporated on November 7, 1955 in New Mexico with a charter membership of 124 nurse-midwives. (New Mexico was found to be the state in which it would be easiest and cheapest to incorporate.) On November 12 and 13, 1955, the first annual meeting of the American College of Nurse-Midwifery was held in Kansas City, Mo. Objectives of the corporation included the development and evaluation of standards for nurse-midwifery care of women and infants, the development and evaluation of standards for nurse-midwifery education, assistance in the development of nurse-midwifery services, accreditation of nurse-midwifery educational programs, determination of the eligibility of individuals to practice as nurse-midwives, establishment of channels for communication with other professional and nonprofessional groups, and promotion and dissemination of research.

One year later, both the American College of Nurse-Midwifery and the American Association of Nurse-Midwives were approved for membership in the International Confederation of Midwives (ICM), providing American nurse-midwives with an international forum for fostering high-quality health care for women and their infants. In 1969 the American Association of Nurse-Midwives and the American College of Nurse-Midwifery merged to form the American College of Nurse-Midwives (ACNM). ACNM has continued to provide leadership in setting standards for nurse-midwifery practice, education, and credentialing (see the ACNM website at www.midwife.org).

In 1981 Sr. Angela Murdoch, President of ACNM, brought together nurse-midwives and other midwives to discuss issues facing midwives in the United States. It was recognized that, although nurse-midwives had national representation in ACNM, there was no similar group for midwives who were not graduates of ACNM-accredited educational programs. Participants in the discussion proposed the formation of a "guild" that would expand communication among midwives, set educational guidelines for the training of midwives, set guidelines for basic competency and safety for practicing midwives, and form an identifiable professional organization for all midwives in the United States (MANA, 2000). In April 1982 almost 100 midwives met to discuss the procedure for creating the organization, and within several days a draft of articles of incorporation was developed, officers chosen, a plan to have a national conference in October 1982 was developed, and the name *Midwives Alliance of North America (MANA)* was approved. MANA has provided leadership in the creation of the Midwifery Education and Accreditation Council and the North American Registry of Midwives (NARM) certification process.

INTEGRATION OF MIDWIFERY INTO HEALTH CARE DELIVERY FOR CHILDBEARING WOMEN

During the last 20 years, midwives have increasingly been integrated into the health care system in the United States. Numerous studies, as well as committees, agencies, and professional bodies, have suggested that increased use of midwives, with their emphasis on health promotion and disease prevention, has the potential to improve the health status of women and their infants. One study exploring the factors associated with the increasing cesarean delivery rate concluded:

> Obstetric care in the United States is burdened by soaring costs and a paradoxic inability to bring rates of infant mortality in line with those of other developed countries. A look at the costs and outcomes of obstetric care demonstrates that a greater reliance on the use of certified nurse-midwives (CNMs) could help solve these problems. Midwifery has a positive track record with regard to quality of care, it represents a good value for health care dollars, and it rates high in client satisfaction (Gabay and Wolfe, 1997, p. 386).

However, even with strong evidence supporting midwifery as the standard of care for childbearing women, the United States has not fully accepted the professional midwife as an autonomous provider of care. Childbirth continues to be primarily a medical event, with 93% of births attended by physicians (most of whom are obstetricians) and 99% of births occurring in hospitals. A move to a midwifery model of care has the potential to decrease costs and the risks associated with inappropriate technologic intervention.

Several categories of midwives continue to practice in the United States. CNMs are individuals who are educated in the two disciplines of nursing and midwifery, have completed an educational program accredited by the ACNM, and are certified by the ACNM Certification Council. Certified midwives demonstrate knowledge and skills equivalent to those of CNMs, have completed an ACNM-accredited educational program, and are certified by the ACNM Certification Council. Certified professional midwives have successfully completed the NARM certification process but are not required to have completed an accredited educational program. Regardless of preparation, all midwives share the belief that there are specific hallmarks of midwifery care, including but not limited to*:

- Recognition that pregnancy and birth are normal physiologic and developmental processes
- Recognition of menses and menopause as normal physiologic and developmental processes
- Promotion of family-centered care
- Promotion of continuity of care
- Promotion of appropriate use of technology rather than routine use of interventions
- Advocacy for informed choice, participatory decision-making, and the right to self-determination

*Adapted from ACNM Core Competencies.

References

Achterberg J: *Woman as healer,* Boston, 1991, Shambhala.

American College of Nurse-Midwifery: *Descriptive data, nurse-midwives—USA,* Washington, DC, 1968, American College of Nurse-Midwifery.

American College of Nurse-Midwives: *ACNM philosophy,* Washington, DC, 1989, American College of Nurse-Midwives.

Borst C: The training and practice of midwives: a Wisconsin study, *Bull Hist Med* 62:606-627, 1988.

Campbell JD et al: Validating a model developed to predict prenatal care utilization, *J Fam Pract* 41(5):457-464, 1995.

Devitt N: The statistical case for the elimination of the midwife—Part I, *Women Health* 4:81-96, Spring 1979a.

Devitt N: The statistical case for elimination of the midwife—Part II, *Women Health* 4:169-186, Summer 1979b.

Emmons AB, Huntingdon JL: The midwife: her future in the US, *Am J Obstet Dis Women Children* 65:393-404, 1912.

Ettinger LE: Nurse-midwives, the mass media, and the politics of maternal health care in the United States, 1925-1955, *Nurs Hist Rev* 7:47-66, 1999.

Gabay M, Wolfe SM: Nurse-midwifery: the beneficial alternative, *Public Health Rep* 112:386-395, 1997.

Kelly M: *Maternity care in ferment: conflicting issues,* New York, 1980, Maternity Center Association.

Kosmak G: Does the average midwife meet the requirements of a patient in confinement? *Trans Am Associate Study Prevention Infant Mortality* 3:238-260, 1913.

Ladd-Taylor M: Women's health and public policy. In Apple RD, editor: *Women, health and medicine in America—a historical handbook,* New Brunswick, NJ, 1992, Rutgers University Press.

Leavitt JW: *Brought to bed: childbearing in America, 1750-1950,* New York, 1986, Oxford University Press.

Leppert PC, Partner SF, Thompson A: Learning from the community about barriers to health care, *Obstet Gynecol* 87(1):140-141, 1996.

Litoff J: *American midwives 1860 to the present,* New York, 1978, Greenwood Press.

MANA: *History of MANA* (web page), 2000, Midwives Alliance of North America, www.mana.org.

Towler J, Bramall J: *Midwives in history and society,* London, 1986, Croom Helm.

Ulrich LT: *A midwife's tale: the life of Martha Ballard based on her diary, 1785-1812,* New York, 1990, Alfred A. Knopf.

Wagner M: *Pursuing the birth machine—the search for appropriate birth technology,* Camperdown, NSW, Australia, 1994, ACE Graphics.

Walsh LV: *Midwife means with woman—an historical perspective,* Washington, DC, 1991, American College of Nurse-Midwives.

Walsh LV: Midwives as wives and mothers, *Nurs Hist Rev* 2:51-66, 1994.

Chapter 2

Clinical Epidemiology in Maternal-Child Health

Catherine A Carr, CNM, DrPH

INTRODUCTION

The word epidemiology means "among (epi) the people (demos)." Epidemiology is the study of the distribution of disease and conditions in the human population and the factors that affect the distribution (Lilienfeld and Stolley, 1994). Clinical epidemiology has a slightly different focus; it examines the outcomes of disease and factors that affect the variance in outcomes. Traditionally the unit of observation or study is groups, and the methodology involves comparison of groups. In this chapter epidemiologic investigation is reviewed, with emphasis on a clinical epidemiologic approach that can be used to enhance clinical decision making. The chapter presents a structured process for midwives to use as they critique clinical practice literature.

The epidemiologic approach is closely related to other more familiar methods of looking at problems or conditions of interest such as the scientific process, the nursing process, the midwifery management process, and clinical management. All are ways that seek to identify, explain, treat, or evaluate the problem or condition of interest. Whereas these other methods focus on the individual, epidemiology focuses on populations or communities. Epidemiology allows the clinician to look at the larger group or population to obtain a better assessment of individual risk.

Epidemiology allows us to describe groups with high or low rates of a condition. It is important to note that "condition" is simply the event of interest and may be positive, negative, or neutral. For example, low birth weight would be a negative condition, progressive labor a positive one, and area of residence may be neutral, depending on any other associated factors such as substandard housing or environmental risk. With better knowledge of group risk, the clinician can assess individual risk, use diagnostic tests more appropriately, and maximize preventive health interventions.

Clinical epidemiology is a relatively new division of epidemiology and is concerned with a defined population of patients rather than community groups. The principles of epidemiology are applied in clinical practice and are used in reading and interpreting literature, understanding the etiology, natural history and prognosis of disease, and improving decision making regarding screening, diagnostic testing, and treatment.

How Epidemiology is Used

Large populations are the traditional unit of interest in epidemiology. In examining the condition of interest, four things are considered:

1. Who has the problem?

Problems may be associated with a particular age

(increase in rates of Down syndrome with older gravidas), ethnicity (sickle cell, Tay-Sachs disease), lifestyle (lung cancer, rate of sexually transmitted infections [STIs]), or occupation (repetitive stress syndrome). The "who" in this criterion is the population group rather than the individual. This first question seeks to identify the attributes of the population group that affect the condition of interest. If the condition of interest is preterm labor, the population group that is most at risk for preterm labor includes women with multiple gestation pregnancies and those who have had previous preterm births. By narrowing the "who" to a more specific group, the clinician may be able to improve care by targeting the most at-risk group for specialized care or by working to change particular risk factors (Research Box 2-1).

2. What is the setting of the problem?

This question seeks to identify whether there is a particular location, environment, or occupational setting in which the problem is more likely to occur. The setting may be site-specific such as "sick buildings" that cause respiratory illness. Environmental risk factors include exposure to secondhand smoke, poor air or water quality, or violence in the home or community. Although work site hazards are much less prevalent than they once were, occupational

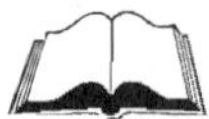

Research Box 2-1

Gribble RK, Meier PR, Berg RL: The value of urine screening for glucose at each prenatal visit, *Obstet Gynecol* 86(3):405-409, 1995.

Background

Glucosuria testing, originally used to assess women for gestational diabetes, is common practice in prenatal care. Serum glucose testing at 24 to 48 weeks identifies women with gestational diabetes in the third trimester if an abnormal 1-hour screening test is followed by an abnormal 3-hour glucose tolerance test. If significant glucosuria in the first and second trimesters is correlated with an elevated 1-hour screen or an abnormal 3-hour test, it would select women who might benefit from early diabetic screening.

Research Question

Does dipstick urinalysis for glucose at prenatal visits predict gestational diabetes and subsequently predict adverse maternal and fetal outcomes?

Methods

A retrospective chart review was performed for all women who received prenatal care at a midwestern clinic and subsequently delivered at the same hospital between July 1, 1991 and September 1, 1993. Prenatal records were reviewed for documented urine dipstick glucose screens and serum diabetes screening and testing. Intrapartum records were reviewed for outcomes, including cesarean delivery, hypertension, fetal heart rate abnormality, APGAR score, and birth weight. Analysis compared women with glucosuria (one or more test results of 250 mg/dl or greater) in the first two trimesters with those who did not have glucosuria (trace or negative results); the two groups were compared for positive serum screening and relevant gestational outcomes.

Sample

Of the 3217 women included in the chart audit, 2965 were included in the evaluation. Women were excluded for multiple gestation, preexisting diabetes, glucosuria at the first prenatal visit (to eliminate the possibility of preexisting but undiagnosed diabetes), failure to complete the standard blood glucose screens between 24 and 28 weeks, or fewer than two documented glucosuria screens during the prenatal period.

Results

Women in the positive urine glucose group had a significantly higher mean value for the 1-hour glucose screen. In addition, gestational diabetes incidence was higher for the positive glucose group. Women with gestational diabetes who also had positive glucosuria were more likely to be insulin dependent. The positive glucosuria group had a significantly higher mean birth weight, although the difference was not clinically important since there were no significant differences in shoulder dystocia, cesarean delivery for dystocia, or infants weighing over 4000 g.

Clinical Application

Urine dipstick results may be used to select women for earlier blood glucose screening for diabetes. However, the authors note that there were no significant differences in perinatal indicators between the two groups. Urine glucose testing in the third trimester after the blood glucose screening results are known is not predictive of pregnancy outcome.

hazards continue to exist for many women. Farm workers are exposed to pesticides, high-tech workers to heavy metals and solvents, health care workers to bloodborne and airborne pathogens, and teachers and child care workers to childhood diseases. Women often have household and childrearing responsibilities in addition to their primary employment. This "second shift" may increase stress and fatigue, leading to increased risk for occupational injuries (Hatch and Moline, 1997).

3. When does the problem occur?

It is important to determine whether the problem occurs only in pregnancy, in relationship to a particular gestational age, or after a specific exposure. Timing of known exposures is critically important. If rubella is contracted in the first trimester, the risk to the fetus of significant congenital anomalies is high. By the third trimester this risk drops to near zero. In contrast, varicella and genital herpes outbreaks are more likely to adversely affect the fetus if contracted close to the time of labor (Research Box 2-2).

4. What factors increase or decrease the problem?

Rest, dietary changes, or changes in stress or activity level may improve or worsen the problem. Adequate folic acid intake in the preconceptual period reduces the risk of neural tube defects. Because the preconceptual and very early pregnancy periods are the critical times, there is renewed emphasis on preconceptual care. Unfortunately this care is most available to the insured, aware consumer who is actively planning a pregnancy. Reduction of risk factors is often not available to most women in the world. Passive interventions such as adding folate to grains and flours may have a far greater effect on reduction of neural tube defects than attempting to provide preconceptual counseling to all women (Research Box 2-3).

By answering these questions, the clinician can begin to examine the problem more closely. The problem or condition is identified and described, and a search for causality and risk factors is begun. Prevention and control measures are sought, and an intervention is planned and then evaluated.

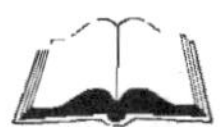

Research Box 2-2

Mellinger AK et al: High incidence of congenital rubella syndrome after a rubella outbreak, *Pediatr Infect Dis J* 14(7):573-578, 1995.

Background

Congenital rubella syndrome (CRS) is most likely to affect infants whose mothers contract rubella in the first trimester and commonly results in profound hearing loss, cardiac anomalies, microcephaly, and other congenital anomalies. As a result of the high rate of CRS (85%), most women who contract rubella in early pregnancy elect to terminate the pregnancy. In 1991 a religious community that did not seek immunization (although it was acceptable to members of the community) experienced an outbreak of rubella. Virtually all susceptible women were infected, and those who were pregnant did not seek abortion. The CRS rate after the outbreak was 2130 per 100,000 live births, compared to a national postoutbreak rate of 1.1 to 49 per 100,000 live births.

Research Question

What is the impact of maternal rubella infection on CRS?

Methods

The prospective study compared rubella serology of women delivering before and after the outbreak and cord blood IgM from infants of both the Amish community and non-Amish infants from the same area. Because the timing of the outbreak was known, the investigators were able to contact physician and midwife providers who served the community. Pregnancy log books and records of prior pregnancies, prenatal records of rubella status, and maternal reports of rubella-like infection were used to determine prior rubella status. Cord blood samples of infants born 8 to 10 months after the outbreak were collected from both groups of newborns. Infants with serologic evidence of rubella infection were followed closely through 18 months of age.

Sample

Amish and non-Amish women delivering during a 3-month period were sampled. Cord blood samples were obtained from 103 Amish infants and 221 non-Amish infants (93 private clients and 128 clinic service clients).

Continued

Research Box 2-2, cont'd

Results

Fifteen of the Amish infants whose mothers were identified as having had rubella during pregnancy had positive cord blood rubella immunoglobulin M (IgM). Nine Amish infants whose mothers were identified as having had rubella during pregnancy did not have cord blood studies but tested positive for congenital rubella. None of the comparison group infants tested IgM positive. Of the 24 infants with congenital rubella infection, 20 (83%) were born to mothers who were infected in the first trimester, and 4 to mothers with second-trimester infection. In the first trimester infections CRS was confirmed in 16 infants, and possible CRS in 2. The 4 infants whose mothers reported second-trimester infection included 1 with confirmed CRS and 3 with possible CRS.

Clinical Application

The rate of CRS in infants of mothers infected in the first trimester was consistent with the literature (80% and 85%). The large number of nonimmune women and the closeness and relative isolation of the community almost guaranteed that nonimmune members would become infected. The authors point out that there were many missed opportunities for discussion about and encouragement of immunization during prior pregnancies. Many in the affected population may have been willing to receive immunization had discussion occurred. In populations in which a large number of people decline immunization, aggressive control measures such as school closings and limitations on social gatherings are necessary during an outbreak.

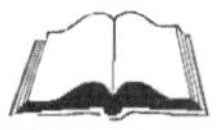

Research Box 2-3

Czeizel AE, Dudas I: Prevention of the first occurrence of neural tube defects by periconceptual vitamin supplementation, *N Engl J Med* 327:1832-1835, 1992.

Background

Women who take folic acid (folate) or multivitamins containing folic acid before conception and in the first trimester have decreased rates of neural tube defects. Both first occurrence and recurrence of neural tube defects are decreased when folate is added to the maternal diet in amounts of 4 mg for women with a prior pregnancy affected by neural tube defect and 0.8 mg for women who have not.

Research Question

To what extent is the rate of first occurrence of defects reduced in women taking folic acid supplements in the periconceptual period?

Methods

Women planning pregnancy were randomly selected to receive a vitamin supplement containing 0.8 mg folic acid or a trace element supplement that lacked folic acid. Supplementation began at least 1 month before conception and continued until the time of the second missed menses.

Sample

Nonpregnant Hungarian women under 35 years of age who were planning a pregnancy and had no history of wanted pregnancy (a history of abortion was not an elimination criterion) volunteered to participate. Pregnancy was confirmed in 4753 women of 7540 who entered the study. The outcome of the pregnancy was confirmed in 2104 women who received folate supplementation and in 2052 who received the folate-lacking supplement.

Results

The folate group had significantly fewer congenital anomalies and no neural tube defects. The trace element group had six neural tube defect cases. Incidence of cleft lip was not affected.

Clinical Application

Women with a history of pregnancy affected by neural tube defect should be counseled to initiate folate supplementation at the level of 4 mg before conception. All women planning pregnancy should receive supplementation at the level of 0.8 mg. Because most pregnancies are unplanned, passive supplementation (adding folic acid to cereals, grains, and other food sources) should be supported as a method to ensure that all women have access to this preventive measure, regardless of their access to preconceptual care, economic situation, or cultural background.

Epidemiology, Research, and the Midwife

When the clinician is providing care to an essentially healthy population, clinical epidemiology can be used to avoid unnecessary intervention, as well as to select treatment plans. Unfortunately epidemiologic research has often been ignored or discounted in maternity care. The use of routine nonstress cardiotocography in post-dated pregnancies, routine electronic fetal monitoring in labor, and denying women food in labor have all been shown to be ineffective at best and potentially harmful. Nonetheless, these interventions remain standard care for childbearing women in the United States (Enkin et al., 1995). The goal of this chapter is to encourage clinicians to critically evaluate existing knowledge and make management decisions based on their analysis. A process to evaluate the research literature on diagnosis and screening tests, interventions, and outcomes is provided so that the clinician is able to effectively apply research findings in clinical practice (Research Box 2-4).

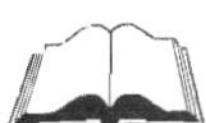

Research Box 2-4

Thacker SB, Stroup DF: Continuous electronic fetal heart monitoring during labor. In Nelson JP et al, editors: *Pregnancy and childbirth module of The Cochrane Database of Systematic Reviews* The Cochrane Collaboration, Issue 1, (updated 02 December 1997), Oxford: update software, 1998, The Cochrane Library.

Background

Electronic fetal monitoring (EFM) in labor is virtually routine in the United States, despite a lack of evidence as to its efficacy. In a 1989 policy statement, the American College of Obstetricians and Gynecologists (ACOG) stated that intermittent auscultation is appropriate in low-risk pregnancies. Both the United States Preventive Services Task Force (1989) and the Canadian Task Force on the Periodic Health Examination (1994) have stated that EFM should be restricted to high-risk pregnancies. Despite the strong evidence that EFM does not improve neonatal outcome in low-risk women, the practice of continuous fetal monitoring in low-risk labor has become a standard of care.

Research Question

Using the results of published randomized controlled trials (RCTs), what is the efficacy and safety of routine continuous electronic fetal monitoring (EFM) during labor with intermittent auscultation?

Methods

Meta-analysis of 12 published RCTs addressing the efficacy and safety of EFM was performed. A search was conducted for published and unpublished studies that compared continuous EFM with auscultation; 12 published and no unpublished studies were discovered. The studies were individually evaluated with selection criteria to assess the quality of the research. Three studies did not meet the criteria and were dropped from the analysis. Data from each study were used to calculate risk elements for eight outcomes, including low APGAR scores, neonatal seizures, neonatal intensive care unit admissions, stillbirth, neonatal death, cesarean delivery, and operative delivery.

Sample

The nine trials included 58,855 pregnant women and 59,324 infants and were conducted in clinical centers in the United States, Europe, and Australia. Both high- and low-risk pregnancies were included.

Results

None of the trials demonstrated an improvement in the EFM group in APGAR scores <7 at 1 minute. With the exception of neonatal seizures (in one trial), there was no difference in neonatal morbidity and mortality. The follow-up of the seizure group is unclear but seems to indicate minimal long-term effects. The cesarean and operative delivery rates were significantly higher in the EFM groups in all studies, particularly for the low-risk women.

Clinical Application

EFM is a classic example of the widespread diffusion of a technology before its efficacy has been determined. Benefits of continuous EFM in normal labor are modest at best and must be weighed against the significant increase in the risk of operative delivery. Efforts to liberalize nursing protocols and increase the use of auscultation as a method of monitoring in labor are supported by the research.

Evidence-Based Practice: Using the Literature

Clinicians must often try to improve the "good" risk factors and decrease the "bad" risk factors that are based on insufficient evidence. Although in many instances evidence is simply not available, all too often research-based evidence is either ignored or underused in favor of intuitive, experiential, or anecdotal data. This has occasionally been referred to as "man-who statistics," as in "I knew a man who . . . ." The traditional approach to medical decision-making involves heavy reliance on clinical experience and the authority of the experience of others.

Even though this time-honored method of clinical problem solving continues to be taught in most practitioner education programs, it is an insufficient basis for appropriate decision making. Knowledge of clinical care and an understanding of pathology are important, but they must be combined with the most current supporting evidence. Grimes (1995) suggests the use of a different paradigm that is based on a critical review of the literature and an explicit evaluation process. This evaluation system was developed by the Canadian Task Force on the Periodic Health Examination (1979) and subsequently adopted by the U.S. Preventive Services Task Force (1989) as a way to evaluate the literature on preventive care (Box 2-1). This approach can be used for the review and evaluation of clinical literature to better ensure that practice is based on appropriate evidence.

Use of this formal system of evaluation requires a greater commitment of the clinician's time and effort. It is more work to seek out and review the literature than it is to simply ask the "authority," whether the authority is the instructor, consultant, or text. The clinician bears additional responsibility for making considered and thoughtful decisions about clinical care. When first using the evaluation system, she or he may be surprised to discover the less than stellar quality of clinical research (Chalmers et al., 1981; Grimes, 1995). However, the reward of finding strong evidence to support clinical care makes the effort worthwhile.

Critical Review of the Literature

Given the clinical reality that convincing evidence for practice is often unavailable, ignored, or undervalued, it is important for all clinicians to develop expertise in critical appraisal of research. To inadequately assess research is hazardous. Without critical assessment, ineffective measures may be used, harmful measures may be applied, resources may be wasted, and opportunities to improve care may be missed. Critical appraisal of literature is first and foremost a systematic approach that has many of the same elements as clinical decision mak-

Box 2-1 *Evaluation of Research Information*

Strength of Recommendations

1. There is strong evidence to support recommendations that the condition be specifically considered in a periodic health examination.
2. There is fair evidence to support the recommendation that the condition be specifically considered in a periodic health examination.
3. There is poor evidence regarding the inclusion of the condition in a periodic health examination, but recommendations may be made on other grounds.
4. There is fair evidence to support the recommendation that the condition be excluded from consideration in a periodic health examination.
5. There is strong evidence to support the recommendation that the condition be excluded from consideration in a periodic health examination.

Quality of Evidence

I. Evidence obtained from at least one properly designed randomized controlled trial.
II-1. Evidence obtained from well-designed controlled trials without randomization.
II-2. Evidence obtained from well-designed cohort or case control studies, preferably from more than one center or research group.
II-3. Evidence obtained from multiple time series with or without the intervention. Dramatic results in uncontrolled experiments (such as the introduction of penicillin treatment in the 1940s) could also be regarded as this type of evidence.
III. Opinions of respected authorities, based on clinical experience, descriptive studies, or reports of expert committees.

Modified from U.S. Preventive Services Task Force: *Guide to clinical preventive services: an assessment of the effectiveness of 169 interventions,* Baltimore, 1989, Williams & Wilkins.

ing or problem solving. These include stating the problem (choosing what to read about), reviewing available information, deciding how compelling the evidence is, and making clinical decisions based on the best evidence available. Considered in this way, critical review of research is yet another clinical tool or skill that can be developed by all midwives.

The method discussed in this chapter was first developed in Ontario, Canada, revised by Newton at the University of North Carolina, and modified for use in midwifery teaching settings by Albers and King (1994). It provides the busy clinician a structured process by which to evaluate the types of research she or he most often needs in practice: screening and diagnosis research, intervention research, and outcomes research. Practical priorities for clinicians in reviewing research include the following:

- Keeping up with the literature in one's field to maintain an awareness of what is and is not known
- Distinguishing strong from weak research
- Evaluating all proposed new interventions, low-tech and low-risk, as well as high-tech, before incorporating them into clinical practice.

Albers (1997) recommends a commonsense approach for busy clinicians to choosing articles for critical review and makes the following suggestions:

- Original research is better than survey articles because the original research contains the details necessary to determine the strength of the evidence.
- Well-known authors may be more likely to pursue an area in which they have developed considerable expertise and experience. Although this is not an absolute, familiarity with an author's work can allow for a faster decision process.
- The topic should be pertinent to the clinician's practice, relevant to her or his practice setting, and include a study population similar to her or his own for best generalizability.

An efficient and quick way to screen articles for further review is to read the abstract. A structured abstract will contain information about the population, sample size, sample selection, and methodology. Sample size will give the reviewer information about the possible strength of statistical relationships, as there are less likely to be "dumb luck" variations with larger numbers. Sample selection, if based on probability methods, will reduce the possibility of selection bias. The sample and its selection should be appropriate for the study (e.g., age, gender, risk status for the condition, confounding factors). Methodology should be evaluated as to where it is on the hierarchy of quality of evidence (see Box 2-1), with the highest or gold standard being a randomized controlled trial (RCT), and the lowest being the opinions of others, clinical experience, or descriptive studies (Boxes 2-2 and 2-3).

However, it is important to be aware of the value of evidence outside of controlled clinical trials. An RCT may be unethical or otherwise unsuitable in a given situation. An example would be examining women's experience of postpartum depression. Not only would it be unethical to induce depression in otherwise healthy women, but the research would be better addressed by a qualitative design that used interviews aimed at discovering nuances of the experience. Observational data can be quite powerful, particularly when the issue involves a threat to health. The association of rubella with congenital anomalies was the result of an observational study. Midwifery has a long tradition of observing and "being with" women. Using evidence-based research to extend the breadth of professional knowledge does not mean that other methods and designs should be ignored. Practi-

Box 2-2 *Example of Unstructured Abstract*

Taylor MC et al: Patient preference for self-collected cultures for group B streptococcus in pregnancy, *J Nurse-Midwifery* 42(5):410-413, 1997.

To determine pregnant women's preference for self-culture technique, 251 women between 24 and 42 weeks' gestation were interviewed after performing self-collected cultures (vaginal and rectal) for group B streptococcus. Patient receptiveness to self-culture, the ability to perform self-culture, and the desire for choice in the future were derived using the Patient Preference Tool. The majority of women (77%, n = 194) gave positive descriptions of self-culture technique over nurse-collected sampling and preferred self-culture technique over nurse-collected sampling (57%, n = 142). Seventy-nine percent (n = 197) stated their desire to have a choice about self-culture in the future when similar testing was needed, and 89% (n = 224) believed that other women would also like to have this choice. In addition, patient samples were highly correlated with nurse-collected samples for accuracy of culture results. This study provides data supporting the belief that women desire active participation in their care.

Box 2-3 *Example of Structured Abstract*

Herbst A, Ingemarsson I: Intermittent versus continuous electronic monitoring in labour: a randomised study, *Br J Obstet Gynecol* 101:663-668, 1994.

Objective

To compare the efficacy in detecting signs of fetal hypoxia in labour of intermittent (I-group) vs. continuous (C-group) electronic fetal monitoring in women with low or moderate risk factors for fetal distress

Design

A prospective, randomised study

Setting

A tertiary referral centre

Subjects

The group consisted of 4044 parturients at low risk for obstetric complications with a reactive fetal heart rate admission test at arrival in labour. During the study period (October 5, 1989 to May 31, 1991), 5647 women were delivered in the labour ward. Of these, 1178 women (20.9%) were excluded because of high risk factors in pregnancy or at admission for labour, including women undergoing elective caesarean section. Of the remaining 4469 women, 4044 (90.5%) were randomised to either intermittent (n = 2051) or continuous monitoring (n = 2029) during the first stage of labour.

Methods

In the C-group the fetal heart rate was recorded continuously with electronic fetal monitoring for 10 to 30 minutes every 2 to 2.5 hours during the first stage of labour, and the fetal heart rate was auscultated every 15 to 30 minutes between recording periods. If complications occurred, recording was changed to continuous. In the second stage of labour all women were monitored continuously. Umbilical cord artery acid-base status was assessed at birth.

Main Outcome Measures

Duration of electronic fetal monitoring, rates of abnormal fetal heart rate patterns, caesarean section for fetal distress, acidosis in umbilical cord arterial blood at birth, APGAR scores of less than 7 at 1 or 5 minutes, and referrals to the neonatal intensive care unit

Results

There were no significant differences between the study groups in the incidence of ominous fetal heart rate recordings: 6.3 (I-group) vs. 6.6 (C-group), or the interval from arrival to first detected abnormal fetal heart rate, although the number of suspicious fetal heart rate patterns was higher in the C-group (28.6%) than in the I-group (24.6%). In the I-group electronic fetal monitoring was performed for 38.8% of the first stage of labour (median monitoring time) as compared with 78.6% in the C-group. The incidence of caesarean section for fetal distress was similarly low in both groups: 1.2% vs. 1%. There were no significant differences in the immediate neonatal outcome in terms of umbilical artery pH, APGAR scores, or admissions to the neonatal intensive care unit.

Conclusions

Intermittent use of electronic fetal monitoring at regular intervals (with stethoscopic auscultation in between) appears to be as safe as continuous electronic fetal monitoring in low-risk labours.

tioners who critically examine all available research will be better prepared to provide the most appropriate care.

STRUCTURED EVALUATION OF CLINICAL LITERATURE

Screening and Diagnosis Testing

Screening is the intervention, test, or tool given to apparently healthy people to identify the presence of an early or latent condition or the presence of a risk factor. For example, pregnant women are commonly screened for the conditions of anemia, glucose intolerance, and syphilis. Lipid screening is done to identify abnormally high cholesterol, a risk factor for heart disease. Screening is typically applied to large groups, and all members of the group are screened.

What is the condition, and is it appropriate to screen for it?

Screening procedures should be used for conditions that are important to discover and for which treatment is available, acceptable, effective, and timely. Test characteristics should include adequate specificity and sensitivity, simplicity of administration, reasonable cost, patient safety, and patient acceptability. For example, it is important to discover asymptomatic urinary tract infection in pregnancy because of its association with both pyelonephritis and preterm labor. If discovered, the infection is easily treated with antibiotic therapy. The screening test commonly used—urine reagent strips that identify the presence of leukocyte esterase, nitrites, protein, and blood—has adequate predictive ability, is easy to perform, is relatively cheap, and is acceptable to patients. Nonpregnant populations are not screened because of the decreased incidence of asymptomatic infection. Conversely, it would make less sense to screen for a disease that has no treatment or perform a screening test that is extremely expensive or causes undue hardship for the patient. For example, using liver biopsy to screen for liver disease would not be appropriate since the procedure is expensive and carries significant risk to the patient.

Diagnosis is the use of an intervention, test, or tool to identify a condition or problem and is done in response to a screening test, presenting complaint, risk assessment, or physical findings. The same test may be used for screening the pregnant population and initial diagnosis in a nonpregnant population (Murphy, 1995). A nonpregnant woman in her 20s would probably not be given a glucose tolerance test unless she had a particular constellation of presenting complaints, risk factors, or physical findings. However, it is community practice to use a glucose tolerance test as a screening tool in pregnancy.

What is the gold standard, and is it reasonable?

For both screening and diagnostic tests, there needs to be a criterion or gold standard. It is important to have a standard in order to have some sort of practice framework. This standard is the single best test or combination of tests for accurate identification of the condition of interest. It is often more expensive, complex, and invasive than a screening test. For example, maternal serum alpha-fetoprotein/human chorionic gonadotropin/estriol is a screening test. Amniocentesis, the standard by which it is measured, is more expensive, more invasive, and more complex. The gold standard for diagnosis may not exist, as in the case of postpartum depression. It may also be unethical or impractical (e.g., liver biopsy for HELLP syndrome).

What are the sensitivity, specificity, and predictive values of the test?

Screening and diagnostic tools are critical to providing reproductive health care, and the introduction of new tests into clinical practice is occurring at an ever-increasing rate. Common screening and diagnostic tools have a wide range of risk, cost, and level of intervention. The use of Leopold's maneuvers to determine fetal position is a simple tool with minimal discomfort to the woman and essentially no risk to the fetus. Conversely, fetal blood sample requires a specially trained professional and special equipment and carries risk to the fetus. Many tools and interventions have become standard of care before they were appropriately evaluated. Classic examples include routine continuous electronic fetal monitoring, routine ultrasonography in normal pregnancies, and routine use of episiotomies to preserve perineal tone.

Not all tests are equally useful in the information that they provide or in the physical or psychologic risk that they pose to the woman, her fetus, and her family. Incorrect diagnosis may lead to inappropriate intervention that can pose physical risk for the woman or her fetus. In addition, incorrectly labeling a mother or fetus as "abnormal" or "at risk" may produce significant psychologic or even physical risk to the woman. It is important for the clinician to understand the efficacy and accuracy of diagnostic and screening tests to provide this information to the client.

Characteristics of screening and diagnostic tests include sensitivity and specificity. Sensitivity is the ability of the tool or test to correctly identify those who have the disease or condition. Specificity is the ability of the tool or test to correctly identify those who do not have the disease or condition. Sensitivity and specificity provide information about the test itself. For example, a very sensitive test would identify all individuals with diabetes in the screened population. Because sensitivity does not consider those who do not have diabetes, the sensitive test may falsely "screen in" women who do not truly have diabetes. Conversely, a very specific test would correctly identify those who do not have diabetes, but may also falsely identify some truly diabetic women as not having the condition. If results are falsely negative, the chance to diagnose and intervene may be lost, potentially increasing the risk of morbidity. False-positive results are likely to subject the woman to unnecessary interventions, with the potential for side effects and accompanying increased stress.

Rates of sensitivity and specificity of the tool or test vary, depending on the ability of the test to identify the phenomenon of interest and the level at which the cutoff points are set. Levels of sensitivity and specificity of laboratory tests can be found in literature accompanying the test, by calling the laboratory that analyzes the test, or by contacting the manufacturer. Tools such as screens for preeclampsia or preterm labor are more difficult to assess for sensitivity and often involve an examination of the literature to discern sensitivity and specificity. Preterm labor screens originally thought to be highly sensitive have been found to be inadequate when used with different population groups.

Some tests are extremely sensitive, such as the Venereal Disease Research Laboratory for syphilis. These tests also have high false-positive rates and are generally followed by a more specific test such as the MHA-TP. The second-line tests are more specific but may be more expensive, more uncomfortable, and more stressful and time consuming for the client.

Predictive values are typically more useful to the health care provider in clinical decision making. They are extremely variable, depending on the prevalence of the condition in the population of interest. A positive predictive value is the level of certainty that the positive test result is correct. Negative predictive value is the level of certainty that a negative test result is correct. As the prevalence (the rate of the condition in the population) rises, the positive predictive value rises, and the negative predictive value declines.

Example:

In a young, urban, sexually active population, the chlamydia rate may be as high as 25%. The health care provider needs to know how to effectively counsel and treat the client with a positive test. If the sensitivity of a chlamydia test is 95% and the specificity rate is 90%, the positive predictive value is 76% (number of true positive results/number of all positive results). The negative predictive value (number of true negative results/number of all negative results) for this particular clientele is 98%. The clinician can appropriately counsel the client with a negative result that her chances of having chlamydia at the time of the test (assuming sufficient incubation time and no reinfection) were extremely low. However, the woman with the positive result has almost a one in four chance of being treated for a sexually transmitted disease that she does not have. Although treatment is relatively cheap and painless, it still subjects the client to antibiotics and stress on her relationship as the couple copes with the issues of an STI (Table 2-1).

In a far more common situation, the incidence of chlamydia would be 10% or lower. With a prevalence of 10%, the positive predictive value would be 51%, and the negative predictive value 99.9%. For the woman with a negative test, this is quite reassuring. It tells a woman with a positive test little other than that she might have chlamydia and may need treatment (Table 2-2).

In terms of the prevalence of the condition, are the study subjects similar to your clients? Will the predictive value of the test be the same for your clients?

In counseling clients the clinician should discuss the prevalence rate and the predictive values, helping each woman to make an informed choice about treatment. In the case example, treatment is simple and inexpensive, and the risks of untreated chlamydia are known and serious. Most clients appreciate the information and

Table 2-1 *Example 1: Predictive Value in Clinical Testing*

Test results	Clients with chlamydia	Clients without chlamydia	Totals
Positive test	238 (true positive)	75 (false positive)	313 with positive test
Negative test	12 (false negative)	675 (true negative)	687 with negative test
	250 (25% of total)	750	1000 total population

In this hypothetic example the population has a chlamydia incidence of 25%. The test used has a sensitivity of 95% and a specificity of 90%. Positive predictive value = true positive/all positive = 238/313 = 76%; negative predictive value = true negative/all negative = 675/687 = 98%.

Table 2-2 *Example 2: Predictive Value in Clinical Testing*

Test results	Clients with chlamydia	Clients without chlamydia	Totals
Positive test	95 (true positive)	90 (false positive)	185 positive test
Negative test	5 (false negative)	810 (true negative)	815 negative test
	100 (10% rate)	900	1000 total population

In a more common situation with a chlamydia incidence of 10% and using the same test with the same sensitivity and specificity. Positive predictive value = true pos/all pos = 95/185 = 51%; negative predictive value = true neg/all neg 810/815 = 99%.

choose treatment "just in case." Knowing that a positive test may not be 100% accurate may prevent additional stress and emotional turmoil for the couple.

Using Testing Information

1. Know the characteristics of your clinical population. Some populations are at higher risk for specific conditions. For example, women of African descent are more at risk for sickle cell anemia than women of northern European descent. A particular population may need earlier diabetic screening, the addition of hemoglobin electrophoresis to the prenatal panel, or other risk-appropriate screening.
2. Consider selective screening.
   Predictive values increase as the prevalence rate increases. It is sometimes helpful to determine whether certain subpopulations in a clinician's practice have higher prevalence rates of a condition to more appropriately target screening and diagnostic testing. For example, it is known that women over 35 years of age have a higher rate of conceptions with genetic abnormalities. Thus it makes sense to target that group of women for genetic counseling and testing. By pooling women with higher risk, the predictive value of the testing improves. Amniocentesis, the gold standard for identifying genetic abnormalities, is expensive, stressful, and carries risk to the woman and her fetus; thus enhancing the efficacy of the test is important.
3. Practice guidelines should reflect the population.
   A practice that serves mostly adolescents or young adults may have different guidelines for STI screening and treatment, depending on the prevalence of disease in the community and the likelihood of follow-up.
4. Counseling should be appropriate.
   Although improved screening and diagnostic tools assist in providing more accurate information, we are still far from being able to definitively inform women of positive diagnoses. To avoid coercion, clinicians must be aware of and knowledgeable about the limitations of tools that are used in practice.

Evaluating Interventions and Outcomes

A wide range of interventions is commonly used in maternity care in clinical practice, including treatments, therapies, and measures of care. Examples include social support, diet and exercise advice, childbirth education, use of comfort measures in labor, and medications. All interventions should be critically examined to prevent doing harm, using resources unnecessarily, or providing care that is of no benefit.

Becoming expert in critical evaluation of literature requires practice and a consistent method of review. Albers (1997) recommends that the midwife ask the following questions:

Were the intervention and control groups similar?

The researcher should provide information that allows the reader to determine whether the size of the group was sufficient to support the conclusions that have been drawn. In general, larger samples provide more powerful evidence. The larger the sample size, the less likely it is that the results will be due to chance. Television commercials offer classic examples of insufficient sample size. "Four out of five dentists/doctors/exterminators recommend Brand X toothpaste/medication/pest control!" However, the number from which this 80% is derived could be anything from five to many thousands.

How the groups are selected is important in assessing the role of bias in the results. Randomization assigns members of the groups randomly so that confounding factors or biases are equally distributed. When randomization is used, the method used should be described. Preassigned numbers in sealed envelopes, notification of group from a central clearing office, or use of a table of random numbers are all recognized methods of randomization. Using the patient's date of birth, using the day of the week, or assigning every other person to a particular group is subject to bias and is not an acceptable method of assignment (Weiss, 1996; Grimes and Schultz, 1996; Schulz et al., 1996).

Although randomization is the gold standard, it may not be possible, depending on the condition of interest. For example, it would be unethical to intentionally expose women to known or suspected toxins, such as assigning women to a group exposed to various levels of secondhand smoke to study the effect of smoking on placental perfusion. It would also be unethical to deny treatment or care known or believed to be beneficial, such as denying care to women to evaluate the effect of lack of prenatal care. When randomization cannot be used and the members of the group cannot be assigned to treatment, observational studies may be appropriate (Murphy and Albers, 1992). Although observational studies are considered weaker than experimental studies, they are the most common studies in health care. Often observational studies are the results of natural experiments that occur when a group is exposed to a treatment due to changes in the workplace, legislation, or policy. This occurred when air carriers banned in-flight smoking and flight attendants were no longer exposed to secondhand smoke, giving researchers an opportunity to examine the effects of removing an exposure on groups of workers. A natural experiment will take place in California if undocumented immigrant women are denied prenatal care but have intrapartum care available. State health policy has been to provide care to all low-income women, regardless of legal documentation status, since 1988. Policy makers on both sides of the decision have argued about the potential effect of denying prenatal care to women. This natural experiment would never take place under the aegis of research but may occur because of changes in the political climate that affect the health care of noncitizens.

In observational studies the group members are examined in their natural state, without assignment to experimental groups. Because there is no randomized assignment, there is increased opportunity for bias if the members of the groups differ. For example, women who seek midwifery care may be different in other ways from those who do not. The comparison groups should be alike in the relevant ways, and inclusion and exclusion criteria should be discussed. Age, economic circumstance, ethnicity, geographic location, and gravida/parity are all potential biases.

Were all clinically relevant outcomes assessed?

In maternity care studies particularly it is important to examine the end points or study outcomes. In a treatment designed to decrease preterm labor rates, a common evaluation is cervical change and admission in labor. However, the number of women who actually deliver prematurely compared to the control group is more clinically relevant. If the outcome is the number of women admitted with a diagnosis of premature labor, it may be biased in favor of the intervention if women are aggressively diagnosed. The treatment to reduce the incidence of preterm labor is irrelevant if the woman in consideration would not have delivered prematurely anyway.

Treatments used in the intrapartum should incorporate discussion of both maternal and fetal outcomes in the postpartum period. Although epidural anesthesia may relieve intrapartum pain, other relevant intrapartum outcomes that are important to assess are use of pitocin to strengthen the contractions, length of second stage of labor, and incidence of assisted and cesarean deliveries. Longer-term postpartum outcomes that should be addressed include headaches, back pain, breast-feeding problems, and neonatal outcomes. Studies that end with the birth of the infant may miss important postpartum and neonatal events. Failure to adequately assess all clinically relevant outcomes may lead to the use of an intervention the side effects of which are unknown and possibly detrimental.

Were all the subjects accounted for?

Virtually all clinical studies have a certain attrition or dropout rate. The rate may vary considerably, but reasons for attrition and its influence on the study should be discussed. Attrition can influence sample size, particularly if the rate is higher in either the control or treatment group. If the study is one that is demanding on the participants, such as keeping a daily journal or attending a certain number of classes or meetings, the characteristics of those who continue the treatment may be quite different from those of clients who drop out. This could affect the results of the study, making the treatment seem more or less effective than it really is.

In any study beginning preconceptually or very early in pregnancy, there will be a number of participants who experience spontaneous abortions. However, it would be anticipated that, unless there were confounding variables, the rate would be similar in each group. A high attrition rate on one or more groups often indicates that some other factor is at work. The participants' tolerance for frustration, their concern about a specific perinatal issue, or even the amount of time they have to participate rather than the condition of interest may be the source of attrition rather than the variable of interest.

Were other factors that could influence the outcome considered?

There may be other factors that influence the outcome of the study:

1. Pregnant women tend to be an unusually young and healthy group who by and large are very interested in the health of their pregnancies and fetuses.
2. It is difficult to control all aspects of a study. Participants in a preterm labor study may self-treat with anything from extra rest to homeopathic remedies. If this occurs, the outcomes may be influenced by the self-treatment, as well as by the treatment under examination.
3. Sometimes influences are societal, as with population-wide reductions in smoking and drinking. Evaluation of smoking cessation programs must consider the influence of societal pressure on pregnant women to avoid tobacco use.

Studies should attempt to ascertain what other factors may be simultaneously influencing the participants.

Are the results both clinically and statistically significant?

In extremely large studies outcomes may be statistically significant but still lack clinical importance. If the intervention results in shortening the active stage of labor in healthy primiparas by 30 minutes, the findings may be statistically significant. However, the clinical importance of a 30-minute difference in length of active labor is debatable. Conversely, in small studies, the difference in outcome in control and treatment groups must be extremely large to detect a difference statistically, particularly if the condition in question is uncommon.

Are the participants similar to your clients?

If the study participants are not similar to your clients in ways that may influence the outcome, the differences in the populations may make generalizations inappropriate. Factors in the population itself, such as age, ethnicity, clinical conditions, parity, and economic situation, may make a significant difference in the outcome.

How were outcomes assessed?

Outcomes should be assessed objectively or blindly to prevent bias. Structured and validated questionnaires, data collection by personnel unaware of the client's participation in the study, and blinded analysis of results are all ways to improve validity of the results.

Summary

In summary, critical appraisal of clinical literature is another skill for the practicing midwife and, like any skill, it improves with practice. Midwifery practice improves when it is based on the best information available. Reading and using research literature is the most meaningful and effective way to ensure that the women and families cared for by midwives continue to receive the best of both the art and science of midwifery care.

References

Albers LL: To believe or not to believe: Key concepts for critical analysis of journal articles, Presentation, Annual Meeting, American College of Nurse-Midwives, Boston, Mass, May 27, 1997.

Albers LL, King VJ: Critical appraisal of journal articles, Presentation, Annual Meeting, American College of Nurse-Midwives, Nashville, Tenn, May 25, 1994.

Canadian Task Force on the Periodic Health Examination: The periodic health examination, *Can Med Assoc J* 121:1193-254, 1979.

Canadian Task Force on the Periodic Health Examination: *The Canadian guide to preventive health care,* Ottawa, 1994, Health Canada.

Chalmers TC et al: A method for assessing the quality of a randomized control trial, *Control Clin Trials* 2:31-49, 1981.

Enkin M et al: *A guide to effective care in pregnancy and childbirth,* ed 2, Oxford, 1995, Oxford University Press.

Grimes DA: Introducing evidence-based medicine into a department of obstetrics and gynecology, *Obstet Gynecol* 86(3):451-457, 1995.

Grimes DA, Schulz KF: Methodology citations and the quality of randomized controlled trials in obstetrics and gynecology, *Am J Obstet Gynecol* 174(4):1312-1315, 1996.

Hatch M, Moline J: Women, work and health, *Am J Intern Med* 32(3):303-308, 1997.

Lilienfeld DE, Stolley PD: *Foundations of epidemiology,* ed 3, New York, 1994, Oxford University Press.

Murphy PA: Primary care for women: screening tests and preventive services recommendations, *J Nurse Midwifery* 40(2):74-87, 1995.

Murphy PA, Albers LL: Evaluation of research studies. Part II: Observational studies, *J Nurse Midwifery* 37(6):411-413, 1992.

Schulz KF et al: Blinding and exclusions after allocation in randomised controlled trials: survey of published parallel group trials in obstetrics and gynaecology, *Br Med J* 312:742-744, 1996.

US Preventive Services Task Force: Guide to clinical preventive services—an assessment of the effectiveness of 169 interventions: report of the U. S. Preventive Services Task Force, Baltimore, 1989, Williams & Wilkins.

Weiss NS: Clinical epidemiology: *The study of the outcome of illness,* ed 2, New York, 1996, Oxford University Press.

Resource

Evidence-Based Health Care: *Highlights of research regarding nurse-midwifery practice in the US,* American College of Nurse-Midwives, 1998, Washington, DC.

Unit II

Healthy Pregnancy

Chapter 3

Anatomy of the Female Reproductive Tract

EXTERNAL GENITALIA

The external reproductive structures include the mons pubis, the labia majora, the labia minora, the clitoris, the hymen, the vestibule, and the urethral and gland openings. They are commonly referred to as the vulva (Figure 3-1).

Mons Pubis

The mons pubis (mons veneris) lies directly over the anterior surface of the symphysis pubis and is composed of fatty tissue. Pubic hair covers the area in a distinct triangular pattern, the base of which aligns with the upper aspect of the symphysis. This differs from male distribution in which the hair pattern extends from the pubic region to the umbilicus and downward over the inner aspect of the thighs.

Labia Majora

The labia majora, extending from the mons to the posterior fourchette, are two folds of adipose tissue covered by skin. Embryologically the labia majora and scrotum arise from the same cells. The size and appearance of the labia majora vary among women, depending on race, age, and parity. Generally the labia are 7 to 8 cm in length, 2 to 3 cm wide, and 1 to 1.5 cm thick. Before puberty the external surface of the labia majora is similar to that of adjacent skin. After puberty the surface is covered with varying amounts of coarse pubic hair, and the skin color becomes darker than adjacent skin. In nulliparous women the labia majora tend to conceal the underlying structures. In multiparous women the labia majora may relax open somewhat, exposing other structures. Directly beneath the skin there is a layer of connective tissue composed of elastic fibers and adipose tissue. Sebaceous, apocrine, and eccrine glands are present. Varying amounts of pubic hair may also be present. The fatty mass that accounts for the bulk of the labia majora contains a plexus of veins that may bleed heavily or form a hematoma if traumatized. The labia majora include the terminal extension of the round ligament.

Labia Minora

When the labia majora are separated, two smaller folds of tissue are seen running from the anterior aspect of the clitoris to the lower third of the introitus. Similar to the labia majora, their size varies dramatically. In nulliparous women they tend to be small and visible only with the labia majora retracted. They may extend beyond the labia majora in multiparous women. The labia mi-

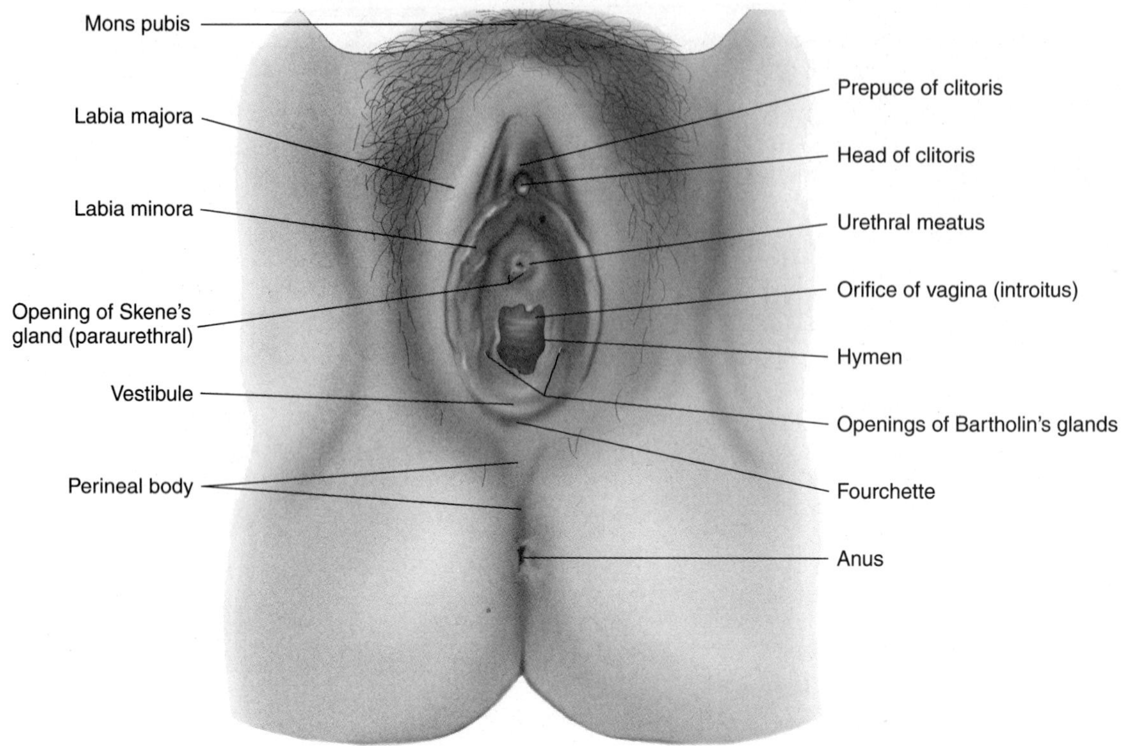

Figure 3-1 External genitalia.

nora, covered by squamous epithelium, tend to be pink and moist when protected by the labia majora. They are rich with sebaceous follicles and apocrine and eccrine glands. Connective tissue, blood vessels, and smooth muscle fiber make up the internal labia minora. They function as erectile tissue and are extremely sensitive because of the many nerve endings that are present.

The anterior aspect of the labia minora come together to form the prepuce and frenulum of the clitoris. Their anatomic structure and innervation contribute to female sexual response. Posteriorly the labia minora of nulliparous women decrease in size and meet to form the fourchette. In multiparous women they appear to fuse with the labia majora at the posterior vaginal opening (Figure 3-2).

Clitoris

The clitoris is composed of the glans, the corpus (body), and two crura. The body of the clitoris is comprised of two corpora cavernosa surrounded by smooth muscle fibers. The crura run from the inferior aspect of the ischiopubic rami and insert below the middle of the pubic arch to form the corpus. The clitoris is less than 2 cm long, even in the erect state. The glans, less than 0.5 cm, is covered by stratified squamous epithelium with numerous nerve endings that make it extremely sensitive. When traction is put on the labia minora, the clitoris becomes angled toward the vaginal opening. The clitoris is considered to be the primary erogenous organ in women.

Vaginal Vestibule

The diamond-shaped area that is surrounded by the clitoris anteriorly, the labia minora laterally, and the fourchette posteriorly is often referred to as the vaginal vestibule. The urethral orifice lies approximately 2 to 3 cm posterior to the clitoris and anterior to the vaginal orifice. It appears as a slit and can be distended to 4 to 5 mm in diameter. The urethra in women averages 3 to 5 cm in length, and the distal two thirds of the urethra lies along the anterior vaginal wall. Stratified transitional epithelium lines the proximal two thirds of the urethra; the distal third is lined with stratified squamous epithelium.

In most women the paraurethral ducts (ducts of the Skene's glands) are apparent on either side of the urethral opening. Occasionally they may open posteriorly

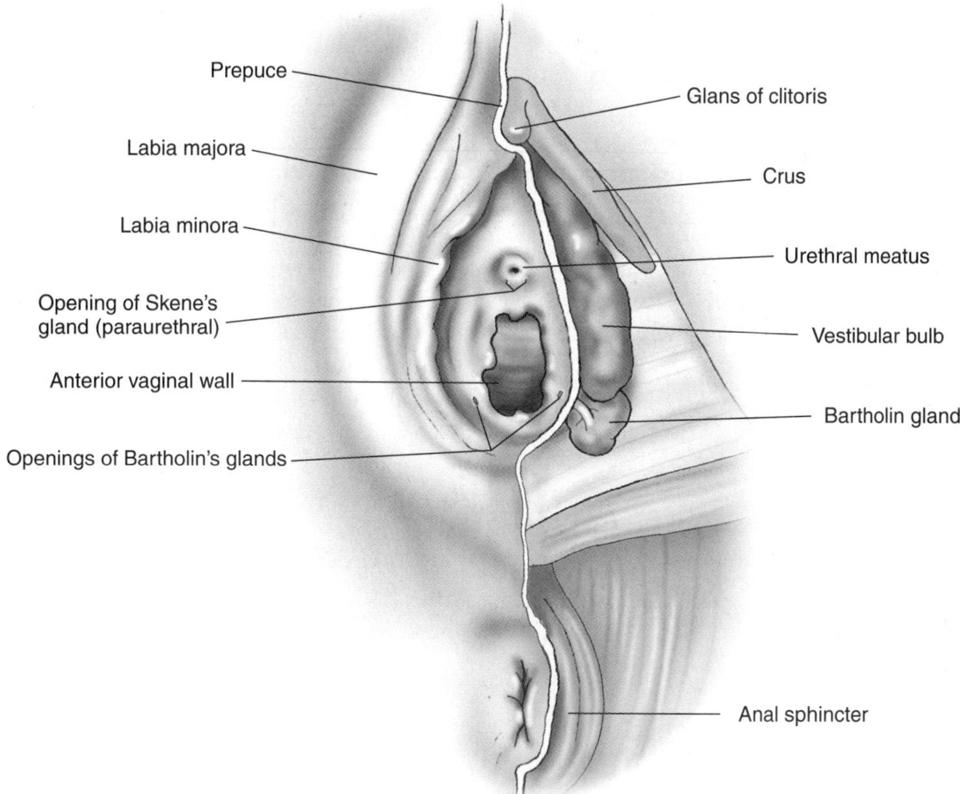

Figure 3-2 Anatomy of structures underlying the external genitalia.

to the urethra. They are 0.5 mm in diameter and vary in length. The paraurethral glands secrete mucus into the vestibule or urethra. The prostate gland in males is homologous to the paraurethral glands.

The greater vestibular glands (Bartholin's glands) lie at the posterior aspect of the vaginal opening, lateral to the midline. They are approximately 0.5 to 1 cm in diameter, with ducts that average 1.5 to 2 cm in length and produce mucoid secretions during sexual arousal. The male Cowper's glands are homologous to the greater vestibular glands.

The vestibular bulbs lie bilaterally under the mucous membrane of the vestibule and the bulbocavernosus muscle. They are vascular bulbs that serve an erectile function during sexual arousal. Embryologically they are similar to the corpus spongiosum of the penis.

The vaginal opening varies in size and shape, as does the hymen. The hymen is comprised of elastic and collagenous connective tissue, with both the internal and external surfaces covered by stratified squamous epithelium. In virginal women the hymen is a membrane that surrounds the vaginal opening and has an opening that may admit up to one or two fingers. The hymenal opening is usually circular or crescent in shape. Typically the hymen is torn with athletic activity, tampon use, and intercourse, usually posteriorly. The edges heal so that the hymen becomes a structure composed of several portions separated by narrow sulci. After childbirth the hymen becomes nodular, and the remnants are called myrtiform caruncles.

Vagina

The vagina is a muscular, tubelike structure that extends from the vulva to the uterus just above the cervix. The areas between the vaginal wall and the cervix are termed the anterior, posterior, and lateral fornices. It is through the lateral fornices that the internal pelvic organs can be palpated during the bimanual pelvic examination. The functions of the vagina include excreting uterine secretions and menstrual flow, providing sexual excitation and response, and active stretching to facilitate birth. The internal part of the vagina evolves from the müllerian ducts, whereas the more distal part is formed from the urogenital sinus. When a woman is in the dorsal lithotomy position, the vagina is angled directly posteriorly; but when she is upright, its axis is horizontal. Because of the anatomic curve to the vagina and its insertion to the uterus at a higher point posteriorly than anteriorly, the posterior wall is approximately 3 cm longer than the anterior wall. Anteriorly the vagina is separated from the bladder and urethra by the vesicovaginal septum, which is comprised of connective tissue. Posteriorly similar connective tissue forms the rectovaginal septum. The most internal, posterior part of the vagina is separated from the rectum by the rectouterine pouch (Douglas cul-de-sac).

The vaginal canal, when not distended, tends to be H-shaped since the anterior and posterior walls lie in contact with each other. This transverse slit formation is influenced by the vaginal attachment to the lateral pelvic wall between the pubic bone and the ischial spine (arcus tendineus). The lateral aspect of the vaginal walls where the anterior and posterior walls meet is the vaginal sulcus.

The lower portion of the vagina is attached to the pelvic diaphragm, the urogenital diaphragm, and the perineal body. The middle third of the vagina is attached to the pelvic diaphragm and the cardinal ligaments. The upper third is supported by the levator ani and the car-

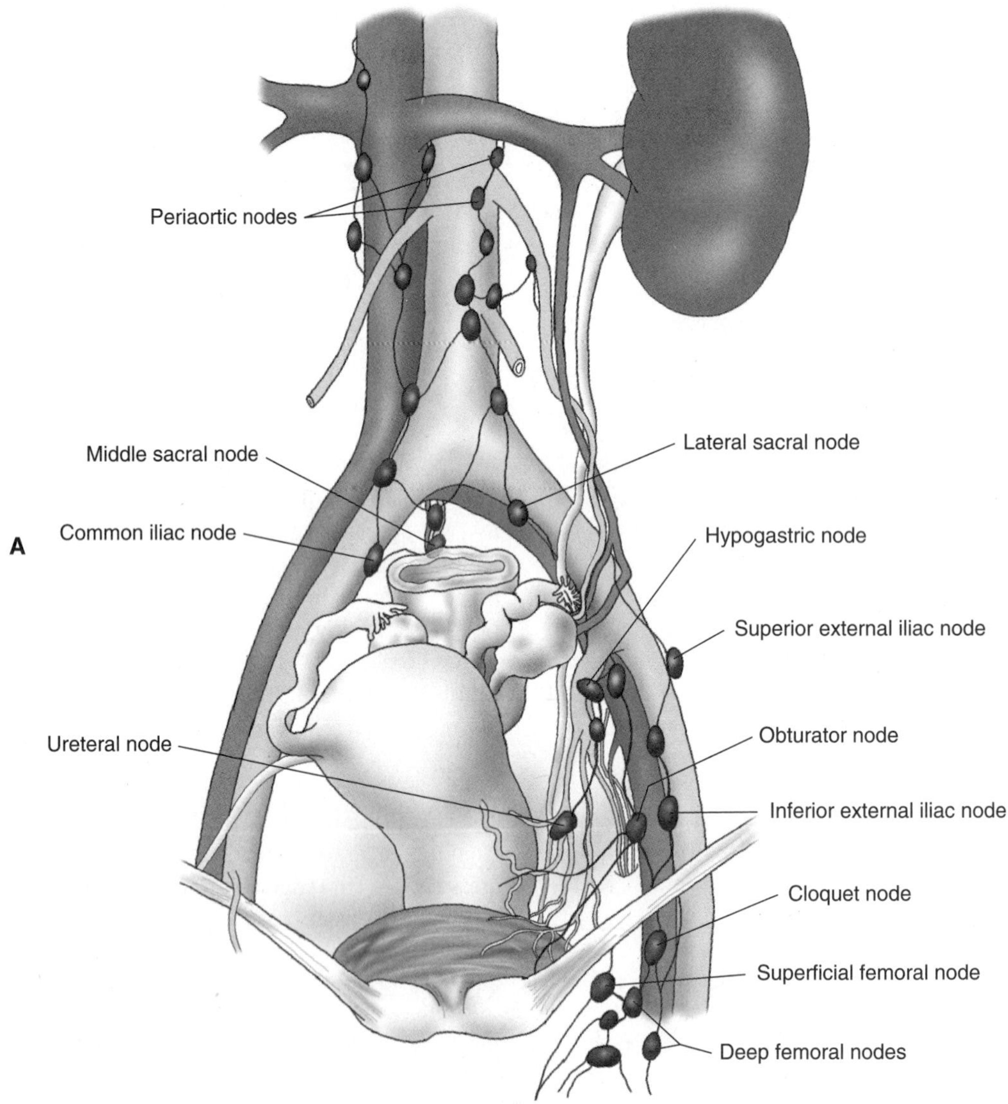

Figure 3-3 Vascular and lymphatic and neurologic anatomy of the vaginal vault. **A,** Lymphatic systems of the pelvis.

Continued

dinal and uterosacral ligaments. The fascial sheath of the vaginal merges with the fascia of the cardinal ligaments, resulting in the a supportive network that includes the levator ani.

The vagina has a rich blood supply, with the upper third served by the cervicovaginal branches of the uterine arteries, the middle third by the inferior vesical arteries, and the lower third by the middle rectal and internal pudendal arteries (Figure 3-3). Extensive venous plexes surround the vagina, emptying into the internal iliac veins. The lymphatics of the lower third of the vagina empty into the inguinal lymph nodes, those of the middle third empty into the internal iliac nodes, and those of the upper third empty into the iliac nodes.

The sympathetic innervation of the vagina arises from the hypogastric plexus. Parasympathetic innervation arises from the sacral region of the spinal cord through the pelvic nerve. The lower third of the vagina is more sensitive because of the sensory branches of the pudendal nerve.

The vagina maintains its normal cellular and bacterial balance through production of vaginal secretions that vary under hormonal influence. The pH of secretions before puberty averages from 6.8 to 7.2. Following puberty the range for pH is 4.0 to 5.0.

PERINEUM

The perineum is usually described as having two distinct parts—the urogenital triangle and the pelvic diaphragm. The urogenital triangle is bordered anteriorly by the symphysis pubis and lateroposteriorly by the ischial tuberosities and contains the external genitalia. It is divided into the superficial space and the deep perineal space. The superficial perineal space is made up of the ischiocavernosus, bulbocavernosus, and superficial transverse muscles (Figure 3-4). These muscles develop in pairs bilaterally. The superficial space also contains the vestibular glands and the vestibular bulbs.

The midline between the vagina and anus is reinforced by the central tendon of the perineum and serves as an insertion point for the bulbocavernosus muscles, superficial transverse perineal muscles, and levator ani. This area is referred to as the perineal body. These muscles provide much of the support for the perineum and deeper organs. The superficial transverse muscles have their origin at the anterior part of the ischial tuberosities and insert in the central tendon. Fibers may also insert into the external anal sphincter and the bulbocavernosus muscles. The ischiocavernosus muscles have their origin at the medial surface of the ischial tuberosities and insert into the pubic arch on each side of the crus of the

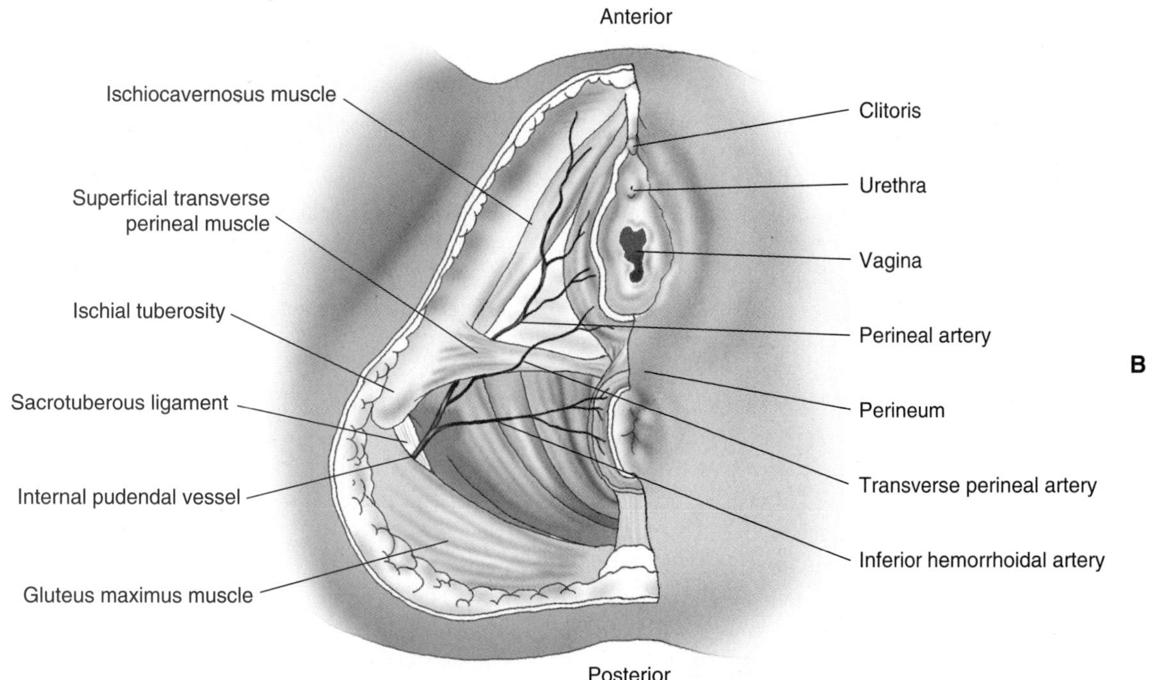

Figure 3-3, cont'd B, Vascular supply of the perineum.

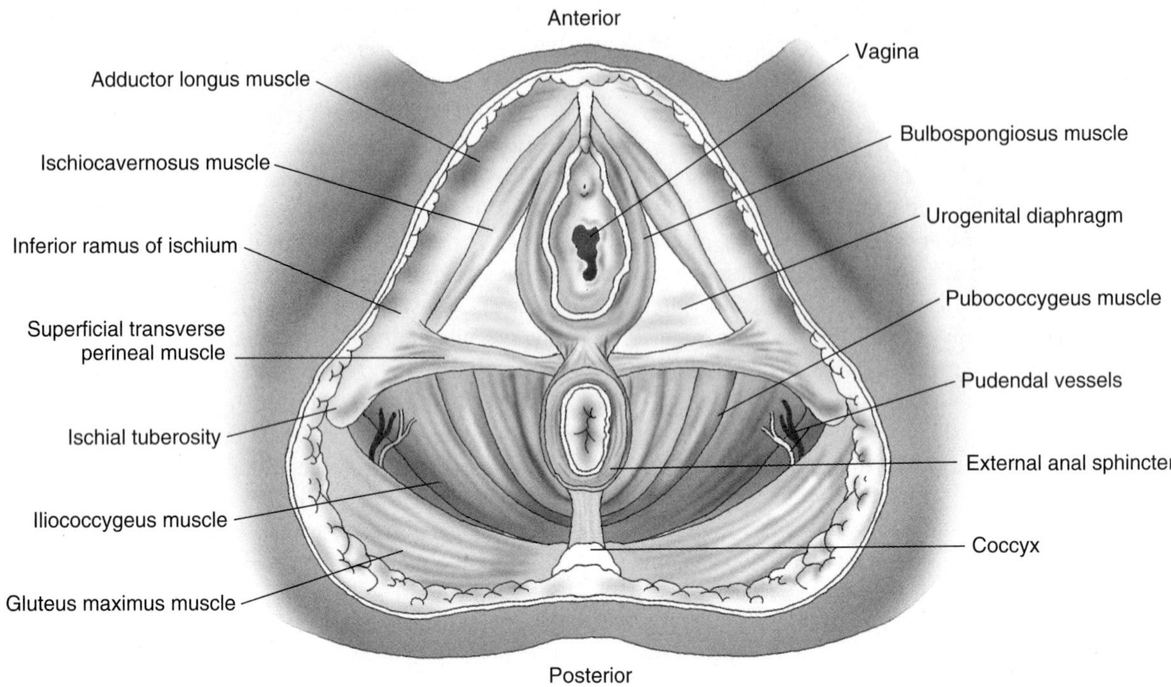

Figure 3-4 Muscles of the perineum.

clitoris. The bulbocavernosus muscles originate posteriorly at the central tendon of the perineum and insert into the dorsum of the clitoris and the inferior fascia of the urogenital diaphragm. It is helpful to conceptualize these muscles as forming a sling of support around the vaginal and its surrounding structures.

The deep transverse perineal muscles, the urethral sphincter, and the internal and external fascial coverings make up the deeper structures of the urogenital diaphragm. The deep transverse perineal muscles serve a function in urinary continence in the male, but it does not appear that they serve a similar function in the female.

The pelvic diaphragm includes the levator ani and coccygeus muscles and the fascial coverings of these muscles. The levator ani muscles originate from the posterior surface of the superior rami of the pubis, the inner aspect of the ischial spines, and the obturator fascia. The levator ani is composed of the pubococcygeus muscle, which includes the pubovaginalis, puborectalis, and iliococcygeus muscles. The muscle provides a slinglike appearance, stretching from the pubis to the coccyx and from one side of the pelvis to the other. The urethra, vagina, and anal canal perforate it. Its origin is at the arch extending from the pubis to the ischial spine, and its insertions include the central tendon of the perineum, the wall of the anal canal, the anococcygeal ligament, the coccyx, and the vaginal wall. The levator ani, along with the abdominal muscles, is essential for supporting the abdominal and pelvic organs. It provides support for the posterior wall of the vagina, and during birthing it supports the fetal head during dilation. The levator ani is innervated by the inferior rectal nerve.

The internal pudendal artery and its branches, the inferior rectal and posterior labial arteries, provide the majority of the perineal blood supply. Perineal innervation is via the pudendal nerve and its branches, the perineal branch of the posterior femoral cutaneous nerve, and the ilioinguinal and genitofemoral nerves.

INTERNAL PELVIC ORGANS

The internal organs included in the pelvis include the uterus, fallopian tubes, ovaries, bladder, and rectum (Figure 3-5).

Uterus

The uterus is a flattened, pear-shaped, muscular organ maintained in place in the pelvis by five sets of bilateral ligaments—the broad, cardinal, round, uterosacral, and

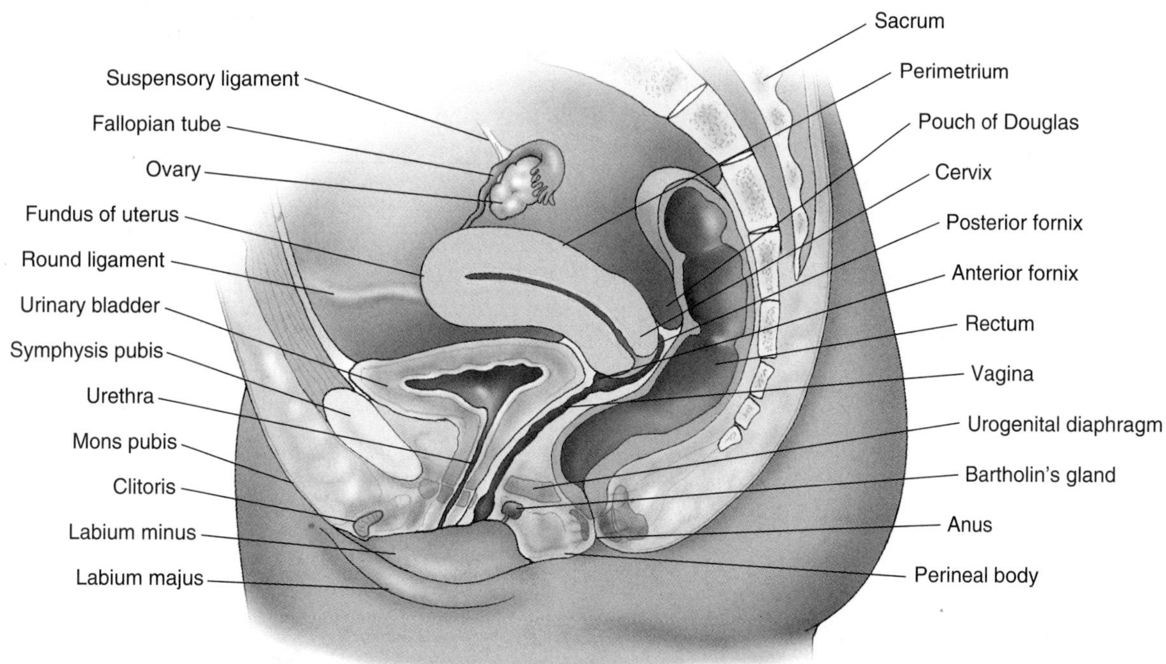

Figure 3-5 Internal pelvic organs.

uterovesical ligaments. It is bordered by the bladder anteriorly and the rectum posteriorly. The lower anterior part is attached to the bladder wall. Peritoneal epithelium covers the rest of the uterus, except at the lateral margins, where it extends to cover the broad ligaments, and at the area immediately above the bladder, where it forms the anterior boundary of the recto-uterine cul-de-sac (Douglas cul-de-sac).

The uterus is divided into three parts: the body (corpus), the isthmus, and the cervix. The anterior of the body is flattened, whereas the posterior part is rounded. The fallopian tubes insert at the cornua, the upper lateral areas of the organ. The area of thick musculature between the insertions of the tubes is the fundus. The isthmus is at the level of the internal os of the cervix where the cells change from the classical stratified mucosa of the endometrium to the simple columnar, mucus-secreting cells of the endocervix. In the nonpregnant state the isthmus is essentially merged with the cervix. In pregnancy, however, it develops into the lower uterine segment. The cervix is the lowest part of the uterus that junctions with the vagina.

The size and shape of the uterus varies by age and parity of the woman. Before puberty the uterus is 2.5 to 3.5 cm in length. After menarche the nulliparous uterus averages 6 to 8 cm in length, with a weight of 50 to 70 g. Multiparous uteri average 9 to 10 cm in length, with a weight of 80 g or more.

The body of the uterus is primarily muscle fibers. The anterior and posterior walls lie almost in contact with minimal space or cavity. The walls of the body of the uterus are comprised of three distinct layers—serosa, myometrium, and endometrium. The peritoneal layer that covers most of the uterus and the posterior cervix is the serosa. Directly beneath the external serosal layer lies the myometrium, which makes up the bulk of the uterine mass and ranges from 1.5 to 2.5 cm in thickness. The myometrium is comprised of smooth muscle cells, fibroblasts, blood and lymphatic vessels, immune cells, and connective tissue. The outer layer of myometrium is a network of fiber bundles arranged in a longitudinal pattern, generally following the long axis of the uterine body. The innermost layer of myometrium is a circular network that form sphincters around the tubal insertions and internal os of the cervix. The middle layer of myometrium forms a distinct interlacing around the many blood vessels and is sometimes referred to as the "figure-of-eight" pattern of fibers.

The muscle fibers are most concentrated in the fundus, where there is only a small proportion of connective tissue cells in relation to the muscle. The proportion of muscle cells to connective tissues decreases toward the isthmus and cervix so muscle only makes up about 10% of cervical tissue. There are increased fibers in the anterior and posterior walls, with fewer fibers in the lateral walls. In the thick muscular area of the fundus, the individual muscle bundles are surrounded by connective tissue sheaths that contain elastic tissue. The pattern of muscle and elastic fibers provides an excellent system for ligating blood vessels following birth to decrease blood loss.

The internal layer of the uterus is the endometrium, a mucosal layer with a pink velvetlike appearance in the nonpregnant female. It is comprised of epithelium, glands, and interglandular mesenchymal tissue in which there are numerous blood vessels. The epithelium is a single layer of closely packed columnar cells. Cilia have been identified in some endometrial epithelial cells in many mammals, including humans, and appear to be in discrete areas separate from secretory cells. The cilia maintain a current that continues from the fallopian tubes downward to the external os of the cervix.

The vascular system of the endometrium is of importance for both menstruation and pregnancy (Figure 3-6). Arterial blood is supplied to the uterus via the uterine and ovarian arteries. Branches of these vessels penetrate the uterine wall and in the myometrium develop a network of arteries parallel to the endometrium (arcuate arteries). Radial arteries branch off the arcuate arteries at

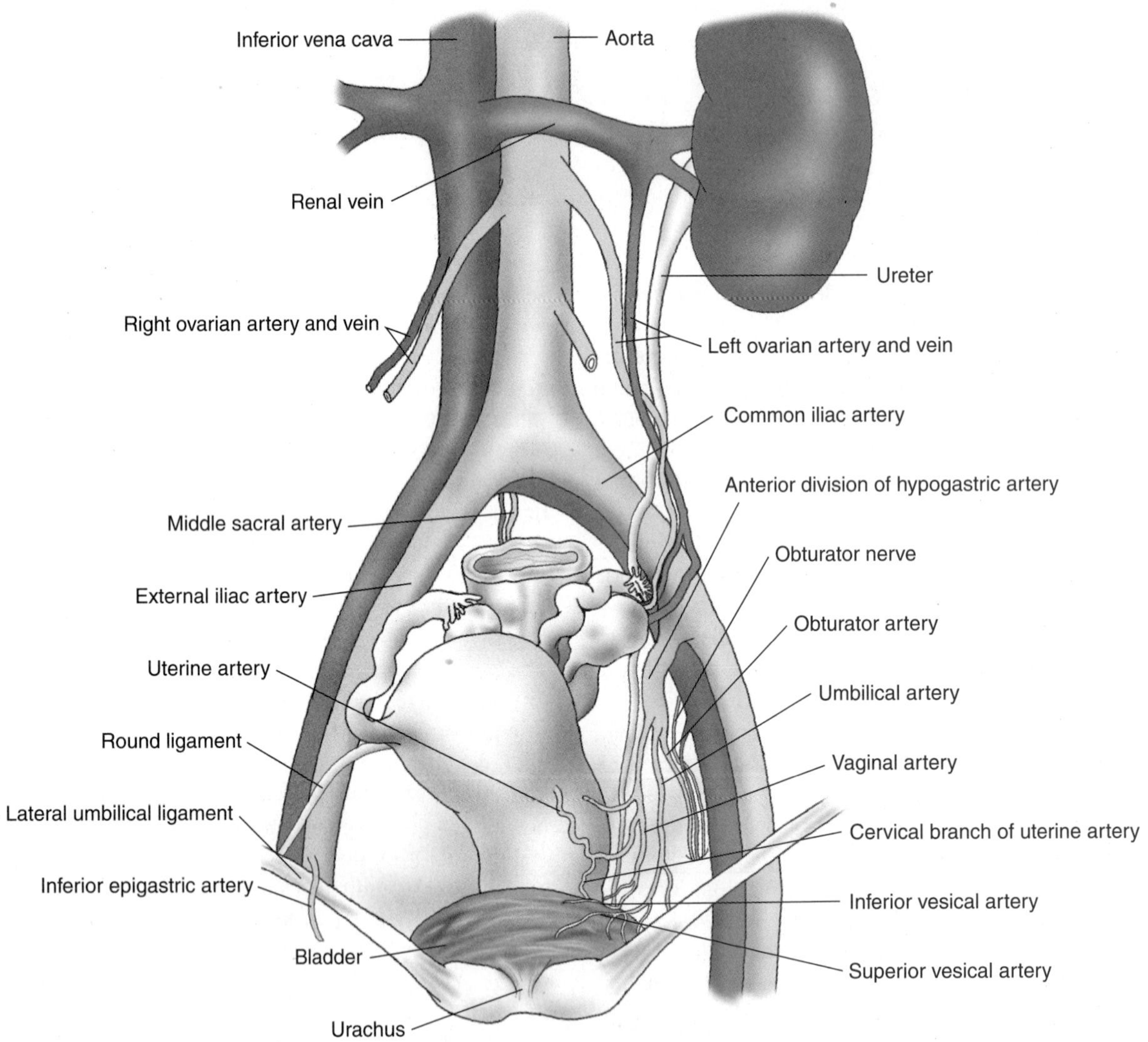

Figure 3-6 Uterine vasculature.

right angles and become the basal and coiled (spiral) arteries of the endometrium. The coiled arteries, which are highly sensitive to several hormones, provide the blood supply for the middle in superficial parts of the endometrium. The basal arteries provide the blood supply for the basal layer of the endometrium and are not influenced by hormonal activity.

The cervix is a distinct portion of the uterus that extends from the internal os to the external os. The lower portion of the cervix extends into the vagina and is referred to as the portio vaginalis. In prepubescent females the cervix makes up approximately two thirds of the uterus, whereas the uterine body makes up about one third. In nulliparous women the cervix and body are about the same length. The cervix in multiparous women makes up about one third of the uterus. The cervix is approximately 2 to 3 cm in length.

The cervix is primarily composed of collagenous tissue, elastic tissue, and blood vessels, with a relatively small amount of smooth muscle cells. It is estimated that only about 10% of cervical tissue is smooth muscle. The internal canal of the cervix is lined with a single layer of high columnar epithelium that rests on a thin basement membrane. The cells have abundant cilia. Numerous cervical glands extend from the endocervical mucous membrane to the connective tissue cells. These glands produce a thick, tenacious mucoid discharge. Occasionally the ducts for these glands become occluded and form nabothian cysts or follicles. The vaginal part of the cervix is covered with squamous epithelium. The line of demarcation where the vaginal and endocervical cells meet, the squamocolumnar junction, is usually at the external os in adult women. However, in pregnancy, with oral contraceptive use, and in early childhood the columnar epithelium may extend into the exocervix, a condition referred to as actopy or eversion. After menopause the junction usually recedes into the endocervical canal.

Fallopian Tubes

The fallopian tubes arise from the müllerian ducts in embryonic life. In mature females they vary in length from 8 to 14 cm. The functions of the fallopian tubes include retrieval of the ovum, provision of an environment conducive for fertilization, and transport and nourishment of the fertilized ovum. The tubes have four distinct parts. The interstitial part runs from the uterine cavity through the uterine wall. The isthmus is the narrowest part and is at the junction of the tube and the uterine wall. The ampulla is the widest part of the tube, running from the isthmus to the fimbriated end of the tube. The infundibulum is the funnel-shaped fimbriated end that opens into the abdominal cavity. The fimbria provide a wide surface for pickup of the ovum. The wall of the tube is composed of a muscular outer layer of longitudinal smooth muscle and a middle muscular layer of circular fibers. The muscle fibers produce rhythmic contractions of the tubes that vary throughout the menstrual cycle and pregnancy. The strongest waves of contractions occur midcycle, and the weakest contractions occur during pregnancy. The inner layer of mucous membrane is ciliated columnar epithelium. The mucous membrane is continuous with the lining of the uterus.

The fallopian tubes are covered by peritoneum. The uterine and ovarian arteries provide their blood supply, and they are innervated by the uterovaginal plexus and the ovarian plexus.

Ovaries

The ovaries are the sites of development and release of ova and the synthesis and secretion of steroid hormones. They lie bilaterally adjacent to the uterus and are almond-shaped with diameters of 2.5 to 5 cm in length, 1.5 to 3 cm in width, and 0.6 to 1.5 cm in depth during the childbearing years. Their size is influenced by the levels of endogenous and exogenous hormone levels. Before puberty and after menopause the ovaries are significantly smaller in size.

Each ovary is attached inferiorly to the broad ligament by mesentery (mesovarium). The uteroovarian ligament (ovarian ligament) connects the lateroposterior part of the uterus to the lower pole of the ovary. The infundibulopelvic ligament of the ovary extends from the upper pole of the ovary to the pelvic wall. The ovarian vessels and nerves are surrounded by this ligament, and vessels and nerves enter the ovary through the mesentery.

The ovary consists of the cortex, the outer part, and the medulla, the internal structure. The cortex is the site of the ova and graafian follicles. The medulla is composed of connective tissue, arteries, veins, and a small amount of smooth muscle. The ovary is covered with a single layer of flattened cuboidal to low columnar epithelium that is continuous with the peritoneum.

THE BONY PELVIS

During labor the fetus must negotiate through the bony pelvis to accomplish birth. Birth attendants must have a thorough understanding of the characteristics of pelvic architecture to appreciate the mechanisms of birth and understand the problems encountered during labor.

The bony pelvis consists of four bones: the sacrum, the coccyx, and two innominate bones (Figure 3-7). The innominate bones are made up of three fused bones—the pubis, the ischium, and the ilium. There are four joints, the symphysis pubis anteriorly, the sacrococcygeal joint, and the two sacroiliac joints posteriorly. The symphysis pubis and sacrococcygeal joints are cartilaginous symphyseal joints, joints that are surrounded by strong ligaments anteriorly and posteriorly and are affected by relaxin during pregnancy. The sacroiliac joints are synovial joints that are supported by the sacroiliac ligaments, the iliolumbar ligament, the lateral lumbosacral ligament, the sacrotuberous ligament, and the sacrospinous ligament.

The pelvis is divided into the true pelvis and the false pelvis. The false pelvis lies above the arcuate and pectineal lines, consists of the broad iliac crests, and is of little obstetric significance during labor. However, it does provide a degree of support to the growing uterus as pregnancy progresses. The true pelvis contains the passage through which the fetus must negotiate.

Understanding the characteristics of the bony pelvis and the influence of specific landmarks on the diameters of the pelvis is essential in predicting and assessing the course of labor. Formal assessment of the pelvis during the physical examination (clinical pelvimetry) gives the clinician information that is helpful in educating the patient about anticipated labor patterns and planning management strategies for labor.

The two pubic bones join anteriorly with the ischiopubic rami, forming the subpubic arch. The arch is typically equal to or greater than a 90-degree angle. A narrow arch decreases the usable space in the anterior pelvis for the descending fetus and is associated with converging sidewalls of the pelvis. The thickness and inclination of the pubis gives further information used in determining the pelvic type (Table 3-1). The rami extend posteriorly to the ischial tuberosities. Posterior and superior to the ischial tuberosities are the ischial spines, which are the landmarks for the midpelvis. The ischial spines are usually blunt and may be difficult to palpate. Prominent spines are associated with a decreased transverse diameter of the midpelvis.

The ileum stretches from the ischial spines superiorly, where it adjoins the sacrum. The sacrosciatic notch can be estimated by either assessing the length of the sacrospinous ligament or palpating the borders of the notch. The width of the notch suggests the inclination of the sacrum. The sacrum consists of five fused vertebrae and terminates with the coccyx. The anterior aspect of the sacrum is typically concave with a slight backward inclination. If the sacrum is short and inclined forward at the level of the spines, it may compromise the anterio-posterior (AP) diameter of the midpelvis. If it is long and inclined forward with termination below the level of the spines, the mechanism of labor is not usually affected. The coccyx is a fusion of four rudimentary vertebrae, and its mobility usually moves it out of the way of the descending fetal part. However, the coccyx may be fixed in place, either congenitally or from previous injury, in which case it may impede descent.

Pelvic Axis

The inclination of the human pelvis reflects the adjustments that were necessary to accomplish bipedal ambulation. Pelvic inclination is normally 55 to 60 degrees of true horizontal when the individual in the erect position. The axis of the pelvis (curve of Carus) is the hypothetic line formed by connecting the center point of each of the planes of the pelvis (Figure 3-8).

The fetal presenting part enters the pelvis and descends at right angles to the plane of the inlet (pelvic brim). In the midpelvis, the axis turns 90 degrees anterior following the sloping pelvic floor. This change in direction places the fetal presenting part into the axis of the outlet. The pelvic axis must be considered when assessing the progress of second stage or assisting the birth of the baby's body and the placenta and when instrumental delivery is necessary.

Pelvic Planes

It is helpful to think of the pelvis as funnel shaped with four distinct planes. Diameters of the planes are measured or estimated anteroposteriorly, transversely, and obliquely. Oblique diameters are described as left or right, depending on their posterior terminus. Sagittal diameters are AP diameters that are estimated from an imaginary line determining the transverse diameter either anterior or posterior to the bony pelvis. For example, the posterior sagittal diameter of the midplane extends from the point of the imaginary line between the ischial spines to the S4 to S5 vertebrae.

The plane of the inlet marks the entry to the true pelvis and is bordered by the upper posterior symphysis pubis, the ridge of the iliac bones (linea terminalis), and the sacral promontory. The AP diameter of the inlet is called the obstetric conjugate and is the shortest diame-

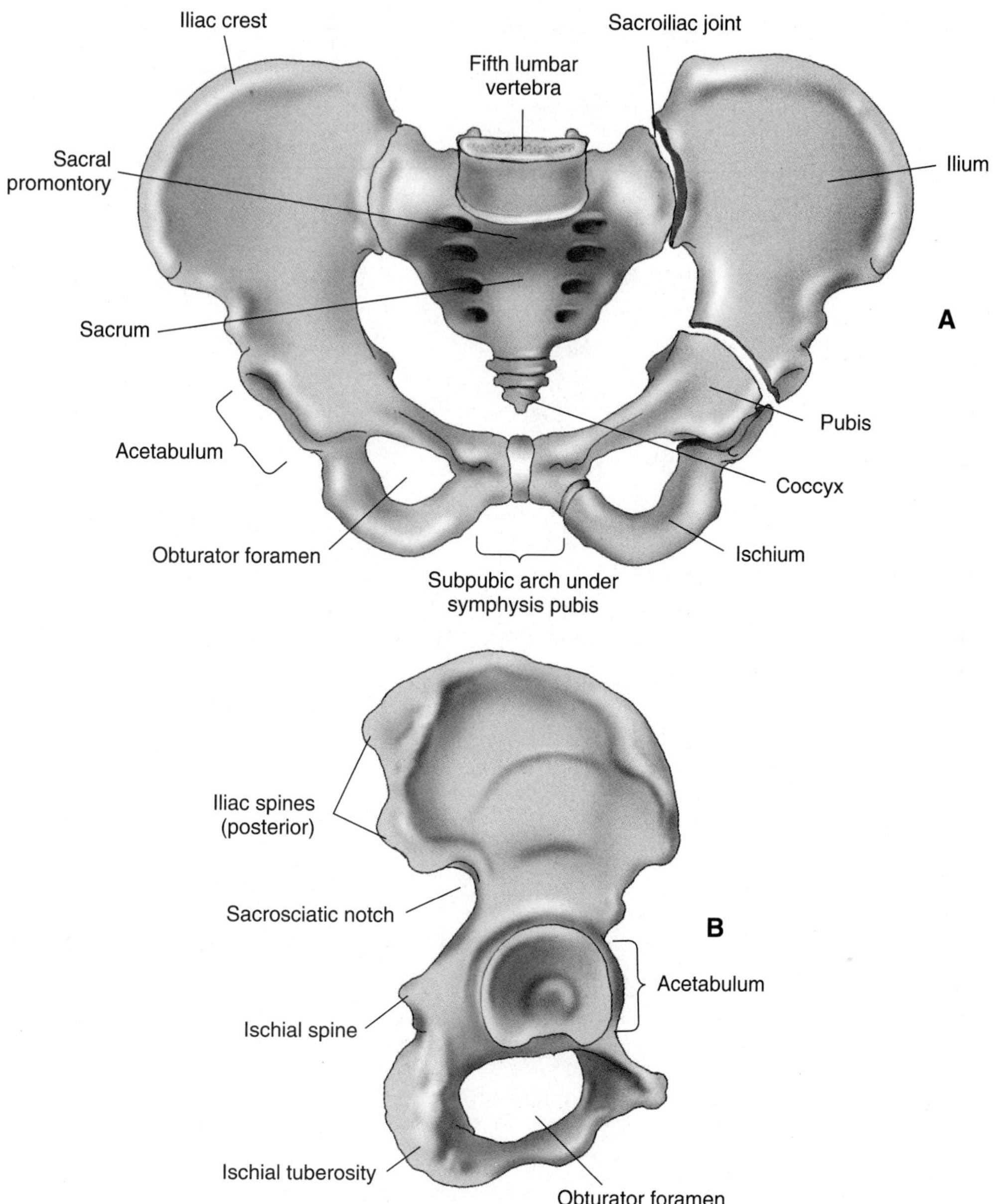

Figure 3-7 Bony pelvis. **A,** Anterior view. **B,** External view of right innominate bone.

ter between the upper posterior symphysis pubis and the sacral promontory. The average AP diameter of the inlet is 11. Since the obstetrics conjugate cannot be directly measured, it is estimated by measuring the diagonal conjugate. The transverse diameter of the inlet represents the greatest diameter between the ileopectineal lines on either side of the pelvis and is estimated to be 13.5 cm.

The plane of greatest diameter corresponds to the imaginary plane at the level of the middle of the symphysis pubis and the junction between the second and third sacral vertebrae. Since this plane does not have any characteristics that impede descent, it is of little obstetric significance.

The plane of the midpelvis is referred to as the plane of least dimensions. It is bordered by the lower edge of the symphysis pubis, the ischial spines, and the lower vertebrae of the sacrum. As the name implies, the transverse diameter of this plane is the narrowest part of the

Table 3-1 *Characteristics of Pelvic Types*

	Gynecoid	Android	Anthropoid	Platypelloid
Pelvic Inlet				
Incidence	85%	4.5%	7.3%	3.1%
Shape	Round or ovoid	Triangular; "heart-shaped"	Ovoid with elongated anteroposterior diameter	Transverse oval
Bone structure	Medium; delicate	Heavy	Medium to heavy	Medium to delicate
Forepelvis	Rounded	Narrow with sharp angulation	Rounded and deep	Shallow and wide
Posterior segment	Deep and roomy	Shallow; pronounced sacral promontory	Long and deep	Shallow
Diagonal conjugate	Adequate; average: 12.5 cm	Adequate to short	Long	Short
Obstetric conjugate	Average: 11 cm	Average	Long	Short; critical diameter: 10 cm
Anterior sagittal diameter	Adequate	Long	Long	Short
Posterior sagittal diameter	Average	Very short	Very long	Very short
Transverse diameter	Adequate; average: 13.5 cm	Adequate	Adequate to somewhat narrowed; critical diameter: 12 cm	Wide
Midpelvis				
Sidewalls	Straight	Convergent	Straight	Straight; slightly divergent
Ischial spines	Blunt	Prominent; encroaching	Blunt to prominent	Variable
Sacrum	Average length; straight to slightly posteriorly inclined; roomy, bowl-shaped	Long, heavy, straight with forward inclination	Long and narrow; straight	Short
Sacrosciatic notch	2-3 fingerbreadths wide	Narrow; <2-3 fingerbreadths	Wide; >3 fingerbreadths	Wide; >3 fingerbreadths
Anteroposterior diameter	Average: 11.5 cm	Shortened; critical diameter: 11.5 cm	Long	Short; critical diameter: 11.5 cm
Anterior sagittal diameter	Adequate	Short	Adequate	Short

Adapted from Whitley N: *A manual of clinical obstetrics,* Philadelphia, 1985, JB Lippincott; and Caldwell WE, Moloy HC: Anatomic variations in the female pelvis and their effect on labor with a suggested classification, *Am J Obstet Gynecol* 26:479, 1933.

Continued

Table 3-1 *Characteristics of Pelvic Types—cont'd*

	Gynecoid	Android	Anthropoid	Platypelloid
Midpelvis—cont'd				
Posterior sagittal diameter	Adequate	Short	Adequate	Short
Transverse diameter	Average: 10.5 cm	Average	Adequate to slightly shortened; critical diameter: 12 cm	Wide
Outlet				
Subpubic arch	Rounded; >90 degrees; >2-3 fingerbreadths	Deep; narrow; angulated	Deep; slightly narrow; slightly rounded	Wide; shallow
Inferior pubic rami	Short, concave inward; fine-boned	Long and straight	Long, narrow	Short; straight
Anterior sagittal diameter	Average: 6 cm	Short	Long	Short
Posterior sagittal	Average	Short	Long	Short
Transverse diameter diameter	Adequate; average: 11 cm	Short; critical diameter: 8.5 cm	Adequate	Wide

pelvis. The transverse diameter in an average gynecoid pelvis is 10.5 cm.

The plane of the outlet can be conceptualized as two triangular planes sharing a common base. The anterior triangle is bordered by the inferior border of the symphysis pubis and an imaginary line drawn between the ischial tuberosities. The posterior triangle is bordered by the ischial tuberosities and the coccyx. The anatomic AP diameter is measured from the lower margin of the symphysis pubis to the tip of the coccyx; but, since the coccyx usually is pushed posteriorly as the fetus descends, the more useful diameter is the obstetric AP diameter, which is measured from the lower edge of the pubis to the sacrococcygeal joint. The obstetric AP diameter of the outlet should measure at least 11.5 cm.

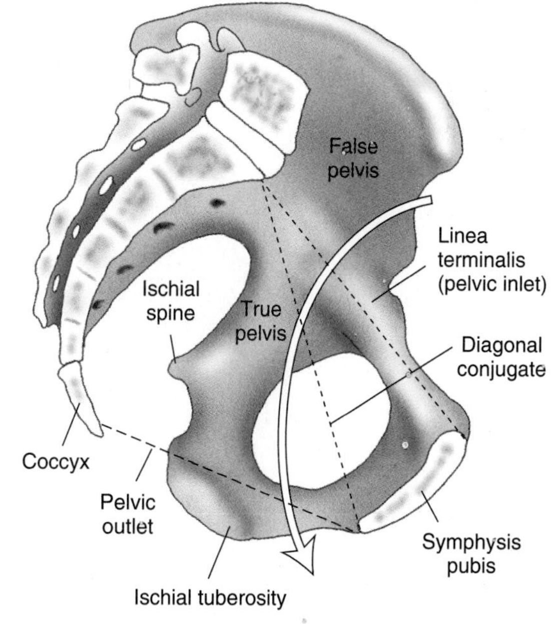

Figure 3-8 Pelvic axis.

Pelvic Diameters

The AP diameters of the planes increase from the inlet to the outlet, whereas the transverse diameters decrease. The greatest diameters of each plane assist with the rotation of the fetal presenting part as it negotiates the pelvic axis (Figure 3-9).

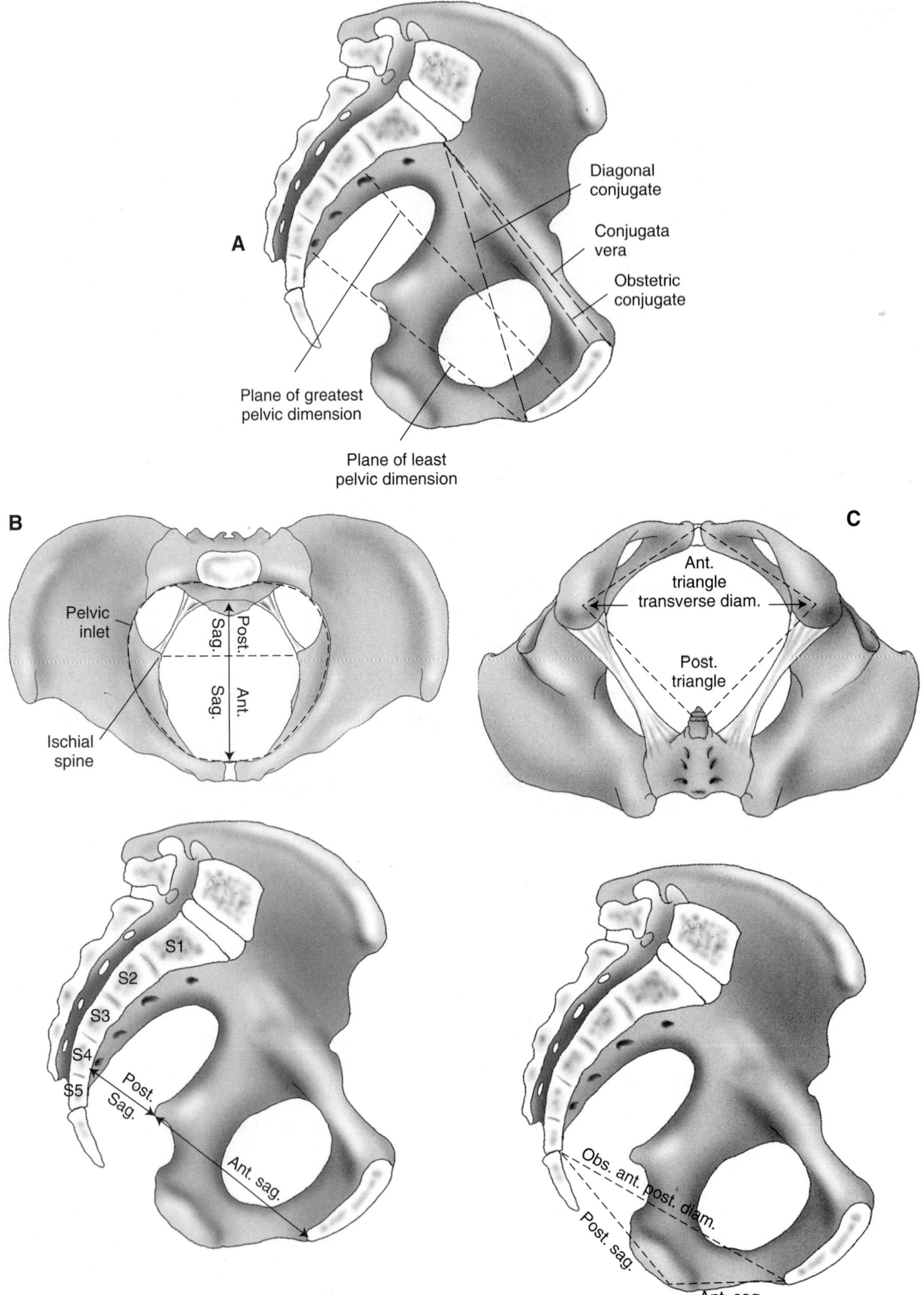

Figure 3-9 Diameters of the **A,** pelvic inlet, **B,** midpelvis, and **C,** pelvic outlet.

Pelvic Types

The variety of pelvic shapes have been grouped into four classifications based on certain characteristics of the pelvic architecture (Caldwell and Moloy) (Figure 3-10). Since the "pure" pelvic type is rare, the Caldwell-Moloy classification is applied to the posterior characteristics of the pelvis, and the anterior characteristics are further described as the tendency. Hence a pelvis with a round roomy posterior segment and a constricted anterior segment would be described as a gynecoid pelvis with an android tendency (Figure 3-11).

The most common pelvic type in women is the gynecoid pelvis. Its rounded inlet, straight side walls, blunt ischial spines, and wide pubic arch make it ideal for childbearing.

The android pelvis is more similar to the male pelvis. The bony structure is heavier than the gynecoid, and the inlet is a distinct heart shape. The narrow forepelvis,

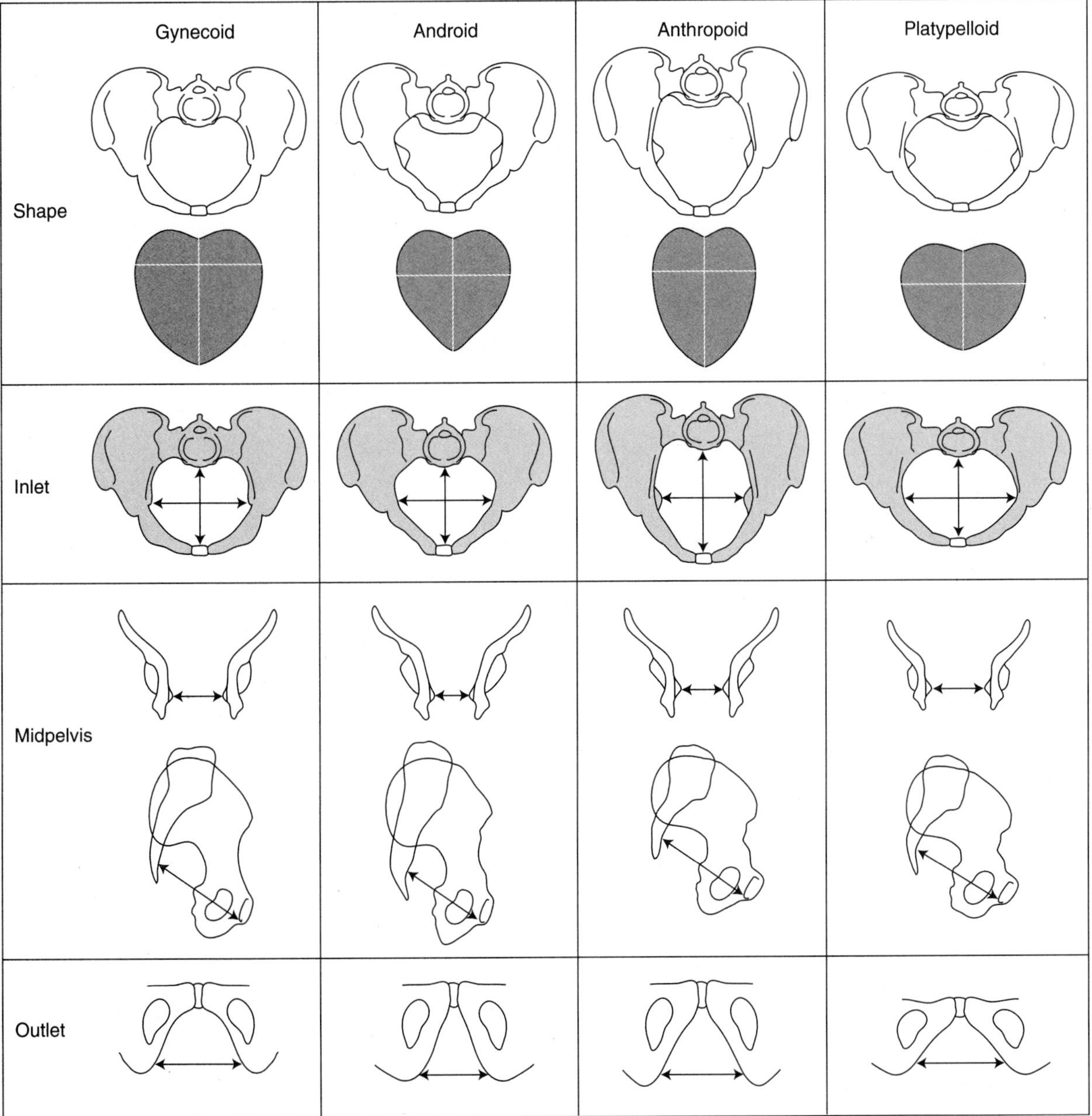

Figure 3-10 Caldwell-Moloy classification.

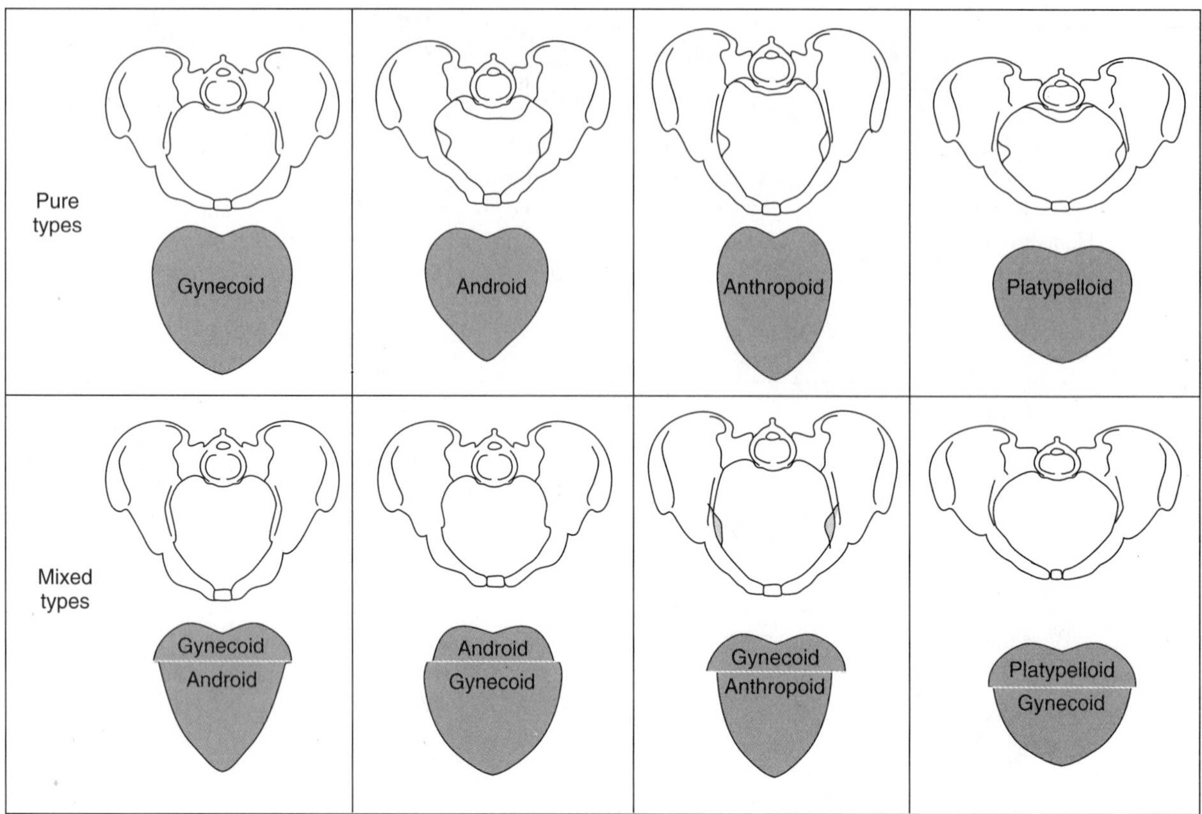

Figure 3-11 Mixed pelvic types.

converging sidewalls, narrow subpubic arch, and prominent ischial spines contribute to a poor prognosis for successful vaginal delivery.

The anthropoid pelvis has an oval inlet with an AP diameter longer than the transverse diameter. The forepelvis may be narrowed, and the spines may be prominent. However, the sacrum is often posteriorly inclined, creating a roomy posterior pelvis that facilitates descent of the fetus in a posterior position. This type of pelvis is more common in women who are of African descent.

The platypelloid pelvis is the least common type. It is characterized by an oval inlet with a narrow AP diameter and an extremely wide subpubic arch. In its pure state the fetus would most likely not be able to enter the inlet, so that prognosis for vaginal delivery is poor. However, the platypelloid tendency is common in Native American women, and delivery is facilitated by roomy posterior pelves.

Chapter 4

Menstrual Cycle and Conception

Conception requires the completion of complex physiologic functions in both the male and female. This chapter will explore the development of female and male germ cells, the normal physiology of the menstrual cycle, and the process of fertilization.

EMBRYONIC AND FETAL DEVELOPMENT OF THE REPRODUCTIVE SYSTEM

Structures related to reproduction differentiate into male and female systems in the embryonic period (Figure 4-1). Genetic sexual identity is established at the time of fertilization and is defined by the complement of X and Y chromosomes. Gonadal sex is determined by the structure and function of the gonads, whereas somatic sex is determined by the structure and function of the other sexual organs. Social sex and psychologic sex define the roles adopted by the individual and expressed in society (Blackburn and Loper, 1992). These definitions become interwoven as a description of the sexual identity of the individual as she or he develops through the life span.

Human gonads arise from three types of cells: (1) primordial germ cells, (2) underlying mesenchyme, and (3) coelomic epithelium. The primordial germ cells are primitive sex cells that can be identified by the fourth week of gestation (Spiegelman and Bennett, 1973). These originate in the primitive ectoderm cells of the wall of the yolk sac, but the specific cells of origin cannot be identified (Speroff, Glass, and Kase, 1999). The cells "migrate" from the yolk sac along the dorsal mesentery of the hindgut to the gonadal ridge (Blackburn and Loper, 1992). These cells continue to divide during the migration by mitosis and will eventually become oogonia or spermatogonia. By the sixth week mitosis has produced 10,000 primordial germ cells, and the gonads contain both the germ cells and the somatic cells.

Two theories of development of the gonadal cells exist. In one, the gonadal ridge arises from the coelomic epithelium on the medial side of the mesonephros during the fifth week of gestation. Invading cells from this ridge grow downward into the mesenchyme, forming the primary sex cord, which contains germ cells surrounded by somatic cells. A newer model proposes that the somatic cells arise from the mesonephros, separate from the cells that arise in the coelomic epithelium (Speroff, Glass, and Kase, 1999). The gonads then separate from the mesonephros, and two layers form—the cortex and the medulla. At 6 weeks' gestation the gonads of females and males are not morphologically distinguishable. In the XX embryo the cortex differentiates into ovarian tissue, and the medulla regresses. Conversely, in the XY embryo the medulla differentiates into testicular tissue while the cortex regresses.

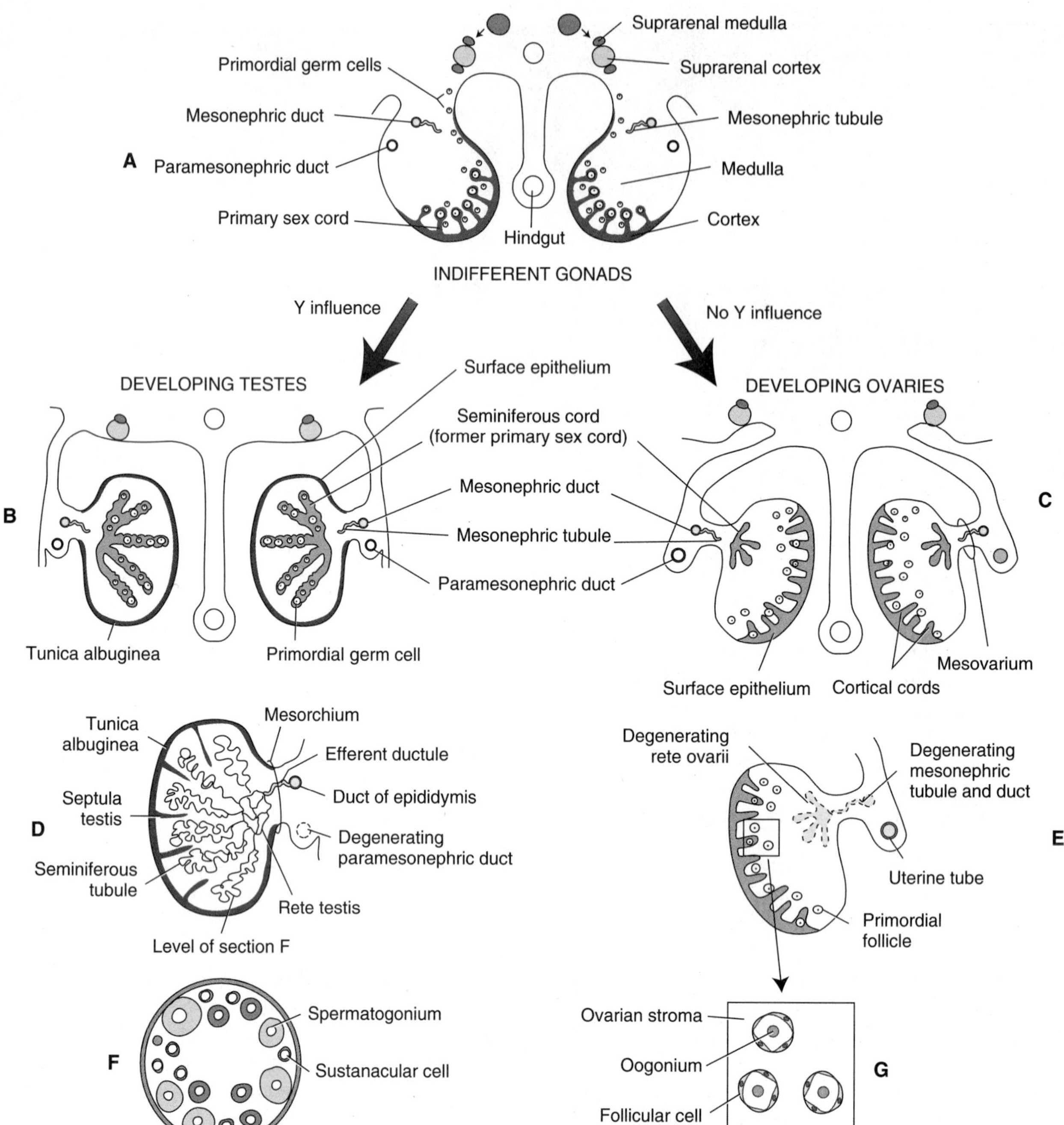

Figure 4-1 Differentiation of ovaries and testes. **A,** 6 weeks, showing the indifferent gonads composed of an outer cortex and an inner medulla. **B,** 7 weeks, showing testes developing under the influence of a Y chromosome. Note that the primary sex cords have become seminiferous cords. **C,** 12 weeks, showing ovaries beginning to develop in the absence of a Y chromosome. Cortical cords have extended from the surface epithelium, displacing the primary sex cords centrally into the mesovarium, where they form the rudimentary rete ovarii. **D,** Testis at 20 weeks, showing the rete testis and the seminiferous tubules derived from the seminiferous cords. An efferent ductule has developed from a mesonephric tubule, and the mesonephric duct has become the duct of the epididymis. **E,** Ovary at 20 weeks, showing the primordial follicles formed from the cortical cords. **F,** Section of a seminiferous tubule from a 20-week fetus. Note that no lumen is present at this stage and that the seminiferous epithelium is composed of two kinds of cells. **G,** Section from the ovarian cortex of a 20-week fetus, showing three primordial follicles containing oogonia. (Adapted from Blackburn ST, Loper DL: *Maternal, fetal and neonatal physiology,* Philadelphia, 1992, WB Saunders, p. 14.)

Differentiation of the sexual organs is thought to begin with the action of histocompatibility-Y (H-Y) antigen genes (testes-determining factor) that are located on the Y chromosome. The SR-Y locus on the short-arm of the Y chromosome is thought to be the primary regulator of testicular development. By week 6 to 7 an increase in H-Y antigens as the cells increase and join with each other contributes to the development of the testicular cords. The primordial germ cells in the testicular cords will develop into the tubules that are the site of the Sertoli cells and spermatogonia. The Sertoli cells are responsible for producing androgen-binding proteins that are important in maintaining the high androgen environment necessary for spermatogenesis (Speroff, Glass, and Kase, 1999). The mesenchyme produces interstitial cells (Leydig cells) that produce testosterone almost immediately. Testosterone induces the masculinization of the external genitalia. Testosterone level rises along with the proliferation of Leydig cells and reaches peak levels at 15 to 18 weeks' gestation. Thereafter there is a decrease in the number of Leydig cells and testosterone production. The rise and fall of androgen secretion by the Leydig cells parallels the levels of human chorionic gonadotropin (hCG), suggesting a regulatory role of hCG. Fetal Leydig cells respond to high levels of hCG and luteinizing hormone (LH) by increasing steroidogenesis and cell multiplication. This is in contrast to adult Leydig cells, which respond to high levels of hCG and LH by decreasing steroidogenesis. The relationship between the functioning of the fetal and adult Leydig cells remains unknown.

As gonadal differentiation proceeds, the primordial germ cells in the testicular cord develop into spermatogonia, which are surrounded by Sertoli cells (Speroff, Glass, and Kase, 1999). The male germ cells remain dormant until puberty when they begin meiotic division.

Ovarian development occurs more slowly than testicular development. At 6 to 8 weeks' gestation the primordial germ cells begin rapid mitotic divisions, producing 6 to 7 million oogonia by 16 to 20 weeks' gestation. The ovary is identifiable by 10 weeks' gestation, and by the twelfth week the medulla is primarily connective tissue with few cells that will mature into follicular cells. Around 12 weeks' gestation oogonia begin the first meiotic division, and during pregnancy the cells progress to the diplotene stage of meiosis when arrest of meiosis occurs. The exact mechanism for this arrest in the meiotic process is not understood, but it is thought that the granulosa cells may secrete an inhibiting substance (Speroff, Glass, and Kase, 1999).

During the fourth month of gestation cortical cords (secondary sex cords) extend into the gonad from the germinal epithelium. Primordial germ cells become incorporated into the cords, and during the sixteenth week of gestation the cords separate into groups of cells consisting of a primitive ova surrounded by a single layer of follicular cells that are derived from the cortical cords. This grouping is termed the primordial follicle and will later develop into a primary follicle if an oocyte is formed. Within these cell clusters mesenchymal cells secrete an outer basement membrane (membrane propia) that will provide nutrients to the developing oocyte. During the period of primary follicle formation, the oogonia begin the meiotic process.

In contrast to the male process of germ cell differentiation, the female process does not rely on steroid production. Estrogen production does not begin until late pregnancy, and steroidogenesis is not at a significant level until puberty. Continued development of the reproductive system in the female occurs independent of ovarian control.

Male and female embryos have two pairs of genital ducts—the mesonephric (wolffian) duct and the paramesonephric (müllerian) duct. The mesonephric ducts arise from the urinary system and develop into the ductus deferens (vas deferens), the epididymis, and the ejaculatory ducts in the male. The mesonephric ducts regress in the female because of a lack of locally produced testosterone. The paramesonephric ducts develop parallel to the mesonephric ducts and then cross and fuse to form a single canal. The paranephronic ducts develop into the fallopian tubes, uterus, and upper portion of the vagina in the female and regress and degenerate in the male. It has also been proposed that the Sertoli cells of the fetal seminiferous tubules secrete a müllerian-inhibiting substance that acts locally to cause regression of the paramesonephric duct. This inhibiting process occurs even before the tubules are completed and before Leydig cells appear and produce testosterone.

Differentiating characteristics of male and female embryos are not noticeable until the ninth week of gestation (Figure 4-2). The genital tubercle begins developing during the fourth week of gestation, and the tubercle grows similarly in both sexes for the next 4 weeks. Labioscrotal swelling and a urogenital fold develop during this time. By the eighth week the anus and urogenital orifice are formed when membranous tissue ruptures to produce the orifices.

Androgens secreted by the male embryo result in the elongation of the tubercle into a penis and the fusion of the labioscrotal swellings into a scrotum. As the urogenital folds pull together, the lateral walls of the urethral

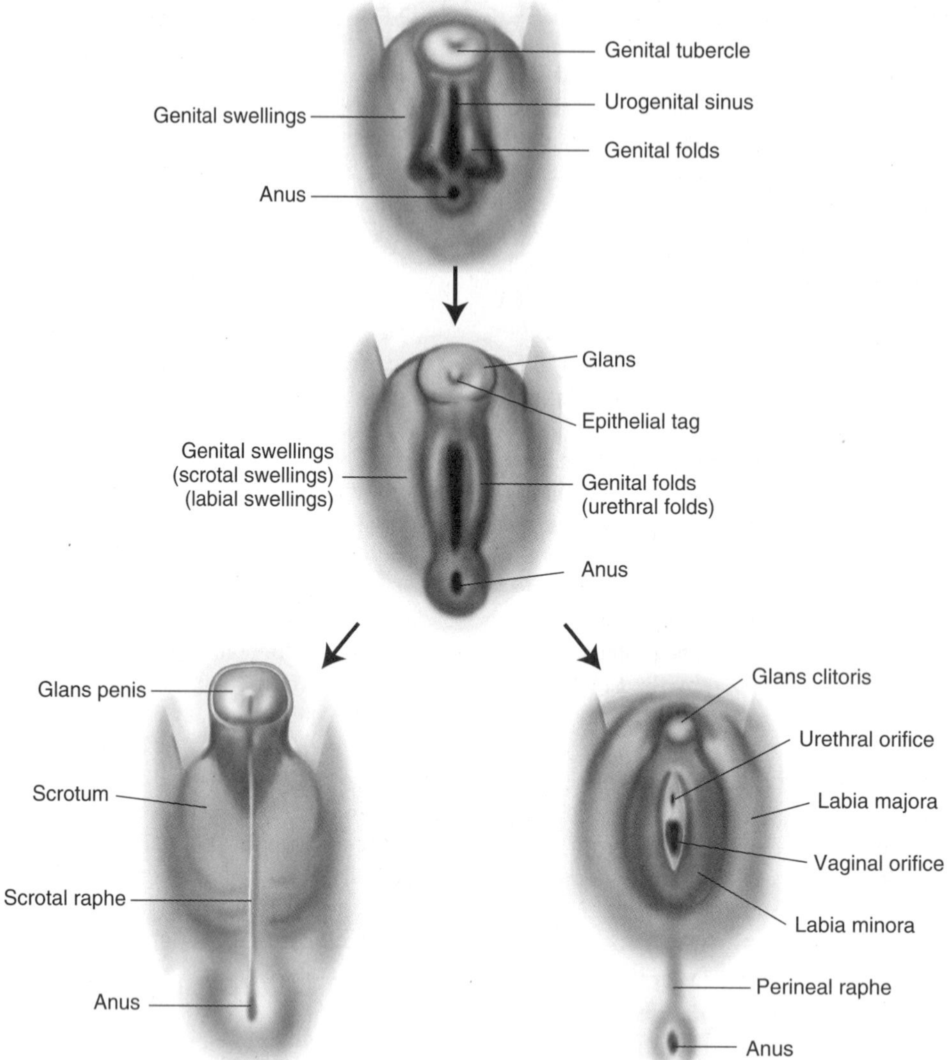

Figure 4-2 Differentiation of external genetalia. *Top,* Undifferentiated stage. *Middle,* Initiation of differentiation at about 10 weeks' gestation. *Bottom,* Final differentiation of external genitalia in both sexes. (Adapted from Blackburn ST, Loper DL: *Maternal, fetal and neonatal physiology,* Philadelphia, 1992, WB Saunders, p. 19.)

groove form, and posterior-to-anterior fusion shifts the urethral orifice to the glans of the penis. Ectodermal tissue grows from the tip of the penis backward to the urethra to join the two systems. Once the penile urethra has formed, the connective tissue surrounding the canal forms the corpus cavernosum. Numerous blood vessels are incorporated into this structure to eventually allow for swelling and erection of the penis.

In female embryos the initial growth of the genital tubercle slows, and the resulting structure is the relatively small clitoris. The urethra and vagina open into a common introitus with the rupturing of the membranes of those structures, and the urogenital folds develop into the labia minora and majora.

GAMETOGENESIS

Oogenesis and spermatogenesis are accomplished by meiosis—the reduction and division of the germ cells to form haploid cells (23 chromosomes) (Figure 4-3). The normal diploid number of 46 chromosomes is restored

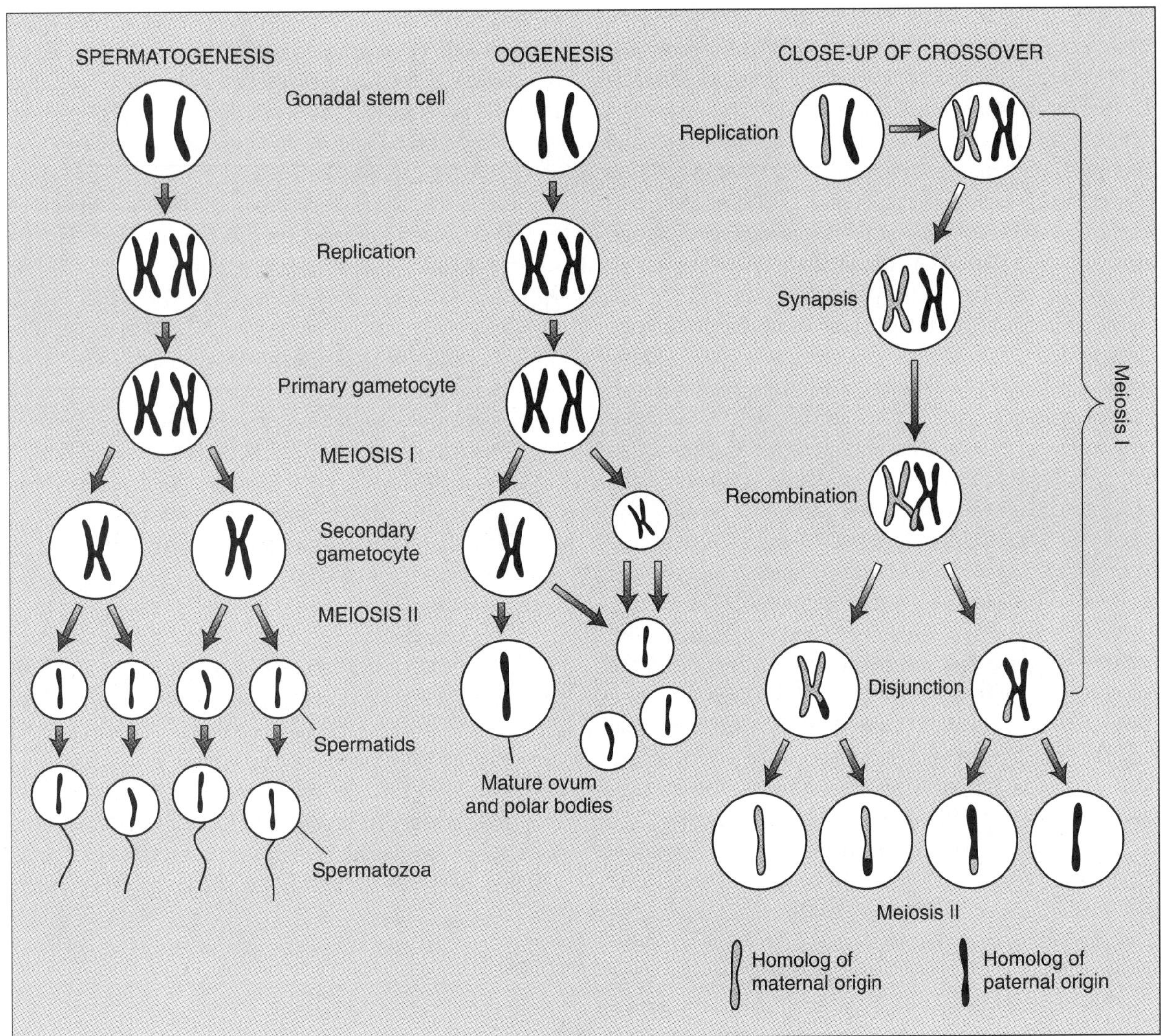

Figure 4-3 Meiosis.

following fertilization. The process differs between the sexes in that gametogenesis in the male produces four sperm from one primary spermacyte, whereas the female produces one mature ovum from the primary oocyte.

Meiosis differs from mitosis in both the outcome of the cell division and the preparation for division. During meiosis the cell experiences a prolonged prophase, during which time there is preliminary pairing of the homologous chromosomes before the first division. It is during this pairing that the genetic material is often translocated or fractured away from the chromatid, leading to fatal errors in development. During metaphase of the first division, the two chromatids that comprise each chromosome in the homologous pairs are pulled by spindle fibers toward opposite poles of the daughter cells, resulting in a haploid number of chromosomes still comprised of chromatid pairs. Therefore the daughter cells differ from the parent cell at the end of this first phase of meiosis. Each oocyte contains 22 paired autosomes and an X chromosome, whereas each spermacyte contains 22 paired autosomes and a Y chromosome. During the second phase of meiosis, the chromatid dyads split, resulting in sperms or an ovum with 23 single-strand chromosomes.

Oogenesis occurs in three phases. During the first phase the germ cells multiply rapidly through mitosis in the developing gonad, becoming oogonia. The second phase continues the rapid mitotic divisions from the eighth through the twentieth weeks of gestation. It is estimated that 6 to 7 million ova are formed by 20 weeks. Because of atresia occurring during fetal life and throughout the life span, only about 300,000 to 400,000 will remain when the female enters puberty. After 20 weeks' gestation the mitotic divisions slow and permanently cease at birth. The third phase involves the movement of the cells into the prolonged prophase of the first meiotic division, and the oocytes form within the primary follicles. Primary oocytes increase in size, and the previously flattened follicular cells surrounding each one become cuboid to form a thick covering. The follicular cells secrete a glycoprotein substance onto the ovum; this will develop into the zona pellucida. The follicular cells elongate and surround the zona pellucida, forming the corona radiata. Each grouping of follicular cells around an ovum averages 6 to 12 mm in diameter, and the cell clusters lie beneath the ovarian epithelium. The further maturation of the ova remains suspended until ovulation occurs. When the first meiotic division is complete, the daughter cells will each have 23 chromosomes, with one daughter cell receiving most of the cytoplasm. The smaller cell, the first polar body, will lie between the zona pellucida and the vitelline membrane of the secondary oocyte but will be cast off before ovulation.

Spermatogenesis involves three stages. The first stage includes ongoing reproduction of spermatogonial cells by mitosis. This occurs during fetal life and through the individual's life span. The second and third stages, meiosis to produce haploid cells and spermiogenesis to mature the cells into functional spermatozoa, occur once the male enters puberty and continue until later life, when decreasing production of testosterone leads to involution of the testes.

The hormones that control spermatogenesis arise from the hypothalamus, anterior pituitary, and testes. Gonadotropin-releasing hormone (GnRH) is secreted from the hypothalamus every 70 to 90 minutes in the mature male. GnRH stimulates the anterior pituitary to release LH and follicle-stimulating hormone (FSH), which stimulate the production of testosterone in the testes, as well as the process of spermatogenesis. LH stimulates the Leydig cells, which in turn secrete testosterone. LH works in collaboration with FSH to initiate spermatogenesis in the Sertoli cells of the seminiferous tubules.

Stem cells, spermatogonia, make up the basal layer of the seminiferous tubule. These continue to undergo mitosis to maintain an appropriate number of stem cells, whereas others separate from the basal layer and begin maturation as spermacytes. Immediately after separation from the basal layer, these cells are termed preleptotene spermacytes. First and second meiotic divisions will result in the formation of secondary spermacytes and spermatids. As the spermatids move through the lumen of the tubules, they undergo morphologic changes that result in the final form of mature sperm.

1. The head of the sperm is formed from the nucleus of the spermatid, with the acrosome forming to supply enzymes necessary for fertilization.
2. The midpiece, located immediately beneath the head, contains the mitochondria necessary for nourishment during transport. The mitochondria are tightly held around the base of the tail, supplying adenosine triphosphate that is necessary for motility.
3. The tail forms from contractile microtubules in the spermatid.

Maturation in the tubules takes approximately 70 days. When the sperm moves from the tubules to the epididymis for storage, the tail remains immature. By the time the sperm reaches the proximal end of the epididymis (14 to 21 days), it is capable of forward motility. Adult males can produce 200 to 300 million sperm per day, which has been estimated to represent 300 to 600 mature sperm per gram of testis per second (Sweet, 1997).

PUBERTY

The menstrual cycle includes cyclic changes in the endocrine system, the ovary, and the uterus. Both individual physiologic factors and environmental factors can influence these cyclic changes. The primary stimulus for the onset of menarche (the first menstrual cycle and menstruation) is not well understood. The production of gonadotropins indicating the functioning of the hypothalamus and anterior pituitary during fetal life is well documented. FSH and LH reach peak circulatory levels at 28 weeks' gestation, and the increasing sensitivity of the pituitary to inhibition by steroids leads to decreased secretions of gonadotropins in the third trimester. Immediately after birth the sudden drop in maternal estrogen and progesterone circulating in the neonate's body may trigger a transient rise in gonadotropin secretion, but negative feedback is quickly achieved, and ovarian and gonadotropic steroid levels remain low for 6 to 8 years. The first steroids related to reproductive function to increase in the blood during childhood are dehydroepiandrosterone (DHA) and dehydroepiandrosterone sulfate (DHAS), adrenal androgens that stimulate the growth of pubic and axillary hair (andrenarche or pubarche) (Speroff, Glass, and Kase, 1999). At about the same time, FSH levels begin to rise. Estrogen and LH levels begin to increase at 10 to 12 years of age. These hormonal changes produce a somatic growth spurt; development of glandular tissue in the breasts (thelarche); growth and development of the uterus, fallopian tubes, vagina, external genitalia; increased vaginal secretions; and increased deposits of fat in the breasts, hips, and buttocks. The appearance of breast tissue changes is the first indicator of activation of the pituitary-gonadal axis in girls (Kaplowitz, Oberfield, and the Drug and Therapeutics and Executive Committees of the Lawson Wilkins Pediatric Endocrine Society, 1999). Since andrenarche precedes that growth spurt, the rise in gonadotropins and estrogen, and the onset of menarche, some researchers theorize that the adrenal gland is the initiator of the pubertal process.

The age of puberty is influenced by genetic factors, socioeconomic conditions, and general health. There has been a decrease in the age of menarche over the last few decades in North America, with recent research finding that the mean age of onset of menarche was 11.5 years in both white and black girls. Earlier menarche is associated with heavier weight and Hispanic, Asian/Pacific Island and African-American ethnicity (Koprowski et al., 1999; Wattigney et al., 1999). Data collected by the American Academy of Pediatrics suggests that black girls begin pubertal changes earlier than white girls (age 8 vs. age 10) (Herman-Giddens et al., 1997). Recent research suggests that the trend toward decreasing age at menarche has leveled off (Speroff, Glass, and Kase, 1999). Landmarks in female pubertal development are noted in Table 4-1.

Before the onset of pubertal changes, low levels of pulsatile gonadotropins are present. Increase in the pulses of GnRH occurs first during sleep cycles, with resulting increases in FSH and LH pulses. These nighttime pulses are unique to puberty, and by full maturation of the woman, there is an increase in daytime pulsatility and a decrease in nighttime pulsatility. Estradiol pulses also become established, and menarche is experienced. The first menstrual cycles tend to be anovulatory until the positive feedback relationship between estradiol and LH promotes regular ovulation.

Table 4-1 *Landmarks in Female Pubertal Development Types*

	Mean (years)
Breast bud	9.96
Onset of pubic hair	10.51
Maximal growth	11.4
Menarche	12.8
Adult breast	14.6
Adult pubic hair	13.7

MENSTRUAL CYCLE

The menstrual cycle is regulated by an intricate interaction of hormone secretion by the hypothalamus, the anterior pituitary gland, the adrenal glands, and the ovaries. The hypothalamus produces neuroendocrine agents that stimulate the production of growth hormone, thyroid-stimulating hormone, adrenocorticotropin hormone, and the gonadotropins. GnRH is the neurohormone that controls secretion of FSH and LH from the anterior pituitary. The superior hypophyseal arteries form a dense network of capillaries that drain into the portal vessels that traverse the pituitary stalk to the anterior pituitary gland (Speroff, Glass, and Kase, 1999). Thus the hypothalamus directly influences the functioning of the anterior pituitary gland, and retrograde flow from the anterior pituitary to the hypothalamus allows for pituitary feedback (Speroff, Glass, and Kase, 1999).

A variety of feed-back mechanisms are necessary for effective reproductive functioning. The long feedback loop refers to the feedback effects of circulating target gland hormones (e.g., estrogen, progesterone) and influences both hypothalamic and pituitary function. The short feedback loop refers to the negative feedback of pituitary hormones on their own secretion, most likely through the inhibition of releasing hormones from the hypothalamus. Ultrashort feedback loops refers to the inhibition of releasing hormone on its own synthesis (Speroff, Glass, and Kase, 1999). Dopamine, norepinephrine, endorphins, serotonin, and melatonin actively influence the feedback loops.

GnRH secretion is controlled by a complex interplay among GnRH, FSH, LH, estrogen, and progesterone. Gonadotropin secretion is stimulated by release of GnRH in pulsed action with specific frequencies and amplitudes. The gonadotropins are also released in a pulsatile pattern. LH pulse mean amplitude ranges from 6.5 IU/L in early follicular phase to 14.9 IU/L in early luteal phase to 7.6 IU/L in late luteal phase. Although FSH has a longer half-life than GnRH and LH, it follows a similar pattern. Pulsatile release of GnRH is stimulated by norepinephrine and inhibited by dopamine and seratonin.

FOLLICULAR PHASE

The first phase of the ovarian cycle is considered the follicular or preovulatory phase. At the time of menarche, approximately 500,000 primordial follicles remain in the ovaries. During the reproductive years the follicles are depleted at the rate of approximately 1000 per month through a process of atresia termed apoptosis. During a woman's life only about 400 follicles will reach maturation and ovulate (Macklon and Fauser, 1998). Initiation of growth of primordial follicles occurs as a random process and is continuous in nature. Complete maturation of a follicle takes at least 85 days.

It is not well understood how selection of a follicle for maturation occurs. The first maturational change is that the oocyte contained within the follicle enlarges and the surrounding layers of granulosa cells proliferate to support the primary follicle. The stroma of the follicle differentiates into internal and external theca layers. The theca interna develops LH receptor sites, and the granulosa cells develop FSH receptor sites. This developmental process takes several months, ending when the follicle reaches its preantral stage. The follicle continues to mature from the early antral to preovulatory stage over a period of 3 months. Early development of the follicle appears to occur without direct stimulation of gonadotropins, but final development into the preovulatory stage depends on FSH (Macklon and Fauser, 1998).

During any cycle many follicles may be ready for stimulation by FSH, but usually only one becomes a dominant follicle destined for ovulation. In young women approximately three to eleven follicles will respond to the rise in FSH that occurs a few days before the onset of menses. This group of cells enters that preantral stage of development, in which the granulosa cells proliferate and secrete estrogens, androgens, and progestins. Estrogens are the prominent steroid produced, and FSH both stimulates the growth of granulosa cells and initiates the steroidogenesis in the cells. FSH and estrogen work synergistically to promote the accumulation of FSH receptor sites, creating a sensitive system for response to even low levels of FSH. Androgens act to both enhance and inhibit the development process. At relatively low levels they enhance the aromatization of androgens into estrogens. At higher levels they inhibit aromatase activity and FSH stimulation of LH receptor sites. Hence successful follicular maturation depends on a delicate estrogen-androgen balance that then shifts to an estrogen-dominated environment (Speroff, Glass, and Kase, 1999).

Further development of the follicle involves the increase of follicular fluid that lies between the ovum and the granulosa cells. When FSH is present, estrogens become the dominant steroid in the fluid. In the absence of FSH, androgens dominate the fluid, and the follicle is destined for atresia. With continued development the theca cells surrounding the follicle develop LH receptor sites and androgens that can be aromatized into estrogens. The follicle that develops a highly estrogenic environment becomes the dominant follicle for ovulation. Through an intricate feedback mechanism, FSH stimulation of less dominant follicles decreases, and those follicles are no longer able to aromatize androgens into estrogens. Further decrease in estrogen environment leads to atresia of the less dominant cells. Even as FSH levels decrease in the latter half of the follicular phase, the dominant follicle is able to survive because of its increased numbers of FSH receptor sites with the resulting increased estrogen secretion.

As estradiol levels increase, they produce an inhibitory effect on FSH secretion. At the same time, the rising estradiol levels stimulate the release of LH. As LH levels rise in the latter part of the follicular phase, they stimulate further androgen production in the theca cells in the dominant follicle, further assisting with the estrogen production necessary for maturation. A further inhibitor to FSH secretion is inhibin, a peptide that works in synchrony with estradiol to decrease FSH levels. FSH stimulates the secretion of inhibin from the granulosa cells, which in turn leads to its suppression as inhibin levels rise. This process specifically decreases the FSH effect on the nondominant follicles while sparing the dominant follicle. Another peptide, activin, is also secreted by the granulosa cells, but differs from inhibin in that it augments FSH activity, including aromatization of androgens into estrogens. An imbalance that favors activin action prevents the normal decrease of FSH levels at this point in the ovulatory process.

Immediately before ovulation the oocyte progresses through its meiotic division, although the process won't be complete until fertilization when the second polar body is extruded. The granulosa cells continue to enlarge, resulting in increased estrogen levels. Approximately 36 to 48 hours before ovulation the mature ovum completes the first meiotic division, creating the primary oocyte and first polar body. Estrogen levels peak about 24 to 36 hours before ovulation, and it is believed that the estrogen feedback to the anterior pituitary promotes an LH surge. LH stimulates the production of progesterone by the granulosa cells of the dominant follicle. This low level of progesterone further stimulates LH secretion and also stimulates an FSH surge that is necessary for full expression of LH receptors on the dominant follicle.

Ovulation occurs approximately 10 to 12 hours after the LH surge. The peak level of LH must continue for 14 to 24 hours for full maturation of the oocyte to occur. The usual LH surge experienced in healthy, fertile women is 48 to 50 hours. The LH surge tends to occur at approximately 3 AM (range midnight to 8 AM) in 85% of women (Cahill et al., 1998). In the northern hemisphere approximately 90% of women ovulate between 4 to 7 PM from July through February (autumn and winter). During spring 50% of women ovulate between midnight and 11 AM (Speroff, Glass, and Kase, 1999). Cahill et al. (1998) found that the LH surge almost always occurs when the serum estradiol level is >600 pmol/L and the follicular diameter is greater than 15 mm.

Immediately before ovulation the follicle wall increases distensibility, and there is a rapid increase in the volume of fluid in the follicle. FSH, LH, and progesterone stimulate the production of proteolytic enzymes that break down the collagen in the follicle wall. Research has demonstrated that prostaglandins increase significantly in the follicular fluid and are essential in both the secretion and activity of the proteolytic enzymes and in stimulating the smooth muscle cells of the ovary to enhance the extrusion of the oocyte. In addition, FSH is necessary to free the oocyte from the follicular attachments and to ensure that there are sufficient LH receptors to maintain an adequate luteal phase. The mechanism that contributes to the drop in LH levels following the surge is not well understood. Ovulation occurs when the ovarian surface membrane covering the follicles ruptures and extrudes the secondary oocyte surrounded by follicular fluid and cells.

LUTEAL PHASE

Once ovulation has occurred, the follicle walls collapse. Under the influence of LH the site becomes vascularized, and the corpus luteum forms. For 3 days following ovulation, the granulosa cells continue to enlarge, and theca lutein cells may differentiate from the stroma to become part of the corpus luteum. Capillaries penetrate the granulosa layer and may fill the remaining central area with blood. This vascularization is necessary to ensure that ovarian steroid levels are maintained to support possible conception. The corpus luteum secretes progesterone, 17 alpha-hydroxyprogesterone, estradiol, and androstenedione for approximately 7 to 8 days. Progesterone appears to be the primary steroid necessary for continuation of early pregnancy since exogenous progesterone given to agonadal women with implanted donated embryos maintains viability until the progesterone of the placenta is sufficient. Progesterone inhibits that growth of other follicles through local inhibitory action. In addition, progesterone, in concert with estrogen and inhibin, provides negative feedback, resulting in continued low levels of gonadotropins. The luteal phase of the menstrual cycle averages 14 days, with a range of 11 to 17 days considered normal.

If fertilization does not occur, thereby stimulating continued functioning of the corpus luteum, the corpus luteum regresses, and progesterone and estrogen levels fall. The mechanism for the process of degradation is not well understood.

UTERINE CHANGES THROUGH THE MENSTRUAL CYCLE

Like the ovary, the endometrium undergoes changes under the influence of the gonadotropic and ovarian hormones. The proliferative phase of the endometrial cycle begins with the end of menses and continues until ovulation. The endometrium increases in thickness from 1 mm to 3 to 5 mm under the influence of the estrogen that is secreted by the follicle. Increased thickness is the result of lengthening of the epithelial cells rather than generation of new cells. Estrogen also influences the proliferation of endometrial glands and vascularization of the endometrium.

Following ovulation, progesterone secreted by the corpus luteum stimulates further thickening of the endometrium and hypertrophy of the endometrial glands. The endometrial glands secrete a substance rich in glycogen in anticipation of implantation of the fertilized ovum. This secretory phase averages 14 days (range 12 to 16), and if conception does not occur, it ceases with the onset of menstruation. The menstrual phase of the endometrium includes vasospasm of vessels and resulting ischemic necrosis. After the initial vasospasm, vessels dilate and the menstrual discharge of blood and sloughed tissue occurs.

Several other structures are affected by the cyclic hormone changes during the menstrual cycle. Cervical mucus tends to be scant and thick during the proliferative phase of the endometrial cycle. The estrogen peak immediately before ovulation causes the mucus to become more watery and thin. Women may note that they feel "wetter" during the ovulatory phase. Spinnbarkeit is the term describing the elasticity of the mucus when it is stretched between the thumb and forefinger. Maximum spinnbarkeit can be noted at the time of ovulation. This thinning of the cervical mucus creates a more hospitable environment for sperm. Increased sodium chloride in the muous will also lead to a mechanism called ferning. The higher salt content results in the formation of salt crystals in a typical "fern" pattern when cervical secretions are dried on a slide and examined under the microscope. Vaginal epithelial cells become larger and cornified at the time of ovulation. Breast tissue undergoes changes under the influence of estrogen, progesterone, and prolactin. Women may experience breast tenderness premenstrually as a result of the increased fluid retention in breast tissue.

Menstrual cycle length is determined by the rate of follicular growth, since the luteal phase remains fairly constant through a woman's reproductive life. Most women experience cycles of 24 to 35 days in length. A 28-day cycle is usually considered "average." Cycles during the first 5 years following menarche tend to be more irregular and longer in length. After age 40 menstrual cycles tend to become longer and more irregular and to have an increasing proportion of anovulatory cycles.

FERTILIZATION

Following ovulation the oocyte, surrounded by the zona pellucida and corona radiata (granulosa cells), is captured by the fimbriae of the fallopian tube. It is theorized that the additional cell mass, as well of the cellular makeup of the zona pellucida and corona radiata, enhances the uptake by the fimbriae. Movement of cilia lining the fallopian tube and peristalsis of the tube move the oocyte into the ampulla of the tube, where fertilization occurs. If fertilization does not occur within 24 hours, the oocyte dies.

Mature sperm that have reached the proximal end of the epididymis and the vas deferens are mixed with seminal fluid that is alkaline and high in fructose. The ejaculate contains approximately 2 to 5 ml of semen containing 50 to 100 million sperm per milliter. Only mature sperm with strong motility make it into the cervical mucus. Prostaglandins in semen are thought to stimulate uterine contractions that facilitate sperm movement through the uterus and into the fallopian tubes. Sperm have been identified in the tubes within 5 minutes of ejaculation, and most viable sperm reach the ampulla of the tube in 1 to 6 hours. There may be a chemical attraction to the ovum that facilitates the sperm transport to the ampulla.

The sperm must complete maturational changes before fertilization can occur. Capacitation represents the removal of glycoproteins and seminal plasma proteins from the membrane over the acrosome. This process decreases the stability of the plasma membrane and the membrane immediately beneath it (acrosomal membrane). When the capacitated sperm comes in contact with follicular fluid or the oocyte, the plasma membrane and the outer acrosomal membranes break down further, allowing the enzymes of the acrosome to be released. This acrosomal reaction is a release of hyaluronidase for penetration of the corona radiata, an enzyme similar to trypsin for digestion of the zona pellucida, and a lysin for penetration of the zona pellucida. Capacitation also results in hypermotility of the sperm, a characteristic that is necessary for penetration of the oocyte.

The inner acrosomal membrane of the sperm attaches to the plasma membrane of the oocyte, fusing the plasma membranes. The head and tail penetrate the cell wall, and the oocyte responds to penetration by completing the second meiotic division. The second polar body is extruded into the perivitelline space. The female nucleus increases in size and is termed the female pronucleus. The tail of the sperm degenerates, and the head enlarges to become the male pronucleus. The two pronuclei move toward each other, the nuclear membranes dissolve, and the chromatin strands combine. The diploid number of chromosomes (46) is achieved with 22 pairs of autosomal chromosomes and one pair of sex chromosomes. Genetic determination of sex is accomplished at this time (Figure 4-4). Immediately after fertilization a platelet-activating factor–like substance can be identified in maternal circulation. It is presumed that it is released from the fertilized ovum (Buster and Carson, 1996).

The fertilized egg is termed a zygote from the first mitotic division through the formation of a blastocyst. The first division occurs about 30 hours after fertilization. These two cells continue dividing into smaller cells. The entire mass is contained by the zona pellucida, and, even as the cells multiply, there is no increase in the mass of the zygote. Cells divide approximately every 12

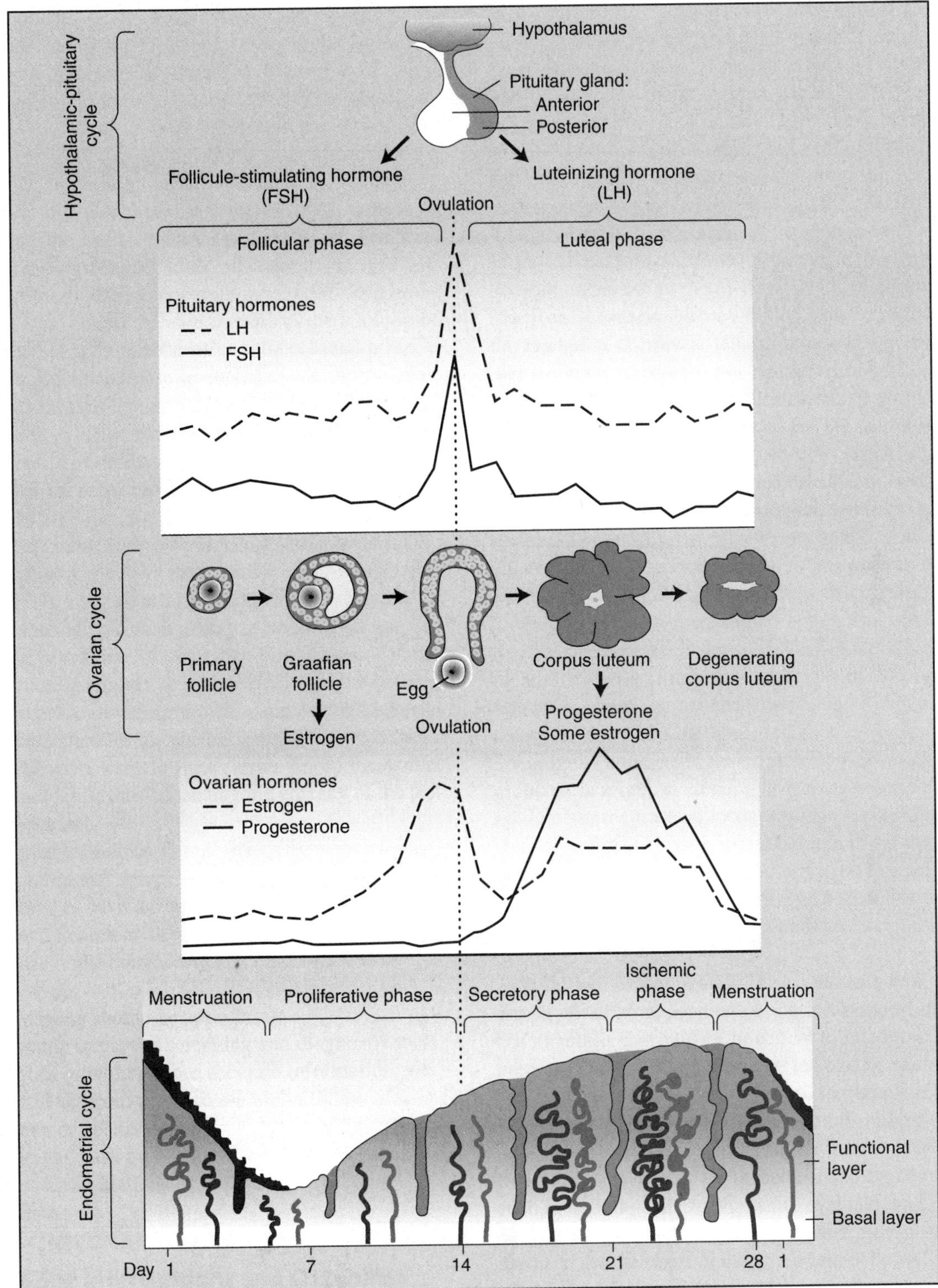

Figure 4-4 Hormone levels during the menstrual cycle.

hours; by 4 days after fertilization the mass consists of 16 blastomeres and is called the morula.

Action of the cilia and peristalsis continue to move the zygote through the fallopian tube to the uterus. The ovum spends about 80 hours in the tube and then takes about 10 hours to pass through the isthmus into the uterus. Fluid in the uterine cavity is absorbed into the mass of cells, creating a fluid-filled sphere called a blastocyst. The blastocyst is comprised of the zona pellucida, which is beginning to stretch with increasing size of the mass; trophoblastic cells, which are a one-cell layer of cells that will form the placenta; an inner cell mass of one to two cells that will form the embryo; and the fluid-filled cavity. The blastocyst remains free-floating in the uterus for 90 to 150 hours after fertilization. Although human chorionic gonadotropin (hCG) is present in the blastocyst, it is not detectable in maternal circulation until implantation allows for transport into the maternal vascular system (Figure 4-5).

Implantation occurs during the fifth to sixth day following fertilization when the blastocyst attaches to the endometrium. The mechanism of site selection for implantation is not well understood, but it may include signals from proteins or enzymes in the endometrial lining. The side of the blastocyst containing the inner cell mass orients itself to the endometrium, and by day 6 to 7, trophoblastic cells produce fingerlike projections that actively invade the endometrial epithelium. On day 7 the trophoblast differentiates into two layers. The inner layer, the cytotrophoblast, rapidly divides through mitosis to develop the syncytium, the chorionic villi, and the amnion. The syncytiotrophoblast is a multinucleated mass that develops the fingerlike projections that actively lyse the endometrial cells. The syncytiotrophoblasts line the fetal side of the intervillous space opposite the decidua basalis. When the syncytiotrophoblast invades blood vessels, small amount of bleeding may occur. This can be noted at the time of the missed period and is referred to as implantation bleeding.

The syncytiotrophoblasts synthesize placental steroids and protein hormones. The cells have a large

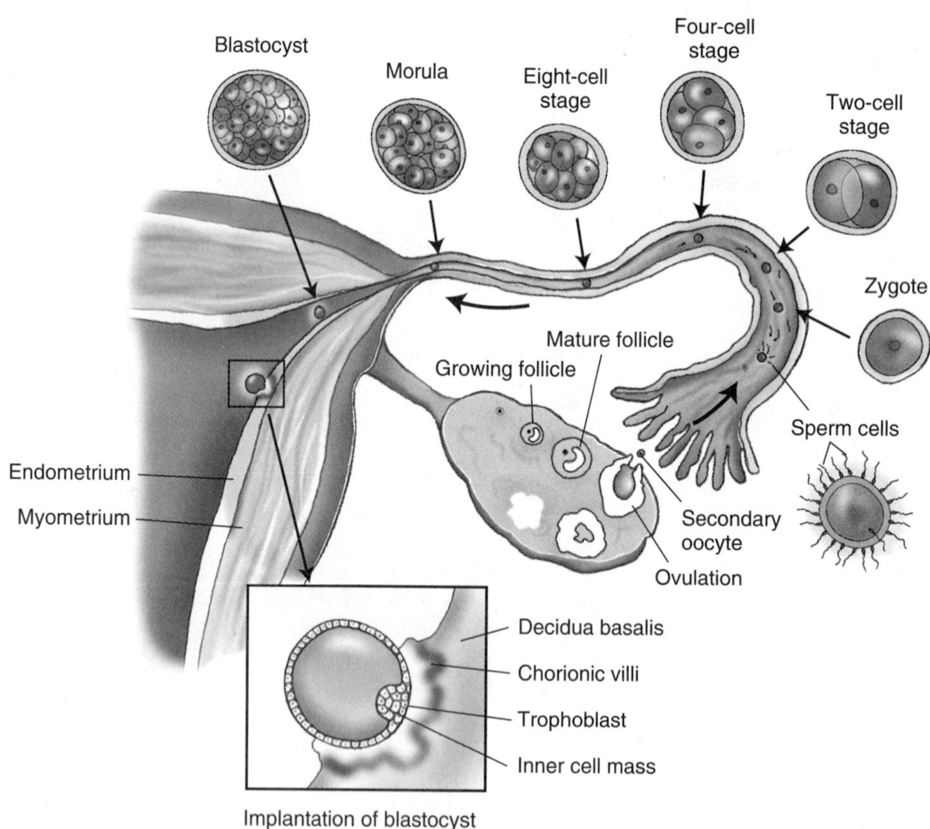

Figure 4-5 Summary of ovulation, fertilization, and implantation.

surface area that lines the intervillous space. Only the maternal blood vessel endothelium and the basement membrane separate them. This arrangement provides for efficient transfer of nutrients and hormone from the fetal to the maternal system. The trophoblastic cells produce hCG, which signals the corpus luteum to continue production of progesterone. It is also believed that the trophoblasts secrete SP1, an immunosuppressive substance to prevent rejection of the blastocyst. SP1 and hCG can be detected in maternal serum 6 to 14 days after ovulation.

It is estimated that one third to one half of fertilized ova do not complete implantation. Those that do not successfully implant and are aborted usually have a genetically abnormal makeup. Implantation is completed 10 days after fertilization. At this time the blastocyst is completely embedded in the endometrium, and by 12 days after fertilization the endometrial epithelium has regenerated over the site. Estrogen and progesterone stimulate the epithelium and stromal cells to hypertrophy. Subnuclear vacuoles that are rich in glycogen and lipids are created (Blackburn and Loper, 1992). These endometrial alterations are termed the decidual reaction, which is necessary for initial nutrition of the embryo. The decidua capsularis covers the growing blastocyst/embryo. As the chorion develops, the decidua capsularis disappears. The vascular bed of endometrium immediately below the blastocyst is called the decidua basalis, which will become the uterine junction with the placenta. The remaining endometrial lining is known as the decidua vera, which will fuse with the chorion as the embryo develops and the products of conception fill the uterine cavity.

References

Blackburn ST, Loper DL: *Maternal, fetal and neonatal physiology,* Philadelphia, 1992, WB Saunders.

Buster JE, Carson SA: Endocrinology and diagnosis of pregnancy. In Gabbe SG, Niebyl R, Simpson JL, editors: *Obstetrics: normal and problem pregnancies,* ed 3, New York, 1996, Churchill Livingstone.

Cahill DJ et al: Onset of the preovulatory luteinizing hormone surge: diurnal timing and critical follicular prerequisites, *Fertil Steril* 70(1):56-59, 1998.

Herman-Giddens ME et al: Secondary sexual characteristics and menses in young girls seen in office practice: a study from the pediatric research in office settings network, *Pediatrics* 99:505-511, 1997.

Kaplowitz PB, Oberfield SE, The Drug and Therapeutics and Executive Committees of the Lawson Wilkins Pediatric Endocrine Society: Reexamination of the age limit for defining when puberty is precocious in girls in the United States: implications for evaluation and treatment, *Pediatrics* 104(4):936-941, 1999.

Koprowski C et al: Diet, body size and menarche in a multiethnic cohort, *Br J Cancer* 79(11-12):1907-1911, 1999.

Macklon NS, Fauser BC: Follicle development during normal menstrual cycle, *Maturitas* 30(2):181-188, 1998.

Speroff L, Glass RH, Kase NG: *Clinical gynecologic endocrinology and infertility,* ed 6, Baltimore, 1999, Lippincott Williams & Wilkins.

Spiegelman M, Bennett D: A light- and electron-microscope study of primordial germ cells in the early mouse embryo, *J Embryol Exp Morphol* 30:97-100, 1973.

Sweet BR: *Mayes' midwifery,* London, 1997, Bailliére Tindall.

Wattigney WA et al: Secular trend of earlier onset of menarche with increasing obesity in black and white girls: the Bogalusa heart study, *Ethn Dis* 9(2):181-189, 1999.

Chapter 5

Growth and Development of the Fetus and Placenta

DEVELOPMENT OF THE PLACENTA

The placenta is defined as the fusion of fetal membranes with the uterine mucosa for the purpose of maternal-fetal exchange of nutrients, gases, and waste substances (Kaufmann and Scheffen, 1998) (Table 5-1). Placental development begins at the time of implantation. The blastocyst is comprised of an inner mass called the embryoblast and an outer layer called the trophoblast. Cells in the embryoblast differentiate into the fetus, umbilical cord, and mesenchyme of the placenta. The trophoblast cells differentiate into the placenta and membranes. The functions of the trophoblasts include (1) invasion of maternal tissue in the decidual layer of the endometrium so that communication between the fetal and maternal systems is possible and (2) production of hormones that are responsible for maintenance of the pregnancy. The most important hormone secreted from the inner cytotrophic cells in early pregnancy is human chorionic gonadotropin, which maintains the corpus luteum for estrogen and progesterone production for 4 to 6 weeks, when the syncytium can take over.

To prepare for implantation, the endometrium undergoes changes that enhance implantation. The endometrial lining is composed of three functional zones. The deepest layer is adjacent to the myometrium and is stimulated by progesterone to develop during the secretory phase of the menstrual cycle. It is also responsible for regeneration of endometrial tissue after menstruation. The outer compacta and middle spongiosa layers contain blood vessels and endometrial glands that increase under the stimulation of estrogen and progesterone. The endometrium becomes edematous; and uterine glands that secrete mucopolysaccharides, lipids, and glycogen support the blastocyst before and during the implantation process. These changes are termed the decidual reaction. Implantation usually occurs on the anterior or posterior wall of the uterus but may occur at other sites. Once it occurs, the decidua differentiates into distinct areas (see Figure 5-6, p. 71). The decidua basalis lies directly under the site of implantation and contributes to the formation of the maternal part of the placental bed. The decidua capsularis is the part that covers the implanted ovum and separates it from the uterine lining. The remaining uterine lining becomes the decidua vera.

As implantation proceeds, the parts of the trophoblast that actively invade the uterine wall proliferate into a two-layer trophoblastic wall that develops into the syncytiotrophoblast. Rapid proliferation of the cells increases the thickness at the point of contact with the uterus, and by day 8 after fertilization confluent vacuoles (lacunae) develop. From day 8 to day 13 these lacunae continue to form in the central part of the syn-

Table 5-1 *Placental and Organ System Functions in Extrauterine Life*

Fetal function	Extrauterine organ system
Gas exchange	Lungs
Excretion, water balance, and pH regulation	Kidneys
Catabolism and resorption	Gut
Synthesis and secretion on hormones	Endocrine glands
Metabolism of food and drugs	Liver
Hematopoiesis (early pregnancy)	Bone marrow
Heat transfer	Skin
Immunology	Immune system

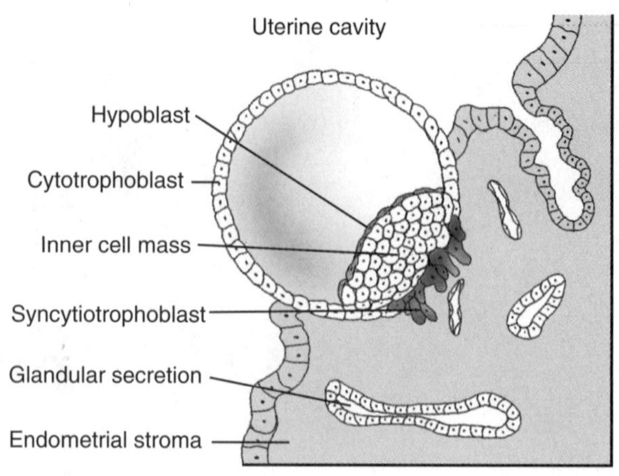

Figure 5-1 Early implantation.

cytiotrophoblast. Lacunae fill with maternal blood as capillaries are invaded (Figures 5-1 and 5-2). Cytotrophoblastic cells begin to invade the syncytial site, and the cells that invade the lacunae become the primary villi. These cytotrophoblastic cells proliferate laterally, eventually forming a continuous shell around the conceptus (Sweet and Tiran, 1997). The shell provides the point of contact between the fetal cells and the maternal basal plate. The basal plate consists of the compact and spongy layers of the maternal decidua basalis, trophoblastic remnants, and fibrinoid material (Blackburn and Loper, 1992). Villi that extend beyond the trophoblastic shell are termed extravillous trophoblasts, and it is these villi that invade the endometrial capillaries and spiral arteries. The syncytiotrophoblast cell membranes begin to disappear, and eventually the syncytiotrophoblast becomes a continuous uninterrupted layer that lines the intervillous space. Implantation is complete 10 days after fertilization (Figure 5-3).

Placental villi consist of connective tissue cells, connective tissue fibers, macrophages, occasional mast cells, and fetal vessels. The endothelium of the villous vessels provides the site for transfer of molecules and secretion of enzymes. It is clear that there must be immunologic system alterations that inhibit rejection of the products of conception since the syncytiotrophoblast, which is in contact with maternal blood, and the amniochorion, which is in contact with the decidua, are tissues that would be expected to promote an immune response. Research has suggested that the syncytiotrophoblast lacks transplantation antigens—human leukocyte antigens (HL-As) A, B, C, DR, or DC—so cannot be identified as "other" by the maternal system (Galbraith, Kantor, and Ferra, 1981; Sutherland, Naiem, and Mason, 1981). In addition, antigens in the paternal genes are not recognized as foreign by the maternal system (Cross, Werb, and Fisher, 1994). The syncytiotrophoblast does manifest unique antigens called trophoblast antigens and trophoblast-lymphocyte cross-reactive antigens. These are thought to influence the formation of antibodies that may regulate trophoblast growth (Beer, 1988). Local suppression of lymphocyte activation in the decidua may also play a role in the prevention of rejection of the conceptus.

Chorionic villi cover the entire chorionic sac until the eighth week of gestation. With the growth of the sac, the chorion comes into contact with the decidua. Blood flow to the chorion decreases, and the villi degenerate. This smooth chorionic membrane is the chorion laeve, which adjoins the amnion between 7 to 10 weeks' gestation. The chorion laeve is composed of a fibroblast layer that is contiguous with the amnion, a reticular layer, and 2 to 10 layers of trophoblastic cells that are contiguous to the decidua capsularis. Even without a direct blood supply, the chorion laeve produces enzymes that synthesize prostaglandins, oxytocin and platelet-activating factor, thereby decreasing the contractility of the myometrium.

When implantation is complete, the decidua covering the site of implantation, the decidua capsularis, bulges into the uterine cavity. As the chorionic sac enlarges, the decidua capsularis expands into the uterine cavity. Between 15 and 20 weeks' gestation the capsular decidua

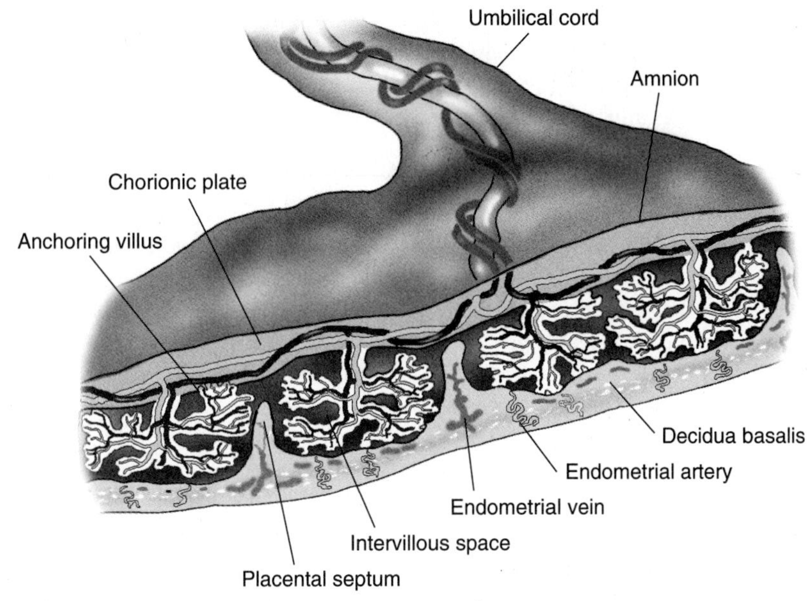

Figure 5-2 Formation of lacunar network.

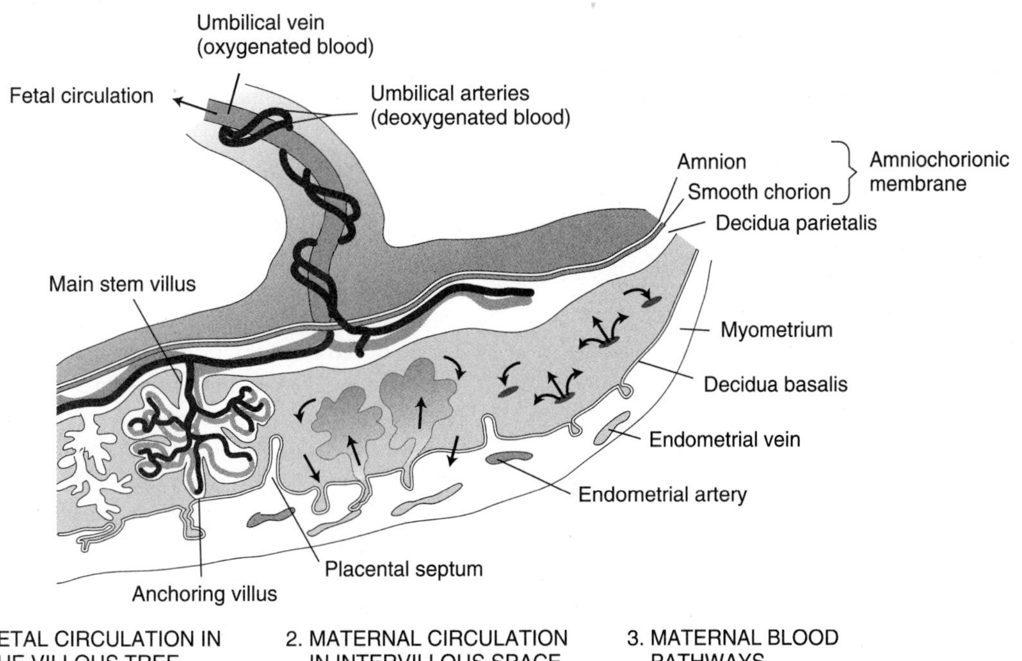

Figure 5-3 Development of maternal-fetal placental circulation.

fuses with the decidua vera on the opposing uterine wall, causing the uterine cavity to be totally filled with the products of conception.

The chorionic villi over the decidua basalis develop into the mature placenta. By midsecond trimester, the cytotrophoblastic shell regresses and is replaced by fibrinoid material and cytotrophoblastic cells. Fibrinoid material also forms along the level of the spongy zone of the decidua basalis, and it is at this plane that the placenta separates following delivery of the infant. Branch villi continue to grow from the primary villi, and by term they make up approximately 60% of the villi. Approximately 60 to 70 of these branching villi are present in a mature placenta. By 8 to 10 weeks after conception, the placenta is considered functionally mature, and no new lobules or primary villi are formed after the first trimester. Continued growth occurs with branching of the primary villi, growth of the mesenchymal core, and growth of additional capillaries (Blackburn and Loper, 1992). These changes increase the surface area available for exchange of oxygen, nutrients, and waste products. The rate in growth slows after 34 weeks' gestation.

During the third trimester the syncytium forms "knots" that are several cell layers thick. This shifting of cell material creates a vasculosyncytial membrane, a thin anuclear membrane that is thought to enhance gas exchange (Khong and Pearce, 1987). Thinning of the syncytium and increase in placental surface area increase the efficiency of placental functioning. Near term the placenta may develop intervillous thrombi, fibrin deposits, infarcts, and calcification that decrease transfer efficiency.

The placental bed is composed of 50 to 60 cotyledons, or lobes, that have arisen around a primary villus and that appear adherent to each other. These cotyledons receive arterial blood via the spiral arteries (uterine arteries). Each lobe develops into one to five units called lobules. The vascular bed of the uteroplacental unit consists of the cotyledons, the endometrium, and the myometrium. As pregnancy progresses, there is a steady redistribution of blood flow, and at term the placental lobes receive nearly 90% of total uterine blood flow.

The uteroplacental system is a low-resistance, high-flow vascular bed. Blood enters the uteroplacental system from the uterine arteries. By term there are an estimated 100 to 200 uteroplacental arteries and 75 to 175 veins. Blood entering the intervillous space flows in pressure waves that are mediated by maternal pulse and blood pressure. The blood flows toward the chorionic plate of the placenta, where it bathes the villi. Blood leaves the intervillous space through the uteroplacental veins and the subchorial, interlobular, and marginal venous lakes (Blackburn and Loper, 1992). Any alteration in maternal or fetal blood flow will have an effect on the diffusion of oxygen, carbon dioxide, nutrients, and wastes. The pressure in the uteroplacental arteries is higher than that of the intervillous space, and the intervillous space pressure is greater than the maternal venous pressure during diastole. Pressure gradients are relatively small, with pressure averaging 25 mm Hg in the uteroplacental arteries and 5 to 10 mm Hg in the uterine veins. The intervillous space averages 150 ml of blood, and it is estimated that the rate of blood flow increases from 50 ml/min at 10 weeks' gestation to 500 to 600 ml/min at term.

MECHANISMS OF TRANSFER

Transfer of gases, nutrients, and waste material occurs through trophoblastic tissue and fetal endothelial cells. This transfer of substances across the placenta membranes is influenced by the surface area of the placenta, the biochemical properties of the substance, the electrical potential differences, the permeability of the membranes, and the rates of maternal and fetal blood flow through the intervillous space and villi.

Molecules moving from the maternal intervillous space to fetal capillary lumen system pass through the following cell layers:

1. Microvillous plasma membrane of the syncytiotrophoblast
2. Syncytiotrophoblast cells of the villus
3. Basal membrane of the trophoblast
4. Connective tissue mesoderm of the villus
5. Fetal capillary epithelium

Molecules rely on a variety of forms of transfer to move from maternal to fetal systems and vice versa.

Passive Diffusion

Passive diffusion occurs when there is a higher concentration of a molecule in one system, leading to movement of molecules across a membrane to a system of lower concentration. The amount of diffusion that occurs depends on the concentration of the solution and the surface area involved. Simple diffusion across the uteroplacental membranes is the usual means of transfer for smaller molecules, particularly when molecules are lipid soluble. The cell walls in the uteroplacental unit have a high lipid content, so fat-soluble substances may easily diffuse those layers. Free water crosses at a rate of 180 ml/second. Carbon dioxide, electrolytes, urea, simple amines, and creatinine all diffuse easily. Oxygen requires a higher pressure gradient than carbon dioxide, probably because the placenta and myometrium also extract oxygen from the maternal system. Fat-soluble vitamin, fatty acid, and steroid transfer are enhanced by the lipid content of the membranes. Narcotics, antibiotics, barbiturates, and anesthetics also transfer via simple diffusion.

Facilitated Diffusion

Facilitated diffusion requires a protein carrier system to move molecules across a membrane. Glucose requires facilitated transfer, with fetal levels reaching only 70% to 80% of maternal levels. A human placental glucose transporter has been identified as a component of the microvillous membrane. Research suggests that transfer rates decrease as maternal glucose concentrations increase. Oxygen may also be transported by facilitated diffusion.

Active Transport

Active diffusion requires energy-dependent carrier systems to transport molecules across gradients. Amino acids, including alanine, glutamine, threonine, and serine, require multiple carrier systems. The net transfer of many amino acids appears to be greater than that needed for fetal growth, leading to speculation that they are also used for energy production or synthesis of other amino acids (Blackburn and Loper, 1992). Amino acids have a higher concentration in fetal umbilical cord blood than in maternal blood. Free fatty acids are hydrophobic in nature and insoluble in plasma. Therefore they circulate bound to albumen and have relatively low transfer rates to the fetus.

Endocytosis, Exocytosis, and Pinocytosis

Endocytosis is an outward pouching of the cell surface to form an intracellular, membrane-bounded vesicle containing extracellular fluid. Endocytosis is used to engulf solid substances and transport them across trophoblastic tissues. Exocytosis is the fusion of a plasma membrane–bounded vesicle to the cell surface, followed by release of its contents. Pinocytosis is the engulfing of microdroplets of maternal plasma. Globulins, lipoproteins, and antibodies are transported via these mechanisms.

Water Transfer (Solvent Drag)

As water crosses the placental membranes, the speed of movement may increase the transport of electrolytes to a rate faster than usual simple diffusion. This mechanism provides maintenance of osmotic balances between the maternal and fetal systems.

Accidental Capillary Breaks

Breaks in capillary walls allow intact blood cells to move between maternal and fetal circulations. Small amounts of fetal cells can be found in the maternal system throughout pregnancy. These usually are no more than 0.1 to 0.2 ml. A fetal blood cell mass greater than 1 ml may trigger isoimmunization.

Independent Movement

Certain organisms independently cross the placental membranes. Maternal leukocytes, *Treponema pallidum,* and many viruses cross under their own power.

PLACENTA

The mature placenta averages one sixth the weight of the fetus and measures 18 to 20 cm in diameter. The thickness at term ranges from 1 cm at the edge to 4 cm in the center. Cord insertion is usually central. Variations of insertion include insertion at the edge of the placenta (battledore insertion) or into the membranes (velamentous insertion) (Figure 5-4).

A healthy placenta will be beefy red, a reflection of hemoglobin content. Pale placentas are associated with fetal anemia; and pale, edematous placentas are associated with immune and nonimmune hydrops, twin-to-twin transfusion in the donor twin, fetal congestive heart failure, and infection.

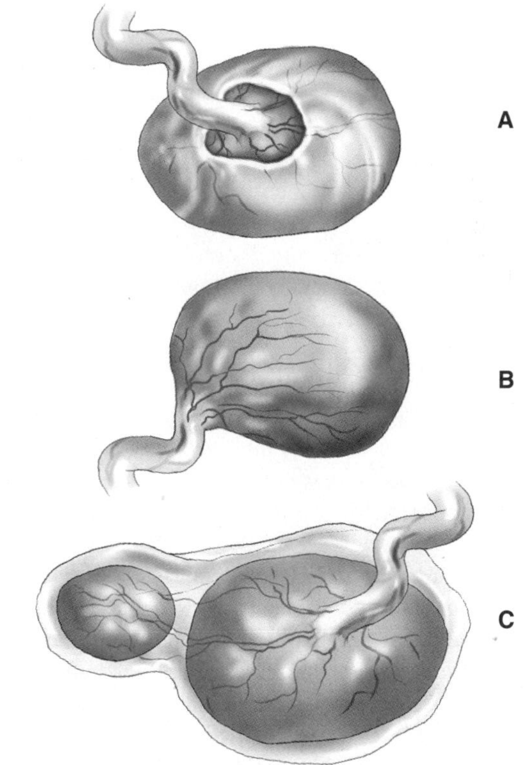

Figure 5-4 Variations of placental development. **A,** Circumvallate; **B,** battledore; **C,** succenturiate lobe.

Placentas that have been exposed to hypoxia or ischemia will demonstrate increased syncytial knots, increased numbers of villous cytotrophoblasts, fibrinoid necrosis of the villi, and thickening of the trophoblast basement membrane (Blackburn and Loper, 1992). Infarctions are associated with pregnancy-induced hypertension and intrauterine growth restriction. Infarctions initially are red or dark brown but develop fibrin deposition with resulting white coloration over time. Meconium-staining of the membranes occurs within 3 hours after passage of the meconium. Hypertrophy of the placenta is associated with maternal smoking and inhalation of secondhand smoke and other hypoxic conditions.

Deviations from Normal Placentation

Succenturiate placenta is the development of one or more additional accessory lobes in the membranes that are attached to the central placenta by vessels. It is thought that this occurs when the distant villi on the chorion laeve fail to degenerate, when implantation is superficial, or when there is a uterine anomaly (e.g., a septum) that alters placental growth. Succenturiate placenta with velamentous insertion of the cord is associated with malrotation of the implanting blastocyst.

In circumvallate placenta the area of the chorionic plate is reduced, causing the fetal membranes to fold back upon themselves. This produces a gray-white ring encircling the central portion of the fetal surface. Fetal vessels stop at the ring, and thus do not cover the entire placenta. When the ring corresponds with the placental margin, the condition may be described as circummarginate placenta. Circumvallate placenta is associated with intrauterine growth restriction.

Umbilical Cord

The expanding amniotic sac joins the connective stalk and allantois to form the umbilical cord. The allantois forms four vessels—two arteries and two veins—but one vein atrophies, and the remaining vein dilates. Occasionally one of the arteries atrophies, leaving a two-vessel cord. This condition is associated with other anomalies. The vessels' fusion with the intravillous vessels establishes fetoplacental circulation by the end of the fifth week of gestation. The umbilical cord grows from 0.5 cm at the time of establishment of circulation to 50 to 52 cm at term (tenth percentile is 40 cm; ninetieth percentile is 70 cm). Cord width averages 1 to 2 cm. Fetal movement leads to twisting of the umbilical vessels, and over 300 spiral turns may develop over the course of the pregnancy. True knots are found in 1% to 1.5% of cords. Wharton's jelly, a substance that contains collagen, muscle, and mucopolysaccharides, protects the vessels against compression.

EMBRYONIC AND FETAL DEVELOPMENT—FIRST TRIMESTER

During the first trimester the embryo develops through the processes of mitotic division, cell differentiation, tissue migration, and reorganization. Two types of metabolism are needed for fetal growth: (1) energy to sustain existing organism, and (2) energy for synthesis of new tissue.

The preembryonic phase of development occurs over the first 2 weeks following fertilization. The inner cell mass of the fertilized ovum (embryoblast) differentiates into a bilaminar disk (or embryonic disk), with an external layer called the primary ectoderm and an inner layer called the primary endoderm. Between 7 to 12 days after conception the inner cell mass differentiates into the embryoblast and the yolk sac. The embryoblast begins gastrulation, a process that produces three layers of cells—ectoderm, mesoderm, endoderm. Cells from the dorsally placed ectoderm differentiate into amnioblasts, which will form the amniotic membranes. Other cells in the ectoderm will develop into the entire nervous system, skin, hair, glands (pituitary, mammary), lens of the eye, lining of the internal and external ear, nose, sinuses, mouth, and anus. The intermediate layer of mesoderm will form the supporting structures—bones and joints, muscles and connective tissue, and the vascular and urogenital systems. The ventrally placed endoderm will develop into the gastrointestinal tract, including liver, gallbladder, and pancreas, and other outpouchings such as the thyroid and parathyroid glands, thymus, and lungs. Once organ differentiation begins, the organism is considered an embryo. The embryonic phase is usually considered to last from 2 to 8 weeks after fertilization.

Growth and development proceeds in a cranial-to-caudal direction. By day 16 after conception, the mesoderm produces a chemical that causes rapid growth in the size of the cells in the ectoderm, and over the next few days the neural plate develops and evolves into the neural groove. At this time two cavities form in the embryonic disk. Dorsally above the ectoderm the amniotic space develops. Ventrally the yolk sac appears from endodermal cells. The primary yolk sac will give rise to blood cells, endothelial cells, and germ cells. During the end of the second week the primary yolk sac begins to degenerate as the secondary yolk sac develops. It is this secondary yolk sac that will provide nutrition to the embryo and eventually be incorporated into the gut. Stem cells for blood cell development are formed in the yolk sac and migrate to the developing liver, thymus, lymph nodes, and bone marrow at about 6 weeks' gestation. The body stalk that develops from these cells provides the connection between the embryo and the trophoblast.

The development of a longitudinal axis and bilateral symmetry begins in the third week of gestation. The human brain begins forming at day 18, becoming the first organ system to differentiate. During days 19 to 21 the end of the organism that will develop into the fetal head grows rapidly to become wider than the remaining structure. The ectodermal layer thickens to produce the primitive streak. Mesoderm cells develop into somites, which align on either side of the neural groove and will develop into bones and other supporting structures. The groove develops into a tube with a lumen that becomes the spinal canal and brain ventricles. Neuroectodermal cells migrate to form an irregular mass on either side of the neural tube, giving rise to the sensory ganglia of the spinal and cranial nerves. The fetal heart begins with organization of mesoderm cells into a primitive cardiac tube, composed of one atrium and one ventricle. The wall is composed of myocardium that is several cells thick and separated from the endocardium by a layer called cardiac jelly. By day 23 cells that will develop into the eyes and ears are present, and neural crest cells that will develop into the skull and face are formed. Over the next 2 days the cardiac structure bends into an S-shaped tube, and primitive contractions of the resulting cells begin the first "beating" of the cardiac system. At the same time an outpouching of the foregut occurs, forming a groove that extends downward and that will eventually be separated from the esophagus by a septum. Over the next 2 to 4 days primitive branching can be seen, creating five divisions—three on the right and two on the left. These will develop into the lungs later in pregnancy.

The primitive blood cells produced in the yolk sac begin migration into the chorionic villi and primitive embryonic circulatory system by day 27. At the same time, upper limb buds form, heart valves and septa differentiate, and digestive epithelium begins differentiation into the locations for the liver, lungs, stomach, and pancreas. Over the next few days the lower limb buds form, and the first layer of skin develops. The eye develops as an outpouching of the forebrain at the side of the facial cleft. Optic vesicles become the eye cup by 6 weeks. The head and neck undergo dramatic changes as the brain differentiates into three parts. The forebrain develops into the cerebral lobes, responsible for the senses, memory, and cognitive functions. The midbrain develops into cells that will relay messages from the peripheral system to the proper part of the brain for translation. The hindbrain develops into the control center for the involuntary cardiac and respiratory systems. As the head develops, the remainder of the cylindrical-shaped embryo bends into a C-shape. By 28 days' gestation the embryo is 2 to 5 mm long.

During weeks 5 to 6 the embryo begins to take on a human likeness. The rapid growth of the brain causes dramatic growth of the head, which flexes onto the thorax. The otic placode invaginates and forms the otic vesicle. The retinal disc develops and presses outward in the embryonic face. A primitive mouth develops. Internal organogenesis proceeds at a rapid pace. In this 2-week span of time the heart chambers further develop and become filled with plasma and blood cells. The mass of the heart and liver approaches the size of the head. The gallbladder, stomach, intestines, and pancreas continue to develop; and the developing liver begins to receive blood from the umbilical vessels.

The face becomes more distinct in the sixth week when the mandible, the dorsal part of the maxilla, and hyoid arches form from the pharyngeal arch. The pharyngeal arch will also differentiate into the muscular and skeletal aspects of the pharyngeal area, the aortic arch, the thyroid bone, laryngeal cartilage, and associated vascular and nerve networks. Pharyngeal pouches also form, and the cells will differentiate into the eustachian tubes, tonsils, thymus, parathyroid, and part of the thyroid. The nares begin to form, and the external pouching of the ear appears.

Internally the esophagus forms from a groove that separates it from the trachea, and the right and left lung sacs develop on either side of the esophagus. The semilunar valves form, along with the pulmonic arch. Early in the fifth week a pair of ureteric buds pouch out from distal part of mesonephric ducts. These grow into a pouch of mesodermal tissue on either side of the sacrum. These metanephric blastema develop into the kidneys. Ureters and collecting ducts differentiate from the ureteric buds. The growth of the bud into the surrounding mesoderm promotes the formation of vesicles that form the primitive tubules. Nephrons differentiate from the metanephric blastema starting in the eighth week of gestation.

During the last 2 weeks of the embryonic period, the head widens, and the nasal pits rotate to face ventrally. The primary cardiac tube has differentiated into aortic and pulmonary channels, and pouches that will develop into the ventricles deepen. Ureters develop and lengthen, and mesentery that attaches the intestines to the rear abdominal wall appears. The gonadal primordium appears, so internal differentiation is present, but external genitalia are not apparent.

At 41 days after fertilization the jaw and facial muscles have further developed, and a distinct nasofrontal groove is present. An olfactory bulb forms in the brain, and the dental laminae (tooth buds) can be identified. The external ear has recognizable form. The pituitary gland begins to form; and the cells that differentiate into the trachea, larynx, and bronchi appear. The heart begins separation into four distinct chambers, and the diaphragm forms. The primitive foregut, midgut, and hindgut are differentiated during the sixth week. The gastrointestinal system is formed by elongation, folding, and pouching of tissues. The distinct abdominal bulging seen in the embryo is the midgut as it herniates into the umbilical cord from 8 to 12 weeks. The intestines develop in the cord and will become incorporated into the abdomen once the embryo enlarges enough to have sufficient abdominal space. Failure of migration to the abdomen results in exomphalos. Primitive germs cells migrate to the genital region.

Eye pigmentation and eyelid development occurs over the next few days. The trunk of the pulmonary artery separates from the aorta. Nipples appear on the chest, and the arms have become proportional length, with recognizable wrists and hand ridges. Nephrons develop from the metanephric tissue surrounding the ampulla, and they differentiate into Bowman's capsule, distal convoluted tubule, and Henle's loop. In the tenth week distal convoluted tubules join to the collecting ducts, and the system produces urine. Urine forms as plasma is filtered in the glomerular capillaries, concentrated in the convoluted tubules and Henle's loop, and passes into bladder and into amniotic fluid. During fetal life the renal system will not be used to clear waste but rather for the production of amniotic fluid. The genital tubercle, urogenital membrane, and anal membranes appear. Ossification of bones begins at this time.

Brain waves are present by day 48 after fertilization. The semicircular canals begin to form in the inner ear. The lower extremities develop further, and knees and ankles are apparent. The gonads begin formation. By day 50 the embryo is 15 to 20 mm long, and spontaneous movements can be observed although not felt by the woman. Primitive nervous reflex activity can be seen at this time. The tip of the nose forms, and the nasal pits appear more like human nares. The urogenital membranes differentiate into male and female at this point, and testes/ovaries are distinguishable. The anal membrane perforates.

Intestinal villi begin to develop at this time and are present throughout the entire small intestine by 14 weeks' gestation.

By the end of the embryonic period (week 8), essentially all external and internal structures have differentiated and are identifiable. The head is well rounded and is held more erect. The eyelids begin to unite and will remain so until late second trimester. The taste buds form, and the caps of primary teeth are present. The bones of the palate begin to fuse. The intestines begin migration into the abdomen. The external genitalia are in primitive formation and difficult to identify as male or female. Over the next 2 weeks sockets for all 20 teeth are completely formed, and the separate folds of the mouth fuse. Early facial hair follicles begin to develop, and the vocal cords form. The intestines are completely in the abdomen, and the liver starts to secrete bile, which is stored in the gallbladder. Enzymes necessary for digestion and absorption develop late in the first trimester and may be essential in preventing bowel obstruction caused by debris found in amniotic fluid and shed cells in the gastrointestinal tract. The glandular development of the thyroid and pancreas is complete, and the pancreas begins to produce insulin. Male and female genitalia become recognizable. Whole body movements can be seen around 10 weeks, and facial grimacing and grasp reflexes can be observed by the end of the first trimester (Figure 5-5).

Amniotic Fluid Production

Amnion is a single layer of cuboidal epithelial cells on a layer of loose connective tissue. The cell structure of the amnion provides channels through which water and solutes can easily diffuse. Transfer rates are mediated by hydraulic, osmotic, and electrochemical factors. By term it is estimated that 250 ml of amniotic fluid is resorbed daily. Up until 20 weeks fluid moves from the maternal vascular system through the placenta and out through the fetal skin. By 25 weeks fetal skin keratinizes, and fluid does not readily pass through. Fetal kidneys and lungs increase fluid production, with the fetal kidneys producing 75 ml/day at 25 weeks and 500 to 700 ml/day at term. Fetal lungs secrete 200 to 400 ml/day at term. Fetal swallowing begins early in the second trimester, and it is estimated that the fetus swallows approximately

AGE (days)	LENGTH mm	STAGE Steeter	GROSS APPEARANCE	CNS	EYE	EAR	FACE
4		III	Blastocyst				
8	0.1	IV	Embryo Trophoblast				
12	0.2	V	Ectoderm Amnionic sac Yolk sac Endoderm				
19	1	IX	Body stalk Heart	Enlargement of anterior neural plate			
24	2	X Early somites	Foregut	Partial fusion Neural folds	Optic evagination	Otic placode	Mandible Hyoid arches
30	4	XII 21-29 somites		Closure neural tube Rhombencephalon mesen., prosen., Ganglia V, VII, VIII, X	Optic cup	Otic invagination	Fusion Mand. arches
34	7	XIV		Cerebellar plate Cervical and mesencephalic flexures	Lens evagination	Otic vesicle	Olfactory placodes
38	11	XVI		Dorsal pontine flexure Basal lamina Cerebral evagination Neural hypophysis	Lens detached Pigmented retina	Endolymphic sac Ext. auditory meatus Tubotympanic recess	Nasal swellings
44	17	XVIII		Olfactory evagination Cerebral hemisphere	Lens fibers Migration of retinal cells Hyaloid vessels		Choana Prim. plate
52	23	XX		Optic nerve to brain	Corneal body Mesoderm No lumen in optic stalk		
55	26	XXII			Eyelids	Spiral cochlear duct Tragus	

Figure 5-5 Timetable of human embryonic development. *Continued*

7 ml daily at 16 weeks, 16 ml daily at 20 weeks, and 200 to 600 ml daily at term.

At 8 weeks' gestation, amniotic fluid volume is approximately 20 ml, causing the amnion to swell and come in contact with the chorion. Fluid increases to 350 to 450 at 20 weeks, 800 to 1000 ml at 36 to 39 weeks, and then declines slightly until birth. The estimated rate of amniotic fluid volume turnover is 95% daily.

Amniotic fluid is necessary for symmetric fetal growth; maintenance of temperature; promoting fetal movement of all extremities; and cushioning the fetus, placenta, and cord. Amniotic fluid provides further protection through its antibacterial features. Fatty acids in the fluid have a detergent effect on bacterial membranes, immunoglobulins and lysozymes protect against infection, and transferrin binds to iron necessary for certain bacterial growth.

EXTREMITIES	HEART	GUT, ABDOMEN	LUNG	UROGENITAL	OTHER
					Early blastocyst with inner cell mass and cavitation (58 cells) lying free within uterine cavity
					Implantation Trophoblast invasion Embryonic disk with endoblast and endoblast
		Yolk sac			Early amnion sac Extraembryonic mesoblast, angioblast Chorionic gonadotropin
	Merging mesoblast anterior to prechordal plate	Stomatodeum Cloaca		Allantois	Primitive streak Hensen's node Notochord, prechordal plate Blood cells in yolk sac
	Single heart tube Propulsion	Foregut		Mesonephric ridge	Yolk sac larger than amnionic sac
Arm bud	Ventric outpouching Gelatinous reticulum	Rupture stomatodeum Evagination of thyroid, liver and dorsal pancreas	Lung bud	Mesonephric duct enters cloaca	Rathke's pouch Migration of myotomes from somites
Leg bud	Auric outpouching Septum primum	Pharyngeal pouches yield parathyroids, lat. thyroid, thymus Stomach broadens	Bronchi	Ureteral evag. Urorect. sept. Germ cells Gonadal ridge Coelom, epithelium	
Hand plate Mesench. condens. innervation	Fusion mid A-V canal Muscular vent. sept.	Intestinal loop into yolk stalk Cecum, gallbladder hepatic ducts, spleen	Main lobes	Paramesonephric duct Gonad ingrowth of coelomic epith.	Adrenal cortex (from coelomic epithelium) invaded by sympathetic cells = medulla Jugular lymph sacs
Finger rays, elbow	Aorta, Pulmonary artery, valves Membrane Ventricular septum	Duodenum lumen obliterated Cecum rotates right Appendix	Tracheal cartilage	Fusion urorect. sept. Open urogen. memb. anus Epith. cords in testicle	Early muscle
Clearing, central canal	Septum secundum			S-shaped vesicles in nephron blastema connect with collecting tubules from calyces	Superficial vascular plexus low on cranium
Shell, tubular bone				A few large glomeruli Short secretory tubules Tunica albuginea Testicle, interstitial cells	Superficial vascular plexus at vertex

Figure 5-5, cont'd For legend see p. 67.

FETAL DEVELOPMENT—SECOND TRIMESTER

During the early fetal period, there is continued differentiation of structures in the various organ systems, with resulting increase in functional ability. At the beginning of the second trimester, the fetus is approximately 8 cm long and weighs about 14 g. The head makes up about one half of the crown-rump length. The neck forms, and the chin is lifted off the chest. The lungs continue to develop, and the fetal heart is pumping about 25 quarts of blood per day. From 3 to 5 months' gestation the liver becomes the primary source of blood cell production. Production by the liver decreases in the third trimester as bone marrow production increases, and some cells are produced by the liver through the first week after birth. The highest proportion of cells produced by the fetal liver are normoblastic erythrocytes. Blood cell production also occurs in the spleen, lymph nodes, and thymus in the second trimester. The spleen primarily produces erythrocytes and lymphocytes; the thymus and lymph nodes produce lymphocytes. The external genitalia now clearly identify whether the fetus is male or female.

Airway branches in the tubules that will become the lungs develop in the late first and early second trimester. Columnar and cuboidal cells form thick epithelial walls that are surrounded by loose mesenchymal tissue. This creates a glandular effect, leading to the term pseudoglandular stage of development.

By 16 weeks' menstrual age, the fetus becomes much more flexible; movement of head, mouth, lips, arms, wrists, hands, legs, feet, and toes can be observed. The face is distinctly human, and the continued growth of the head and neck have shifted the ears higher on the head to the normal placement that will be observed at birth. Ossification of the skeleton allows for identification of bones using radiography. Over the next 2 weeks the eyes have matured, and blinking can be noted. Fingertips and toes develop their unique swirls. Meconium begins to accumulate in the intestines as a result of swallowed amniotic fluid containing cells that have been shed and digestive secretions. At this point the placenta and fetus are approximately the same size.

At 20 weeks' menstrual age the fetus demonstrates sleep and wake cycles. Lanugo appears on the skin; and vernix begins to be formed from secreted oils, dead skin, and lanugo. Brown fat forms in the neck, chest, and groin. The ovaries contain primitive egg cells. Fetal movements can usually be felt by the woman at this time, and the fetal heart sounds are distinct enough that they can be auscultated with a fetoscope by an experienced examiner. From 20 to 24 weeks the fetus grows to 30 cm length and 780 g weight. The bones in the ear harden, and myelination of the auditory fibers occurs at weeks 24 to 26, making sound conduction possible. Voluntary fetal reactions to sound can be noted, but refinement of auditory function continues through the third trimester.

During early second trimester the epithelial cells of the distal air spaces of the developing lungs flatten, and a rich vascular system begins to proliferate. Capillaries develop closer to the epithelium. By 24 weeks' gestation the surface epithelium thins as the vascular proliferation increases. By 26 to 28 weeks the epithelium and vascular bed of the lungs have developed to the point where gas exchange is possible. Surfactant secretion begins in the late second trimester (25 to 28 weeks), although its production will not be sufficient to ensure alveolar stability until 33 to 35 weeks' gestation.

Brain waves are similar to those seen in full-term infants, the eyelids unfuse, and the fetus opens and closes the eyes voluntarily. Eyelashes appear. Subcutaneous fat begins to form, and approximately 2% to 3% of body weight is fat. The central nervous system initiates breathing movements. The testes descend into the scrotum.

Fetal Circulation

Fetal circulation demonstrates modifications to allow for the fact that the placenta is the organ of gas exchange, not the lungs. These modifications include:

- Larger and more numerous red blood cells
- Higher hemoglobin content
- Modified form of hemoglobin (HbF), which is active in the slightly more acid blood
- Ductus arteriosus
- Ductus venosus
- Foramen ovale
- Hypogastric arteries

As noted previously, fetal blood cells are first formed from mesoderm in the yolk sac from 3 to 6 weeks after fertilization. The responsibility for blood cell production is then assumed by the liver, accounting for its relative large size in fetal life. Bone marrow production of blood cells is a late development, occurring in the late second trimester and third trimester. Fetal hemoglobin differs from adult hemoglobin in that it has two alpha and two gamma chains rather than two alpha and two beta chains.

The fetus exists in a state of aerobic metabolism with arterial Po_2 ranging from 20 to 25 mm Hg. Adequate fetal tissue oxygenation is achieved by higher cardiac output and organ blood flow, higher hemoglobin concentration, and greater oxygen-carrying capacity of fetal hemoglobin. These modifications result in a shift in the fetal oxygen dissociation curve so that, at a normal fetal Po_2 of 20 mm Hg, fetal whole blood O_2 saturation can be 50%, in contrast to maternal saturation, which is less than 40% at that Po_2 level.

Oxygenated blood from the placenta goes through ductus venosus in the fetal liver to the inferior vena cava and through vessels to the left lobe of the liver. A major branch joins the portal vein to supply the right lobe of the liver. About one half of the umbilical blood flow is shunted through the ductus venosus after 30 weeks' gestation. Well-oxygenated ductus venosus blood flow combines with left hepatic vein flow in the inferior vena cava. As the blood enters the right atrium, 30% to 50% of the oxygenated blood is shunted through the foramen ovale to the left atrium. Blood with highest oxygen content is shunted to left ventricle and supplies blood to the carotid circulation and upper body and brain. The foramen ovale acts like a one-way valve, allowing only right to left shunting. Right hepatic blood enters the inferior vena cava, lowering the oxygen content to form a stream that is preferentially directed through the tricuspid valve. Small amounts of the well-oxygenated blood enter the right atrium, where it mixes with poorly oxygenated blood from the superior vena cava. The blood that is not shunted through the foramen ovale passes through the tricuspid valve, into the right ventricle, then into the pulmonary arteries, where about 10% of the flow goes to the lungs. The remaining 60% to 90% is shunted through the ductus arteriosis to the aorta. High pulmonary resistance and higher mean pulmonary artery pressure are responsible for the shift. Patency of the ductus arteriosis is thought to be maintained through high levels of prostaglandin (PG) E_2 and local PGI_2. About 60% of the aortic blood volume goes to the placenta, where it undergoes gas, nutrient, and waste exchange with the maternal system. The remainder of the fetal blood flow goes to the trunk and lower limbs.

FETAL DEVELOPMENT—THIRD TRIMESTER

Fetal growth during third trimester includes increases in fat and muscle mass and further functional maturation of organ systems. Increase in skin thickness, coupled with the formation of subcutaneous fat deposits, results in the loss of skin translucency seen earlier in pregnancy. Vernix and lanugo decrease as the fetus approaches term. As the fetus fills the uterine cavity, the extremities are forced into a more constant flexed attitude. The central nervous system fully controls rhythmic breathing movements and body temperature.

Rapid brain growth continues, and increased convolutions provide greater surface area for cognitive function. Head circumference increases to accommodate the growing brain. The eyes develop pupil reflexes to light at 32 weeks' menstrual age, and the iris develops the gray-blue color seen in neonates. Final formation of eye pigmentation requires exposure to light; thus it will not be apparent until about 5 months after the birth. The eyelids are open during awake states and closed during sleep. Fingernails and toenails are present. As white fat continues to be deposited subcutaneously, the skin color appears to lighten, and by 36 weeks about 15% of the fetal weight is fat. The fatty deposits create the typical dimpling in the wrists, elbows, and knees seen in healthy, well-nourished neonates.

Lung maturity that indicates decreased risk for respiratory distress syndrome (RDS) occurs in the third trimester. Maturity can be estimated through assessment of the surfactant phospholipids produced. Sphingomyelin levels remain constant through pregnancy. However, phosphatidylcholine (lecithin) levels rise significantly at 34 to 35 weeks' gestation. Gluck (1971) and Gluck and Kulovic (1973) found that, when the ratio of lecithin to sphingomyelin (L/S ratio) is greater than or equal to 2, the risk for RDS is small. The presence of phosphatidylglycerol also is an indication that synthesis of surfactant is sufficient to decrease the risk of RDS.

At term the fetus can be observed turning toward light sources (orienting process). Although ossification has continued, the bones retain some flexibility, which is a protective factor during the birth process. Tissue growth continues, with a greater proportion due to fat acquisition (82 g/week). Nonfat tissue acquisition is estimated to average 43 g weekly at term.

TERATOLOGY—THE STUDY OF ABNORMAL DEVELOPMENT

Alterations in structure and function of developing fetal organ systems can occur through genetic influence or the influence of external factors such as toxins, heat, or radiation. Genetic transmission accounts for 15% to 20% of anomalies. Chromosomal aberrations account for 5%. Approximately 10% of malformations or anomalies are directly caused by environmental factors, including drugs, chemicals, radiation, infections, and mechanical problems. The remainder are most likely caused by a complex interplay of multiple factors (Sever and Mortensen, 1996).

In considering the effect of genetic or environmental factors on the developing fetus, it is helpful to consider Wilson's six general principles of teratogenesis (1977) when seeking understanding of deviations in fetal growth and development.

1. Genotypes of the conceptus will account for differences in susceptibility to a teratogen. Animal studies have shown variation in structural anomalies when different genetic strains of species are exposed to agents.
2. The susceptibility to a teratogen varies across time during gestation as different organs and systems develop. The term "critical stages of development" refers to the time period during which

an organism is most likely to experience effects from a teratogen. In human gestation the embryonic period (weeks 2 through 8) is considered the most sensitive time since most structural effects are noted in the first trimester.

3. The mechanism of action on the developing organism will effect the susceptibility. Mechanisms include gene mutation, chromosomal abnormalities, mitotic interference, altered nucleic acid integrity or function, lack of normal precursors, altered energy sources, changes in membrane characteristics, osmolar imbalance, and enzyme inhibition.
4. Susceptibility influences the final manifestations of the teratogenic effect. These manifestations include death, malformation, growth retardation and functional disorders. The manifestation is strongly associated with the developmental phase when exposure occurred. In general, exposure during the embryonic period is associated with structural malformations or death, whereas exposure during the fetal period is associated with functional disorders or growth restrictions.
5. The agent that is associated with the teratogenic effect must have access to the developing organism. For example, drugs usually gain access to the fetus through transfer across the placenta. If a molecule is too large for placental transfer, another means of access must be possible to affect the fetus.
6. As the amount of exposure increases (dose), the manifestations of abnormal development must increase.

The study of the effect of agents on the developing embryo/fetus usually uses epidemiologic methodologies to understand risk. Although the development of many anomalies is not well understood, there is an increasing body of knowledge available to the clinician to assess exposure risk preconceptually and during pregnancy. Risk assessment should include the following data collection during the clinical visit.

Genetic Screening

Numerous forms have been developed by professional organizations to identify women at increased risk for genetic problems in the fetus. The American College of Obstetricians and Gynecologists Prenatal Record includes a screening tool that can efficiently be administered at the initial prenatal visit or during a preconception visit. General areas that should be considered when screening are maternal and paternal age, family history of genetic syndromes, and exposure to infections known to affect the developing embryo.

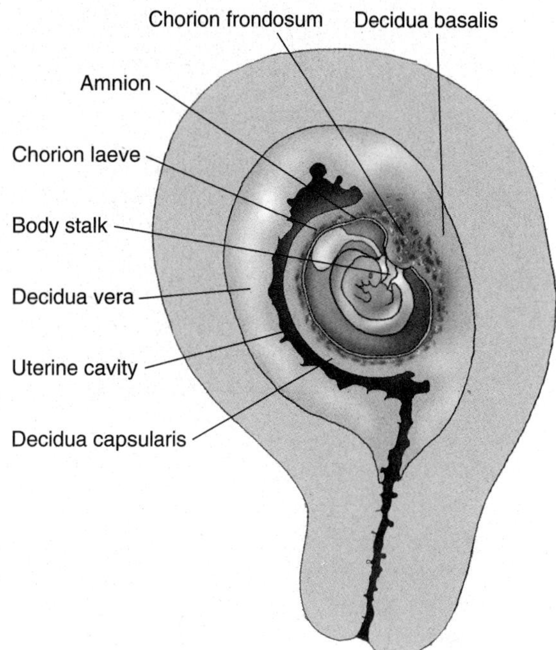

Figure 5-6 Development of membranes and decidua.

Environmental Screening

The clinician should explore both the residential and work environment to identify factors associated with teratogenesis. Examples of these factors include air, water and soil pollutants, chemicals in the home or workplace, radiation, blood products or other body fluids, and high temperatures. Common occupational exposures are listed in Table 5-2.

Lifestyle Behavior Screening

The effects of exposures related to lifestyle behaviors is well documented in the literature. Use of over-the-counter drugs, alcohol, cigarettes, illicit drugs, and inhalants all may lead to structural or functional malformations. Multiple sexual partners or staying with a partner who is not monogamous increases the risks associated with infections. Working long hours, increased stress in the home or workplace, and excess physical exercise may have an effect on the developing fetus.

Table 5-2 *Common Occupational Exposures to Teratogens*

Occupation	Agents
Health personnel	Infectious agents, anesthetic gases, radiation, alcohol, laboratory chemicals, noise
Textile and garment workers	Cotton and fiber dusts, formaldehyde, dyes, heat, solvents, flame retardants
Electronics workers	Lead, tin, antimony, trichloroethylene, methylene chloride, resins
Plastics workers	Acrylonitrile, formaldehyde, vinyl chloride
Printing personnel	Ink mists, methanol, carbon tetrachloride, lead, noise, solvents, trichloroethylene
Photographic processors	Bromides, iodines, silver nitrate
Transportation workers	Carbon monoxide, polynuclear aromatics, lead
Painters	Lead, toluene
Cosmetologists	Solvents, dyes
Clerical workers	Trichloroethylene, carbon tetrachloride, formaldehyde, cigarette smoke
Cleaning personnel	Solvents
Restaurant servers, bartenders	Cigarette smoke
Day care workers, teachers	Infectious agents

In general there are three critical periods of development in human pregnancy. During the first 17 days following fertilization, exposure to teratogens may lead to ineffective implantation and spontaneous abortion. Clinicians can explain to women that the effect is usually considered "all or nothing." If implantation proceeds normally, one can assume that the conceptus has not been affected by the agent. During the embryonic period (days 18 to 55) exposure leads to structural and functional alterations for the organ(s) that is developing at the distinct time of exposure. For example, exposure to an agent in the first 40 days of gestation may cause structural anomalies of the heart, since it is undergoing significant differentiation at that time, but the exposure will not affect the genitals, which do not differentiate until later in the gestation. During the fetal period, exposure may lead to structural anomalies for organ systems that continue differentiation into the second trimester, but it more commonly leads to functional or growth abnormalities.

The balance of the chapter addresses several known exposures that are associated with increased risk of adverse reproductive outcomes.

Infectious Agents

Teratogenic effects of viral infection in pregnancy have been well documented. Rubella, cytomegalovirus (CMV), herpes simplex, parvovirus, and varicella have distinct syndromes, with effects usually being most pronounced when the infection occurs during the first trimester.

Rubella virus easily crosses the placenta, and the fetal effects are most severe when the infection occurs in the first trimester. About 50% of fetuses exposed in the first 4 weeks following conception will manifest abnormalities, including hearing loss, eye defects, cardiac anomalies, microcephaly, mental retardation, growth restriction, hepatosplenomegaly, hemolytic anemia, and thrombocytopenia. The risk of fetal effects decreases to 25% when the infection occurs in the second month following conception and declines to 10% when the fetus is exposed later in the first trimester. Only 1% of fetuses exposed after the first trimester will develop sequelae.

CMV can be transported across the placenta and passed from mother to fetus both in primary and recurrent infections. Approximately 50% to 80% of women have antibodies indicating past exposure to the virus, but the antibodies do not produce lifelong immunity. When women develop primary CMV infection in pregnancy, approximately 40% to 50% of their fetuses will be affected. The greatest risk of congenital infection is when the maternal infection occurs in the third trimester, but infection during the first trimester is associated with the most severe fetal effects. Only 5% to 18% of infected infants will be symptomatic at birth. Of those who are severely affected, 30% will die. Eighty percent of survivors develop severe neurologic morbidity, ocular abnormalities, or neural hearing loss. Of infants whose mothers experience primary CMV infection in pregnancy, 10% to

15% will develop subsequent problems such as hearing loss, vision problems, or dental defects within the first 2 years of life. Clinical signs of congenital infection include hepatosplenomegaly, intracranial calcifications, jaundice, growth restriction, microcephaly, chorioretinitis, and hearing loss (Duff, 1996). Research suggests that infants exposed to recurrent infection are not likely to be symptomatic at birth but may subsequently develop hearing loss or another sequela (Fowler, Stagno, and Pass, 1992). It is estimated that about 1% of infants born in the United States have congenital CMV infection and 1% of those are symptomatic at birth. An additional 1% of infected infants will develop subsequent neurologic or developmental problems.

Severe primary herpes simplex virus infection in pregnancy is associated with spontaneous abortion, preterm delivery, and growth restriction. Although the most common transmission is direct contact with lesions during birth, there are documented cases of intrauterine infection with intact membranes.

Human parvovirus B19 is associated with fetal hydrops resulting from viral infection of the erythroid stem cells of the fetus. The risk of this severe fetal effect when the infection occurs in the first trimester is 5% to 15%.

Congenital varicella is associated with spontaneous abortion, intrauterine fetal death, cutaneous anomalies, limb hypoplasia, muscle atrophy, malformed digits, psychomotor retardation, microcephaly, cortical atrophy, cataracts, chorioretinitis, and microphthalmia. The incidence of fetal effects is small, with epidemiologic studies finding only 1% to 2% of exposed infants manifesting organ or functional effects; highest risk is when infection occurs in the second trimester.

Syphilis infection is associated with fetal demise, intrauterine growth restriction, and preterm birth. *Treponema pallidum* crosses the placenta at any point in pregnancy, and up to one third of infected fetuses are stillborn. Clinical manifestations of infection early in pregnancy include chorioretinitis, iritis, lymphadenopathy, hepatosplenomegaly, and skin lesions. Infection late in pregnancy is associated with dental malformations, deafness, nasal anomalies, mental retardation, hydrocephalus, optic nerve atrophy, and arthritis-like syndromes.

Acute toxoplasmosis infection in pregnancy is associated with chorioretinitis, periventricular calcifications, ventriculomegaly, seizures, mental retardation, ascites, hepatosplenomegaly, and rash. The risk of fetal infection is greater in the third trimester, and, although 40% of exposed infants show evidence of infection, less than half will be symptomatic at birth.

Ionizing Radiation

Studies of the reproductive experiences of women exposed to acute high doses of radiation have found an association between exposure and microcephaly, mental retardation ophthalmic defects, spina bifida, cleft palate, and abnormalities of the extremities. Effects are most pronounced when the exposure occurs before 15 weeks.

They decrease with increasing distance from the source of the radiation. There is currently no solid evidence of effect when the pregnant woman is exposed to chronic low-dose radiation. Exposure to diagnostic radiation has been associated with increased risk for abnormal karyotypes and altered sex ratios at birth (increase in females over proportion expected). There has also been research suggesting an increase in leukemia in children exposed in utero, but the magnitude of risk is relatively small, increasing from 1:3000 to 1:2000 (Sever and Mortensen, 1996).

Lead

Exposure to lead has been associated with increased perinatal mortality, growth and mental retardation, and developmental disabilities. Public health efforts have led to policy changes that have decreased exposure in the air and in paints used in residential buildings. Lead has toxic effects on the nervous system, and it is reasonable to assume that the developing embryo and fetus may be susceptible to the effects. Maternal blood lead levels as low as 10 μg/dl are associated with decreased gestational age at birth and decreased birth weight. Neurologic problems such as lower IQ, attention deficit disorder, hearing deficits, learning disabilities, and shorter stature are associated with higher lead levels.

Herbicides and Pesticides

Although the Environmental Protection Agency has worked to decrease exposure to chemicals known to have teratogenic and fetotoxic effects, there continues to be concern about exposure during pregnancy. Unfortunately there is little research on the effects of exposure to newer agents, and women may be exposed either in the workplace (e.g., nurseries, agriculture) or in their residences when they live near fields that are treated chemically. All employers using chemicals are required to maintain a Material Safety Data Sheet for all chemicals; although the information reported by the manufacturer may be limited, a woman concerned about exposure can at least obtain chemical information that can then be discussed with a genetic counselor or expert committee on teratogens.

Hazardous Waste

Hazardous waste sites have received much press coverage as increasing concerns have been raised about the effect of exposure to the many compounds found in water and soil. Studies have found associations between proximity to waste sites and nervous system, musculoskeletal system, cardiovascular system, and skin anomalies. Unless epidemiologic investigation has been completed at a particular site, the clinician often has limited data on which recommendations can be based.

Commonly Used Pharmacologic Agents

Many commonly prescribed drugs are contraindicated in pregnancy because of the increased risks of fetal effects. Agents associated with effects, particularly when exposure is in the first trimester, include androgens, diethylstilbestrol, isotretinoin, lithium, phenytoin, tetracycline, and valproic acid.

Cigarette Smoke

Exposure to cigarette smoke, both primary and secondary, has been associated with intrauterine growth restriction. Association with delayed neurologic and intellectual development has also been suggested, but these findings most likely have multiple associated factors. Growth restriction is most likely caused by the effect of carbon monoxide, which decreases the oxygen-carrying capacity of hemoglobin, and nicotine, which causes vasoconstriction, resulting in decreased uteroplacental perfusion.

Alcohol

The effects of chronic alcohol use and binge drinking have been well documented. Chronic use is associated with fetal alcohol syndrome, which has characteristics that include growth retardation, microcephaly, delayed cognitive development, attention deficit disorder, and craniofacial abnormalities (small palpebral fissures, flattened maxilla, flat philtrum, and short upturned nose). Exposure in the first trimester leads to structural and functional abnormalities, whereas exposure later in pregnancy contributes to growth restriction.

References

Beer AE: Immunologic aspects of normal pregnancy and recurrent spontaneous abortion, *Semin Reprod Endocrinol* 6:163, 1988.

Blackburn ST, Loper DL: *Maternal, fetal and neonatal physiology—a clinical perspective,* Philadelphia, 1992, WB Saunders.

Cross JC, Werb Z, and Fisher SJ: Implantation and the placenta: key pieces of the development puzzle, *Science* 266:1508-1510, 1994.

Duff P: Maternal and perinatal infection. In Gabbe SG, Niebyl JR, Simpson JL, editors: *Obstetrics—normal and problem pregnancies,* New York, 1996, Churchill Livingstone.

Fowler KB, Stagno S, Pass RF: The outcome of congenital cytomegalovirus infection in relation to maternal antibody status, *N Engl J Med* 326:663, 1992.

Galbraith RM, Kantor RS, Ferra GB: Differential anatomical expression of transplantation antigens within the normal human placental chorionic villus, *Am J Reprod Immunol* 1:331-335, 1981.

Gluck L: Diagnosis of the respiratory distress syndrome by amniocentesis, *Am J Obstet Gynecol* 109:440-444, 1971.

Gluck L, Kulovic M: Lecithin/sphingomyelin ratios in amniotic fluid in normal and abnormal pregnancy, *Am J Obstet Gynecol* 115:539, 1973.

Kaufmann P, Scheffen I: Placental development. In Polin RA, Fox W, editors: *Fetal and neonatal physiology,* ed 2, Philadelphia, 1998, WB Saunders, pp 59-70.

Khong TY, Pearce JM: In Lavery JP, editors: *The human placenta: clinical perspectives,* Rockville, Md, 1987, Aspen, pp 25-45.

Sever LE, Mortensen ME: Teratology and the epidemiology of birth defects: occupational and environmental perspectives. In Gabbe SG, Niebyl JR, Simpson JL, editors: *Obstetrics—normal and problem pregnancies,* New York, 1996, Churchill Livingstone.

Sutherland CA, Naiem M., Mason DY: The expression of major histocompatibility antigens by human chorionic villi, *J Reprod Immunol* 3:323, 1981.

Sweet BR, Tiran D, editors: *Mayes' midwifery—a textbook for midwives,* ed 12, London, 1997, Baillière Tindall.

Wilson JG: Current status of teratology—general principles and mechanisms derived from animal studies. In Wilson JG, Fraser FC, editors: *Handbook of teratology,* vol 1, New York, 1977, Plenum.

Chapter 6

Maternal Anatomic and Physiologic Adaptations in Pregnancy

From conception through the postpartum period, the pregnant woman's body experiences dramatic adaptations that support the growing embryo and fetus and promote the woman's maintenance of health. It is essential that the clinician understand the normal anatomic and physiologic changes to accurately identify deviations from normal.

ADAPTATIONS IN THE REPRODUCTIVE SYSTEM

The Uterus

Uterine changes throughout the pregnancy and birth and after the birth are profound. During pregnancy the uterus supports the developing embryo and fetus and maintains the structures that account for maternal-fetal communication. During the birthing process the muscles of the uterus work in a synchronous way to expel the fetus. After birth the muscles of the uterus control bleeding and involute to the normal nonpregnant state.

Uterine growth. The uterus increases in mass from a prepregnant weight of 70 g to a weight at term of approximately 1100 g (Gabbe, Niebyl, and Simpson, 1996). The volume at term averages 5 L, but it can be as much as 20 L in the case of multiple gestation or hydramnios. Uterine growth begins after implantation and involves both hyperplasia and hypertrophy of cells. Individual myometrial cells increase 100-fold in length by term. In addition to the increase in mass of myometrial cells, the uterine wall has an increase in collagenous connective tissue and intercellular ground substance.

Early uterine growth is primarily stimulated by the increasing estrogen levels. It is clear that early growth is not necessarily in response to the mechanical distention from the growing products of conception, since similar enlargement is seen with ectopic pregnancies. During the first 3 months of pregnancy the uterine wall thickens to about 25 mm. As the pregnancy progresses, stretching of the uterine wall as a result of the growth of the fetus leads to a thinning out of the wall to 5 to 15 mm at term (Blackburn and Loper, 1992; Cunningham et al., 1997). The thinning of the uterine walls allows the clinician to easily palpate the fetus during the third trimester.

Uterine growth is most pronounced in the uterine fundus (Figure 6-1). This asymmetry of growth is best appreciated by noting the positions of attachment of the fallopian tubes and the ovarian and round ligaments as pregnancy progresses. Early in pregnancy the tubes and ligaments insert just below the apex of the fundus. In the third trimester the insertions are at points lightly above the middle of the uterus.

During the first trimester the uterus also changes in shape. Early in pregnancy the uterus retains its pear shape. The uterus gradually changes to a more sphere-

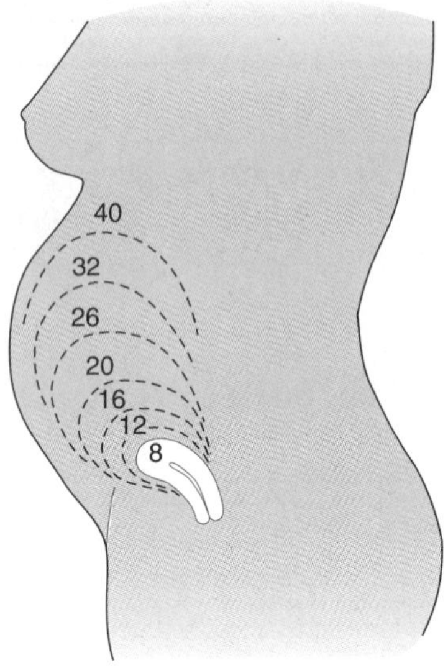

Figure 6-1 Uterine growth by weeks' gestation.

shaped organ by 12 weeks' gestation. After 12 weeks the shape becomes more elliptic or ovoid.

The uterus remains a pelvic organ for the first 12 weeks of pregnancy; after 12 weeks it becomes an abdominal organ. As it rises into the abdomen, it causes distention of the anterior abdominal wall, displaces the intestines laterally and superiorly, and at term is at the level of the liver.

Because of the stretching of the broad and round ligaments, the uterus retains some mobility in the abdomen. When the woman is standing, the long axis of the uterus aligns with the axis of the pelvic inlet. The abdominal muscles maintain this alignment unless the abdominal wall is unusually lax. When the pregnant woman is supine, the uterus shifts posteriorly to rest on the spine and great vessels. The uterus maintains a slight rotation to the right (dextrorotation) through the second and third trimesters, most likely the result of the rectosigmoid on the left side of the abdomen.

Uterine growth leads to increased uterine blood flow, accomplished through increased vessel diameter and decreased vascular resistance (Thaler et al., 1990). The uterine arteries are the primary source of blood supply to the uterus. At term blood flow demonstrates a fourfold increase when compared to the nonpregnant state, and that volume constitutes 12% of cardiac output. Before pregnancy mean uterine artery blood flow is 94 ml/min. By the end of first trimester, the uterine blood flow is 100 ml/min. Flow increases to over 300 ml/min by term.

Contractility. The uterus demonstrates irregular contractile activity in the nonpregnant state. This contractile activity increases and becomes more regular in pregnancy. Early in pregnancy the contractions are mild and irregular and usually not noted by the woman. By the second trimester the contractions may be palpated by the examiner, and as pregnancy progresses they may become noticeable and uncomfortable for the pregnant woman (Ramsey, 1994). The frequency of contractions at 25 weeks' gestation has been found to average 0.32/hr, with an increase at term to 2.33/hr (Zahn, 1984). Named after the individual who first described them, these Braxton-Hicks contractions do not typically lead to cervical change since they are not synchronous and irregular in frequency. Cervical examination with documented cervical change is the only way to accurately identify whether the uterine contractions are Braxton-Hicks contractions or the contractions of active labor.

Several distinct changes occur in the myometrial cells to foster increased contractility in pregnancy. The hypertrophy and hyperplasia of myometrial cells under the influence of estrogen allows for increased contractile proteins to be found in the cells. The increased potential for contractility is further enhanced by an increase in intracellular calcium. Movement of extracellular calcium into the myometrial cell is facilitated by increased transfer through receptor- and voltage-mediated channels and release of calcium from endoplasmic reticulum. Myometrial cells are arranged in a network of bundles, but the individual cells do not have specific contacts until late pregnancy. Gap junctions, the transcellular membrane channels that contain proteins that facilitate transfer of impulses, increase in number during pregnancy (Valenzuela, Germain, and Foster, 1993). By late pregnancy the gap junctions provide sites for efficient transfer of ions between cells, as well as a low resistance pathway for passage of electrical and chemical impulses. These gap junctions are necessary for the development of synchronous uterine contractions. Finally, there are increased numbers of mitochondria and cellular STP, which enhance energy production in the myometrial cells (Blackburn and Loper, 1992).

Cervical changes. The cervix increases in mass and water content in pregnancy. Increased vascularity and edema, as well as hypertrophy and hyperplasia of the cervical glands cause the cervix to soften (Goodell sign) and develop a bluish tinge (Chadwick sign) about 1 month after conception. About 85% to 90% of the cervix is connective tissue; the remaining 10% to 15% is smooth muscle. There is a higher concentration of smooth muscle in the upper part of the cervix (25%), and the proportion of smooth muscle decreases through the middle (16%) and lower (6%) parts of the cervix (Fuchs and Fuchs, 1996) (Figure 6-2).

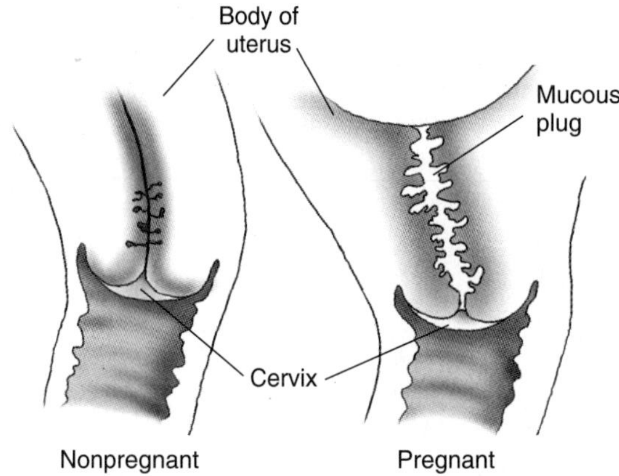

Figure 6-2 Changes in cervix induced by pregnancy.

The connective tissue consists of collagen and elastin fibers that create a dense network in a gel-like proteoglycans. The collagen forms a relatively rigid rod-shaped structure that assists in preventing premature dilation during pregnancy. The elastin is thought to provide elasticity so that the cervix can dilate during birth and return to its normal shape after birth.

The cervical glands occupy only a minimal part of the cervix in the nonpregnant state. At term they occupy about one half of the cervical mass. The glandular spaces become filled with mucus, and shortly after conception the thick mucus plug fills the cervical canal.

The columnar epithelium of the endocervical canal and the endocervical glands proliferate to the point where they extend from the external os onto the portio vaginalis of the cervix. Although this eversion may appear to be erosion, inflammation is rarely identified.

For birth to occur the cervix must undergo softening, effacement, and increased dispensability. This process, called cervical ripening, involves changes in the collagen, proteoglycans, and smooth muscle. Collagenase, elastase, and other enzymes degrade the collagen, leading to greater solubility and increased water content in the cervix. The result is further softening of the cervix.

Cervical ripening occurs primarily because of the influence of hormones, including estradiol, progesterone, relaxin, prostacyclin, and prostaglandin E_2 (PGE_2). Progesterone inhibits collagen breakdown, and it has been suggested that factors that inhibit progesterone may play a role in cervical ripening. Increased cervical relaxin may influence changes in water and mucopolysaccharide content in the cervix, although the role of relaxin in humans is controversial. It is thought that prostaglandins have a localized effect on cervical softening. The amount of PGE_2 in cervical mucus increases in second trimester, suggesting that initial changes to enhance ripening begin well before term (Fuchs, Ivell, and Friedman, 1995).

The Ovaries and Fallopian Tubes

Ovarian function. Fertilization and implantation bring about a cessation of maturation of follicles and ovulation. The corpus luteum functions during the first 6 to 7 weeks of pregnancy, contributing to progesterone production. Removal of the corpus luteum before 7 weeks' gestation will result in a decrease in maternal progesterone and spontaneous abortion. Removal of the corpus luteum later in pregnancy does not cause this effect.

Relaxin is a protein hormone secreted by the corpus luteum and possibly by the uterine decidua during pregnancy. Research findings suggest that relaxin may cause uterine muscle relaxation and cervical softening or "ripening."

The smooth muscle of the tubes undergoes little hypertrophy. The epithelium of the mucosa is flattened when compared to that of the nonpregnant state. Decidual cells may be identified in the endosalpinx, but no continuous decidual membrane develops.

Vagina and perineum. The vulva and perineum demonstrate increased vascularity and hyperemia in pregnancy. The increased vascularity of the vagina leads to development of a bluish color (Chadwick sign), similar to the cervical change noted in pregnancy. Increased levels of estrogen stimulate changes in the vaginal walls, including increase in the thickness of the mucosa, softening of the connective tissue, and hypertrophy of the smooth muscle cells. These changes lead to a lengthening of the vagina. Rugae become more pronounced in nulliparae. In multipara previous stretching of the vagina may result in the rugae being smoother than in nulliparae.

Vaginal secretions increase, and these increased secretions produce a heavy, whitish mucus discharge. Many pregnant women find the discharge so pronounced by the third trimester that they find it helpful to wear a pad to absorb secretions. Under stimulation of estrogen, the vaginal mucosa metabolizes glycogen. Increased lactobacilli in pregnancy enhance this metabolism. A by-product of the glycogen metabolism is lactic acid, which decreases the vaginal pH. The pH ranges from 3.5 to 4.0 in the introitus, midvagina, and anterior and posterior fornices as a result of the increased production of lactic acid from glycogen in the vaginal epithelium. Cervical pH ranges from 5.2 to 6.0. The increased acidity of the vaginal secretions is important in the control of growth of pathogens. Elevated pH values are associated with disturbed vaginal flora (Riedewald et al., 1990).

ADAPTATIONS IN THE CARDIOVASCULAR SYSTEM

During pregnancy there are dramatic changes in the cardiovascular system. These changes are necessary to ensure adequate perfusion of maternal organs and the fetal-placental unit.

Heart

Cardiac output. Cardiac output is determined by heart rate and stroke volume and is affected by arterial blood pressure, vascular resistance, maternal weight, and basal metabolism rate. Studies have demonstrated that, when the pregnant woman is at rest in the lateral recumbent position, cardiac output increases.

Recent studies have demonstrated that the greatest cardiac changes occur during the first trimester and are due to increased stroke volume and heart rate (Capeless and Clapp, 1989; Mabie et al., 1994; Robson et al., 1989). Cardiac output increases 22% by 8 weeks, an increase of 1 L/min over prepregnant output. By 24 to 28 weeks' gestation output has increased by 20% to 50%, and this level is maintained through the rest of the pregnancy. After the first trimester, heart rate increases by 10 to 15 beats/min and accounts for a greater proportion of the increased cardiac output than stroke volume. Stroke volume declines somewhat in the third trimester and is significantly influenced by maternal position. Stroke volume is least when the pregnant woman in third trimester is in the supine position. By 8 weeks' gestation systemic vascular resis-

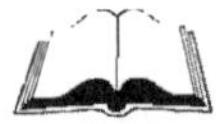

Research Box 6-1

Capeless EL, Clapp JF: Cardiovascular changes in early phase of pregnancy, *Am J Obstet Gynecol* 161(6 part 1):1449-1453, 1989.

Background

Changes in heart rate, cardiac output, and systemic vascular resistance have been well documented during the second and third trimesters of pregnancy. In addition, pregnancy-induced changes have been compared to postpartum adjustment. No previous studies investigated the changes from the prepregnant period through early pregnancy.

Research Question

What is the magnitude and timing of changes in cardiac output, stroke volume, heart rate, mean arterial pressure, and systemic vascular resistance in early pregnancy?

Methods

Subjects were enrolled before conception and evaluated within 3 months of conception and at 6 to 8, 14 to 16, and 22 to 24 weeks' gestation. Heart rate and blood pressure were determined using appropriate monitors. M-mode echocardiography was used for determination of cardiac output. Statistical analysis was performed with repeated measures of analysis of variance with the Bonferroni correction for multiple comparisons.

Sample

Eight subjects completed all study periods. Mean age was 30.8 years, and all were either primigravidae or primiparae. All subjects were nonsmoking, physically active women with no history of heart disease.

Results

Cardiac output increased 1 L/min by 8 weeks' gestation, a 22% change over preconception values. This represents 57% of the total increase in output achieved by 24 weeks' gestation. The increase in stroke volume at 8 weeks' gestation represented a 22% change over preconception values and 78% of the total increase by 24 weeks' gestation. Statistically significant increase in heart rate did not occur until 16 weeks' gestation. End-diastolic heart volume increased significantly by 8 weeks' gestation, with 65% of the total change occurring at that time. Systemic vascular resistance decreased by 8 weeks' gestation to 30% below preconception values. This represented 90% of the total change by 24 weeks' gestation.

Clinical Application

Findings can be used when educating women about the dramatic cardiovascular changes in early pregnancy. However, they may only document the experience of physically fit women who are somewhat older than most primigravidae.

tance has decreased to 70% of prepregnant value, further enhancing cardiac output (Capeless and Clapp, 1989) (Research Box 6-1).

The growing uterus in the second and third trimesters provides the primary influence on the changes in cardiac output in selected maternal positions. In the supine position the uterine mass compresses the inferior vena cava, leading to decreased venous return and a 20% to 30% decrease in cardiac output. This syndrome almost always is associated with increased heart rate in response to the decreased output. There is somewhat less compression of the vena cava in the sitting position, and the lateral recumbent position provides the best venous return (Research Box 6-2).

The increase in cardiac output does not appear to be related to an increase in metabolic needs or increased demands of the fetal-placental unit. The most dramatic changes occur in the first trimester when the fetal mass

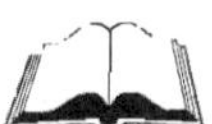

Research Box 6-2

Clark SL et al: Position change and central hemodynamic profile during normal third-trimester pregnancy and postpartum, *Am J Obstet Gynecol* 164:883-888, 1991.

Background

The effect of position changes, particularly supine position, on blood flow through the aorta and inferior vena cava in late pregnancy has been well documented. However, previous studies do not provide data regarding preload of the left and right sides of the heart, pulmonary vascular pressures, and left ventricular functioning.

Research Question

What are the effects of position change on maternal central hemodynamics?

Methods

Subjects underwent pulmonary artery catheterization and radial arterial line placement. After a 30-min stabilization period in the left lateral position, baseline hemodynamic measurements were made. After 10-min stabilization periods between each position change, measurements were also taken in the right lateral recumbent, supine, sitting, standing, and knee-chest positions. Measurements included determination of cardiac output and oxygen consumption. Studies were repeated between 11 and 13 weeks after delivery.

Sample

Volunteers were recruited from physician offices, and the study was done at the Utah Valley Regional Medical Center, altitude 4540 feet. Ten volunteers who met inclusion criteria of primigravity, maternal age less than 26 years, singleton vertex fetus, gestational age between 36 and 38 weeks, and no obstetric or medical complication were studied.

Results

There was a mean fall of cardiac output of 9% in the supine position and 18% in the standing position when compared with the left lateral position. The decrease noted in the sitting position was not significant. No significant differences were seen in mean systemic vascular resistance, mean arterial pressure (MAP), central venous pressure (CVP), or mean pulmonary artery pressure in any position change. After pregnancy there was no change in hemodynamics in the supine position when compared with left lateral position. A 31% fall in cardiac output, 27% increase in heart rate, 42% rise in systemic vascular resistance, and 106% rise in pulmonary vascular resistance was noted in the standing position. No significant differences were found in MAP, CVP, or mean pulmonary artery pressure.

Clinical Application

Findings suggest that the increased vascular volume during pregnancy provides a stabilizing effect, even in light of decreased systemic vascular resistance. This implies greater hemodynamic stability in response to orthostasis when compared to the postpartum period. The significant decrease in cardiac output in late pregnancy when the woman is standing has implications for women who must stand motionless for long periods of time. Women with additional risk factors for uteroplacental insufficiency are particularly at risk for delivering low-birth-weight infants. The authors suggest that ambulation or other exercise may negate the cardiovascular effects of standing. Clinicians should counsel women whose employment requires standing to use exercise and position change to ensure adequate uteroplacental perfusion.

and resultant demand are not as great as in later pregnancy. The increased oxygen demand caused by maternal changes in respiration and cardiac activity also does not occur until the major output changes have occurred.

Several other changes contribute little to the physiologic explanations of increased output. Increase in circulating blood volume does not significantly influence the output since filling pressures in the heart are not elevated. Increased blood uterine blood flow does not parallel the changes in output (Blackburn and Loper, 1992). Studies on the effect of estrogen on the actomyosin-adenosine triphosphatase action in the myocardium suggest that increased contractility may alter the stroke volume. However, further research is needed to assess the actual effect of this hormonal influence.

The increased cardiac output in pregnancy leads to increased flow in several specific organ systems. Obviously the uterine blood flow increases throughout pregnancy to meet the maternal needs of increased muscle mass and the fetal-placental needs of circulation. It is estimated that the uterus receives 10% to 20% of the total maternal cardiac output. The uteroplacental unit is a low-resistance vascular bed that is widely dilated and not capable of autoregulation. Therefore increased demands for oxygen by either the maternal uterine muscle or the fetus are met through increased extraction of oxygen from the blood rather than increased uterine blood flow.

Renal blood flow (RBF) increases in pregnancy to a peak of about 30% over prepregnant flow. Renal flow is altered by maternal position, with decreased flow noted at term when the woman is supine. This is probably caused by compression of the major vessels by the gravid uterus. Concurrent with the increased renal flow is an increase of the glomerular filtration rate (GFR) of 50% over prepregnant rates.

Skin perfusion increases in pregnancy with vasodilation that may be instrumental in dissipating excessive heat generated by fetal metabolism. Increased peripheral blood flow is also associated with the increased vascularity and hyperemia noted in the mucous membranes that contributes to the nasal congestion common during pregnancy.

Heart rate. Heart rate in women of childbearing age ranges from 60 to 200 beats/min. This wide variation is necessary to meet demands from rest to maximal exercise activities. Heart rate changes to maintain blood pressure when changes in vascular resistance and stroke volume occur. Both heart rate and venous return are increased in pregnancy, thus contributing to the need for increased output.

Maternal heart rate increases an average of 15 to 20 beats/min as pregnancy progresses. The early increase in rate (as early as 4 weeks' gestation) is most likely due to hormonal influence on the sinus node and myometrium (Clapp, 1985). Recent research suggests that maternal heart rate variability decreases as pregnancy progresses (Stein et al., 1999). Increased rate increases the myocardial oxygen demand, a demand that is easily met by women without preexisting cardiac disease.

Stroke volume. Stroke volume increases in pregnancy to a level approximately 30% above nonpregnant levels by midsecond trimester. Although earlier studies suggested that stroke volume fell in the last trimester, Mabie and associates (1994) found that stroke volume continued to increase until 36 to 39 weeks' gestation.

Heart size and position. As uterine growth displaces the diaphragm upward, the heart becomes displaced to the left and upward. Therefore the apex moves laterally from its prepregnant position. A resultant perceived increase in size of the heart is often noted during x-ray studies. Studies have also found that left ventricular wall mass and end-diastolic dimensions are increased in pregnancy, although the increased ventricular dimensions are not significant enough to alter output (Mabie et al., 1994). There is some evidence that healthy pregnant women have a small degree of pericardial effusion that may increase the apparent cardiac size on x-ray film. Because of these changes, the diagnosis of cardiomegaly must be made with extreme caution.

Normal anatomic and physiologic changes in pregnancy may alter some cardiac sounds. Over 90% of pregnant women develop a systolic ejection murmur secondary to the increased cardiac blood flow. It is usually heard by 12 weeks' gestation along the left sternal border in the third intercostal space. These common murmurs usually disappear by the eighth postpartum day. A soft, transient diastolic murmur may be heard in 20% of pregnant women. These murmurs are most likely due to the increased blood flow through the tricuspid or mitral valves or to the physiologic dilation of the pulmonary artery (Blackburn and Loper, 1992). Approximately 10% to 14% of pregnant women demonstrate continuous murmurs most likely due to breast vasculature (mammary souffle). Occasionally the mammary souffle can only be heard during diastole and may be misinterpreted as a diastolic murmur.

Pregnancy may also be associated with splitting of the first heart sound in 88% of women. This sound is most easily heard at the left sternal border between the third and fifth intercostal spaces. This change is most likely due to earlier closure of the mitral valve. During the third trimester a split caused by the increased interval between the aortic and pulmonary closure may be noted, most likely because of the reduced diaphragmatic movement. Some pregnant women develop a loud, easily heard third sound (Cutforth and MacDonald, 1966).

Vascular Changes

Blood pressure. Even with the well-documented increases in cardiac output and blood volume, there is no appreciable increase in either arterial or venous blood pressures in healthy pregnancy. Typically blood pressure remains at the woman's nonpregnant norm during the first trimester, then decreases in the second trimester. Blood pressures reach the lowest level in the late second trimester, with a return to the woman's baseline by term. The diastolic pressure decreases an average of 20 to 25 mm Hg, whereas the systolic decreases about 10 to 15 mm Hg. Mean arterial pressure ([systolic BP + diastolic BP × 2]/3) is lowest during the second trimester. Changes in blood pressure are primarily caused by the hormonal influence on peripheral resistance.

Both age and parity have been shown to have an effect on blood pressure. As parity increases, both systolic and diastolic blood pressures decrease, with the greatest difference being noted between nulliparas and primiparas. This effect has been noted even with correction for the influence of increasing age. Maternal age greater than 35 years is associated with no decrease in systolic blood pressure and increase in diastolic pressure.

Research has suggested no change in antecubital venous blood pressure during pregnancy. However, venous pressure below the uterus may be increased as a result of pressure of the gravid uterus and pooling when the woman is in an upright position.

Blood pressure is controlled by the renin-angiotensin-aldosterone system, which is altered in pregnancy. In normotensive pregnant women plasma renin, renin activity, renin substrate, angiotensin II, and aldosterone increase. Research has suggested that prostaglandins probably mediate the effect of angiotensin II on the vessel musculature.

Systemic vascular resistance. Systolic vascular resistance (mean arterial pressure divided by cardiac output) is decreased in pregnancy. The uteroplacental circulation, which serves as a low-resistance receptor of much of the increased flow, accounts for most of the change. The remainder of the change can be accounted for by the hormonal effect of estrogen and progesterone on the vessel walls, as well as increased body temperature, which contributes to vasodilation.

ADAPTATIONS IN THE HEMATOLOGIC SYSTEM

The maternal hematologic system undergoes significant changes to ensure adequate perfusion of the increased vascular space, protect the maternal-fetal unit from postural effects on blood pressure and flow, and protect against the effect of blood loss during delivery.

Blood Volume

Plasma changes. Circulating blood volume increases 30% to 50% in pregnancy, with an average of 1.5 L increase. Blood volume changes begin at approximately 6 weeks' gestation and peak at 30 to 34 weeks. Plasma volume increases an average of 50%, with the increase beginning at about 6 weeks. A further rate of increase is noted in the second trimester. The plasma levels plateau at 32 to 34 weeks' gestation. The relatively faster increase in the plasma, compared to the solid blood components, leads to a normal physiologic hemodilution that is most apparent at 28 to 30 weeks' gestation.

The etiology of plasma expansion in pregnancy is poorly understood. The hormonal effects of estrogen and progesterone on plasma renin activity and aldosterone probably result in retention of sodium, with a resultant retention of water. The vasodilation effect of progesterone increases the capacity of the veins to accommodate the increased volume. Deviation in the normal increase in plasma volume is associated with complications in pregnancy. Decreased plasma expansion is associated with pregnancy-induced hypertension (PIH), intrauterine growth retardation, and fetal demise. Increase in plasma expansion beyond the expected levels is associated with multiparity, maternal obesity, fetal macrosomia, prolonged pregnancy, and multiple gestation.

The hypervolemia of pregnancy leads to a dilution of plasma proteins and blood cellular components. This leads to an approximate 20% decrease in viscosity, which results in decreased flow resistance.

Changes in red blood cells. Total red blood cell (RBC) volume increases in pregnancy by about 33% (450 ml) in women who have iron supplementation, and 18% (250 ml) in women who do not take iron supplements. Increased circulating erythropoietin and increased RBC production account for the increase. Erythropoietin levels begin to rise at the end of the first trimester, following the initiation of plasma changes. The mean age for maternal RBCs is lower in the latter part of pregnancy, reflecting the fact that RBC produc-

Table 6-1 *CDC/IOM Cutoff Values for Anemia in Women*

	Hemoglobin (g/dl)	Hematocrit (%)
Nonpregnant	12.0	36
Pregnant		
First trimester	11.0	33
Second trimester	10.5	32
Third trimester	11.0	33

Adapted from *Nutrition during pregnancy and lactation: an implementation guide*, National Academy Press, Washington, DC, 1992.

tion exceeds destruction. The increased production is also reflected in the increased reticulocyte count found in pregnancy.

Mean cell volume, diameter, and thickness of the RBC change, leading to a more spheric appearance of the cell. Hemoglobin and hematocrit decrease through the second trimester as a result of the plasma volume expansion (Table 6-1). Total hemoglobin increases from 85 to 150 g in pregnancy, but net hemoglobin decreases secondary to hemodilution (Research Box 6-3).

Changes in other blood components. White blood cell (WBC) mass increases slightly early in pregnancy, then levels off during the second and third trimesters. This increase is a result of increased neutrophil production. Total WBC count ranges from 5,000 to 12,000/mm^3 and may increase to 20,000/mm^3 in labor without infection. Changes in the WBCs are similar to those seen with other physiologic stress such as exercise.

There are conflicting reports on platelet changes in pregnancy. Recent research suggests that there is a slight decrease in platelets in the last 2 months of pregnancy. The usual range for platelet counts in pregnancy is 150,000 to 400,000/mm^3. Platelet counts below 100,000/mm^3 are considered abnormal.

Total plasma proteins decrease 10% to 14%, with the decrease mainly occurring in the first trimester. Absolute values of albumin increase in pregnancy, but because of hemodilution there is a decrease in albumin concentration, leading to a net decrease in colloid osmotic pressure.

Globulin levels increase in pregnancy (>2.3 to 3.5 g/dl). Fibrinogen increases 50% to 80%, from a nonpregnant average of 300 mg/dl to an average of 450 mg/dl in late pregnancy. The erythrocyte sedimentation rate (ESR) increases during pregnancy (>20 mm/hr), most likely because of the increased globulin and fibrinogen levels. Alterations in plasma proteins influence the binding powers of calcium and some pharmacologic agents. If drugs are transported by albumin, dosages may need to be adjusted in pregnancy.

Changes in coagulation factors. Changes in coagulation factors increase the risk for thrombosis and consumptive coagulopathies. Data suggest that there is an ongoing activation of the coagulation system within the uteroplacental system from about 11 weeks' gestation. Intravascular and extravascular fibrin is found in the uteroplacental circulation, intervillous spaces, and placental bed (Blackburn and Loper, 1992).

Many factors involved in the clotting cascade are increased in pregnancy. The contact factors associated with the initiation of coagulation are increased (factor XII, prekallikrein, kininogen). Factors I (fibrinogen), VII (proconvertin), VIII (antihemophilic globulin), IX (Christmas factor), and X (Stuart factor) are elevated; factor II (prothrombin) may either be elevated or stable. Factors XI (plasma thromboplastin antecedent) and XIII (fibrin-stabilizing factor) are decreased. These changes in the clotting factors lead to a slight decrease in the partial thromboplastin time and the prothrombin time.

There is evidence that some of the changes in coagulation factors lead to a chronic low-grade intravascular coagulation. Maternal plasminogen (profibrinolysin) increases, probably in response to estrogen activity. Fibrinolytic activity increases until the third trimester, when it decreases until term. The hypercoagulable state of pregnancy is balanced by plasminogen, which is elevated. Tissue plasma inhibitors are decreased, thus maintaining an equilibrium between clotting and clot lysis.

ADAPTATIONS IN THE RESPIRATORY SYSTEM

The respiratory system incurs significant alterations both anatomically and physiologically to meet the increasing oxygen demands of the mother and fetus.

Anatomic and Mechanical Changes

The diaphragm rises about 4 cm by late pregnancy, probably as a result of the pressure of the growing uterus in the abdomen. Softening of the cartilage in the thoracic cage, as well as in the musculature, enhances the widen-

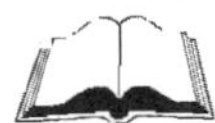

Research Box 6-3

Mashburn J, Graves B, Gillmor-Kahn M: Hematocrit values during pregnancy in a nurse-midwifery caseload, *J Nurse Midwifery* 37(6):404-410, 1992.

Background

Anemia is the most common complication of pregnancy, and it has been estimated that its incidence is 30% of the pregnant population in industrialized countries. The Centers for Disease Control and Prevention (CDC) recommends the following hemoglobin levels for diagnosing anemia in pregnancy: 1st trimester—<11; 2nd trimester—<10.5; third trimester—<11.4. These levels were determined from data pooled primarily from white European women who were supplemented with iron during their pregnancies.

Research Question

What is the range of hematocrit levels of nurse-midwifery patients who are primarily from a black, indigent, inner-city population in the southeast United States?

Methods

Charts were reviewed retrospectively for 111 women who delivered in October 1989, January 1990, and June 1990. Documented hematocrits and the gestational age at the time of the laboratory study were recorded, with an average of 3.5 values per subject. Means and standard deviations of the hematocrits were calculated and compared to the pooled, 4-week interval hemoglobins (converted to hematocrits) as described by the CDC. Further analysis was done among groups in the sample.

Sample

All patients who delivered in the Nurse-Midwifery Service during the above-noted months were included in the chart audit. This yielded 111 subjects with a mean age of 21.9 years. Fifty-nine percent had experienced at least one previous birth, and 86% were black. All women were supplemented with prenatal vitamins containing 60 mg of elemental iron, and women with hematocrits <35% were supplemented with ferrous sulfate, 300 mg TID. Compliance with vitamin and mineral supplementation was not determined.

Results

Sample mean hematocrits did not differ significantly from the CDC 50th percentile until the 21 to 24 week interval. After that gestational age, all sample means were lower than the CDC 50th percentiles. By 36 to 40 weeks' gestation, the sample means were more similar to the CDC fifth percentile values.

Clinical Application

The data suggest that black indigent women enter pregnancy with depleted iron stores that increases the risk for more severe anemia as the pregnancy progresses. Although racial difference in normal hematocrits may account for some of the difference, it would not account for the pattern of hematocrits falling lower in midpregnancy and failing to return to prepregnant values by the end of gestation.

Clinicians need to consider their patients' probable iron stores when considering whether to recommend iron supplementation. When risk factors include poor nutrition, low income, closely spaced pregnancies, and other factors that increase the risk of iron deficiency anemia, iron supplementation may be indicated from the beginning of pregnancy, even when initial hematocrits are in the normal range.

ing of the subcostal angle and flaring of the lower ribs. This results in an increase in the transverse diameter of the thorax of an average of 2 cm. The circumference of the thorax increases about 6 cm. The changes in the bony thorax cannot be attributed to the enlarging uterus, since the flaring occurs before any increase in abdominal pressure on the diaphragm.

The respiratory rate does not change in pregnancy, but the tidal volume, minute ventilatory volume (tidal volume × respiratory rate), and minute oxygen uptake increase as pregnancy progresses. The tidal volume increases 25% to 40%, with a resultant decrease in expiratory reserve volume, residual volume, and functional residual capacity. The maximum breathing capacity (vital capacity) is not changed. The elevation of the diaphragm and the changes in the bony thorax are the major influences on the altered volumes. Total pulmonary resistance may be reduced up to 50%, possibly a result of the effect of progesterone. Progesterone most likely promotes relaxation of the bronchiole smooth muscle, further decreasing resistance.

Increased tidal volume, along with the hormonal effect of progesterone, leads to a decrease in blood CO_2. Data suggest an increased sensitivity to CO_2, along with a decreased CO_2 threshold in the respiratory center of the brain, leads to a feeling of shortness of breath or the maternal perception of an increased need for a deep breath (the "sigh of pregnancy"). Researchers have also suggested that progesterone directly stimulates a local effect on the lung, causing water retention that results in decreased diffusion capacity. Hyperventilation then becomes a means for maintaining normal Po_2 levels.

Changes in Acid-Base Balance

The effect of progesterone on the respiratory system is thought to contribute to a compensatory respiratory alkalosis. This respiratory alkalosis may facilitate CO_2 transfer from the fetus to the maternal system by increasing the arterial CO_2 pressure ($PaCO_2$) gradient.

ADAPTATIONS IN THE URINARY SYSTEM

The renal system is responsible for regulation of fluid and electrolyte balance, control of arterial blood pressure, excretion of metabolic wastes, regulation of vitamin D activity, and erythrocyte production and gluconeogenesis (Blackburn and Loper, 1992). Pregnancy adaptations include sodium retention and increased extracellular fluid volume. Renal system adaptations are necessary to maintain homeostasis in the presence of increased intravascular and extravascular volumes, excrete increased metabolic waste products, and interact with the cardiovascular changes to meet maternal and fetal oxygen demands. Understanding of the blood volume changes, total body water changes, and renal clearance changes is essential as clinicians are faced with clinical decision making regarding pharmacologic interventions during pregnancy and the immediate postpartum period.

Renal System Structure Changes

Kidney. The kidney increases in length by about 1 to 2 cm, most likely in response to increased RBF and vascular volume (Blackburn and Loper, 1992). Dilation of the renal calyces and pelvis begins in the first trimester and becomes more pronounced in the second half of pregnancy. Hydronephrosis occurs in 80% to 90% of women (Beydon, 1985), probably in response to the effects of progesterone and the increased intraureteral pressure superior to the pelvic rim. The hydronephrosis is more commonly seen in the right kidney, most likely reflecting the increase in right ureteral distention described below.

Ureters. The ureters elongate and develop single and double curves that may appear like kinking on x-ray. Once the uterus becomes an abdominal organ, its increasing mass compresses the ureters at the pelvic brim. This compression leads to increased intraureteral tone above the level of the pelvis. The lumen of the ureters increases in diameter, and hypertonicity and hypomotility have been reported . Because of these changes, the volume of the ureters may increase 25 times that found in the nonpregnant state, which corresponds to an increase in volume to 300 ml of urine. The change in length begins early in pregnancy, with hypertrophy of the longitudinal smooth muscles in the distal parts of the ureters. Since this effect may also be seen in women taking oral contraceptives and hormonal replacement therapy, it is most likely hormonally induced by progesterone and estrogen. The right ureter is dilated more than the left in up to 86% of women (Schulman and Herlinger, 1975). This occurs because the right ureter crosses the right ovarian vein rather than running parallel as it does on the left. In addition, the right iliac vein is more rigid on the right than on the left, providing greater compression as the right ureter crosses it.

Bladder. Bladder tone decreases in response to the smooth muscle effect of progesterone. Bladder capacity increases to about 1 L. As the uterus enlarges during the second half of pregnancy, the bladder becomes displaced anteriorly and superiorly. Displacement alters the intravesicular insertion of the ureters, which may lead to urine regurgitation into the ureters during urination (Beydon, 1985). The mucosa lining the bladder becomes hyperemic and edematous, increasing the risk of trauma during labor and birth.

Changes in Hemodynamics

RBF increases 35% to 60% during the first trimester, then decreases from second trimester until delivery. However, this finding is most likely influenced by the supine position used in the studies, a position that decreases blood flow to the kidneys. Increased cardiac output and blood volume and decreased vascular resistance and vasodilation of preglomerular and postglomerular capillaries contribute to RBF changes early in pregnancy.

The GFR increases 40% to 50% in pregnancy, with the increase beginning shortly after conception and peaking at 9 to 16 weeks. The early second trimester level is maintained until term. Increased glomerular blood flow and decreased colloid osmotic pressure contribute to the increased GFR (Blackburn and Loper, 1992).

The increased RBF and GFR results in an increase in the proportion of RBF that is filtered. This results in increased excretion of amino acids, glucose, protein, electrolytes, and vitamins, which leads to a decrease in plasma values of creatinine, urea, blood urea nitrogen, and uric acid levels. Increased GFR may also increase excretion of drugs and alter plasma drug levels.

Increased GFR increases the volume and solutes of the tubules by 50% to 100%. Increased tubular resorption is necessary to prevent depletion of sodium, chloride, glucose, potassium, and water. At times, tubular resorption cannot meet the demands of the increased filtered load, and excretion of glucose and amino acids may occur. Renal glucose excretion remains high throughout pregnancy, resulting in glycosuria, and urinary glucose values may be up to ten times that found in the nonpregnant state (Davison, 1987).

Protein excretion increases from less than 150 mg/24 hr to as much as 300 mg/24 hr (Davison, 1987). There can be significant variation from day to day. Because of this increase in excretion, values of 1+ protein on urine dipsticks are common and should not be interpreted in isolation from other physiologic changes to mean renal disease or pregnancy-induced hypertension.

Uric acid filtration increases up to 30% in the first trimester of pregnancy. With a net decrease in resorption, uric acid excretion is increased, and serum levels are decreased up to 25% as early as 8 weeks' gestation. Levels increase toward nonpregnant levels by the end of pregnancy as tubular resorption increases.

Potassium retention increases as a result of decreased excretion, yet it is rapidly used by maternal and fetal sources, since serum potassium does not increase. This retention is not clearly understood, but it may be influenced by the antagonistic effect of progesterone on renal tubular actions on aldosterone.

ADAPTATIONS IN THE GASTROINTESTINAL SYSTEM

Pregnant women report changes in appetite, amount and type of food consumed, and tolerance of certain foods. Although such changes may be influenced by sociocultural factors, anatomic and hormonal influences on the gastrointestinal tract alter the usual functioning of the gastrointestinal system.

Mouth

Many women report changes in taste soon after conception. This may be a result of hormonal influences on the saliva, as well as a change in olfactory sense. Saliva becomes more acidic in pregnancy. Although early studies suggested an increase in production of saliva, others suggest that there is only a perceived increase secondary to the decrease in swallowing efforts during the period of nausea and vomiting. A few women do have documented ptyalism (excess salivation) that occurs primarily during the day and ends with delivery.

Under the influence of estrogen, the gums become more vascular, hyperplastic, and edematous. Decreased thickness of the gingival epithelial surface contributes to the frequent friable gum diseases seen during pregnancy. Bleeding may occur with chewing or brushing, and the friable surfaces predispose the gums to gingivitis. It is estimated that 50% to 77% of women experience gingivitis during pregnancy. Incidence is higher with preexisting dental problems, increasing maternal age, and increasing parity. In less than 2% of pregnant women, the hyperplasia of the gums leads to the formation of a friable, tumorlike mass called epulis. Epulis usually regresses spontaneously after delivery, but it may need to be excised during pregnancy if excess bleeding or increased periodontal disease develops.

Esophagus

Increased progesterone levels lead to a decrease in tone of the lower esophageal sphincter. This decrease in tone is associated with an increased incidence of acid reflux from the stomach into the esophagus. The changes in the diaphragm further contribute to the problem by changing the usual acute esophageal-gastric angle, thereby enhancing reflux.

Stomach

Progesterone decreases the tone and motility of the stomach. In addition, it may decrease the tone of the pyloric sphincter, leading to reflux of alkaline duodenal contents into the stomach. As pregnancy progresses, pressure on the stomach by the enlarging uterus may decrease the amount of food that can be consumed without discomfort. Reduction in acid and pepsin production may also slow digestion, although the effect of pregnancy on gastric acid secretion is not well understood.

Small and Large Intestines

The smooth muscle relaxation caused by progesterone decreases intestinal tone and motility. Decreased motility may further be influenced by decreased levels of motilin, a hormonal peptide. The decrease in tone leads to delayed transit time, which becomes more prolonged as pregnancy progresses. Studies have suggested that prolonged transit time in late pregnancy is caused by an inhibition of smooth bowel contractions (Lawson, Kern, and Everson, 1985). Delayed transit time, in conjunction with hypertrophy of the duodenal villi, leads to increased absorption capacity. Increased absorption of iron, calcium, lysine, valine, glycine, proline, glucose, sodium, chloride, and water has been demonstrated (Blackburn and Loper, 1992). The influence of progesterone on enzyme transport may contribute to decreased absorption of niacin, riboflavin, and vitamin B_6.

Reduced motility and prolonged transit time in the colon lead to increased absorption of water, with a resulting increased risk for constipation. Increased flatulence has also been documented. As the uterus grows, the appendix and cecum are displaced superiorly and laterally. This anatomic alteration is important to keep in mind when a woman presents with acute abdominal pain and appendicitis is one of the differential diagnoses.

Hemorrhoids are common in pregnancy. They are caused by the vessel wall relaxation secondary to the influence of progesterone, and pressure of the veins by the size and weight of the gravid uterus. Bearing down efforts when constipation is present also contribute to the development of hemorrhoids.

Liver and Gallbladder

Increased estrogen and progesterone levels modify the metabolism and excretion of bilirubin in pregnancy. Increased alkaline phosphatase and lipids tend to mimic symptoms associated with liver disease. Spider angiomata and pruritus are common complaints during pregnancy. Studies suggest an increase in size and decrease in motility in the gallbladder and bile duct. The increase in volume dilutes the bile and decreases its solubility of cholesterol. Cholesterol can then precipitate and form stones and crystals.

ADAPTATIONS IN THE ENDOCRINE SYSTEM

Thyroid

Enlargement of the thyroid gland in pregnancy has long been recognized, and recent research suggests that most women experience an 18% increase in thyroid volume. In addition, investigators found that one fourth of subjects experienced greater than 25% increase in size. This is a result of hypertrophy of the glandular tissue and increased vascularity. Thyroxine (T_4) levels increase in maternal serum beginning in the second month of gestation. Levels plateau at 9 to 16 μg/dl compared to nonpregnant levels of 5 to 12 μg/dl. It is thought that estrogen is influential in increasing the hepatic synthesis of T_4-binding proteins, resulting in a binding capacity that handles the increased levels of T_4. Changes in levels of unbound thyroid hormones remain controversial, with some studies reporting no change, some reporting a decrease, and some reporting an increase. Glinoer and associates (1990) argue that there is a decrease in free triiodothyronine and T_4 in pregnancy when compared to nonpregnant levels, most likely caused by the increase in thyroid-binding proteins (Research Box 6-4).

Thyroid-releasing hormone, which stimulates synthesis and release of thyroid-stimulating hormone (TSH), is not increased in pregnancy. TSH levels may increase slightly in pregnancy, but they remain in the reference range for nonpregnant women. Data suggest that, because human chorionic gonadotropin (hCG) possesses an intrinsic TSH-like activity, it directly stimulates the thyroid to secrete T_4. Indeed, there may a decrease in TSH at the time of peak hCG levels at the end of first trimester, and there is a linear relationship between hCG and free T_4 concentrations in maternal serum.

Parathyroid

Data suggest that there is an increase in parathyroid hormone (PTH), most likely as a result of hyperplasia. It is possible that the glandular change is caused by estrogen and human placental lactogen. PTH levels rise progressively during pregnancy so that levels at term are approximately 30% to 50% above nonpregnant levels.

Adrenal Glands

There is an increase in circulating cortisol during pregnancy, with much of it bound by cortisol-binding globulin. The increased level is most likely a result of de-

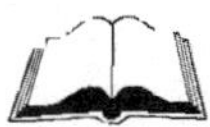

Research Box 6-4

Glinoer D et al: Regulation of maternal thyroid during pregnancy, *J Clin Endocrinol Metabol* 71:276-280, 1990.

Background

Although alterations in thyroid function have been well documented, changes in the levels of free triiodothyronine (T_3), thyroxine (T_4), and thyroid-stimulating hormone (TSH) and the potential role of thyroid stimulators of placental origin are not well understood.

Research Questions

What are the thyroid changes that occur as a result of (1) increased thyroid hormone-binding capacity of serum caused by the increase in thyroid-binding globulin levels; (2) effects of increased human chorionic gonadotropin (hCG) levels on serum TSH; and (3) a marginally low iodine intake?

Methods

Seven hundred and thirty-two consecutive pregnant women were enrolled in the study in 1988. A detailed history of thyroid-related past events was recorded, the thyroid gland was palpated, and the following laboratory studies were done: total and free T_4 and T_3, T_4-binding globulin, serum thyroglobulin, TSH, random urine iodine concentration, thyroid autoantibodies, hCG, and thyroid volume. Patients with identified thyroid problems were then excluded. Second blood laboratory studies were done at 30 to 33 weeks' gestation and 1 to 4 days postpartum. Thyroid ultrasonography was performed during pregnancy and postpartum to determine thyroid volume. Mean values per trimester were calculated, and appropriate statistical analyses were used.

Sample

Mean age of the participants was 28 years, and mean gestational age at enrollment was 17 weeks. Twenty-nine percent of the cohort were primigravidae. The study was conducted in Brussels, Belgium, which suggests that most study participants were white and of European descent.

Results

Data suggest that pregnancy is associated with a decrease in free T_4 and T_3 by about 30% in late pregnancy. There was no correlation between urinary iodine and alterations in thyroid function. There was a decrease in TSH early in pregnancy that corresponds to peak hCG levels, and there was a linear relationship between hCG and free T_4 concentrations. Thyroid size (volume) increased significantly by an average of 20%.

Clinical Application

Findings suggest that clinicians should consider recommending increased iodine intake to meet the demands of increased thyroid activity in pregnancy when patients live in areas with known low intake of iodine.

creased metabolic clearance of cortisol, since there is no apparent increase in cortisol secretion by the maternal adrenals. Levels of adrenocorticotropic hormone are decreased in early pregnancy, whereas levels of free cortisol are increased. This mechanism is poorly understood.

By the fourth month of gestation, the maternal adrenals secrete increased amounts of aldosterone. Aldosterone secretion is increased even more in the face of restriction of sodium intake. Increased production of aldosterone is influenced by the increased levels of angiotensin II, which stimulates the zona glomerulosa of the adrenal to secrete aldosterone. It has been suggested that this mechanism provides a balance to the natriuretic influence of progesterone.

References

Beydon SN: Morphologic changes in the renal tract in pregnancy, *Clin Obstet Gynecol* 28(2):249-256, 1985.

Blackburn ST, Loper DL: *Maternal, fetal and neonatal physiology,* Philadelphia, 1992, WB Saunders.

Capeless EL, Clapp JF: Cardiovascular changes in early phase of pregnancy, *Am J Obstet Gynecol* 161(6 part 1):1449-1453, 1989.

Clapp JF: Maternal heart rate in pregnancy, *Am J Obstet Gynecol* 159:1456-1460, 1985.

Cunningham FG et al: *Williams obstetrics,* ed 20, Stamford, Conn, 1997, Appleton & Lange.

Cutforth R, MacDonald CB: Heart sounds and murmurs in pregnancy, *Am Heart J* 71(6):741-747, 1966.

Davison JM: Overview: kidney function, *Am J Kidney Dis* 9:248-252, 1987.

Fuchs A-R, Fuchs F: Physiology and endocrinology of parturition. In Gabbe SG, Niebyl JR, Simpson JL, editors, *Obstetrics: normal and problem pregnancies,* ed 3, New York, 1996, Churchill Livingstone.

Fuchs A-R, Ivell R., Friedman S: Oxytocin and the timing of parturition: influence of oxytocin receptor gene expression and stimulation of prostaglandin release. In Ivell R, Russell J, editors: *Oxytocin: molecular and cellular approaches in medicine and research,* London, 1995, Plenum.

Gabbe SG, Niebyl JR, Simpson JL: *Obstetrics: normal and problem pregnancies,* ed 3, New York, 1996, Churchill Livingstone.

Glinoer D et al: Regulation of maternal thyroid during pregnancy, *J Clin Endocrinol Metabol* 71(2):276-287, 1990.

Lawson M, Kern FJ, Everson GT: Gastrointestinal transit time in human pregnancy: prolongation in the second and third trimesters followed by postpartum normalization, *Gastroenterology* 89(5):996-999, 1985.

Mabie WC et al: A longitudinal study of cardiac output in normal human pregnancy, *Am J Obstet Gynecol* 170(3):849-856, 1994.

Ramsey EM: Anatomy of the human uterus. In Chard T, Grudzinskas JD, editors: *The uterus,* Cambridge, 1994, Cambridge University Press.

Riedewald S et al: Vaginal and cervical pH in normal pregnancies and pregnancy complicated by preterm labor, *J Perinatal Med* 18(3):181-186, 1990.

Robson SC et al: Serial study of factors influencing changes in cardiac output during human pregnancy, *Am J Physiol* 256:1060-1065, 1989.

Schulman A, Herlinger H: Urinary tract dilatation in pregnancy, *Radiology* 48:638-641, 1975.

Stein PK et al: Changes in 24-hour heart rate variability during normal pregnancy, *Am J Obstet Gynecol* 180(4):978-985, 1999.

Thaler I. et al: Changes in uterine blood flow during human pregnancy, *Am J Obstet Gynecol* 162(1):121-125, 1990.

Valenzuela G J, Germain A, Foster TC-S: Physiology of uterine activity in pregnancy, *Curr Opin Obstet Gynecol* 5:640-646, 1993.

Zahn V: Uterine contractions during pregnancy, *J Perinatal Med* 12:107-111, 1984.

Chapter 7

Diagnosis and Dating of Pregnancy

Midwives and other clinicians working in community-based practices and providing care to women of childbearing age are always faced with consideration of pregnancy as a diagnosis. In an ideal world all women would receive comprehensive preconception care that enhances health status before a planned pregnancy. Unfortunately, our world is far from ideal, and clinicians regularly see women who face unplanned although often wanted pregnancies. A caring clinician will provide an environment that fosters the client's perception that she is an active participant in the examination, and that validates the woman's own feelings and beliefs about her pregnancy. A clinic milieu that limits provider time with the client and values the "efficiency" of technology over the importance of establishment of a strong professional relationship with the client is not consistent with the midwifery philosophy of care.

Essentially all women presenting for prenatal examinations have made the determination that they are pregnant. This assumption may be made by the woman's knowledge of her body and her own cycles or by a positive pregnancy test finding using a home test or a test done in any one of a variety of community clinical sites. One of the primary goals of the initial prenatal examination is the accurate diagnosis and dating of pregnancy, with the client and provider working together toward that goal.

Data necessary for accurate diagnosis and dating of pregnancy are gathered through history taking and physical examination. Biochemical tests and special studies such as ultrasound examination provide additional data that may be essential in accurately dating the pregnancy. Accurate dating of pregnancy reduces the use of unnecessary interventions, including screening, diagnostic, and medical management measures (e.g., induction of labor). Improved dating of pregnancy also reduces infant morbidity and mortality by more accurately identifying the fetus at risk for poor outcomes (Nichols, 1987).

Signs and symptoms of pregnancy are commonly categorized as presumptive, probable, and positive. Presumptive symptoms have traditionally been considered "subjective symptoms observed by the patient herself" (Van Blarcom, 1937, p.100). Early medical texts describe symptoms as those indications of pregnancy that a woman experiences before the physician can diagnose the pregnancy with certainty. Because of their subjective nature, they are often less validated by physicians, particularly in medical cultures that rely primarily on biotechnologic findings. Presumptive signs are characteristics that can be observed by others but that can be commonly found in other conditions. Probable signs of pregnancy are physical characteristics that can be seen or otherwise quantified by the examiner and that are more specific to the physiologic changes caused by the pregnancy. Both symptoms and signs of pregnancy may be found in other conditions; thus they cannot be considered positive indicators of pregnancy. Positive signs of pregnancy are those findings clearly identify the fetus and that cannot be explained by any other health condition.

PRESUMPTIVE INDICATORS OF PREGNANCY

Presumptive Symptoms

Cessation of menses. In healthy, sexually active women who have regular menstrual cycles, the missed period is highly suggestive of pregnancy. Cessation of menses is not a good predictor of pregnancy in women with irregular cycles, in women who are lactating and have not resumed normal cycles, or in young women who conceive before menarche.

Since the first day of the last menstrual period (LMP) in a woman with regular cycles is one of the most reliable clinical estimators for gestational age (Johnson, Walker, and Niebyl, 1996), it is incumbent on the midwife to gather an accurate menstrual history. Research has suggested that 14% to 58% of women have uncertain LMPs (Andersen et al., 1981), but these estimates are limited by the fact that the sample populations may not represent the true characteristics of the childbearing population (convenience samples in teaching institutions) and that the clinicians gathering the data were primarily male physicians. Since research suggests that midwives and nurse practitioners are particularly strong in establishing relationships with their clients, it is possible that these providers may be better able to identify a known or approximate LMP in a higher proportion of clients.

Many women, particularly if they kept menstrual calendars or planned the pregnancy, are extremely accurate in noting their LMP. If a menstrual calendar has not been kept, the clinician can assist the woman in remembering the LMP by using a calendar and "probes" to link the LMP with other life occurrences. With probing, women often remember that the LMP fell around a holiday or other special event. Women may also be more open to discussing menstrual history with a female provider, especially if cultural beliefs influence specific gender roles surrounding sexuality.

Along with establishing LMP, it is helpful to establish last normal menstrual period. Menstrual data should include the woman's perception of whether the last bleeding was typical of her cycle (lighter, normal, or heavier flow), whether the duration was normal, and whether it occurred at the expected time of menses. Establishing previous menstrual period gives further information about the pattern or cycle of menses. A report of a light period may actually be a report of implantation bleeding or other nonmenstrual bleeding unrelated to the LMP.

Since cessation can be caused by many other conditions, cessation of menses must be considered in the context of other health-related factors. The most common cause of a "missed period" is an anovulatory cycle. Other conditions to consider when evaluating missed periods are severe illness, rapid weight loss, eating disorders, incorrect use of oral contraceptives, use of depo-medroxyprogesterone acetate for greater than 1 year, and menopause.

Estimating the Expected Day of Delivery Using Last Menstrual Period Pregnancy begins with the fertilization of the ovum. However, unless extensive biochemical and ultrasonic studies are being done during the menstrual cycle (e.g., with management of women who have a history of infertility), the exact day of fertilization is rarely known. Several methods can be used to estimate the gestational age and therefore the expected day of delivery (EDD). In light of the importance of accurately dating the pregnancy, it is interesting to note that few studies have investigated the accuracy of commonly used methods. Furthermore, few studies have investigated mean gestational age in current populations. The assumption that mean gestational age is 280 days from LMP has gone largely unchallenged, even with recent investigations that suggest that mean gestational age from LMP is 283 to 284 days (Merkatz and Thompson, 1990). Although a variance of a few days may seem to be insignificant, one must consider the impact of the use of technology on pregnancies that are misidentified as preterm or postterm.

Naegle's rule. The calculation of EDD based on this mathematical rule is remarkably accurate, in spite of the fact that Naegle's calculation was developed without sound evidence that the mean length of gestation is 280 days. Spontaneous delivery occurs in approximately 90% of pregnant women by the end of the 41st week as calculated by this method.

Naegle's rule is based on the following assumptions:

1. The average length of pregnancy is 266 days from conception, or 280 days from the last menstrual period
2. The average menstrual cycle is 28 days in length
3. Ovulation and fertilization occurs on day 14 of the menstrual cycle
4. The reported LMP was a true period and not bleeding from other causes

To estimate the EDD, the clinician subtracts 3 months from the LMP, then adds 1 year and 7 days to that date. For example, if a woman's LMP was December 7, 1999, one subtracts 3 months, giving a date of September 7, 1999. One then adds 1 year and 7 days, establishing an EDD of September 14, 2000. It is important to remember that this rule is based purely on a mathematical model and is not meant to correspond with particular landmarks in pregnancy such as fertilization or implantation.

When a woman has a history of regular cycles with an interval different than 28 days, adjustments should be made in calculating the EDD. Adjustments are usually made if the variation is 1 week or more from the average of 28 days. If a woman reports cycles of 35 days, 1 week is added to the EDD. If she reports 21-day cycles, 1 week is subtracted from the EDD.

Maternal perception of pregnancy. Some women report "knowing" they were pregnant at or shortly after conception. Women may experience feelings of ovulation and may be sensitive to the early pelvic and hormonal changes of pregnancy. Women who have experienced previous pregnancies may be especially sensitive to the hormonal influences on their bodies. For example, women who have experienced changes in smell that trigger feelings of nausea may notice those changes within several weeks of fertilization when exposed to common noxious smells such as coffee or cigarette smoke.

To date there has been no scholarly research exploring these symptoms of pregnancy. Future research using qualitative methods would contribute to this underexplored aspect of early pregnancy.

Breast changes. Breast tenderness or tingling similar to that experienced by some women premenstrually is caused by the hormonal changes in pregnancy. It may occur as early as 2 weeks following fertilization, leading to the perception that it is premenstrually induced.

Nausea and vomiting. Hormonal influence on the gastrointestinal system may lead to characteristic nausea and vomiting ("morning sickness") that appears around the fifth or sixth week of pregnancy and continues until about 14 weeks' gestation. Many women report a characteristic change in the olfactory sense, with specific odors triggering the nausea. It has been estimated that about half of pregnant women experience nausea or vomiting in pregnancy. Although the nausea and vomiting is most common in the morning, it can occur at any time throughout the day. It can occur with a variety of disorders, including but not limited to gastrointestinal viruses and stress.

Urinary frequency. Pressure on the bladder caused first by anteflexion of the anteriorly positioned uterus and later in the first trimester by the enlarging uterus leads to urinary frequency. This usually resolves when the uterus rises out of the pelvis at 12 weeks' gestation. Frequency may again become a problem late in third trimester with the pressure exerted on the bladder by the presenting part. Frequency can also be a symptom of infection.

Overwhelming fatigue. Overwhelming fatigue out of proportion to that usually experienced may be noted from about 6 weeks of pregnancy through the first trimester. Fatigue secondary to awakening because of discomfort or the need to urinate returns as a problem late in pregnancy. Sleep habits may be altered in periods of stress, lifestyle changes, or illnesses that interfere with comfort and relaxation.

Maternal perception of fetal movement. Perception of "fluttering" in the lower abdomen is usually noted by primigravidae between 18 and 20 weeks of pregnancy. Multipara may report movement as early as 16 weeks. This first perception of movement is often termed "quickening" and can be used along with other dating parameters to determine gestational age. Used with other dating parameters, evidence of 22 weeks of fetal movement supports the diagnosis of term pregnancy. Similar feelings in the gut may be produced by peristalsis or pockets of gas in the bowel.

Presumptive Signs

Increased basal body temperature. Increased basal body temperature that remains elevated for greater than 3 weeks is a presumptive sign of pregnancy. The temperature must be taken correctly and charted conscientiously. Other factors that may increase basal body temperature include infection or obtaining the temperature after rising and increasing activity.

Breast changes. In primigravidas increase in size and deepening of the coloration of the areola may be noticed by 6 to 8 weeks after the LMP. Fair-complexioned women experience color change to a deep rose color; dark complexioned women may note color change to deep brown or black. Changes in size and coloration are not as apparent in multiparas, since the changes do not regress after the birth. Later in the pregnancy women may notice leaking of colostrum. Similar changes can be present in women with prolactin-secreting pituitary lesions or with the ingestion of drugs that induce hyperprolactinemia.

Vaginal mucosa and vulvar changes. Vasocongestion of the vaginal mucosa causes a characteristic dark rose or bluish-red tint (Chadwick's sign). Occasionally the vulva will also become a darker color. These changes can occur in other conditions that lead to vasocongestion.

Cervical changes. Cervical softening along with vaginal tissue softening, often accompanied by increased leukorrheal discharge, may be present (Goodell's sign).

Skin changes. Increased pigmentation across the face ("mask of pregnancy") is termed melasma or chloasma. Pigmentation in a line running down the center of the abdomen is termed *linea negra* and is more pronounced in women with dark complexions. It is most dramatic in primigravidae since, once the changes have occurred, the pigmentation may fade but never goes away totally. Pigmentation changes may occur with use of medications such as oral contraceptives and in certain illnesses. Striae across the abdomen may become evident but are present in other conditions that cause stretching of the skin (e.g., weight gain).

Probable Indicators of Pregnancy

Uterine changes. The uterus undergoes distinct changes in size, shape, and consistency early in pregnancy. From about 6 weeks after the last menstrual period until 12 weeks' gestation, the uterus changes from a firm pear-shaped organ to a softer, globular shape. Several changes have been described in the literature.

Softening of the uterine isthmus (Hegar's sign). Approximately 6 to 8 weeks after the last period the examiner can determine this change during the bimanual examination. With two fingers in the posterior fornix of the vagina, the examiner then uses the external hand to provide pressure over fundus. The internal fingers are then able to palpate the firm cervix and the softer isthmus. The fundus, like the cervix, feels firm to palpation. Occasionally the fundus may flex dramatically anteriorly or posteriorly because of this softening. The McDonald sign is determined when the uterine fundus and cervix can be easily flexed on each other and depends on the softening of the tissue of the isthmus.

Softening of the cervix (Goodell's sign). At approximately 8 weeks' menstrual age the cervix softens so that it no longer feels like the fibrous, nonpregnant cervix. Other conditions such as use of oral contraceptives can cause a similar softening in the cervical tissue.

Asymmetry of the uterus with implantation near the cornua (Piskacek's sign). When implantation occurs near the cornua of the uterus, a soft prominence may be palpated over the site of implantation.

Uterine enlargement becomes apparent at approximately 7 weeks' gestation. The uterus remains a pelvic organ until approximately 12 weeks' gestation, when the fundus can be palpated just above the symphysis pubis.

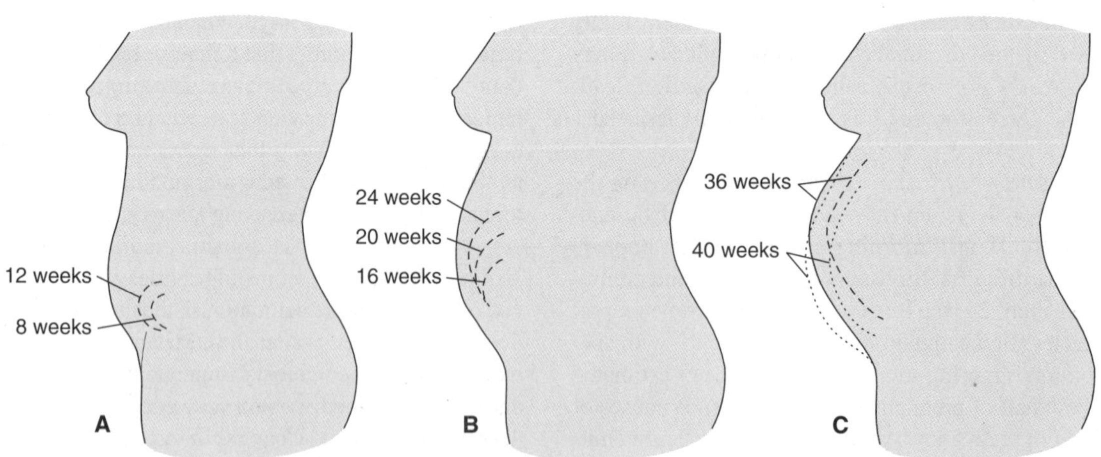

Figure 7-1 Uterine growth. **A,** 8 to 12 weeks; **B,** 16 to 24 weeks; **C,** 36 to 40 weeks.

Enlargement of the abdomen. Enlargement of the abdomen is usually more pronounced in multiparous women then in nulliparous women. Serial sizing of the uterus up to 20 weeks' gestation can provide a fairly reliable method of dating the normal pregnancy. Other anatomic changes, including myomas and other masses, may elevate the uterine fundus (Figure 7-1).

Use of uterine sizing in determining expected day of delivery. Before 12 weeks' gestation, the uterus is sized during bimanual examination of the pelvis. The fundus can be palpated abdominally above the symphysis after 12 weeks' menstrual age. Between 12 and 20 weeks' gestation, gestational age is estimated using the symphysis and umbilicus as landmarks. Typically the fundus is midway between the symphysis and umbilicus at 16 weeks and at the umbilicus at 20 weeks. From 20 to 36 weeks' gestation, measurement of fundal height in centimeters estimates the weeks' gestation, plus or minus 2 cm (Figure 7-2; Table 7-1). From 36 weeks until delivery, fundal height varies greatly as a result of the range of normal fetal weights at term and the effect of descent of the presenting part (Figures 7-3 and 7-4).

Palpation of the fetus. From about 26 weeks through term, the fetal body can be palpated through the abdominal wall. Because myomas can sometimes mimic the fetal parts, this finding cannot be considered a positive sign of pregnancy.

Ballottement of the fetus. Around midsecond trimester the fetal mass is relatively small compared to

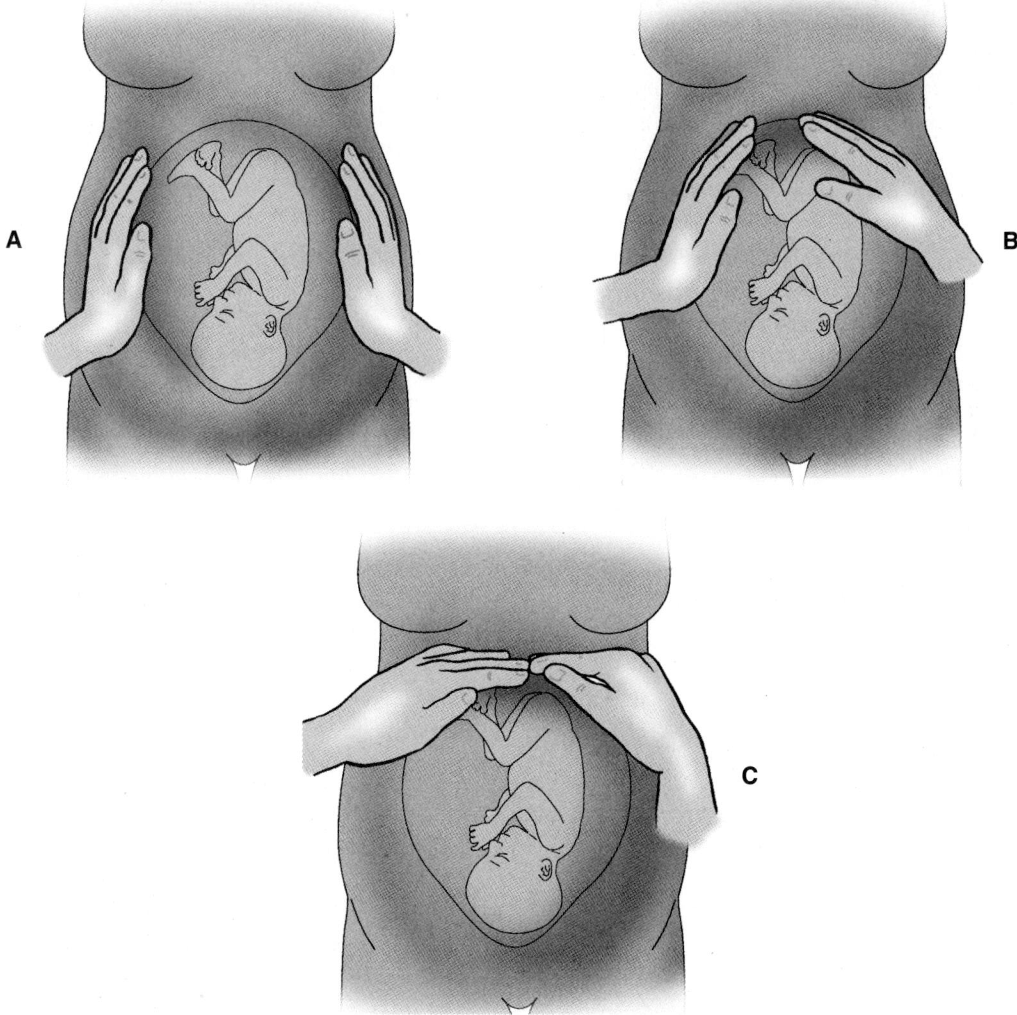

Figure 7-2 Determining the fundal height. **A,** Lateral aspects of uterus palpated by examiner; **B,** examiner moves hands toward fundus; **C,** fundal height palpated accurately.

Table 7-1 *Fundal Height Estimates for Dating*

Weeks' gestation	Fundal height
12	At symphysis or 1-2 cm above symphysis
16	9 cm or midway between symphysis and umbilicus or 3-4 fingerbreadths above symphysis
20	18 cm or at umbilicus
24	24 cm ± 2 cm or 1-2 fingerbreadths above umbilicus
28	28 cm ± 2 cm or midway between umbilicus and xiphoid process or 3-4 fingerbreadths above umbilicus
32	32 cm ± 2 cm
36	36 cm ± 2 cm or at 1 fingerbreadth below xiphoid process

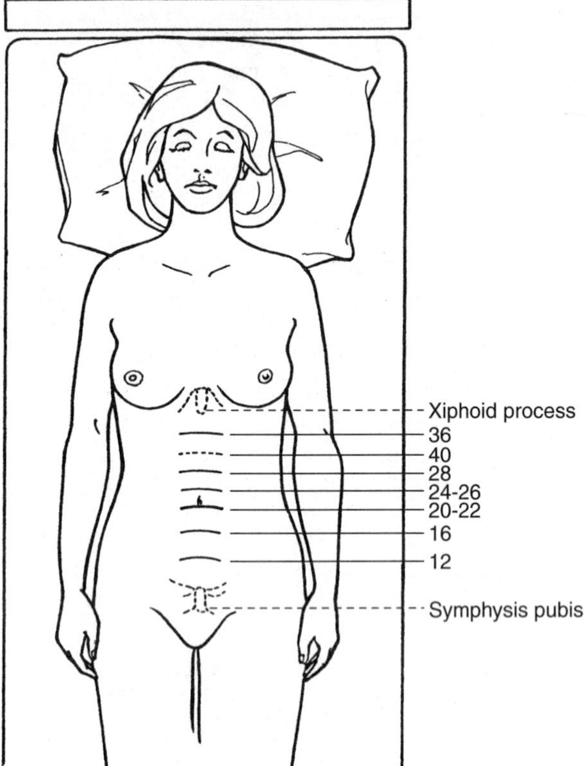

Figure 7-4 Line drawing of fundal heights.

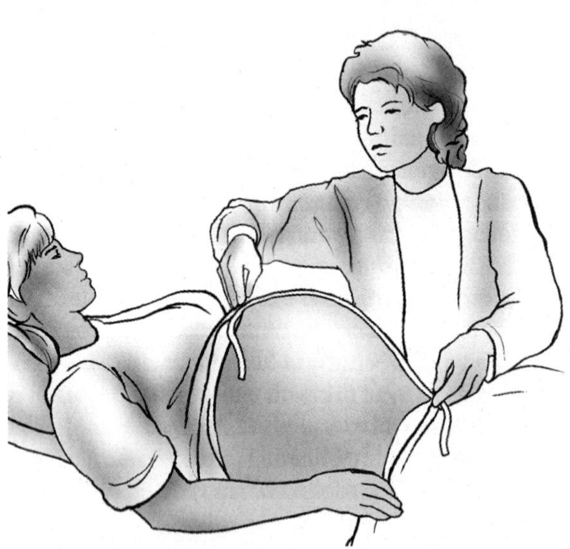

Figure 7-3 Fundal height measurement using measuring tape.

the volume of amniotic fluid. When sudden pressure is exerted over the uterus, the fetus sinks in the fluid and rebounds to its original location. The rebound (ballottement) can be felt by the experienced examiner.

Braxton-Hicks contractions. Throughout pregnancy the uterus undergoes contractions that may or may not be felt by the woman. These contractions do not cause cervical change. The examiner may palpate these contractions during assessment of the abdomen. Since they can occur in other conditions such as uteri with pedunculated submucosal myomas, they are not a positive sign of pregnancy.

Endocrine tests of pregnancy. Pregnancy tests determine the presence of human chorionic gonadotropin (hCG) in maternal serum or urine. Because elevated hCG is present in other conditions such as trophoblastic disease, it cannot be considered a positive sign of pregnancy.

hCG is produced by the anterior pituitary gland and the syncytiotrophoblast in the placenta. Nonpregnant levels of hCG are well below the sensitivity detectable by most clinical assays used for pregnancy monitoring. hCG is detectable in serum by 8 days after fertilization in 5%

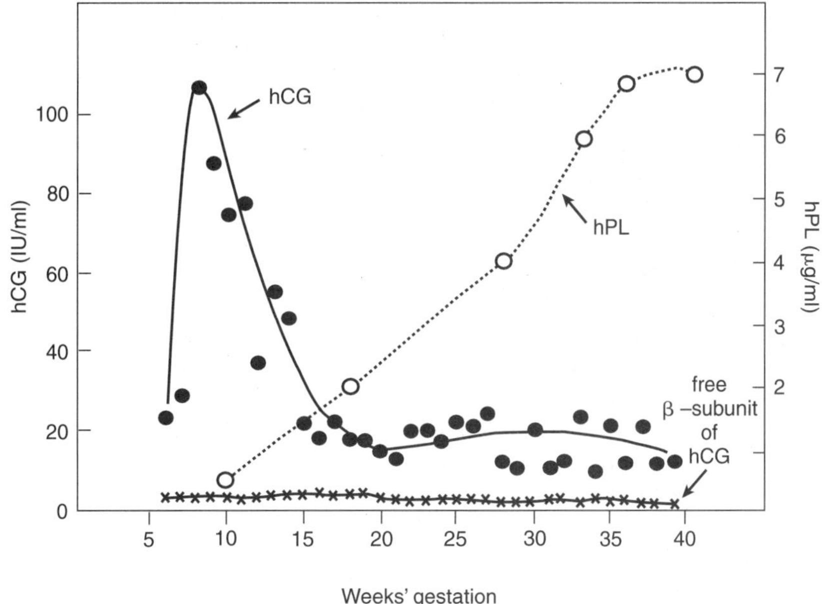

Figure 7-5 hCG levels in pregnancy. *hCG*, human chorionic gonadotropin; *hPL*, human placental lactogen.

of women, and almost all women will have detectable serum hCG by 11 days following fertilization (Buster and Carson, 1996). It has both alpha and beta subunits. The alpha subunit is almost identical to those of the luteinizing hormone, follicle-stimulating hormone, and thyroid-stimulating hormone and therefore is not useful in identifying elevation caused by pregnancy. However, the beta subunit is distinct and forms the basis for a sensitive biochemical test. hCG levels double every 1.3 to 2 days in early pregnancy, rising sharply until about 70 days' gestation, when the serum level begins to fall. After 120 days' gestation the hCG level remains at 5 to 20 mIU/ml. The levels of hCG in maternal serum and urine are consistent, with hCG level in 1 L of maternal serum equivalent to hCG level in 24 hours of urine (Figure 7-5).

Numerous pregnancy tests are available for use in commercial laboratories and clinics, as well as tests that can be done by consumers in their homes. All of these tests are based on the principle of identification of hCG through recognition of an antibody to the beta-subunit of the molecule.

Radioimmunoassay Radioimmunoassay (RIA) is the traditional laboratory technique for identifying the beta-subunit of hCG. In this process a radioactive substance and hCG are linked and used to identify displacement of the radio-labeled material by nonradio-labeled hCG in the pregnant woman's urine or serum. If none is displaced, there is no detectable hCG in the woman's sample. The biologic hCG can be quantified with great accuracy using this method; thus it is useful for following serial specimens. Disadvantages of the RIA technique include its limited sensitivity (5 mIU/ml) when compared to newer techniques, and the time necessary to complete the test (4 hours).

Immunoradiometric Assay (IRMA) Immunoradiometric assay (IRMA) uses anti-hCG antibodies that are bound to the walls of a test tube. Serum is added to the tube, and then a second radioactive antibody is added. The amount of the second antibody bound to the tube allows for an estimation of the amount of hCG in the serum sample. Advantages of the IRMA include that it can be completed in 30 minutes and it is sensitive to 150 mIU/ml.

Enzyme-linked Immunosorbent Assay (ELISA) The enzyme-linked immunosorbent assay (ELISA) process is sensitive to low levels of hCG, having the ability to detect as little as 10 mIU/ml in serum. A monoclonal antibody binds with the hCG present in the sample. When a second antibody linked with an enzyme is added, there is a color change, indicating presence of hCG. Advantages of the ELISA include its ease of use, its ability to diagnose up to 5 days before the missed period, and its fast time to complete (5 to 15 minutes).

Fluroimmunoassay Fluroimmunoassay (FIA) is similar to the ELISA and IRMA in that an antibody is labeled for identification, but the FIA uses a fluorescent label. The degree of fluorescence emitted allows for detection of as little as 1 mIU/ml. Advantages include its superior sensitivity and the fact that it can be done in 2 to 3 hours.

Agglutination Inhibition Pregnancy testing kits available to clinical sites and laboratories may continue to use a process that identifies hCG through inhibition of agglutination when the patient's urine is exposed to latex particles bound to hCG and a solution with hCG antibody. One drop of urine is mixed with one drop of antibody-containing solution on a black slide. One drop of agglutinate with hCG-coated latex particles is then added. If hCG is not present in the urine, the antibody will cause agglutination or flocculation of the latex particles, which is easily seen when the slide is exposed to a bright light. In other words, if agglutination occurs, the pregnancy test is negative. If hCG is present in the urine, it binds to the antibody and prevents antibody-induced agglutination of the latex particles. The solution remains a milky white color with no evidence of flocculation. A test without agglutination is read as positive.

Serial hCG levels. Since beta hCG levels rise in a predictable fashion during the first weeks of gestation, serial serum levels under 10,000 on two separate occasions at least 2 days apart provide a good estimation of gestational age. Date of conception can be calculated, and from that EDD extrapolated. Similarly, use of daily urine hCG tests when there is a negative test(s) with a conversion to positive can be used if the clinician knows the sensitivity level of the test.

Positive Indicators of Pregnancy

There are three accepted positive signs of pregnancy: (1) identification of fetal heart tones distinct from maternal heart rate; (2) palpation of fetal movement by the examiner; and (3) imaging of the fetus through the use of ultrasound or radiographic techniques.

Fetal heart tones. The identification of fetal heart tones detected by auscultation by fetoscope or Doppler or ultrasonographic visualization of heart motion provides a sound diagnosis of pregnancy. The earliest that fetal heart motion can be identified using transvaginal ultrasound is 4 weeks after conception (6 weeks' menstrual age). Transabdominal real-time ultrasound can identify fetal heart tones by 8 weeks' menstrual age. Depending on the sensitivity of the equipment and the maternal size, Doppler instruments can usually identify fetal heart tones at 10 to 12 weeks' menstrual age. If the uterus is retroverted or if there is significant adipose tissue, fetal heart tones may not be identified with doptone until 14 weeks' gestation. Auscultation of fetal heart tones with a fetoscope is usually possible between 17 and 19 weeks in nonobese women (Jimenez, Tyson, and Reisch, 1983). Auscultated heart tones for 22 weeks is an indication of term gestation, although this dating parameter is seldom used in light of the frequency of ultrasound dating.

Auscultation of the fetal heart tones may also identify other sounds. The umbilical (funic) souffle is produced by the movement of blood through the umbilical arteries and sounds like a whishing sound that is synchronous with the fetal heart rate. The uterine (maternal) souffle is a soft whishing sound produced by the blood cursing through the dilated uterine vessels and is synchronous with the maternal pulse. Uterine souffle may be heard in other conditions in which the uterine blood flow is increased, such as with large myomas. Maternal pulse in other large vessels in the abdomen, including the aorta, can often be heard during pregnancy. Fetal movements are usually heard as distinct kicks or turbulence while the clinician is listening to the fetal heart rate.

Palpation of fetal movements. Fetal movement may be identified by the examiner as early as 20 weeks' gestation, although it is more usual to feel distinct movements from 26 weeks to term. By identifying the position of the fetus, the experienced examiner can usually make the differentiation between arm and leg movements late in pregnancy. During the third trimester the examiner is often able to visualize the movement through the abdominal wall, particularly when the fetus is in a posterior position.

Visualization of the fetus. The normal intrauterine pregnancy can usually be identified by sonography by 5 to 6 weeks' menstrual age. A ringlike echo pattern, the gestational sac, noted intrauterinely, confirms the presence of the pregnancy, and absence of the sac after 6 weeks' gestation suggests the absence of a viable pregnancy. By 8 weeks' menstrual age, fetal poles can be identified, and measurement of the crown-rump length can be used to diagnose and date the pregnancy. The crown-rump length is predictive of gestational age ±4 days until 12 weeks' gestation.

The loss of clarity of the gestational sac or lack of identification of the fetal pole after 8 weeks is consistent with the diagnosis of blighted ovum. In this case the embryo has ceased to develop, and abortion will eventually occur. Women are often given the option of surgical intervention to abort a nonviable pregnancy rather than waiting for spontaneous expulsion.

By 11 weeks' gestation, the gestational sac is no longer visible as a distinct entity. By 14 weeks the fetal head and thorax are easily identifiable, and the placental site can be noted. As the pregnancy progresses, a variety of sonographic studies can identify major organs and skeletal development; fetal movement, including breathing efforts; development and maturation of the placenta; and volume of amniotic fluid (see Chapter 12).

Although radiologic studies have been replaced by sonography for diagnosis and assessment of pregnancy, it should be noted that fetal skeleton can be identified by x-ray after 16 weeks' gestation. This finding may be an unexpected finding on radiographic studies done for other reasons.

Use of Ultrasound in Estimation of Gestational Age

Transvaginal and transabdominal ultrasonic examinations are able to identify products of conception approximately 5 weeks after the missed period when the gestational sac can be visualized. At 6 weeks' gestation the fetal yolk sac becomes visible. Fetal heartbeats and breathing efforts can be identified as early as 7 weeks' gestation, and limb movement can be identified by 9 weeks' gestation. First trimester ultrasounds for dating use crown-rump length in calculating the gestation age. After 12 weeks crown-rump measurements are more variable due to the flexion and extension of the fetal body. Biparietal diameter, head circumference, abdominal circumference and femur length are used to estimate gestational age after 12 weeks.

Dating the gestation using ultrasound examination is most accurate in the early first trimester when variation is ±7 days. As pregnancy progresses, the standard error increases to ±4 weeks (Table 7-2).

Table 7-2 *Accuracy of Gestational Age Estimates Using Transabdominal Ultrasound*

Gestational age	Accuracy	Parameters
5-6.5 weeks	±7 days	Mean sac diameter
7-13 weeks	±5-7 days	Crown-rump length
14-20 weeks	±7-10 days	Biparietal diameter Head circumference Abdominal circumference Femur length
20-40 weeks	±2-4 weeks	Biparietal diameter Head circumference Abdominal circumference Femur length

SUMMARY

The increase in biotechnical studies to diagnose and date pregnancy has increased dramatically in the past two decades. All types of data collection need to be assessed for effectiveness in accurately identifying and dating the pregnancy. In addition, the impact on care, including cost and use of resources, needs to be assessed before new technologies are broadly accepted. It is important that the clinician continue to recognize the wisdom of considering the sound data that are often available when the time is taken to obtain a detailed menstrual, sexual, and social history.

After extensive review of the literature, Nichols (1987) has proposed the following Levels of Dating Criteria for use when comparing and contrasting sometimes differing estimates of gestational age:

Level 1 (margin of error, 5 to 14 days)

1. Basal body temperature chart with coital record demonstrating ovulation and sustained temperature elevation
2. Ultrasound between 7 and 10 weeks' menstrual age, using crown-rump length to calculate gestational age
3. Serum hCG levels under 10,000 on two separate occasions rising appropriately
4. Urine pregnancy testing, which may initially be negative, but becomes positive as soon as detectable levels of hCG are present in maternal urine
5. Two ultrasounds obtained before 25 weeks' gestational age, which estimate dates of delivery within 2.6 weeks of each other; use of the EDD based on the earlier ultrasound
6. Last menstrual period, which is normal, regular, and certain

Level 2 (margin of error, 2.6 weeks)

1. One ultrasound obtained by an experienced ultrasonographer between 13 and 27 weeks

Level 3 (margin of error, 3 weeks)

1. Uterine sizing

Level 4 (margin of error, greater than 3 weeks)

1. Ultrasound obtained after 28 weeks' gestational age
2. First fetal heart tones by either fetoscope or doptone
3. Quickening
4. Other signs and symptoms of pregnancy

References

Andersen HF et al: Gestational age assessment. II. Prediction from combined clinical observations, *Am J Obstet Gynecol* 140(7):770-774, 1981.

Buster JE, Carson SA: Endocrinology and diagnosis of pregnancy. In Gabbe SG, Niebyl JR., Simpson JL, editors: *Obstetrics: normal and problem pregnancies,* ed 3, New York, 1996, Churchill Livingstone.

Jimenez JM, Tyson JE, Reisch JS: Clinical measures of gestational age in normal pregnancies, *Obstet Gynecol* 61(4): 438-443, 1983.

Johnson TRB, Walker MA, Niebyl JR: Preconception and prenatal care. In Gabbe SG, Niebyl JR., Simpson JL, editors: *Obstetrics: normal and problem pregnancies,* ed 3, New York, 1996, Churchill Livingstone.

Merkatz IR, Thompson JE: *New perspectives on prenatal care,* New York, 1990, Elsevier.

Nichols C: Dating pregnancy: gathering and using a reliable data base, *J Nurse-Midwifery* 32(4):195-204, 1987.

Van Blarcom CC: *Obstetrical nursing,* ed 3, New York, 1937, Macmillan.

Chapter 8

Components of Prenatal Care

Care provided during pregnancy has undergone dramatic changes in the latter half of the twentieth century. These changes are most noted in two areas: (1) the move from providing care by a physician generalist or community midwife to providing care by an obstetric specialist or subspecialist, and (2) the increasing use of biotechnology in care practices. Numerous studies have explored the relationship between prenatal care and perinatal outcomes, usually by looking at time of initiation of care and number of visits. Review of the literature reveals that women who participate in prenatal care experience lower maternal and perinatal mortality and that there is an association between number and timing of prenatal visits and pregnancy outcomes (Villar and Bergsjo, 1997). Few studies have attempted to identify ways in which specific care practices influence the outcome of pregnancy for the woman and her babies (Klerman, 1990). Therefore, for as much as prenatal care has been shown to be associated with improved outcomes, we have limited understanding about the specific factors that truly have an effect on outcomes and the interrelationships among the multiple factors that seem to influence maternal and infant health.

Prenatal care is not just medical care offered in a selected site by a specialized provider. A broader definition of prenatal care includes care and support offered to the pregnant woman in her family, her community, and her workplace, as well as the organizational care received in her site of health services. When women conceive, they have already been exposed to numerous beliefs and practices surrounding childbearing. The beliefs held by a woman will influence her concept of pregnancy (healthy state vs. sick state), her reaction to normal physiologic changes in her body, her acceptance of care practices offered in the dominant medical system in her community, and her preparation for birth and mothering (Research Box 8-1).

Traditionally, formal, institutionalized prenatal care has been shaped by experts' (obstetricians') opinions regarding practices that will positively influence the outcome of pregnancy. Physician specialists have remained central in defining the expected components of care. Since physician care reflects a paradigm grounded in identification and treatment of pathology, it is not surprising that medical recommendations for components of care are primarily biomedical interventions thought to ameliorate pathologic aspects of pregnancy. When other professionals have had input into prenatal program designs or recommendations, their contributions have usually been in the area of "expanded" services such as patient education, nutrition counseling, and social support services.

Women consumers of care are rarely included in planning prenatal services. When research has explored

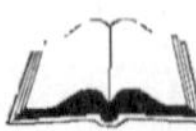

Research Box 8-1

Goldenberg RL, Patterson ET, Freese MP: Maternal demographic, situational and psychosocial factors and their relationship to enrollment in prenatal care: a review of the literature, *Women Health* 19(2-3):133-151, 1992.

Background

A substantial amount of literature has documented the association between little, late, or no prenatal care and increased risk for poor pregnancy outcomes. Most programs that have been developed to increase the use of prenatal care have reduced only slightly the number of women receiving little or no prenatal care. Relatively little is known about the personal factors that influence a woman's decision to seek prenatal care.

Research Question

What information about the initiation of prenatal care is found in the published literature?

Methods

The authors conducted a literature review to identify demographic, situational, and psychosocial variables associated with care seeking behavior in pregnancy. The method of obtaining published studies for review is not identified.

Sample

Not applicable

Results

Six demographic variables were found to be associated with inadequate prenatal care: age less than 20 years, high parity, low level of education, low income, unmarried status, and nonwhite race. Situational variables associated with inadequate prenatal care include lack of child care, financial problems, transportation problems, distance from the caregiver, rural residence, difficulty in scheduling during clinic hours, and lack of knowledge of community resources. Psychosocial variables associated with inadequate prenatal care include unwanted pregnancy, delayed diagnosis of pregnancy, feeling healthy and not identifying a medical problem associated with the pregnancy, and past experience of dissatisfaction with the provision of health care.

Clinical Application

Providers who are in a position to develop prenatal programs can use these findings to target populations that have increased risk factors for inadequate prenatal care. Future evaluation research should address factors not well understood rather than the commonly studied demographic variables associated with inadequate care.

women's perceptions of components of prenatal care, several consistent themes emerge. Omar and Schiffman (1995) categorized factors identified as important to women in their sample into three areas—provider-, staff-, and system-related factors. Their findings suggest that women desire providers who are caring and respectful and who spontaneously offer information and education. Continuity of provider is also seen as important, and women identify dissatisfaction when they have to see a different provider at each visit (Graveley and Littlefield, 1992; Omar and Schiffman, 1995). In addition, women prefer care in sites where staff are caring and respectful. Preference for providers who share gender and ethnicity is not consistent in the literature (Delgado, Lopez-Fernandez, and Luna, 1993; Handler et al., 1996; Omar and Schiffman, 1995).

Women want to receive care in systems that offer clean environments, child-friendly areas, efficient scheduling, and minimal waiting times (Handler et al., 1996; Thomas et al., 1987). In both private and public settings, women receiving prenatal care often have difficulty scheduling initial appointments in the first trimester (Omar and Schiffman, 1995). Although women are encouraged to obtain prenatal care early in pregnancy, some physicians and medical systems continue to tell patients to wait until they have missed two periods or until 12 weeks' gestation. Women also desire flexibility of appointment times, including the availability of evening hours. One focus group participant who was receiving care in a private physician setting stated, "My doctor doesn't have after-hours, so I have to rearrange my lunch hour; otherwise I lose the leave time I need after the baby comes" (Omar and Schiffman, 1995) (Research Box 8-2).

Standards and guidelines for prenatal care have been promulgated in the United States since 1925 when the Children's Bureau recommended standards to decrease maternal and infant mortality. Most studies of prenatal care now cite the *Guidelines for Women's Health Care* (American College of Obstetricians and Gynecologists,

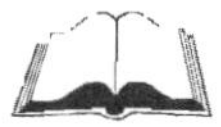

Research Box 8-2

Handler A et al: Women's satisfaction with prenatal care settings: a focus group study, *Birth* 23:31-37, 1996.

Background

The United States continues to have low-birth-weight and infant mortality rates higher than those of other developed countries. It has been suggested that ensuring early and continuous prenatal care for all women will improve perinatal outcomes. There is a known relationship between patient satisfaction and use of health care services, yet relatively little attention has been paid to women's perceptions of the quality of care given during their pregnancies. The authors argue that exploration of the characteristics of care and related satisfaction is important as managed care systems evolve in order to maximize characteristics that most positively affect women's satisfaction.

Research Question

What are the characteristics of care that affect women's satisfaction with prenatal care?

Methods

This qualitative study used focus groups to obtain information about the characteristics of care that led to increased satisfaction. A preliminary self-administered questionnaire that explored the importance of various characteristics of prenatal care was completed by participants. Focus groups were guided by a previously tested guide of questions. Discussion was audiotaped, and tapes were transcribed and coded to identify themes for each ethnic group. Themes were independently validated by a research team skilled in qualitative methods.

Sample

Fifty women participated in eight focus groups. Two groups were conducted with second-generation Mexican women, two with second-generation Puerto Rican women, two with black women, and two with white women. Participants were recruited from free-standing women, infants, and children nutrition program sites and were receiving prenatal care in a variety of settings.

Results

The questionnaire results indicated that 94% of the women thought it was very important that the prenatal care provider explain what he or she was doing and answer any questions that the woman had. Other characteristics identified as important by more than 50% of the respondents were the availability of 24-hour access to care, the ability to see the same provider at each visit, and scheduling so that there was "enough time" for the visit. Only 16% of the respondents thought it was important to have a provider who shared race/ethnicity with the woman. The focus group results found that motivation to seek care rested with a universal belief that care made a difference in outcome of the pregnancy. Specific care practices identified as valued were hearing the baby's heart beat and seeing the baby on ultrasound. Participants also valued being treated with respect by the provider, technical expertise in the provider, and seeing the same provider at each visit. Women became angry if they had to wait for long periods of time and then had a short prenatal visit with a provider who did not answer questions or talk with them.

Clinical Application

Findings from this study can be used in designing or revising health delivery systems to meet the needs of both the women and the provider. Limitations of the study include the fact that the sample may not have been representative of the population groups studied and that the participants were all low-income, urban women. Further study in other populations should be able to evaluate whether the themes that were identified are universal.

1996) and the *Guidelines for Perinatal Care* (American College of Obstetricians and Gynecologists, 1996; ACOG and American Academy of Pediatrics, 1997) as the accepted standards for clinical services for women and infants. Not until the U.S. Public Health Service Expert Panel on the Content of Prenatal Care evaluated all identified research regarding prenatal care practices was there an organized attempt to identify those factors for which there is evidence of effectiveness of prenatal care (Expert Panel, 1989). One of the significant aspects of the panel's work is that a multidisciplinary team with a public health focus explored the issue, thus generating a report with greater depth than would have been achieved if only medical specialists had been represented.

AN OVERALL ASSESSMENT

From its introduction into health service delivery, the goal of prenatal care has continued to be the promotion of optimum health status for both mother and baby. It is believed that early identification of problems or potential problems that may have a negative effect on the mother and/or infant and development of a management plan to address those problems will contribute to improvement of pregnancy outcomes. The Expert Panel expanded the goal of prenatal care beyond the immediate promotion of well-being for the woman and her infant in the perinatal period to include the promotion of the health and well-being of the family from preconception through the first year of the infant's life.

Prenatal care begins when conception is first considered and continues until labor begins. It consists of health promotion, risk assessment, and interventions linked to the risks and conditions uncovered. These activities require the cooperative and coordinated efforts of the woman, her family, her prenatal care providers, and other specialized providers. The objectives of prenatal care for the mother, infant, and family relate to outcomes through the first year following birth (Expert Panel, 1989).

During the second half of the century, maternal and infant mortality decreased significantly, largely in part to factors external to the medical system. Women were delivering fewer babies, and nutrition and social conditions had improved. Availability of safe blood replacement products and antibiotics addressed common medical problems encountered during pregnancy and the postpartum period. Prenatal care programs that were introduced after 1965 sought specifically to address the problems of low birth weight and preterm birth as a means to improve infant health. Many studies link lack of prenatal care or inadequate prenatal care to increased low birth weight and preterm birth rates; however, other studies have failed to support this association (Groutz and Hagay, 1995).

Relatively few studies have examined the components of care in a way that associations with outcomes can be identified. Intuitively, it seems reasonable that a combination of interventions that lead to improved health and lifestyle behaviors along with biomedical interventions to identify problems or potential problems is a comprehensive approach to meeting the goals of prenatal care. Although practitioners in prenatal clinics and provider offices are likely to routinely include commonly accepted biomedical interventions in prenatal care (e.g., blood pressure determinations, measurement of fundal height, auscultation of fetal heart rate), they less frequently provide health behavior advice. Studies also suggest that certain subgroups of women, including adolescents and women of color, may be less likely to receive appropriate counseling and education during their prenatal care encounters (Kogan et al., 1994b).

Early and Continuing Risk Assessment

Risk assessment includes the gathering of data through history-taking, physical examination, and use of laboratory tests and special studies as appropriate to identify factors that may increase the risk or chance of poor pregnancy outcome (Box 8-1). Risk assessment is "a dynamic process that includes concepts of relative risk and attributable risk" (Expert Panel, 1989). It is recognized that risk status may change as the pregnancy progresses. For that reason, risk assessment continues through each visit, with the plan of care revised as necessary when factors that change risk status are identified. Risk factors are characteristics that are associated with specific pregnancy outcomes. They are often interrelated and may have indirect relationships with outcomes (see Chapter 2). Sophisticated statistical analyses can estimate the degree of risk that is attributed to a specific factor.

Perinatal risk factors include medical and psychosocial factors. Medical risk factors can be further divided into five areas—genetic factors, nutrition and anthropometric characteristics, medical conditions that preceded pregnancy, reproductive history, and medical conditions specific to the pregnancy (Expert Panel, 1989).

Genetic abnormalities contribute to fetal and neonatal morbidity and mortality. When women and their partners are identified as carrying increased risk for genetic disorders, they can make reasoned decisions regarding reproduction before conception and early in pregnancy. Genetic disorders that can be identified prenatally include Tay-Sachs disease; Duchenne muscular dystrophy; alpha and beta thalassemia; sickle cell disease; sex chromosome abnormalities (e.g., XXY, XXX, XXY); and trisomies 13, 18, and 21 (Cirigliano et al., 1999; Heckel et al., 1999; Kazazian, 1991; Lebo et al., 1990; Nevo et al., 1999; Wood et al., 1993). Genetic risk assessment includes identification of health status of first- through third-degree relatives, evaluation of abnormal pregnancy outcomes, identification of exposure to agents that contribute to genetic disorders, identification of advanced parental age(s), and identification of ethnic status associated with specific risk for genetic problems (Groutz and Hagay, 1995).

Box 8-1 *Data Necessary for Risk Assessment*

Sociodemographic Data
Menstrual history
Past obstetric history
Contraceptive history
Sexual history
Medical/surgical history
Infection history
Family and genetic history
Nutrition history
Substance use
Social support
Stress abuse
Psychologic (mental illness, pregnancy readiness)
Environment (housing, finances, extremes of activity, exposure to teratogens)

Physical Examination
General physical examination
Blood pressure/pulse
Height
Weight
Pelvic examination, including clinical pelvimetry
Breast examination

Laboratory Tests

Hemoglobin/hematocrit	Hepatitis B
Rh factor	Toxoplasmosis
Rubella titer	Cytomegalovirus
Urine dipstick (protein/sugar)	Herpes
	Varicella
Pap smear	Human immunodeficiency virus
Infection screens	
Tuberculosis	Hemoglobinopathies
Gonorrhea	Tay-Sachs
Chlamydia	Parental karyotype
Syphilis	Illicit drug screen

From Expert Panel on the Content of Prenatal Care: *Caring for our future: the content of prenatal care,* Washington, DC, 1989, US Public Health Service.

Nutrition and anthropometric characteristics may reflect underlying medical conditions, as well as long-term nutritional status. Poor nutrition with resulting underweight or overweight status can contribute to neonatal and maternal morbidity. Underlying medical disorders related to these characteristics may be associated with specific perinatal problems. For example, a woman who is obese with underlying diabetes is at greater risk for fetal loss and specific fetal organ malformations. Risk assessment for problems related to nutritional and anthropometric characteristics include identification of extremes in maternal age, race, or ethnicity associated with increased risk for specific nutritional or anthropometric deviations from normal, family history of nutritionally related abnormalities, and social/environmental factors that influence nutritional status.

Preexisting maternal medical disease may increase the risk of maternal and fetal/neonatal mortality and morbidity. Hypertension, diabetes, cardiac disease, history of clotting disorders, thyroid disorders, renal disease, and cancer all may increase the risk of poor perinatal outcomes. Chapter 25 discusses medical complications in pregnancy. Risk factors associated with underlying medical disorders include advanced maternal age, racial or ethnic groups with increased prevalence of specific diseases, and family history of specific medical conditions.

Previous experience in pregnancy is strongly associated with the course of the current pregnancy. Women who have a history of preterm birth or delivery of a low-birth-weight infant are at increased risk of similar outcomes unless there is a known causative agent that has been eliminated (Bakewell, Stockbauer, and Schramm, 1997; Raine, Powell, and Krohn, 1994). For example, a woman who previously abused cocaine during pregnancy but who is now clean and has made significant other lifestyle changes has decreased her risk for complications associated with drug use. Likewise, a woman with a history of a preterm birth secondary to a severe motor vehicle accident may not be at increased risk with the current pregnancy unless she experiences similar trauma. Risk assessment for past obstetric factors that are associated with increased risk in the current pregnancy includes identification of previous pregnancy losses, preterm labor and birth, and deviations in fetal growth in previous pregnancies.

Medical or obstetric conditions that develop with the current pregnancy may increase the risk of poor perinatal outcomes. Examples include preeclampsia, development of abnormal maternal antibodies, multiple gestation, and exposure to infectious agents known to affect the fetus. Risk factors for these medical or obstetric conditions include extremes in maternal age, extremes in parity, paternal factors, maternal medical history, and social and environmental factors. Screening to assess risk or diagnosis of infectious diseases is recommended. Because of the known neonatal effects, screening for syphilis, gonorrhea, chlamydia, herpes, group B streptococcus, and hepatitis B should be done early in pregnancy. Screening for maternal human immunodeficiency virus (HIV) infection is recommended, and screening for tuberculosis is recommended in populations at increased risk for the disease.

Numerous studies have identified psychologic, emotional, social, and environmental factors that are associated with positive and negative outcomes of pregnancy. The strong association between poverty and poor pregnancy outcome reminds us that pregnancy is not just a biomedical event. Many psychosocial factors are interrelated with stress, and in recent years studies have validated the previously held belief that stress may be associated with maternal and neonatal morbidity (Orr et al., 1996; Pritchard and Teo, 1994).

A variety of risk assessment instruments have been developed to identify women at increased risk of poor pregnancy outcome through a quantitative method. Four main reasons for use of risk assessment instruments emerge in the literature:

1. To assist in clinical decisions regarding screening, diagnosis, and interventions, thereby improving quality of care
2. To identify women who will benefit from referral to special "high risk" clinics
3. To identify women who will benefit from referral to a more acute level of care in a regionalized system of health care delivery
4. To identify women who are most appropriate for receiving perinatal services in an alternative site or with an alternative provider

Risk assessment instruments have typically been developed to identify women at increased risk for perinatal mortality, low birth weight, or preterm birth. Sensitivities of instruments tend to be higher when attempting to predict increased risk for perinatal mortality and low birth weight than for those that attempt to predict risk of preterm labor and birth. Risk assessment instruments tend to be more sensitive for multiparous women, since many of the factors that are weighted are related to previous experience in pregnancy. One should keep in mind that an instrument developed for one population will need to be re-evaluated before use in other populations, since the influence of risk factors and the interaction of factors will vary from community to community. At best, an adequate risk assessment instrument will identify women at increased risk for a given outcome so that interventions can be introduced to decrease the risk (Research Box 8-3).

Health Promotion

To obtain the most appropriate care for the pregnant woman's needs, health promotion activities include education and counseling to promote healthful behaviors, to increase knowledge about pregnancy and parenting, and to increase the individual's comfort and ability in negotiating the health and medical care system. Health education activities during pregnancy have moved from community-sanctioned beliefs passed through the oral tradition to formalized instruction from health care professionals to the pregnant woman and her family. Common areas included in health education efforts include information on fetal growth and development, nutrition, exercise, self-help strategies for common discomforts, and danger signs for which the woman should seek immediate medical attention. In addition, preparation for childbirth and parenting are often offered in formal classes apart from the clinician's office.

Although it is commonly accepted that health education leads to improved health outcomes, there are few rigorous studies that evaluate specific educational interventions in pregnancy. Thompson (1990) found no studies that examined the effectiveness of nutritional counseling on eating habits, teaching self-help measures for common problems encountered in pregnancy on problem resolution, or parenting and infant care education on parenting skills. A recent review using MEDLINE failed to identify any studies evaluating the effects of health education on pregnancy since 1990. The few studies that have been done in the area of health education are hampered by small sample size and lack of appropriate control groups. Preterm birth prevention programs, fetal movement counting to identify infants at risk for asphyxia, and breast-feeding promotion and preparation provide examples of education interventions that may improve pregnancy outcomes in some populations. Further research is needed to establish not only the effect of such programs, but also the methods that are most effective in promoting learning.

Medical and Psychosocial Interventions

Medical interventions have been the core of prenatal care since the 1920s. These interventions initially included assessing blood pressure and maternal weight gain, measuring fundal height, determining presentation and position of the fetus after 30 weeks, and ascertaining fetal heart rate. Through the decades, other medical interventions such as clinical pelvimetry, general physical

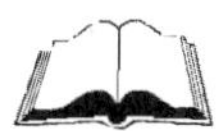 Research Box 8-3

Kogan MD et al: Relation of the content of prenatal care to the risk of low birth weight, *JAMA* 271(17):1340-1345, 1994.

Background

Previous studies exploring the association of prenatal care and pregnancy outcome have used indices that quantify prenatal care by number of visits and/or gestational age at entry into care. There has been little exploration of the relationship of content of care and pregnancy outcome.

Research Question

What are the associations among prenatal procedures and advice and low birth weight?

Methods

The 1988 National Maternal and Infant Health Survey (NMIHS) database was used to identify the following prenatal procedures recommended by the Expert Panel on the Content of Prenatal Care for inclusion at the initial prenatal visit: blood pressure measurement, urine culture, hemoglobin or hematocrit, recording of height and weight, and health history. The NMIHS was also used to identify health behavior advice recommended by the Expert Panel: breast-feeding, reducing or eliminating alcohol, reducing or eliminating smoking, not using illegal drugs, eating proper foods, taking vitamin and mineral supplements, and gaining an appropriate amount of weight. Maternal age, parity, race/ethnicity, educational level, household income, marital status, employment, prior poor outcome, hypertension, and smoking were control variables. The outcome variable was low birth weight. Data analysis included bivariate associations between low birth weight and prenatal procedures; associations among low birth weight, prenatal procedures, and prenatal counseling while stratifying for covariates; and logistic regressions to isolate the contributions of procedures and advice to low birth weight.

Sample

The NMIHS sample consisted of 9953 women who had a live birth in 1988 and who reported receiving prenatal care for a singleton pregnancy. The sample was nationally represented but excluded South Dakota and Montana, and oversampled for blacks and low-birth-weight infants. The sample was identified using state vital records, and then a questionnaire was completed and merged with the vital record data. Response rate for the questionnaire was 74%.

Results

Significantly lower percentages of low-birth-weight infants were found for women who reported that they received advice on vitamin use, breast-feeding, proper weight gain, and avoidance of alcohol. The only procedure associated with increased low birth weight was lack of determination of maternal weight. The positive impact of advice was strongest in high-risk groups: household income less than $6000, primiparas, teenagers, hypertensives, inadequate users of prenatal care, women using publicly funded sites, smokers, and women with a previous poor pregnancy outcome. Regression analysis identified the following factors associated with low-birth-weight infants: black race, smoking, not married, primipara, Asian ethnicity, less than 12 years of completed school, hypertension, and prior poor outcome.

Clinical Application

The findings that lack of advice regarding behaviors during pregnancy was associated with low birth weight and that lack of prenatal procedures was not associated with increased risk of low birth weight emphasizes the importance of the health promotion and disease prevention aspects of prenatal care. Programs that attempt to cut costs by decreasing time for counseling and advice may be inadvertently contributing to increased risk of low birth weight. The findings are limited by the fact that the data were self-reported and that not all factors recommended by the Expert Panel could be measured. In addition, women who experience a low-birth-weight outcome may recall procedures and advice differently from those who deliver appropriate- and large-for-gestational-age babies. The finding that women at higher risk for a low-birth-weight infant experience the greatest benefits of advice and counseling provides support for ensuring that these components of care be maintained in clinical services that target that population.

Table 8-1 *Suggested Risk Assessment Activities and Schedule of Visits*

Activity	6-8 wks	14-16 wks	24-28 wks	32 wks	36 wks	38 wks	39 wks	40 wks	41 wks
Medical history	x*								
Psychosocial history	x*								
Update histories		x	x	x	x	x	x	x	x
General physical examination	x*								
Blood pressure/pulse	x		x	x	x	x	x	x	x
Height	x*								
Weight	x	x	x	x	x	x	x	x	x
Height/weight profile	x*								
Pelvic examination/ pelvimetry	x								
Breast examination	x								
Fundal height		x	x	x	x	x	x	x	x
Fetal position/heart rate			x	x	x	x	x	x	x
Cervical examination									x
Hemaglobin/hematocrit	x			x					
Rh factor	x*								
Antibody screen	x*			x					
Pap smear	x*								
Diabetic screen			x						
Triple screen (MSAFP)		x							
Urine culture	x								
Rubella titter	x*								
Syphilis test	x*				x†				
GC culture	x				x†				
Hepatitis B	x*								
HIV (offered)	x								
Illicit drug screen (offered)	x								
Chlamydia screen	x				x†				
TB screen	x*								
Hemoglobinopathies	x*‡								

Adapted from Expert Panel on the Content of Prenatal Care: *Caring for our future: the content of prenatal care,* Washington, DC, 1989, US Public Health Service.
* Do at first prenatal visit if not done at preconception visit.
†Repeat in women at increased risk for sexually transmitted infections.
‡Do in populations at increased risk.

examination, and biochemical testing and ultrasound screening and diagnosis were introduced. By the 1960s evaluation of psychosocial interventions such as smoking cessation programs, drug intervention programs, and expanded services, including nutritional counseling and childbirth education, appeared in the literature, prompting the federal government to include "expansion of services" in medical assistance regulations by the 1980s. Peoples-Sheps, Hogan, and Ng'andu (1996) completed a retrospective review of records for initial prenatal visits and found that adherence to expected physical examination, history taking, and selected laboratory tests was high in their sample. However, inclusion of components that addressed behavioral risk factors and health promotion and education was low. Kogan and colleagues (1994a, 1994b), in exploring data collected in the 1988

National Maternal and Infant Health Survey, found that black women were less likely to receive counseling regarding smoking cessation, alcohol use, and breastfeeding. In addition, the team was able to identify that women who reported not receiving all types of advice recommended by the Expert Panel were more likely to have a low-birth-weight infant. The literature suggests that the medical model of prenatal care continues to place greater emphasis on medical intervention or management than on a broader multidisciplinary approach to care.

SCHEDULING OF CARE

The original suggestion of timing of visits made by the Children's Bureau in the 1920s is strikingly similar to the patterns of visits used in most clinical settings today. The concept of evaluating pregnant women every month until the seventh month, then every 2 weeks until the ninth month, then weekly until delivery was proposed in response to the recognized problem of preeclampsia, a problem that usually presents in the third trimester. The Expert Panel recommended a somewhat different schedule based on their determination of the most effective way to address medical and psychosocial needs in pregnancy. The suggested core visit schedule is outlined in Table 8-1.

This alteration in scheduling of visits has been explored in a variety of health delivery systems to determine whether the decreased number of visits will affect maternal and neonatal outcomes. Many of these studies have been done in health maintenance organizations (HMOs), where cost control and preventive health care have traditionally been important factors in delivery of services. McDuffie and colleagues (1996) conducted a randomized controlled study in a group-model HMO to determine whether an appointment schedule of fewer visits would be associated with an increase in adverse perinatal outcomes. Their findings suggest that good perinatal outcomes and patient satisfaction were similar between women receiving traditional prenatal services and those receiving a reduced number of visits. The McDuffie team also explored whether there would be a difference in use of services, including maternal serum alpha-fetoprotein screening, ultrasound examinations, hematocrit testing after 20 weeks, diabetic screening, visits to nonobstetric providers or emergency rooms, numbers of telephone calls for advice, and hospitalizations when women received a reduced number of prenatal visits. Data were collected on 2328 low-risk women, and the investigators found no significant differences between those with traditional care (mean 14 visits) and those with the experimental schedule (mean 9 visits) in all categories except obstetric ultrasound at 15 to 24 weeks. A statistically significant higher percentage of women in the control (traditional care) group underwent obstetric ultrasound at 15 to 24 weeks' gestation (McDuffie et al., 1997). Walker and Koniak-Griffin (1997) similarly found no difference in perinatal outcomes when women were randomly assigned into an alternative prenatal visit schedule or a traditional prenatal care schedule. In addition, the women assigned to the alternative schedule reported increased satisfaction with the provider and the prenatal care system

PRECONCEPTION CARE

One of the problems with initiating pregnancy care after conception is that the opportunity to reduce factors that may be associated with increased risk of perinatal problems may be missed before effects on the developing fetus or the woman. Preconception care includes risk assessment, with appropriate medical or psychosocial interventions before conception. During the preconception risk assessment, one identifies risks that can be modified, while recognizing that not all risk factors can be changed. For example, short stature and advanced maternal age cannot be modified. However, even when modification is not possible, other screening or medical interventions may be appropriate to decrease the degree of risk or assist with decision making when there are several options for management. Preconception care is particularly useful in determining conditions in which early or preconception intervention is optimal (e.g., treatment for chronic hypertension, anemia, infections) and behavior or lifestyle factors that can be modified through education or counseling (e.g., smoking, drug use, poor nutrition, unsafe sexual practices). Preconception care should be routinely incorporated into primary care services, including routine annual examinations, family planning services, and school-based clinics.

Risk Assessment

Medical history should include identification of menstrual, obstetric, contraceptive, medical, and surgical factors that may influence conception, fetal development, and maternal health status with pregnancy. Psychosocial history should identify behaviors that may have a negative effect on the woman and her fetus, including the use of tobacco, alcohol, and other substances; increased stress in her environment; extremes of physical work or exercise; and presence of physical abuse.

Screening tests that provide baseline information on maternal status include tests to identify infection status (HIV, cytomegalovirus, herpes simplex, hepatitis, syphilis, toxoplasmosis, rubella, and varicella). Screening tests for cervical cytology abnormalities, chlamydia, gonorrhea, and other cervical infections allow for prompt treatment as problems are identified. Assessment for hemoglobinopathies, Tay-Sachs disease, and parental karyotype may be offered when family and personal history suggest genetic disorders.

Health Promotion

Education regarding the wisdom in avoiding smoking, alcohol, and drugs should be offered. The importance of good nutrition, including vitamin and mineral supplementation, should be discussed. Education and counseling regarding safer sex practices to decrease risk of sexually transmitted infections should be reviewed.

Medical and Psychosocial Interventions

When factors that increase risk of perinatal problems are identified, interventions can be proposed to modify risk. Common interventions include:

1. Folic acid supplements when dietary sources are not adequate to decrease risk of neural tube defects
2. Iron supplements when iron deficiency anemia is identified
3. Immunization for rubella or varicella when the woman is found to be nonimmune
4. Immunization against hepatitis B for women at risk for infection
5. Treatment for sexually transmitted infections
6. Further evaluation and treatment for abnormal Pap smear
7. Referral to smoking cessation programs
8. Referral to weight loss programs
9. Referral for genetic counseling when increased risk is identified in the woman's or her partner's families
10. Referral for further evaluation and treatment when medical conditions such as hypertension, diabetes, or asthma are identified

INITIAL PRENATAL VISIT (6 TO 8 WEEKS)

One of the primary goals of the first prenatal visit is the diagnosis and dating of pregnancy. In addition, the clinician must assess health status to identify medical or psychosocial problems or potential problems. Counseling regarding pregnancy options may be indicated if the woman has not determined whether she will continue the pregnancy. Following the complete initial assessment, the clinician, in collaboration with the pregnant woman, creates a plan of care that meets the needs of the woman, her fetus, and her family.

Risk Assessment

History of present pregnancy. Beginning the initial prenatal visit with a review of the present pregnancy provides a solid base for diagnosing and dating the pregnancy and identifying pregnancy-related risk factors. A complete menstrual history is obtained, noting whether the reported last menstrual period was normal in timing and duration. Documentation of the previous normal menstrual period will help in determining menstrual regularity. Contraceptive history and sexual history may also provide relevant information on the timing of conception, increased risks for implantation problems, and increased risks for infections that will affect the pregnancy. History of signs of pregnancy, as well as common discomforts, may assist the clinician in confirming the gestational age and evaluating whether the problems are consistent with the expected gestational age. Identification of danger signs, including vaginal bleeding, cramping, or loss of pregnancy signs, should be noted.

Medical and surgical history. When the pregnant woman is not an established patient in the practice with a previously documented medical history, a complete medical/surgical history must be obtained. Periodic update of this data is necessary in established patients. Areas of particular interest in pregnancy include the following.

Cardiovascular History Previous identification of cardiac murmur or deviations from normal should be noted, and efforts should be made to obtain copies of any cardiac workups that have been completed. Any history of hypertension, particularly during previous pregnancies and/or while on hormonal contraception, should be noted. Presence of varicose veins and any history of phlebitis must be noted.

Respiratory History Any history of asthma should be explored, with documentation of medications currently taken or taken as needed. Other respiratory problems that may be exacerbated with the increased demands of pregnancy should be identified.

Thyroid History Any workup and/or treatment for hyperthyroidism or hypothyroidism should be noted. Current medication should be noted, and baseline thyroid panel should be ordered to establish increased risk because of thyroid disorders.

Liver Disease History Any history of liver disease, including hepatitis, should be noted, with baseline liver function tests ordered as necessary.

Gastrointestinal History History of gastric irritability or bowel problems should be noted. Digestive problems that affect the woman's ability to tolerate specific foods should be identified. Screening for history of anorexia and bulimia should be included.

Neuromuscular History Any history of seizure activity should be noted, and current intake of antiepileptic medications must be documented.

Urinary History Any history of kidney disease or frequent urine infections must be noted. History of urinary tract infections (UTIs), particularly upper tract infections, in previous pregnancies, increases the risk of UTI in the current pregnancy and requires screening throughout the pregnancy.

Gynecologic History Any history of abnormal pap smears, vaginal infections, sexually transmitted infections, uterine or adnexal surgeries, or pelvic pain should be noted. History of infertility and use of assisted reproductive technologies to achieve conception should be identified. Contraceptive history, including side effects, is essential for dating the pregnancy, identifying the possibility of fetal exposure to hormonal agents, and counseling for postpartum choice of contraceptive method.

Previous Pregnancy History Numbers and outcomes of all pregnancies and complications, including infection and hemorrhage, should be obtained. Care should be taken to ensure that risk factors such as low birth weight, preterm birth, and preterm labor are identified. Method of infant feeding should be noted to offer appropriate counseling, particularly regarding breastfeeding during this pregnancy.

Psychosocial History Current relationship status and support system should be documented. Any history of physical or sexual abuse should be explored, and, if the woman is currently with an abusive partner or previously abusive partner, the clinician should ascertain whether she is safe and whether she has plans for escape if necessary. Daily habits, including exercise, should be explored. Work in and outside the home should be noted, with particular attention to exposure or activity that may affect the woman or fetus. Habits such as smoking, alcohol consumption, and drug use should be identified. History of depression or other mental health problems and treatment used should be obtained.

Physical examination and special studies Physical examination data obtained from healthy women during the initial prenatal visit and the associated rationale are noted in Table 8-2. Physical examination data that identify or suggest increased risk for perinatal problems in most cases will confirm suspicions that arose during history taking. Laboratory data collected at the initial visit are noted in Table 8-1.

Health Promotion

Health promotion counseling during the initial visit aims to provide information that will help the pregnant woman make lifestyle changes associated with improved pregnancy outcomes. Nutrition counseling includes a dietary assessment with recommendations for changes if indicated (see Chapter 11). Avoidance of teratogens should be addressed, recognizing that the woman may need to initiate changes in her work or home environment in order to decrease exposure. The importance of smoking cessation and avoidance of alcohol and drugs should be reviewed. Seatbelt use should be reviewed with instruction regarding the proper placement of the belt as pregnancy progresses. Review of normal physiologic and emotional changes in pregnancy will provide the woman with a baseline to identify changes that might indicate problems. Numerous patient education materials offer visual aids to explain fetal growth and development.

Discussion of sexuality in pregnancy in a way that is sensitive to the woman's cultural beliefs assists her in understanding the physiologic and emotional changes that may be experienced in pregnancy. Often "permission-giving" is necessary for she may have been told that sexual activity in pregnancy may harm the baby. If risk assessment identified factors

Table 8-2 *Physical Examination Data Collected During Initial Prenatal Visit*

Data	Rationale/association with complications
General assessment	Women who appear fatigued, acutely ill, disoriented, or distracted may have underlying medical problems or psychosocial problems.
Blood pressure (BP)	Elevated BP may indicate chronic hypertension or, if identified after 20 weeks' gestation, may indicate pregnancy-induced hypertension.
Pulse	Elevated pulse may indicate underlying thyroid disorder. Irregular pulse may indicate underlying cardiac disease.
Skin	Pale skin and mucous membranes may indicate anemia. Lesions may indicate chronic or acute infection, benign growth, or melanoma.
Head	Pale skin and limp hair may indicate underlying nutritional deficiencies. Identification of parasites may be associated with poor living conditions. Nasal mucous membranes may be inflamed with infection, pale with allergies, and inflamed and excoriated with cocaine use. Poor dentition may be related to poor dental hygiene, poor nutrition, and/or lack of access to dental care.
Neck	Enlargement may indicate thyroid disorder; nodule(s) may indicate benign or malignant lesion.
Thorax and lungs	Dyspnea may be a sign of underlying respiratory disease. Rales and rhonchi may indicate bronchitis. Wheezing is associated with asthma or obstructed pulmonary disease.
Heart	Abnormal heart sounds may indicate underlying cardiac disease.
Breasts	All breast lumps require diagnostic workup. Women with flat or inverted nipples need specific counseling regarding breast-feeding.
Abdomen	After 12 weeks' gestation, sizing of uterus identifies deviation in uterine/fetal growth. During third trimester, estimated fetal weight and fetal presentation and position are necessary in planning for delivery. Identification of fetal heart tones establishes fetal viability. Irregularities in fetal heart rate may indicate cardiac pathology. Before third trimester, identification of abdominal masses and/or tenderness necessitate further workup to determine whether pathology exists.

that increase the risk of sexually transmitted infections, discussion of lifestyle changes to decrease risk is in order. The clinician should offer HIV counseling and testing to all women, regardless of apparent risk of exposure.

Discussion of common discomforts of pregnancy and self-help strategies for those discomforts enables the woman to understand normal changes and identify those changes that may deviate from normal.

Orientation to the practice should include the usual pattern of prenatal visits, and the typical screening and diagnostic tests recommended during the pregnancy. It is critical that the clinician discusses danger signs necessitating immediate contact with the practice. Written instructions explaining how to contact the clinician after office hours are essential, and can be effectively printed on a business card or form that can be kept with the patient at all times.

Medical and Psychosocial Intervention

Medical and psychosocial interventions are dependent upon the data collected as part of risk assessment. Examples of medical and psychosocial interventions that have been found to be effective in improving outcomes include directed nutritional interventions for women with poor nutrition, smoking cessation programs in pregnancy, initiation of vitamin and mineral supplements in women who are anemic or are at risk for poor nutritional intake, and treatment of infections that are associated with amnionitis with preterm rupture of membranes (Bergsjo and Villar, 1997).

Table 8-2 *Physical Examination Data Collected During Initial Prenatal Visit —cont'd*

Data	Rationale/association with complications
Extremities	Edema may indicate underlying cardiovascular disease. Varicosities may increase risk of phlebitis in pregnancy.
Pelvic examination—external examination	Lesions and discharge may be associated with sexually transmitted infections or deviations in vaginal flora. Vulvar varicosities may increase discomfort during pregnancy. Scar tissue from previous episiotomy or lacerations may increase risk of laceration during birth. Hemorrhoids may increase discomfort in pregnancy.
Pelvic examination—speculum examination	Abnormalities of the vaginal and cervix may be associated with congenital abnormalities that may preclude vaginal delivery. Lesions and discharge may be associated with sexually transmitted infections or deviations in vaginal flora. Lesions of the cervix may be associated with cancer or precancerous cells.
Pelvic examination—bimanual examination	Sizing of uterus not compatible with dates may indicate inaccurate dating, fetal demise, multiple gestation, trophoblastic disease, or large fibroids. Cervical motion tenderness may indicate ectopic pregnancy or pelvic inflammatory disease (PID). Adnexal fullness or tenderness may indicate PID. Nodules or enlargement of the ovary requires further workup for diagnosis. Poor vaginal tone may be associated with urinary stress incontinence and increased discomfort in late pregnancy.
Rectal examination	Enlarged hemorrhoids may increase discomfort and bleed during pregnancy. Recto-vaginal examination may reveal weakened recto-vaginal wall, scar tissue, and/or fistulas.

REVISITS—FIRST TRIMESTER

Risk Assessment

Interval history is necessary to determine any changes in the woman's health status, any acute illnesses that may have occurred since the previous visit, and any changes in the woman's home or work environment that may have an effect on her health and well-being. Physical examination data for risk assessment recommended by the Expert Panel are noted in Table 8-3.

Health Promotion Activities

The clinician should review of all of the areas covered in the first visit. Support should be given for positive lifestyle and behavior changes made by the woman. Further counseling exploring employment issues and general health habits can be initiated to expand the clinician's understanding of the woman's life experiences.

Medical and Psychosocial Interventions

Interventions will reflect the increased risk for problems or the identified medical or psychosocial problems identified at the first visit. If initial screening and diagnostic tests identify conditions usually responsive to treatment (e.g., UTI, iron deficiency anemia, genital infections), interventions can be introduced appropriately.

REVISITS—SECOND TRIMESTER

Risk Assessment

Interval history should include the woman's own perception of how she feels the pregnancy is progressing, the identification of danger signs such as vaginal bleeding, the continuation or resolution of any first trimester discomforts, and the identification of maternal perception of fetal movement (quickening). Physical assessment areas for risk factors are noted in Table 8-4. Recommended laboratory tests are noted in Table 8-5.

Health Promotion Activities

In addition to continuing the counseling initiated in the first trimester, the clinician should review the signs and symptoms of preterm labor with the woman, noting particularly when she should contact the practice should

Table 8-3 *Physical Examination Data for Prenatal Revisits in First Trimester*

Data	Rationale/association with complications
General appearance	Common discomforts such as nausea and vomiting of pregnancy and excessive fatigue may leave her with little energy or feelings of general malaise. These signs may also indicate underlying medical disorder(s).
Weight	Nausea and vomiting of pregnancy may lead to weight loss and dehydration. Change in eating habits to control nausea may lead to weight gain.
Fundal height	Lack of expected uterine growth may indicate missed abortion. Excessive growth may indicate trophoblastic disease.
Fetal heart tones (FHTs)	Identification of FHTs with portable Doppler devices is possible between 10 and 12 weeks unless the uterus is retroverted and retroflexed or the women is obese. Lack of FHTs by 12 weeks may indicate inaccurate dating, missed abortion, or normal variation.

Table 8-4 *Physical Assessment for Risk Factors in Second Trimester*

General appearance	Women who appear fatigued, acutely ill, disoriented, or distracted may have underlying medical problems or psychosocial problems.
Blood pressure (BP)	Systolic and diastolic levels decrease in mid-pregnancy. Lack of decrease in BP may indicate increased risk for pregnancy-induced hypertension.
Weight	Weight gain less than 10 pounds by 20 weeks' gestation is associated with increased risk for a low-birth-weight infant.
Fundal growth	Growth greater than expected may indicate multiple gestation, inaccurate dating, polyhydramnios, or fibroids. Growth less than expected may indicate intrauterine growth restriction, preterm labor resulting in the presenting part deep in the pelvis, or fetal demise.
Fetal heart rate (FHR)	Irregular rate may indicate cardiac pathology; lack of FHR may indicate fetal demise.

Table 8-5 *Laboratory Tests for Screening in Second Trimester*

Test	Rationale
Triple marker screen	Screens for increased risk for neural tube defects, abdominal wall defects, trisomy XVIII and trisomy XXI; done at 15-20 weeks
Glucose screen	Screens for diabetes; done between 24-26 weeks
Hemoglobin/ hematocrit	Screens for anemia that has developed since first visit or is used to evaluate response to iron therapy in anemia diagnosed earlier in pregnancy; done along with the glucose screen to minimize number of blood draws
Ultrasound for anatomy scan	Screens for anatomic anomalies; confirms dating

preterm labor be suspected. In preparation for the birth and parenting, the clinician should review the childbirth education and parenting education opportunities available in the community. If none exists, recommendations for reading or instructional videos should be given with a plan to assess the woman's knowledge as the pregnancy progresses. Counseling regarding breast-feeding should be done with recommendations for opportunities for classes, support groups, and readings and videos given.

REVISITS—THIRD TRIMESTER

Risk Assessment

Interval history includes review of general well-being and third-trimester danger signs. Sudden excessive weight gain due to edema, visual changes, and abdominal pain should be noted. Identification of signs of preterm labor should be noted.

Physical examination for risk factors continues in the third trimester and includes the procedures noted in Table 8-6. Risk assessment data for third trimester obtained through laboratory tests and/or special studies, rationale for the testing, and association of abnormal findings with problems or potential problems are noted in Table 8-7.

Health Promotion Activities

Follow-up on counseling done in first and second trimester continues through the third trimester. Review of seat belt use as well as discussion about the importance of use of infant car seats should be done. The clinician should review employment status and assist with decision-making regarding for disability and family leave. Assessment of the woman's readiness for labor and delivery as well as the family's readiness for the new baby is essential.

Table 8-6 *Physical Examination Data Collected During Third Trimester*

Data	Rationale/association with complications
Blood pressure	Elevation may indicate pregnancy-induced hypertension.
Weight	Excessive weight gain associated with edema may indicate pregnancy-induced hypertension. Poor weight gain is associated with increased risk of a low-birth-weight infant.
Fundal height	Fundal height less than expected may indicate intrauterine growth restriction, inaccurate dating, preterm labor with presenting part deep in pelvis, or fetal demise. Fundal height greater than expected may indicate polyhydramnios, macrosomia, presence of a factor that prevents the presenting part from descending into pelvis (contracted pelvis, placenta previa, large soft tissue masses), or fibroids.
Fetal lie/presentation	Identification of abnormal lie or presentation may make it necessary to make appropriate plans for delivery.
Fetal heart tones	Abnormal rate and rhythm may indicate fetal cardiac problems.
Cervical examination	Cervical check at 41 weeks is recommended by some clinicians to assess readiness for induction.

Table 8-7 *Laboratory Tests and Special Studies Recommended in Third Trimester*

Test	Rationale and timing
Antibody screen in women who are Rh negative	Screens for development of antibodies in the case of previous fetal-maternal transfusion; done at 28 weeks
Repeat RPR	Screens for syphilis; recommended for women with increased risk for exposure since initial prenatal visit; done at 34-36 weeks
Repeat GC/CT	Screens for gonorrhea and chlamydia; recommended for women with increased risk for exposure since initial prenatal visit; done at 34-36 weeks
Repeat HIV	Screens for HIV; recommended for women with increased risk for exposure since initial prenatal visit; done at 34-36 weeks.
Beta strep culture	Screens for colonization of beta-hemolytic streptococcus; done at 34-38 weeks

GC/CT, Gonorrhea/*Chlamydia trachomatis; HIV,* human immunodeficiency virus; *RPR,* rapid plasmin reagin.

Medical and Psychosocial Interventions

As in the first and second trimesters, interventions depend on findings as a result of risk assessment.

References

American College of Obstetricians and Gynecologists: *Guidelines for women's health care,* Washington, DC, 1996, American College of Obstetricians and Gynecologists.

American College of Obstetricians and Gynecologists and American Academy of Pediatrics: *Guidelines for perinatal care,* Elk Grove, Ill, and Washington, DC, 1997, American Academy of Pediatrics and American College of Obstetricians and Gynecologists.

Bakewell JM, Stockbauer JW, Schramm WF: Factors associated with repetition of low birthweight: Missouri longitudinal study, *Paediatr Perinatal Epidemiol* 11:119-129, 1997.

Bergsjo P, Villar J: Scientific basis for the content of routine antenatal care. II. Power to eliminate or alleviate adverse newborn outcomes; some special conditions and examinations, *Acta Obstet Gynecol Scand* 76:15-25, 1997.

Cirigliano V et al: Rapid detection of chromosomes X and Y aneuploidies by quantitative fluorescent PCR, *Prenat Diagn* 19(12):1099-1103, 1999.

Delgado A, Lopez-Fernandez LA, Luna JD: Influence of doctor's gender in the satisfaction of the users, *Med Care* 31(9):795-800, 1993.

Expert Panel on the Content of Prenatal Care: *Caring for our future: the content of prenatal care,* Washington, DC, 1989, US Public Health Service.

Graveley EA, Littlefield JH: A cost-effectiveness analysis of three staffing models for the delivery of low-risk prenatal care, *Am J Public Health* 82(2):180-184, 1992.

Groutz A, Hagay ZJ: Prenatal care: an update and future trends, *Curr Opin Obstet Gynecol* 7:452-460, 1995.

Handler A et al: Women's satisfaction with prenatal care settings: a focus group study, *Birth* 23(1):31-37, 1996.

Heckel S et al: In utero fetal muscle biopsy: a precious aid for the prenatal diagnosis of Duchenne muscular dystrophy, *Fetal Diagn Ther* 14(3):127-132, 1999.

Kazazian HH: Prenatal diagnosis of beta-thalassemia, *Semin Perinatol* 15(3):15-24, 1991.

Klerman LV: The need for a new perspective on prenatal care. In Merkatz IR, Thompson JE, editors: *New perspectives on prenatal care,* New York, 1990, Elsevier.

Kogan MD et al: Racial disparities in reported prenatal care advice from health care providers, *Am J Public Health* 84(1):82-88, 1994a.

Kogan MD et al: Relation of the content of prenatal care to the risk of low-birth-weight: maternal reports of health behavior advice and initial prenatal care procedures, *JAMA* 271:1340-1345, 1994b.

Lebo RV et al: Prenatal diagnosis of alpha-thalassemia by polymerase chain reaction and dual restriction enzyme analysis, *Hum Genet* 85(3):293-299, 1990.

McDuffie RS et al: Effect of frequency of prenatal care visits on perinatal outcome among low-risk women: a randomized controlled trial, *JAMA* 275(11):847-851, 1996.

McDuffie RS et al: Does reducing the number of prenatal office visits for low-risk women result in increased use of other medical services? *Obstet Gynecol* 90(1):68-70, 1997.

Nevo Y et al: Fetal muscle biopsy as a diagnostic tool in Duchenne muscular dystrophy, *Prenat Diagn* 19(10):921-926, 1999.

Omar MA, Schiffman RF: Pregnant women's perceptions of prenatal care, *Matern Child Nurs* 23(4):132-142, 1995.

Orr ST et al: Psychosocial stressors and low birthweight in an urban population, *Am J Prev Med* 12(6):459-466, 1996.

Peoples-Sheps MD, Hogan VK, Ng'andu N: Content of prenatal care during the initial workup, *Am J Obstet Gynecol* 174(1):220-226, 1996.

Pritchard CW, Teo PY: Preterm birth, low birthweight and the stressfulness of the household role for pregnant women, *Soc Sci Med* 38(1):89-96, 1994.

Raine T, Powell S, Krohn MA: The risk of repeating low birth weight and the role of prenatal care, *Obstet Gynecol* 84(4):485-489, 1994.

Thomas H et al: Evaluation of an integrated community antenatal clinic, *J R Coll Gen Pract* 305(37):544-547, 1987.

Thompson JE: Health education during prenatal care. In Merkatz IR, Thompson JE, editors: *New perspectives on prenatal care,* New York, 1990, Elsevier, pp 549-582.

Villar J, Bergsjo P: Scientific basis for the content of routine antenatal care. I. Philosophy, recent studies, and power to eliminate or alleviate maternal outcomes, *Acta Obstet Gynecol Scand* 76:1-14, 1997.

Walker DS, Koniak-Griffin D: Evaluation of a reduced-frequency prenatal visit schedule for low-risk women at a free-standing birthing center, *Nurse Midwifery* 42(4):295-303, 1997.

Wood N et al: Diagnosis of sickle-cell disease with a universal heteroduplex generator, *Lancet* 8886-8887(342):1519-1529, 1993.

Chapter 9

Screening for Maternal Risk Factors During Pregnancy

Prenatal care includes procedures and interventions to screen for and diagnose perinatal problems or potential problems. Screening includes activities that assess the psychosocial and physical status of the pregnant woman. It is essential that the clinician understand the rationale for these recommended screening practices, as well as the limitations inherent in their use. Screening and diagnostic measures used to directly assess fetal status are addressed in Chapter 13.

SCREENING FOR PSYCHOSOCIAL FACTORS THAT INFLUENCE MATERNAL AND INFANT HEALTH

Psychosocial factors have been recognized as direct influences on pregnancy outcome (e.g., the association between stress, low birth weight, and preterm labor) and indirect influences on the woman's experience during pregnancy (e.g., the association between poverty and access to prenatal care). The majority of births that result in a preterm or low birth-weight infant are to women who have no "medical" risk factors but who are at high risk because of "social" factors (Misra and Guyer, 1998). Research suggests that women who are screened for psychosocial risk factors once each trimester are half as likely to have a low-birth-weight baby when compared to women who were not screened (Wilkinson, Korenbrot, and Greene, 1998). Numerous panels and professional organizations have recommended routine screening for psychosocial risk factors during pregnancy (Expert Panel on the Content of Prenatal Care, 1989). Research suggests that such routine screening is not consistently done, with one study estimating that only about half of pregnant women receive assessment and counseling regarding health and lifestyle behaviors during the initial prenatal visit (Peoples-Shep, Hogan, and Ng'andu, 1996). Many physicians have little training in identifying and managing psychosocial issues, and this fact may explain the lower rates of assessment for these risk factors (American College of Obstetricians and Gynecologists, 1999).

Although it is considered important to routinely assess for psychosocial risk factors, there are no screening tools that have demonstrated satisfactorily high degrees of sensitivity and specificity (American College of Obstetricians and Gynecologists, 1999). Until research has identified a valid and reliable screening mechanism, providers will continue to obtain psychosocial data through personal interviews.

Demographic Factors

Family income and maternal age, parity, education, marital status, and race are all associated with inadequate prenatal care (Goldenberg, Patterson, and Freese, 1992).

Women younger than 20 years of age are less likely to obtain early and consistent prenatal care, often because of access problems. Women older than 35 years of age also are at increased risk for inadequate prenatal care, often because the healthy multiparous woman does not perceive the need to have frequent provider visits to establish that the pregnancy is progressing normally. Likewise, women who are already mothering several children may have fewer visits because of the perception that prenatal care is not necessary or because of access barriers such as lack of child care or transportation. Lower level of education, particularly when associated with young age, is strongly associated with inadequate prenatal care. Even with the creation of expanded medical assistance programs for pregnant women, women living below the poverty level have increased rates of inadequate care. Poverty continues to be a co-variable with numerous other factors that are associated with poor pregnancy outcome. Race as a risk factor also is strongly related with factors associated with poverty, although some research findings suggest that physiologic differences among races may also play a role in indicators such as low birth weight.

Community Factors

Nonfinancial barriers to care include lack of transportation (especially in rural areas), limited clinical hours or hours that conflict with women's typical work schedules, and lack of child care. When these factors are identified, referral to appropriate community resources is warranted. Community assessment should also include consideration of the influence of environmental factors on the woman and her infant. Substandard housing, poor sanitation, industrial pollution, and exposure to toxins all may have a negative effect on maternal and fetal/neonatal health and development.

Lifestyle Behaviors

Psychosocial assessment should include exploration of the woman's usual lifestyle, including nutrition and exercise; household and workplace activity; and use of tobacco, alcohol, and drugs. Nutritional assessment is discussed in Chapter 11. Exploration of activity should identify whether the woman participates in regular, planned exercise or in activities that may increase the risk for her and her fetus. Exercise that is vigorous enough to inhibit normal weight gain is associated with intrauterine growth restriction of the fetus. Lack of exercise may be associated with increased weight gain, decreased tolerance to the work of labor, and decreased sense of well-being.

The provider should not assume that, because a woman is not employed outside the home, she doesn't "work." Caring for small children, particularly several under the age of six, is demanding work. Women providing child care for children other than their own also are at increased risk for exposure to infectious diseases.

The effects of tobacco, alcohol, and drug use in pregnancy have been widely reported. All women should be screened for prepregnancy and current use of these substances. Women who smoke or use alcohol or drugs should be offered referrals to cessation programs. The clinician should also identify whether the woman's partner or other householders use these substances. Exploration of the physical environment in which she lives, as well as the relationship status and family culture, will assist in identifying other factors that will have direct and indirect influences on the woman's substance use.

Sexual behaviors should be assessed to identify risk factors, including number of current and past partners, history of sexually transmitted infections, and participation in activities that increase risk for injury to the woman or her fetus. Women who are not in mutually monogamous relationships should be counseled regarding the risk of infections and use of safer sex practices.

Violence in the Community and Home

Community assessment should identify threats to individuals and groups, including gang activity and increased incidence of violent crimes. Although the provider most likely is not in the position to change community attributes, she or he can explore strategies to increase the safety of the woman in her environment.

The incidence of physical abuse during pregnancy ranges from 1% to 20% (Cokkinides et al., 1999), and many professional groups have advocated screening all women for intimate partner violence. Research suggests that intimate partner violence may escalate during pregnancy and the postpartum period. Because of this, screening should be done at the initial prenatal visit and at least once during each trimester. Screening is also indicated when a woman has bruising or improbable injury or is in a depressed mood (American College of Obstetricians and Gynecologists, 1999). The three-question Abuse Assessment Screen has been shown to be effective in identifying women at increased risk for injury at the hands of the intimate partner (McFarlane, Parker, and Soeken, 1995) (Figure 9-1).

ABUSE ASSESSMENT SCREEN

1. Have you ever been emotionally or physically abused by your partner or someone important to you?
☐ Yes ☐ No

2. Within the last year, have you been pushed, shoved, slapped, hit, kicked or otherwise physically hurt by someone? If yes, by whom?
☐ Yes ☐ No

☐ Husband/ex-husband ☐ Parent/Step-parent
☐ Boyfriend/ex-boyfriend ☐ Other relative
☐ Stranger ☐ Sibling ☐ Multiple

3. Since the pregnancy began, have you been pushed, shoved, slapped, hit, kicked or otherwise physically hurt by someone? If yes, by whom?
☐ Yes ☐ No

☐ Husband/ex-husband ☐ Parent/Step-parent
☐ Boyfriend/ex-boyfriend ☐ Other relative
☐ Stranger ☐ Sibling ☐ Multiple

4. Within the last year, has anyone forced you to have sex? If yes, by whom? ☐ Yes ☐ No

☐ Husband/ex-husband ☐ Parent/Step-parent
☐ Boyfriend/ex-boyfriend ☐ Other relative
☐ Stranger ☐ Sibling ☐ Multiple

Additional data can be gathered by asking the following:
How long have you been in the relationship?
How many times have you been pushed, shoved, slapped, hit, kicked or otherwise physically hurt by someone?
Can you mark the area of injury on this figure of the body?

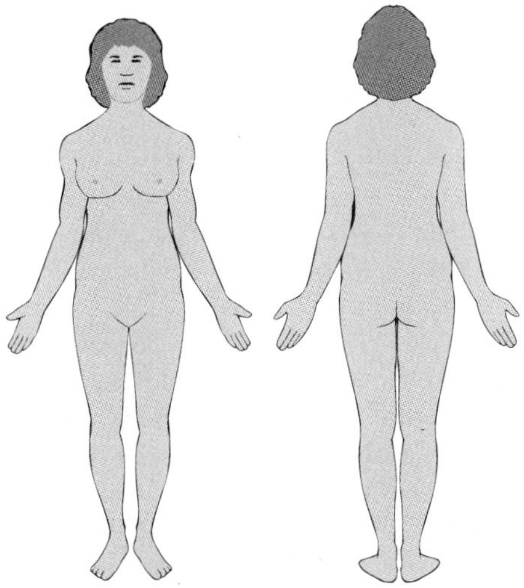

Figure 9-1 Abuse assessment screen. Redrawn from McFarland J, Parker B: Preventing abuse during pregnancy: an assessment and intervention protocol, *MCN* 19(6):321, 1994.

SCREENING USING PHYSICAL ASSESSMENT

Complete Physical Examination

Since many women use their nurse-midwife or obstetrician-gynecologist as their primary care provider, reproductive care visits provide a unique opportunity for general health screening (Nagey, 1989). Health deviations not associated with pregnancy and those that may affect the course of pregnancy or may be affected by pregnancy can be identified through the physical examination. Examples of primary care problems that are commonly identified during prenatal examinations include enlarged lymph nodes, thyroid enlargement or nodules, breast masses, cardiac murmurs, skin lesions, and vascular disorders.

Maternal Blood Pressure

Determining blood pressure, particularly in the last trimester of pregnancy, was one of the early screening measures incorporated into prenatal care to identify women with preeclampsia. Following the trend of blood pressure throughout pregnancy continues to be a tool to identify hypertensive disorders in pregnancy that require further intervention.

The practitioner needs to ensure that the procedure used for obtaining blood pressure in pregnant women is consistent in both the optimal positioning of the arm and the use of an appropriate size cuff. Study findings suggest that the mean blood pressure is lowest when the arm is supported at heart height and highest when the arm is dependent (Terent and Breig-Asberg, 1994; Wall-Manning and Paulin, 1987). The pregnant woman should be seated in a way that the arm can be comfortably rested on a table or arm of the chair. Taking blood pressure when the arm is in a dependent position will lead to overdiagnosis of hypertensive disorders.

It is essential that an appropriate-size cuff be used. Too narrow or too short a cuff bladder causes overestimation of blood pressure (undercuffing), whereas too wide or too long a cuff causes underestimation of blood pressure (overcuffing) (Sprafka et al., 1991). When a size other than the average cuff routinely used in the clinic setting is necessary, the size should be noted in the woman's record so that all staff checking the blood pressure are consistent in sizing the cuff.

It is common for staff to have the woman rest on her left size if an elevated blood pressure is noted. The blood pressure is then repeated while she is still in the left lateral position. This practice leads to false reassurance and inaccurate comparisons of blood pressure readings. Repeat blood pressures may be appropriate when a woman's activity or emotional status immediately before the blood pressure determination was known to be a factor associated with transient increases in pressure. However, it is essential that the repeat measure be done with the same appropriately-size cuff in the same sitting position with a supported arm.

! Clinical Alert

Medical consultation and/or referral is recommended for the following findings:

- Blood pressure 140/90 on two separate occasions at least 6 hours apart
- Increase in systolic pressure of >30 mm Hg above baseline (prepregnant or first trimester level)
- Increase in diastolic pressure of >15 mm Hg above baseline (prepregnant or first trimester level)
- Immediate consultation recommended for diastolic pressure >110 mm Hg

Maternal Height, Weight, and Body Mass Index Assessment

Establishing weight at each prenatal visit was also an early component of prenatal care. Rapid weight gain of greater than 2 pounds per week was associated with edema and therefore used as a further sign of preeclampsia. However, as the medical model of care increasingly influenced prenatal care, weight became a proxy indicator for nutrition. It has been suggested that medical recommendations regarding restrictive weight gain in pregnancy were used as a method of control by physicians rather than an intervention based on sound scientific evidence of benefit (Wertz and Wertz, 1977).

Weight should be obtained in a standardized way, using a balanced scale. Effort should be made to obtain weight at similar times of day in similar dress. Because of variation in weight of shoes, it is reasonable to obtain weights in stocking feet. When there is more than one scale in the clinical setting, efforts should be made to use the same scale for each measurement. In many practices women weigh themselves and record findings on the record. When this is done, a staff member can review the procedure to ensure consistency in the process. It is also essential to ensure that scales are situated in a place that allows privacy for the woman.

At the initial visit the woman's height and prepregnant weight should also be obtained. With height and

Table 9-1 *Weight Gain Recommendations by BMI*

Weight/height category	Pounds	Kilograms
Recommended Total Weight Gain		
Low (BMI <19.8)	28-40	12.5-18
Normal (BMI 19.8-26.0)	25-35	11.5-16
High (BMI > 26.0-29.0)	15-25	7.0-11.5

Adapted from National Academy of Sciences: Nutrition during pregnancy, Washington, DC, 1990, National Academy Press.
BMI, Body mass index.

weight, initial body mass index (BMI) can be determined. When prepregnant weight is unknown, weight at initial visit in first trimester may be substituted. BMI is defined as prepregnant weight/height^2 and is considered a better indicator of nutritional status than weight alone. Table 9-1 illustrates the recommended weight gain for each BMI category. Figure 9-2 is an example of one form to establish BMI.

Women with a history of eating disorders may be either very uncomfortable with obtaining weights or obsessive about weight determination. The practitioner may offer the option of not obtaining weights at every visit and substituting more frequent nutritional reviews to establish that adequate calories are being consumed.

Healthy patterns of weight gain are discussed in Chapter 11.

! Clinical Alert

Medical consultation is recommended for weight loss secondary to nausea and vomiting of pregnancy or secondary to weight loss caused by eating disorders.

Nutritional consultation is recommended for weight gain <10 pounds by 20 weeks' gestation, inconsistent weight gain, or excessive weight gain.

Uterine Sizing (Conception Through 12 Weeks' Gestational Age)

Uterine growth begins after implantation, and serial sizing of the uterus during the first trimester provides a systematic way to date the pregnancy and determine whether the growth is normal or not. Serial uterine sizing in the first trimester is done using bimanual examination of the pelvis. Expectant size of the uterus is illustrated in Figure 9-3. Accuracy of uterine sizing is enhanced when the client is relaxed and has an empty bladder and an anterior-positioned uterus. Sizing of the uterus provides data that either confirm the menstrual dating or raise suspicions regarding the expected date of delivery.

! Clinical Alert

Medical consultation is essential for diagnosis of missed abortion, ectopic pregnancy, multiple pregnancy, and trophoblastic disease.

Measurement of Fundal Height (12 Weeks Through Term)

Use of fundal height measurement to estimate gestational age is a skill that has been used by birth attendants for several centuries. Description of estimating uterine size using anatomic landmarks can be found in early texts published since the eighteenth century. By the early twentieth century, it became clear that there was significant variation in the landmarks used, so efforts were made to develop more accurate means for assessment. Measuring the distance between the symphysis pubis and the uterine fundus using calipers or a measuring tape measure became integrated into practice to obtain more reliable measurements.

MacDonald first described the use of a measuring tape in the first decade of the twentieth century. He described using the fingers of one hand to hold the end of the tape on the upper border of the symphysis while the fingers of the second hand are placed perpendicular to the uppermost part of the uterine fundus. The tape grasped by the fundal hand is pressed into the palm of the hand so that the tape is in contact with the maternal abdomen for the length of the uterus except for the "last dip" (Engstrom and Sittler, 1993). Spalding used a similar method of tape measurement; but he had the superior hand rest at the ensiform cartilage while reading the measurement corresponding to the upper most border of the fundus. Neither of these methods included the uppermost curve of the fundus, which is usually easily palpable.

The use of calipers to measure fundal height was introduced to increase accuracy. One tip of the instrument is placed on the superior aspect of the symphysis pubis, and the other is placed at to uppermost central aspect of the fundus. Research suggests that the use of calipers may improve reliability (Engstrom, McFarlin, and Sittler, 1993), but the instrument is less portable and more awkward than a tape measure.

Fundal height measurement using a tape measure most commonly uses one of two techniques. The first (Figure 9-4, *A*) involves holding the zero-mark of the tape measure on the superior aspect of the symphysis pubis and stretching the tape measure longitudinally along the central aspect of the uterus to the top of the fundus. The tape is held in contact with the skin and follows the superior curve of the fundus. Data suggest that this method may have improved intraexaminer and interexaminer reliability (Engstrom, McFarlin, and Sittler,

Body Mass Index (BMI)

Weight	Height (ft., in.)																
(lb.)	4'10"	4'11"	5'0"	5'1"	5'2"	5'3"	5'4"	5'5"	5'6"	5'7"	5'8"	5'9"	5'10"	5'11"	6'0"	6'1"	6'2"
125	26	25	24	24	23	22	22	21	20	20	19	18	18	17	17	17	16
130	27	26	25	25	24	23	22	22	21	20	20	19	19	18	18	17	17
135	28	27	26	26	25	24	23	23	22	21	21	20	19	19	18	18	17
140	29	28	27	27	26	25	24	23	23	22	21	21	20	20	19	19	18
145	30	29	28	27	27	26	25	24	23	23	22	21	21	20	20	19	19
150	31	30	29	28	27	27	26	25	24	24	23	22	22	21	20	20	19
155	32	31	30	29	28	28	27	26	25	24	24	23	22	22	21	20	20
160	34	32	31	30	29	28	28	27	26	25	24	24	23	22	22	21	21
165	35	33	32	31	30	29	28	28	27	26	25	24	24	23	22	22	21
170	36	34	33	32	31	30	29	28	28	27	26	25	24	24	23	22	22
175	37	35	34	33	32	31	30	29	28	27	27	26	25	24	24	23	23
180	38	36	35	34	33	32	31	30	29	28	27	27	26	25	25	24	23
185	39	37	36	35	34	33	32	31	30	29	28	27	27	26	25	24	24
190	40	38	37	36	35	34	33	32	31	30	29	28	27	27	26	25	24
195	41	39	38	37	36	35	34	33	32	31	30	29	28	27	27	26	25
200	42	40	39	38	37	36	34	33	32	31	30	30	29	28	27	26	26
205	43	41	40	39	38	36	35	34	33	32	31	30	29	29	28	27	26
210	44	43	41	40	38	37	36	35	34	33	32	31	30	29	29	28	27
215	45	44	42	41	39	38	37	36	35	34	33	32	31	30	29	28	28
220	46	45	43	42	40	39	38	37	36	35	34	33	32	31	30	29	28
225	47	46	44	43	41	40	39	38	36	35	34	33	32	31	31	30	29
230	48	47	45	44	42	41	40	38	37	36	35	34	33	32	31	30	30
235	49	48	46	44	43	42	40	39	38	37	36	35	34	33	32	31	30
240	50	49	47	45	44	43	41	40	39	38	37	36	35	34	33	32	31
245	51	50	48	46	45	43	42	41	40	38	37	36	35	34	33	32	32
250	52	51	49	47	46	44	43	42	40	39	38	37	36	35	34	33	32
255	53	52	50	48	47	45	44	43	41	40	39	38	37	36	35	34	33
260	54	53	51	49	48	46	45	43	42	41	40	38	37	36	35	34	33
265	56	54	52	50	49	47	46	44	43	42	40	39	38	37	36	35	34
270	57	55	53	51	49	48	46	45	44	42	41	40	39	38	37	36	35
275	58	56	54	52	50	49	47	46	44	43	42	41	40	38	37	36	35
280	59	57	55	53	51	50	48	47	45	44	43	41	40	39	38	37	36
285	60	58	56	54	52	51	49	48	46	45	43	42	41	40	39	38	37
290	61	59	57	55	53	51	50	48	47	46	44	43	42	41	39	38	37
295	62	60	58	56	54	52	51	49	48	46	45	44	42	41	40	39	38
300	63	61	59	57	55	53	52	50	48	47	46	44	43	42	41	40	39
305	64	62	60	58	56	54	52	51	49	48	46	45	44	43	41	40	39
310	65	63	61	59	57	55	53	52	50	49	47	46	45	43	42	41	40
315	66	64	62	60	58	56	54	53	51	49	48	47	45	44	43	42	41
320	67	65	63	61	59	57	55	53	52	50	49	47	46	45	43	42	41
325	68	66	64	62	60	58	56	54	53	51	50	48	47	45	44	43	42

Figure 9-2 Body mass index. (Redrawn from Mayo Clinic.)

1993). The second approach (Figure 9-4, *B*) involves using the ulnar surface of the superior hand to identify the uppermost part of the fundus, then bringing the tape over the fundal hand or between the middle and index fingers while holding the opposite end of the measure in place on the superior symphysis (Varney, 1997; Engstrom and Chen, 1984; Engstrom and Sittler, 1993). Variability between examiners in both methods may account for differences in measurement of ±1 to 2 cm.

Maternal position affects the measurements obtained by tape method. Measurements in the supine position are the greatest, whereas measurements with knee flexion are the smallest (Engstrom et al., 1993). Maternal bladder volume can also affect measurements. Research findings suggest that prevoid fundal height measurements are significantly larger than postvoid measurements (Engstrom et al., 1989). Women should be instructed to void within 30 minutes of the examination to obtain more accurate measurements.

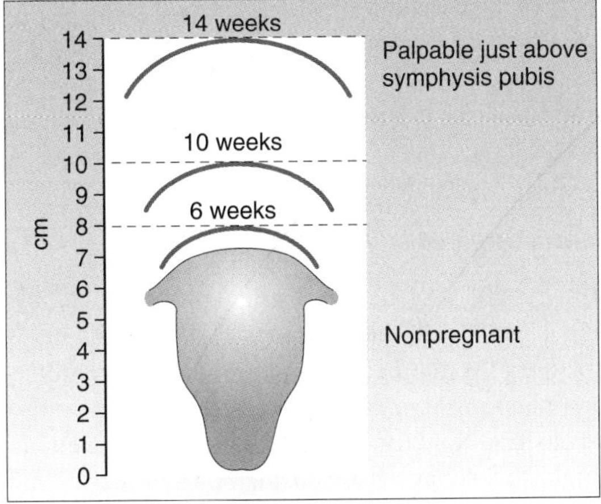

Figure 9-3 Uterine growth in first trimester.

Other factors that affect fundal height measurements include maternal obesity, maternal abdominal tone, parity, fetal lie, fetal position, amniotic fluid volume, and myomata. In interpreting the fundal height measurement, the clinician must always consider those factors in order to make a reasoned judgment regarding the accuracy of the findings. Ideally fundal height measurements should be obtained by the same clinician using the same technique at each prenatal visit. Realistically this is not possible in most of the current health delivery systems. Therefore, to decrease errors in interpretation of fundal height measurement findings, practices should consider developing guidelines to ensure uniform procedures for obtaining fundal height measurements.

! Clinical Alert

Further diagnostic studies are warranted if fundal height is greater than ±2 cm of the weeks' gestation between 20 and 36 weeks without other indication for discrepancy (e.g., transverse lie).

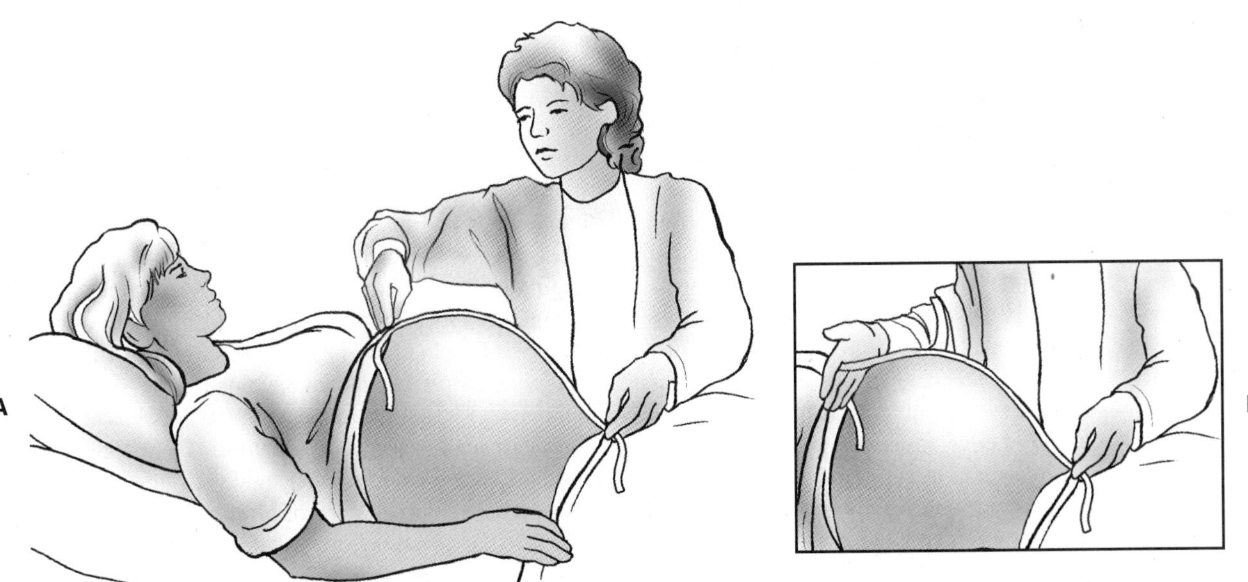

Figure 9-4, **A** and **B**, Hand positions for fundal height measurement.

Abdominal Examination of the Pregnant Uterus

Abdominal examination of the pregnant uterus involves a comprehensive examination that assesses maternal and fetal characteristics. Examination begins with inspection of the abdomen, with particular notation of scars or other lesions. Inspection also allows for a general appraisal of contours and may identify fetal movement. A longitudinal ovoid shape of the uterus suggests a longitudinal lie, whereas a more transverse ovoid appearance suggests a transverse or oblique lie. A smooth contour suggests that the fetal back is anterior; irregular contour, particularly with a slight depression superior to the symphysis pubis, suggests that the fetal back is posterior.

Before palpation the examiner rests one of the examining hands on the woman's abdomen. This serves to help the woman relax for the examination and provides information on uterine tone. During the late third trimester, the uterus may be sensitive to touch, and palpation may produce contractility. The examiner should await relaxation of the uterus before palpating the fetal lie, presentation, and position.

Abdominal examination also includes the performance of Leopold maneuvers (see below), estimation of fetal weight, and auscultation of fetal heart rate.

Leopold Maneuvers for Lie, Presentation, Position, and Attitude

Palpation of the uterus to determine fetal lie, presentation, position, and attitude is possible starting in late second trimester. A systematic scheme of abdominal palpation (Leopold maneuvers) allows the clinician to assess these fetal characteristics. Palpation of the uterus may also allow the examiner to perceive fetal movement and estimate fetal weight (Research Box 9-1).

Evaluation of the accuracy of Leopold maneuvers has yielded mixed results. Thorp, Jenkins, and Watson (1991) compared findings from palpation with determination of fetal presentation by ultrasound and concluded that the technique performed poorly. Sensitivity, specificity, positive predictive value, and negative predictive value were 28%, 94%, 24%, and 95%, respectively, in a population with a prevalence of noncephalic presentation of 7%. The study findings reflect the skill of one physician considered to be at the skill level of a beginning resident in obstetrics and one perinatologist. No differences were noted in accuracy of findings when comparing the inexperienced and experienced clinicians. Conversely, Lydon-Rochelle and colleagues (1993) described the accuracy of Leopold maneuvers when used by experienced certified nurse-midwives and concluded that the technique was an effective tool for screening for malpresentation. Their data found that sensitivity, specificity, positive predictive value, and negative predictive value were 88%, 94%, 74%, and 97%, respectively, in a population with a 17% frequency of fetal malpresentation.

Leopold maneuvers are illustrated in Figure 9-5. Table 9-2 on p. 125 describes the maneuvers.

! Clinical Alert

Further diagnostic studies should be considered with persistent malposition in third trimester or when the presenting part remains out of the pelvis at term in a nullipara to rule out placenta previa, fetal anomalies, or uterine anomalies.

Estimating Fetal Weight

Estimation of fetal weight is a care process that may influence management decisions when assessing fetal growth during the late second and third trimesters and when planning for delivery. Palpation of the fetal outline has traditionally been used to estimate weight, although studies have also considered the effectiveness of symphysis-fundal height measurements and abdominal girth measurements. Neither of these has proven useful because of low sensitivity, specificity, positive predictive value, and negative predictive value. More recently, ultrasound studies have been used to estimate fetal weight when small-for-gestational-age and large-for-gestational-age fetuses are suspected.

Studies have suggested that there is no advantage to using ultrasound estimations of weight in late third trimester, particularly in the identification of macrosomic infants (Pollack, Hauer-Pollack, and Divon, 1992). Clinical estimation of weight using palpation and ultrasound imaging has been shown to have no significant difference in accuracy of findings (Raman, Urquhart, and Yusof, 1992; Chauhan et al., 1992; Watson, Soisson, and Harlass, 1988). Even when the woman is obese, there is no advantage to ultrasound estimations of fetal weight when compared to clinical estimations (Field, Piper, and Langer, 1995). There is also evidence that postterm parous women's predictions of birth weight are comparable to clinical estimation, and both estimates may be more accurate than ultrasound estimations (Chauhan et al., 1995). These results suggest that clinicians would be

Research Box 9-1

Lydon-Rochelle M et al: Accuracy of Leopold maneuvers in screening for malpresentation: a prospective study, *Birth* 20(3):132-135, 1993.

Background

Leopold maneuvers are commonly used to screen for malpresentations in late pregnancy. Two previous studies reported poor sensitivity (28% and 53%) and specificity (94% in each). The gold standard for determining fetal presentation is ultrasound scanning, but this requires special equipment and operator training, and its use increases the costs of prenatal care.

Research Question

What is the accuracy of Leopold maneuvers in screening for malpresentations in the third trimester?

Methods

Women arriving in a perinatal ultrasound unit for a third-trimester scan were invited to participate in a study of the use of Leopold maneuvers for determining position of the baby. A prospective comparative design was used in which each woman served as her own control. All women who participated had completed at least 27 weeks' gestation. Women were instructed not to discuss the reason for the ultrasound with the midwife doing the abdominal examination. The hospital's on-call midwife performed Leopold maneuvers and noted whether the fetus was cephalic or noncephalic. Additional data on parity, height, weight, and medical indication for ultrasound were collected after the abdominal examination. Presentation findings as determined by Leopold maneuvers were compared with presentation findings during the ultrasound examination.

Sample

One hundred women were receiving care in a southwest teaching hospital in which a disproportionate number of women enrolled for care after the first trimester. The mean gestational age for the participants was 33.9 weeks, the mean height was 63.9 inches, and the mean weight was 164.1 pounds.

Results

Four experienced midwives performed Leopold maneuvers on 150 women. Four participants had incomplete data and were excluded from analysis. Seventeen percent of the fetuses were in noncephalic positions. Sensitivity of Leopold maneuvers as a screening test for abnormal presentation was 88%; specificity was 94%. Positive predictive value was 74%, and negative predictive value was 97%.

Clinical Application

The relatively high sensitivity decreases the likelihood of missing a malpresentation, and the high specificity lowers the likelihood of excess ultrasound procedures for validation of presentation. Further procedures that increase the sensitivity and specificity of Leopold maneuvers include pelvic examination and having a second clinician assess the abdomen. Findings are limited by the fact that the four midwives who did the examinations were very experienced. The high levels of sensitivity and specificity may not be replicated in samples of clinicians who are less experienced or clinicians who tend to depend more on technology than on their hand skills.

wise to listen to the woman's perception of fetal weight during assessment of the fetus.

Recently there have been recommendations to consider elective cesarean section when the estimated fetal weight is greater than 4000 or 4500 g to decrease the risk of fetal trauma during vaginal birth. However, since ultrasound prediction of macrosomia has low positive predictive value and since the rate of shoulder dystocia is low even in large infants, this does not appear to be a sound approach (Benacerraf, Gelman, and Frigoletto, 1988; Pollack, Hauer-Pollack, and Divon, 1992). Some clinicians have called for elective induction when macrosomia is suspected in an attempt to prevent shoulder dystocia and other problems encountered with delivery of a large infant. Research findings suggest that use of induction of labor when ultrasound-determined findings of macrosomia are present is associated with increased cesarean section rate without decrease in shoulder dystocia (Combs, Singh, and Khoury, 1993). The conflicting findings of studies, along with the lack of evidence of benefit of making labor management decisions based on estimated birth weights determined by ultra-

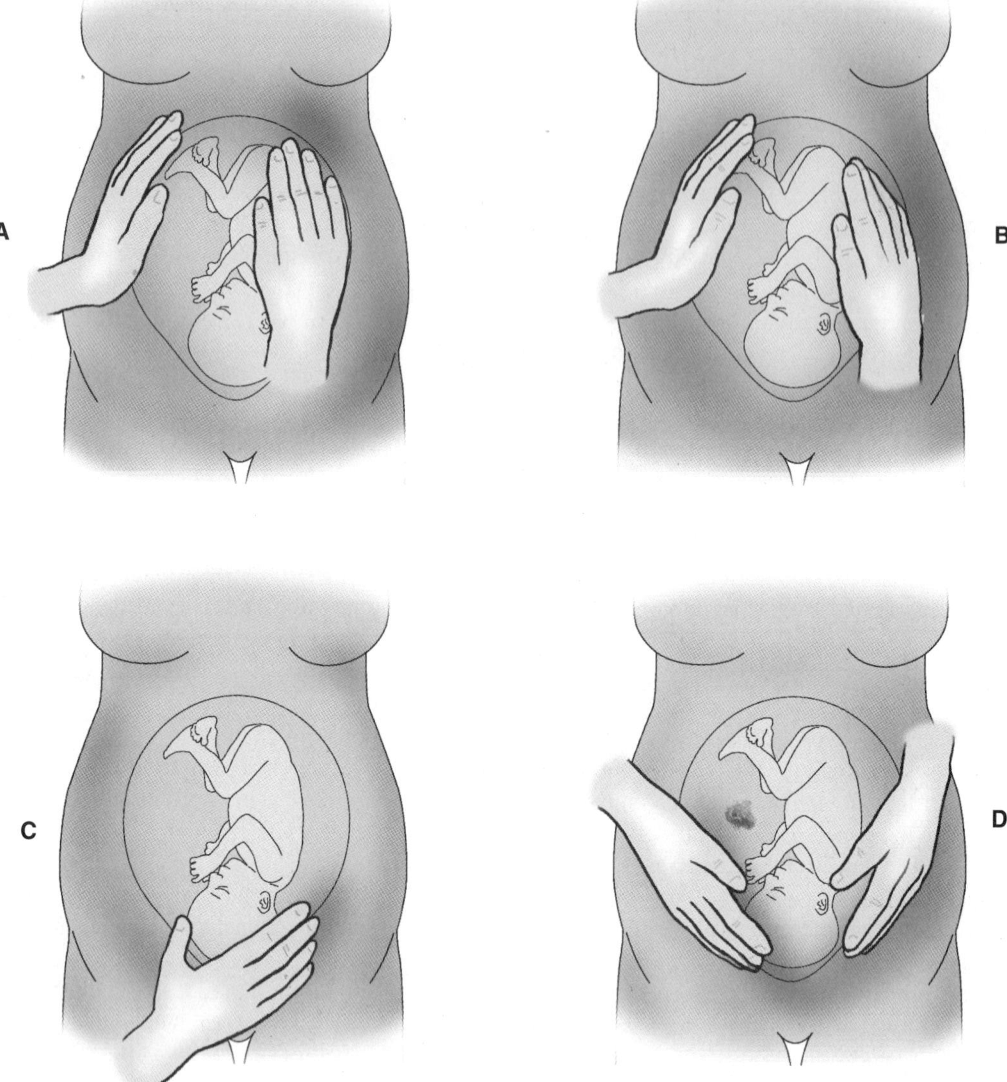

Figure 9-5 Leopold maneuvers. **A,** Determination of fetal part in fundus; **B,** determination of location of fetal back and "small parts"; **C,** determination of ballotability of presenting part; **D,** determination of degree of descent of pelvis.

sound alone, should remind the clinician to consider multiple techniques for estimation of birth weight rather than relying on technology alone.

Becoming accurate in estimation of fetal weight by palpation requires practice and on-going use of the skill. The beginning clinician can use several techniques to develop the skill of assessing fetal size.

1. Palpate the size of the fetus in early labor and compare with birth weight.
2. Palpate swaddled babies in the nursery and compare estimate with the daily weight or birth weight.
3. Make bags of flour or sugar in weights of 3 to 10 pounds in 1-pound increments. Close your eyes and palpate the bags, paying attention to bulk as well as the absolute weight.

! Clinical Alert

Further diagnostic investigation is warranted when clinical assessment raises suspicion of a small-for-gestational-age or large-for-gestational-age fetus.

Table 9-2 *Leopold Maneuvers*

First Maneuver	
Palpate upper part of uterus with both hands to identify fetal part(s) in fundus.	Determines lie and presentation; the fetal head (vertex) is a hard, ballotable sphere; the breech is irregularly shaped and softer than the head
Second Maneuver	
With one hand push the fetus toward the opposing hand. Use the opposing hand to palpate the opposite side of the uterus with firm, circular motions. A smooth, firm surface indicates the fetal back; knobby parts indicate fetal "small parts" such as knees, feet, elbows. A skilled clinician can also identify fetal thighs and shins. Repeat maneuver, examining contents of opposite side of uterus.	Determines the position of the fetal landmarks that identify whether the fetus is in a left or right position (e.g., LOA, ROA, LOT, ROT, LOP, ROP)
Third Maneuver	
Use the thumb and fingers of one hand to grasp the fetal part just above the symphysis pubis. Attempt to move it side to side to ascertain whether it moves independently of the body of the fetus (fetal head). This move also identifies whether the presenting part is firm and globular (fetal head) or softer and more irregular (breech). In addition, this provides information on whether the presenting part is beginning to descend into the pelvis. Some clinicians stabilize the fetal part in the fundus with the other hand to better appreciate whether the presenting part is ballotable.	Confirms findings of first maneuver
Fourth Maneuver	
Face the woman's feet. Take both hands and slide them down the sides of the uterus, noting the degree to which the presenting part is descending into the pelvis. In a vertex presentation the examiner may also identify the cephalic prominence.	Provides information about fetal attitude (flexion or extension of the fetal head) and descent of the head into the pelvis

Auscultation of Fetal Heart Tones

Auscultation of fetal heart rate has traditionally been done with a stethoscope, but more recently, portable Doppler devices have been introduced to clinical use. Evaluating the rate and rhythm of fetal heart movements has been used not only to establish viability but also as an indicator of general fetal health status. Antepartum assessment of fetal heart rate patterns is an indirect measure of placental function, the integrity of the fetal nervous system, and cardiac function. Developmental maturity of the fetal system also allows the clinician to assess the fetus's reaction to stimuli. A fetus that is well oxygenated through normal uteroplacental function, that has an intact central nervous system, and that has normal cardiac structures will demonstrate an increase in heart rate with fetal movement. Fetal heart acceleration associated with fetal movement depends on integration of peripheral receptors, spinal cord, brain, autonomic nervous system, and myocardial fibers (Druzin, 1992).

As noted in Chapter 7, fetal heart tones can first be heard using a stethoscope between 17 and 19 weeks' gestation. Depending on sensitivity of the equipment and maternal habitus, fetal heart tones may be heard as early as 10 to 12 weeks' menstrual age with a doptone device.

Early auscultation of fetal heart tones indicates viability but can only give a crude indication of dating because of variances in maternal size and instrument sensitivity. Use of rate and rhythms to assess fetal status is not possible until central nervous system maturity develops in the late second trimester.

Fetal heart tones should be auscultated for 30 to 60 seconds to determine periodic changes in rate or rhythm. Normal range of fetal heart rate is 110 to 160 beats/min, with the rate more consistently in the high range of normal in the first half of pregnancy. Irregularities may indicate cardiac structure anomalies that can be identified through ultrasonographic anatomic scans and fetal echocardiography.

! Clinical Alert

Referral for further perinatal evaluation is indicated when the clinician auscultates abnormal fetal heart rhythms or rate.

Assessment for Edema

Assessment for edema is done at each visit after 20 weeks' gestation. Although some dependent edema is normal in pregnancy, generalized edema and edema concurrent with proteinuria and/or increased blood pressure is not normal and needs further evaluation.

Inspection for edema should be done in a systematic way to decrease interexaminer and intraexaminer variation.

1. Inspect the woman's general appearance for signs of edema.
2. Apply pressure on the woman's hands, pretibial area, and ankles with thumb or index finger for several seconds. Release pressure and assess the depth of the depression and the amount of time it takes for the depression to disappear.
3. Grade the edema on the following scale:

Trace	Minimal edema of the lower extremities with no residual depression after release of pressure
1+	Minimal edema of the lower extremities with minimal residual depression after release of pressure
2+	Marked edema of lower extremities
3+	Edema of lower extremities, face, and hands
4+	Generalized massive edema (Nichols and Zwelling, 1997)

When increasing edema is noted or when the woman presents with a new finding of marked edema, deep tendon reflexes (DTRs) should be assessed. Determination of baseline DTRs is essential when following a woman at risk for preeclampsia.

! Clinical Alert

Medical consultation is recommended for dependent edema not responsive to elevation of the extremities and for generalized edema.

SCREENING USING LABORATORY OR SPECIAL PROCEDURES

Urine Screening for Protein and Glucose

Evaluation for proteinuria at prenatal visits was recommended as early as 1903 as a way to identify preeclampsia. It has become routine to check for proteinuria with reagent dipsticks, but there are little data to indicate that this practice is necessary in women without risk factors for or signs of hypertensive disorders (Gribble, Fee, and Berg, 1995).

Most urine reagent strips for identification of proteinuria rely on a process that uses a buffered chemical indicator (e.g., tetrabromophenol blue) that reacts in the presence of protein. Results are reported as Negative, Trace, 30 mg/dl (1+), 100 mg/dl (2+), 300 mg/dl (3+), and >2000 mg/dl (4+). The few studies that have evaluated the use of reagent strips as a screening tool have found that there is no correlation of proteinuria without other signs of preeclampsia (hypertension, edema) and development of preeclampsia in low-risk women. In women with known hypertensive disorders, it is suggested that the reagent strip may be used as a diagnostic test as opposed to a general screen (Gribble, Fee, and Berg, 1995).

Screening for proteinuria as an indicator of urinary tract infection has also become a routine practice. Data suggest that other tests are available on reagent strips that are much more sensitive and specific and have greater positive and negative predictive value than protein alone. Etherington (1993) found that presence of a positive nitrite screen has a 90% positive predictive value. Using multiple measures (leukocyte esterase/nitrite/protein, leukocyte esterase/nitrite/blood, nitrite/protein/blood, or leukocyte esterase/nitrite/protein/blood) produces a greater than 99% negative predictive value (Etherington, 1993).

Many clinical sites continue to use a urine culture as a diagnostic test for urinary tract infection. An advantage of this approach over screening is the identification of specific organisms. Although a disadvantage of this approach is the increased cost, identification of group B streptococcus (GBS) bacteriuria provides data that will influence clinical intrapartum management and measures to decrease the risk of neonatal GBS infection.

Although the routine for testing glucosuria as a means of diagnosing diabetes dates back to the early twentieth century, the correlation between urine and blood glucose is poor in pregnancy (Gribble, Meier, and Berg, 1995). Women who have positive glucose screens using reagent strips in the first two trimesters of pregnancy are more likely to have a diagnosis of gestational diabetes when blood glucose screening is done at 24 to 28 weeks' gestation. However, it is important to remember that only a small proportion of women who are diagnosed with gestational diabetes have glucosuria. Data suggest that glucosuria in third trimester is not associated with shoulder dystocia, cesarean section for dystocia, or rate of birth weight >4000 g, leading to a recommendation to eliminate glucosuria screening in the third trimester for women with a normal 24- to 28-week glucose screen (Gribble, Meier, and Berg, 1995).

! Clinical Alert

Further diagnostic testing for hypertensive disorders should be done when proteinuria is accompanied by hypertension and/or edema.

Further diagnostic testing should be done when repeated glucosuria is noted in the first and second trimesters.

Routine Screening for Perinatal Infections

Identification of women at risk for perinatal infections that have the potential for poor outcomes for both the woman and her fetus/newborn is an important component of prenatal care. Management of perinatal infections is discussed in depth in Unit 4, Collaborative Care of Complications in Pregnancy. This section will review the current recommendations for screening during prenatal care.

Syphilis. The early identification of maternal syphilis was a goal of the prenatal initiatives in the early twentieth century. The impact of the disease on the newborn was widely recognized, and once antibiotic therapy was determined to be effective in preventing many of the neonatal sequelae, it was thought that congenital syphilis could be eliminated. Unfortunately this goal has not been met, and the United States is experiencing an increase in the incidence of syphilis in some geographic areas (American Academy of Pediatrics. and American College of Obstetricians and Gynecologists, 1997). The Centers for Disease Control and Prevention (CDC) recommends serologic screening for syphilis for all women at the first prenatal visit, with a repeat screen in the third trimester and at delivery for women at increased risk for infection (Centers for Disease Control and Prevention, 1998a). This subgroup includes women with new or multiple sexual partners, women diagnosed with other sexually transmitted infections, and women living in communities with high prevalence of the disease.

Gonorrhea. Screening for gonorrhea in pregnant women also became an early public health effort to decrease neonatal morbidity. The CDC recommends that women at increased risk for sexually transmitted infections or living in communities with high prevalence be screened for gonorrhea at the initial prenatal visit. Women at increased risk for the disease should also be rescreened in the third trimester (Centers for Disease Control and Prevention, 1998a).

Chlamydia trachomatis. Screening for *Chlamydia* is a relatively recent prenatal intervention. The CDC recommends that women at risk for the disease, including women under 25 years of age and women with new or multiple sex partners or a sex partner with other partners, be screened in the third trimester to decrease the chance of neonatal morbidity. Women with a diagnosis of *Chlamydia* in early pregnancy have an increased risk of testing positive in late pregnancy (Allaire et al., 1998). Many professional organizations also recommend screening at-risk women at the initial prenatal visit. Universal screening for *Chlamydia* in pregnant women is not recommended (American Academy of Pediatrics and American College of Obstetricians and Gynecologists, 1997).

Hepatitis B virus. Routine screening for hepatitis B surface antigen (HBsAg) is well incorporated into prenatal care in the United States (Centers for Disease Control and Prevention, 1994). Infants born to mothers who have been infected with hepatitis B virus (HBV) are at high risk for perinatal HBV infection and chronic liver disease as adults. The American College of Obstetricians, Academy of Pediatrics, American Academy of Family Practice, and Advisory Committee on Immunization Practices all have recommended routine screening for HBsAg early in pregnancy to identify newborns who will need immunoprophylaxis. Women who screen negative but who are at increased risk for exposure to HBV during pregnancy should be rescreened in the third trimester (Centers for Disease Control and Prevention, 1998b). Pregnant women who screen negative may be offered the vaccination if they are at risk for exposure.

Hepatitis A virus. Since hepatitis A virus has little effect on pregnancy and is rarely transmitted to the fetus/neonate, routine screening in pregnancy is not warranted. Women living or traveling in areas in which the infection is common should consider hepatitis A vaccine as a preventive measure. Since the vaccine is produced from inactivated virus, the risk to the fetus is low (American Academy of Pediatrics and American College of Obstetricians and Gynecologists, 1997).

Hepatitis C virus. Screening for hepatitis C virus (HCV) is a serological test for HCV antibodies, with diagnostic enzyme immunoassay and radioactive immunoblock assay done when the individual screens positive. Routine screening for HCV is not recommended (American Academy of Pediatrics and American College of Obstetricians and Gynecologists, 1997; Centers for Disease Control and Prevention, 1998b). Pregnant women with a history of intravenous drug use, blood transfusion, or repeated exposure to blood products should be screened.

Herpes simplex virus. Routine screening for herpes simplex virus (HSV) is not warranted. Diagnostic cultures should be limited to suspected primary cases of HSV. Routine serial cultures in the third trimester are no longer recommended (Centers for Disease Control and Prevention, 1998a).

Human immunodeficiency virus. Since there are established medical benefits to screening, including reduction of perinatal transmission through the use of zidovudine, routine testing for all pregnant women should be offered (Centers for Disease Control and Prevention, 1998a). Because universal testing has not become a reality for a variety of legal and ethical reasons, the Institute of Medicine has recommended a national policy of universal human immunodeficiency virus (HIV) testing as a routine component of prenatal care (ACOG Executive Board, 1999; McCormick, Davidson, and Stoto, 1999). Until routine testing becomes incorporated into prenatal care, all women should be offered screening for HIV infection, with the option of anonymous testing when disclosure of the testing would have negative ramifications for the woman.

Human papillomavirus. Certain types of human papillomavirus are associated with the development of genital lesions, and, although transmission is rare, neonates are at risk of developing laryngeal papillomatosis following exposure to the virus during the birth process. Asymptomatic cases can be identified through the use of DNA diagnostic techniques. Pap smears are less sensitive in identifying subclinical cervical infection (American Academy of Pediatrics and American College of Obstetricians and Gynecologists, 1997). Since the risk to the fetus is small, there are currently no organizational recommendations for routine screening using laboratory methods. Physical examination identifies lesions in the infected woman.

Rubella. Screening for immune status for rubella is well incorporated into prenatal care. Since the public education system in the United States requires immunization against the disease, most adult women who were raised in this country are seropositive. The public health effort to eliminate the disease through immunization has dramatically decreased the incidence of congenital rubella. When a seronegative woman is exposed to rubella or develops symptoms suggestive of the disease during pregnancy, further testing is indicated to determine active infection. Serial serum testing for antibodies should be done at the time of exposure and 2 weeks following the first screen. In some cases an additional screen at 4 weeks after exposure is useful in determining infection status.

Varicella. Varicella is a relatively mild and self-limiting disease in childhood, but adults who acquire the disease may experience serious sequelae, including pneumonia and encephalitis (Centers for Disease Control and Prevention, 1996). When a pregnant woman develops varicella, the fetus may be affected. Further, when the disease occurs between 5 days before and 3 days after delivery, 20% of exposed newborns will develop neonatal varicella. Neonatal varicella is associated with a case fatality rate of 30% to 50% (Smith et al., 1998). Current immunization recommendations include the vaccination of all infants at 1 year of age, with "catch-up" of susceptible children up to 13 years of age. Most women of childbearing age are immune to varicella virus. However, if a woman gives a history of not having the disease previously and if she is seronegative, she should be counseled that she is at risk for developing the disease if she is exposed to the virus. Since the effects of the varicella vaccine virus on pregnancy are not known, vaccination during pregnancy is not recommended (Centers for Disease Control and Prevention, 1996). Vaccination on nonimmune women during the postpartum period appears to be a cost effective intervention (Smith et al., 1998).

Tuberculosis. Routine screening for tuberculosis in low-risk populations is not recommended. Screening for high-risk populations identifies women who will need treatment during the postpartum period. Individuals at increased risk for the infection include those with close contacts with infected persons; those foreign-born persons from areas in the world where tuberculosis is endemic (Asia, Africa, Latin America); medically underserved, low-income persons; intravenous drug users; and individuals in substandard and/or crowded living conditions (Centers for Disease Control and Prevention, 1995; U.S. Department of Health and Human Services, 1994).

Other Routine Screening Tests

Maternal serum alpha-fetoprotein/triple marker. An elevated maternal serum alpha-fetoprotein (MSAFP) in the second trimester is associated with neural tube defects and ventral wall defects in the fetus. Unexplained elevations in MSAFP are also associated with intrauterine fetal death, intrauterine growth restriction, fetal distress, placental abruption, oligohydramnios, and preeclampsia (Yaron et al., 1999). Decreased MSAFP levels are associated with trisomy 21 and trisomy 18. In an attempt to create a more sensitive screening test, hCG and estriol have been added to the screen, yielding the triple marker or expanded MSAFP test. Increased levels of human chorionic gonadotropin (hCG) in the second trimester are associated with an increased risk of preeclampsia and poor pregnancy outcomes. It appears that elevated values of MSAFP and serum hCG in women at low risk for poor perinatal outcomes are more predictive than elevated values in women with a priori increased risk (van Rijn et al., 1999). There is little in the literature addressing the significance of second trimester levels of estriol as a predictor of pregnancy outcome. One theory of the relationship of the triple marker levels and pregnancy outcome is that the abnormal findings may reflect placental abnormalities that contribute to the poor pregnancy outcomes (Yaron et al., 1999).

MSAFP screening has become a routine component of prenatal care, and most states provide state funding to follow up on abnormal screenings. However, because of concern over the relatively high false-positive rate, providers vary in the routine use of the screening. Findings of one study suggest that a high proportion patients cared for by obstetrician-gynecologists are screened (77% to 80%), and a lesser proportion are screened if they are cared for by nurse-midwives (64%) or family practice physicians (62%) (Yaron et al., 1999).

Triple marker screening should be offered to all women between 15 to 20 weeks' gestation. Counseling regarding use of the test as a screening tool should include an explanation of the possibility of a false positive and the further testing that is recommended when there are "screen positive" findings. In some settings a repeat of the screen will be done, whereas in others, women who screen positive will be offered immediate genetic counseling and further testing to rule out neural tube/ventral wall defects and chromosomal abnormalities.

Glucose screening. Screening for gestational diabetes mellitus (class A_1 gestational diabetes, GDM) has become standard practice in prenatal care. GDM is associated with increased perinatal morbidity, although there is not agreement on specific outcomes associated with the diagnosis. The most common outcome noted in the literature is excessive fetal growth (large for gestational age), which is usually defined as birth weight greater than the ninetieth percentile for gestational age. Some researchers have suggested that excess perinatal mortality and morbidity is found in a small subgroup of women whose fasting glucose levels are elevated and that GDM without fasting hyperglycemia is not a significant contributor to fetal and neonatal morbidity (Casey et al., 1997). Although screening for GDM has become a routine procedure in the United States, it is not clear whether its identification and the resulting interventions improve perinatal outcome (Khine, Winklestein, and Copel, 1999).

The American College of Obstetricians and Gynecologists (1994) has recommended selective screening for GDM in women younger than 30 years of age and routine screening for those older than 30 years of age. The Third International Workshop and Conference on Gestational Diabetes recommended universal screening of all pregnant women, and the American Diabetes Association (1999) recommends selective screening for women under 25 years of age and routine screening of all other pregnant women (Khine, Winklestein, and Copel, 1999). Risk factors for GDM used in selective

Table 9-3 *Cut-off Values for the 3-Hour Glucose Tolerance Test*

Fasting	> 95 mg/dl
1 hour	> 180 mg/dl
2 hour	>155 mg/dl
3 hour	>140 mg/dl

screening include glucosuria, random serum glucose greater than 130 mg/dl, history of gestational diabetes, macrosomia, polyhydramnios, strong family history of diabetes, history of large infants, and unexplained pregnancy losses. The use of selective screening in young populations (adolescents or women less than 25 years of age) is supported in the literature (Khine, Winklestein, and Copel, 1999; Kieffer et al., 1999).

Initial screening is done using a 50-g oral glucose test with a serum glucose drawn 1 hour after ingestion of the solution. Most institutions set the cutoff point at 140 mg/dl, although some physicians have called for determination of a positive screen when the value is greater than 125 mg/dl or 130 mg/dl. A diagnostic 100-g, 3-hour oral glucose tolerance test is used to evaluate those who screen positive, and a diagnosis of GDM is made when there are two abnormal values. Cutoff values for the 3-hour glucose tolerance test are noted in Table 9-3.

References

Allaire AD et al:. Initial and repeat screening for *Chlamydia trachomatis* during pregnancy, *Infect Dis Obstet Gynecol* 6(3):116-122, 1998.

American Academy of Pediatrics and American College of Obstetricians and Gynecologists: *Guidelines for perinatal care,* ed 4, Elk Grove, Ill, and Washington, DC, 1997, American Academy of Pediatrics and American College of Obstetricians and Gynecologists.

ACOG Executive Board: *Joint statement on human immunodeficiency virus screening (ACOG Statement of Policy),* Washington, DC, 1999, American College of Obstetricians and Gynecologists.

American College of Obstetricians and Gynecologists: *Management of diabetes in pregnancy (Technical Bulletin No. 200),* Washington DC, 1994, American College of Obstetricians and Gynecologists.

American College of Obstetricians and Gynecologists: *Psychological risk factors: perinatal screening and intervention (Educational Bulletin 255),* Washington, DC, 1999, American College of Obstetricians and Gynecologists.

American Diabetes Association: Gestational diabetes mellitus, *Diabetes Care* 22(suppl 1):S74-S76, 1999.

Benacerraf BR, Gelman R, Frigoletto FD: Sonographically estimated fetal weights: accuracy and limitation, *Am J Obstet Gynecol* 159(5):1118-1121, 1988.

Casey BM et al: Pregnancy outcomes in women with gestational diabetes compared with the general population, *Obstet Gynecol* 90(6):869-873, 1997.

Centers for Disease Control and Prevention: Epidemiologic notes and reports of maternal hepatitis B screening practices—California, Connecticut, Kansas, and United States, *MMWR* 43(17):311, 317-320, 1994.

Centers for Disease Control and Prevention: Essential components of a tuberculosis prevention and control program: recommendations of the Advisory Council for the Elimination of Tuberculosis, *MMWR* 44(RR-11):1-16, 1995.

Centers for Disease Control and Prevention: Prevention of varicella: recommendations of the Advisory Committee on Immunization Practices (ACIP), *MMWR* 45(RR 11):1-25, 1996.

Centers for Disease Control and Prevention: Guidelines for treatment of sexually transmitted diseases, *MMWR* 47 (RR1):1-118, 1998a.

Centers for Disease Control and Prevention: Recommendations for prevention and control of hepatitis C virus (HCV) infection and HCV-related chronic disease, *MMWR* 47(RR-19):1-39, 1998b.

Chauhan SP et al: Intrapartum detection of a macrosomic fetus: clinical versus 8 sonographic models, *Aust NZ J Obstet Gynecol,* 35(3):266-270, 1992.

Chauhan SP et al: Parous patients' estimation of birth weight in postterm pregnancy, *J Perinatol* 15(3):192-194, 1995.

Cokkinides VE et al: Physical violence during pregnancy: maternal complications and birth outcomes, *Obstet Gynecol* 93(5):661-666, 1999.

Combs CA, Singh NB, Khoury JC: Elective induction versus spontaneous labor after sonographic diagnosis of fetal macrosomia, *Obstet Gynecol* 81(4):492-496, 1993.

Druzin ML, editor: *Antepartum fetal assessment,* Boston, 1992, Blackwell Scientific Publications.

Engstrom JL, Chen EH: Prediction of birthweight by the use of extrauterine measurements during labor, *Res Nurs Health* 7(4):315-323, 1984.

Engstrom JL, Sittler CP: Fundal height measurement. Part 1: Techniques for measuring fundal height, *J Nurse Midwifery* 38(1):5-16, 1993.

Engstrom JL, McFarlin BL, Sittler CP: Fundal height measurement. Part 2: Intra- and interexaminer reliability of three measurement techniques, *J Nurse Midwifery* 38(1):17-22, 1993.

Engstrom JL et al: *Br J Obstet Gynaecol* 96(8):987-991, 1989.

Engstrom JL et al: Fundal height measurement. Part 3: The effect of maternal position on fundal height measurements, *J Nurse-Midwifery* 38(1):23-27, 1993.

Etherington IJ: Reagent strip testing of antenatal urine specimens for infection, *Br J Obstet Gynaecol* 100:806-808, 1993.

Expert Panel on the Content of Prenatal Care: *Caring for our future: the content of prenatal care,* Washington, DC, 1989, US Public Health Service.

Field NT, Piper JM, Langer O: The effect of maternal obesity on the accuracy of fetal weight estimation, *Obstet Gynecol* 86(1):102-107, 1995.

Goldenberg RL, Patterson ET, Freese MP: Maternal demographic, situational and psychosocial factors and their relationship to enrollment in prenatal care: a review of the literature, *Women Health* 19(2/3):133-151, 1992.

Gribble RK, Fee SC, Berg RL: The value of routine urine dipstick screening for protein at each prenatal visit, *Am J Obstet Gynecol* 173(1):214-217, 1995.

Gribble RK, Meier PR, Berg RL: The value of urine screening for glucose at each prenatal visit, *Obstet Gynecol* 86(3):405-410, 1995.

Khine ML, Winklestein A, Copel JA: Selective screening for gestational diabetes mellitus in adolescent pregnancies, *Obstet Gynecol* 93(5):738-742, 1999.

Kieffer EC et al: Glucose tolerance during pregnancy and birth weight in a Hispanic population, *Obstet Gynecol* 94(5):741-746, 1999.

Lydon-Rochelle M et al: Accuracy of Leopold maneuvers in screening for malpresentation: a prospective study, *Birth* 20(3):132-135, 1993.

McCormick MC, Davidson EC, Stoto MA: Preventing perinatal transmission of human immunodeficiency virus in the United States, *Obstet Gynecol* 94(5):795-798, 1999.

McFarlane J, Parker, B, Soeken K: Abuse during pregnancy: frequency, severity, perpetrator, and risk factors of homicide, *Public Health Nurs* 12(5):282-289, 1995.

Misra DP, Guyer B: Benefits and limitations of prenatal care, *JAMA* 279(20):1661-1662, 1998.

Nagey DA: The content of prenatal care, *Obstet Gynecol* 74(3):516-528, 1989.

Nichols FH, Zwelling E: *Maternal-newborn nursing—theory and practice,* Philadelphia, 1997, WB Saunders.

Peoples-Shep MD, Hogan VK, Ng'andu N: Content of prenatal care during the initial workup, *Am J Obstet Gynecol* 174(1 pt 1):220-226, 1996.

Pollack RN, Hauer-Pollack G, Divon MY: Macrosomia in postdates pregnancies: the accuracy of routine ultrasonographic screening, *Am J Obstet Gynecol* 167(1):7-11, 1992.

Raman S, Urquhart R, Yusof M: Clinical versus ultrasound estimation of fetal weight, *Aust NZ J Obstet Gynaecol* 32(3):196-199, 1992.

Smith WJ et al: Prevention of chickenpox in reproductive-age women: cost effectiveness of routine prenatal screening with postpartum vaccination of susceptibles, *Obstet Gynecol* 92(4):535-545, 1998.

Sprafka JM et al: The effect of cuff size on blood pressure measurement in adults, *Epidemiology* 2(3):214-217, 1991.

Terent A, Breig-Asberg E: Epidemiological perspective of body position and arm level in blood pressure measurement, *Blood Press* 3(3):156-163, 1994.

Thorp JM, Jenkins T, Watson W: Utility of Leopold maneuvers in screening for malpresentation, *Obstet Gynecol* 78(3):394-396, 1991.

US Department of Health and Human Services: *Core curriculum on tuberculosis: what every clinician should know,* ed 3, Atlanta, Ga, 1994, US Department of Health and Human Services.

van Rijn M et al: Adverse obstetric outcome in low- and high-risk pregnancies: predictive value of maternal serum screening, *Obstet Gynecol* 94(6):929-934, 1999.

Varney H: *Varney's midwifery,* ed 3, Boston, 1997, Jones and Bartlett Publishers.

Wall-Manning HJ, Paulin JM: Effects of arm position and support on blood pressure readings, *J Clin Hypertension* 3(4):624-630, 1987.

Watson WJ, Soisson AP, Harlass FE: Estimated weight of the term fetus: accuracy of ultrasound vs. clinical examination, *J Reprod Med* 33(4):369-371, 1988.

Wertz RW, Wertz DC: *Lying in,* New York, 1977, The Free Press.

Wilkinson DS, Korenbrot CC, Greene J: A performance indicator of psychosocial services in enhanced prenatal care of Medicaid-eligible women, *Matern Child Health J* 2:131-143, 1998.

Yaron Y et al: Second trimester maternal serum marker screening: maternal serum alpha-fetoprotein, beta-human chorionic gonadotropin, estriol, and their various combinations as predictors of pregnancy outcome, *Am J Obstet Gynecol* 181(4):968-974, 1999.

Chapter 10

Common Discomforts and Behavior Modifications in Pregnancy

Women experience a variety of discomforts throughout pregnancy. Most are related to the anatomic and physiologic changes that occur; others are related to the emotional aspects of pregnancy. Many self-care measures have been passed down through generations and often reflect the cultural meaning of pregnancy in the community. It is important for the clinician to recognize the likelihood that the woman has used self-care remedies before seeking the advice of the health care professional.

There is a paucity of research investigating the effectiveness of interventions used to relieve common discomforts. When research has been conducted, it has focused primarily on interventions based in the biomedical approach to care. This chapter offers suggestions found in a variety of sources with many recommending "alternative" or "natural" interventions. It is important to keep in mind that these time-held remedies need to be evaluated as fully as biomedical approaches before we can assure women that they are safe and effective.

When possible, discomforts are presented in terminology commonly used by women rather than medical terminology to reflect the usual presentation of the problem.

BACKACHE

Cause

Low backache is the most frequent muscular-skeletal problem reported in pregnancy. The progesterone- and relaxin-induced softening of joints, particularly along the spinal column, as well as the changing center of gravity as pregnancy progresses, contributes to the common complaint of backache. Upper backache is associated with the increased weight of the breasts and postural factors often associated with employment conditions. Lower backache is associated with the lordosis created when the increasing weight of the uterus pulls the spine out of alignment. Another type of pain, described by women as occurring in the posterior part of the pelvis distal and lateral to the lumbosacral junction, radiates to the posterior part of the thigh. This condition differs from sciatica in that it is not specific to the nerve root distribution and does not extend to the ankle or foot (Ostgaard, Andersson, and Miller, 1993). Relaxation of the sacroiliac joints may contribute to this type of pain (Heckman and Sassard, 1994).

The prevalence of low backache increases with parity and age. There is no association between maternal height, weight, pregnancy-induced weight gain, or fetal weight and backache (Heckman and Sassard, 1994).

Data Collection

Subjective

Description of onset, timing, character of the pain
Description of associated activity
Description of interventions that have improved or worsened the pain
Identification of history of back problems
Identification of history of recent trauma
Identification of associated danger signs such as urinary tract infection symptoms, contractions, increased pelvic pressure

Objective

Observation of posture when standing and sitting
Inspection of skin for signs of trauma
Abdominal palpation to identify uterine contractions
Identification of fetal station
Identification of cervical status (if signs of preterm labor)
Palpation for identification of suprapubic tenderness and costovertebral angle tenderness
Urine reagent strip or culture

Differential Diagnosis

Normal musculoskeletal changes of pregnancy
Preterm labor
Urinary tract infection
Muscle strain or bruising secondary to trauma, including physical abuse

Interventions

When assessment determines that the backache is associated with the usual pregnancy weight and postural changes, education regarding causative factors should be offered. Exercises, including pelvic rocking and general stretching may be helpful for low back pain. Attention to posture with correction of exaggerated lordosis should be demonstrated. Women should be counseled to wear low-heeled, comfortable shoes, since higher heels lead to further exaggeration of the lordosis. Warm baths or showers may be comforting, especially before sleep. Positions that enhance relaxation of the back muscles during rest can be suggested, described, or demonstrated. Supportive pillows between the legs and under the abdomen while in a side-lying position is usually helpful. Arising from the supine position should be done by rolling onto the side and raising oneself gradually, using the arms for support.

Massage has been shown to relieve muscle tension. The woman's partner can be taught to apply firm pressure with the heel of the hand over the sacral area, with the woman guiding the amount of pressure and location to gain maximum effect. Specific essential oils (e.g., lavender and chamomile) may be used to further increase relaxation and decrease pain in the third trimester. Some sources report that their use in the first trimester is contraindicated (Sweet, 1997). Acupressure, acupuncture, and chiropractic manipulation may also be of benefit.

When lordosis is associated with lax abdominal tone, an abdominal binder or girdle may offer relief. Use of an abdominal support such as "Loving Lift" has been shown to relieve symptoms for some women. These can be purchased in stores specializing in maternity apparel. If analgesia becomes necessary, acetaminophen is the drug of choice since aspirin is contraindicated in pregnancy and ibuprofen is contraindicated in the second and third trimesters (Heckman and Sassard, 1994).

Upper back pain related to the increased weight of the breasts may be alleviated by attention to good posture and wearing a well-fitting bra. Characteristics of a well-fitting bra are noted under Interventions for Breast Tenderness.

Indications for Referral

Backache associated with signs and symptoms of urinary tract infection or preterm labor require further evaluation. Lower urinary tract infection may be treated independently according to practice policies. Upper urinary tract infection and preterm labor require collaborative care or referral to medical care according to practice policies.

BREAST TENDERNESS

Cause

During the first trimester the breasts undergo dramatic changes. Estrogen stimulates the proliferation of the ductile system of the breasts. The glandular system is stimulated by human placental lactogen, human chorionic gonadotropin, and prolactin; progesterone stimulates growth of the lobules (Blackburn and Loper, 1992). The hormones further stimulate the alveoli to increase in size and deepen in color. The tenderness almost always diminishes at the end of the first trimester, although some women may continue to experience tenderness throughout the pregnancy.

Data Collection

Subjective

Description of onset, frequency, duration, and character of tenderness
Identification of any specific sites of tenderness
Identification of current lactation status

Objective

Inspection of breasts for signs of infection or nipple irritation
Palpation of breasts for masses

Differential Diagnoses

Normal breast changes in pregnancy
Mastitis
Mastalgia of undetermined etiology

Interventions

The clinician should offer reassurance regarding the normalcy in pregnancy caused by hormonal changes. Tenderness may be alleviated by wearing a well-fitting bra. Women should look for the following characteristics when buying brassieres for pregnancy and lactation:

- The bra should be made of cotton or other porous, easily washable material that will absorb perspiration.
- The bra should be shaped to give firm support to the entire breast.
- There should be no seams or underwires that put increased pressure on distinct areas of the breast.
- The shoulder straps and back should be wide enough to prevent tension over the shoulders and under the arms.

In addition, the clinician should discuss the implications for sexual expression and the wisdom of sharing the fact that the breasts are tender with her partner. Sexual play that includes the breasts may need to be deferred until the tenderness subsides.

Indication for Referral

There is rarely need for referral for normal breast tenderness in pregnancy. Mastitis can be treated independently according to practice policies. Patients with breast masses or mastalgia beyond normal pregnancy changes should be referred for medical evaluation.

CONSTIPATION

Cause

Progesterone-induced smooth muscle relaxation leading to decreased motility in the bowel predisposes women to constipation in pregnancy. Delayed motility, along with increased levels of aldosterone and angiotensin, leads to increased water absorption with resulting hard stools. Straining often becomes necessary for evacuation. Changes in diet and activity, lack of adequate fluids, and use of iron supplements also contribute to the development of this problem. In addition, the increasing size of the gravid uterus may prevent the natural leaning forward during evacuation, thereby decreasing the urge to evacuate.

Data Collection

Subjective

Description of usual bowel pattern
Description of current pattern
Identification of prior and current laxative use
24-hour diet recall, including all fluids consumed
Identification of self-care activities that have improved or worsened the condition
Identification of characteristics of any abdominal pain

Objective

Abdominal palpation to identify masses, bloating, tenderness

Differential Diagnoses

Normal bowel changes of pregnancy exacerbated by diet or decreased fluid
Constipation related to gastrointestinal pathology

Interventions

Explanation of the normal changes in pregnancy that predispose women to constipation should be offered. Preventive measures, including dietary inclusion of fluids (at least six to eight 8-ounce glasses daily), increased dietary fiber, increased fresh fruits and vegetables, and identification of particular foods that stimulate bowel activity (prunes, prune juice, hot drinks) should be explored. When necessary, occasional use of a fiber laxative may be recommended. Dosage depends on the product, and instruction on the packaging should be followed. Docusate sodium (100 mg BID) for short-term use may be appropriate. Mineral oil is contraindicated since it prevents absorption of fat-soluble vitamins. Discussion of preventing dependence on laxatives should be included in the counseling. Discussion regarding daily routines may identify behaviors such as ignoring an urge to defecate, which inhibits normal bowel functioning.

Firm abdominal massage in a clockwise direction may stimulate peristalsis (Sweet, 1997). Acupressure applied intermittently for about 10 seconds at the point midway between the pubic and umbilicus over approximately 10 minutes may also stimulate bowel activity (Sweet, 1997).

Indications for Referral

Constipation that is unrelieved with dietary changes and laxatives may require further medical evaluation. Changes in bowel habits accompanied by severe abdominal pain or rectal bleeding requires a consultation or referral for medical evaluation.

FAINTING/LIGHTHEADEDNESS

Cause

Lightheadedness or actual fainting is most commonly caused by postural hypotension in the latter half of pregnancy. Rapid changes in position such as standing quickly or bending over and then straightening up, as well as standing in one position for prolonged periods of time, interfere with cerebral circulation. Lightheadedness can also be caused by hypoglycemia throughout pregnancy. Late in pregnancy women may experience faintness when lying in the supine position (supine hypotensive syndrome). The weight of the gravid uterus compresses the inferior vena cava and the aorta, resulting in decreased cardiac output and decreased uteroplacental perfusion. In early pregnancy nausea and vomiting may contribute to lower blood glucose; later, fetal demand may affect maternal glucose levels.

Data Collection

Subjective

Description of onset, frequency, and character of episodes of faintness
Description of related activity
Description of associated dietary status (e.g., lack of food or fluids)
Description of associated environmental factors, including heat or lack of ventilation
Description of loss of consciousness or seizure activity

Objective

Inspection for signs of injury
Blood pressure
Pulse

Differential Diagnoses

Normal pregnancy changes in cerebral blood flow
Normal pregnancy changes in glucose metabolism
Hypotension

Interventions

Client education should include the probable cause and interventions that address that cause. For lightheadedness associated with postural changes, the client should be reminded to change position slowly. Women should be instructed to avoid the supine position during the second half of pregnancy. For problems related to dietary intake, the client should be reminded to have small frequent snacks and maintain hydration.

Indication for Referral

When actual loss of consciousness has occurred with possible injury, the client should be referred for further medical evaluation.

FATIGUE

Cause

Fatigue during the first trimester is thought to be caused by increased basal metabolism rate, increased demands on the cardiovascular and renal systems, and loss of sleep caused by urinary frequency and emotional factors (Pugh and Milligan, 1993). Fatigue lessens in the second trimester and increases late in pregnancy as a result of increased maternal weight, difficulty finding a comfortable position, fetal factors, and urinary frequency (see Sleep, Difficulty With). Psychologic factors that are associated with fatigue are stress, anxiety, and depression (Research Box 10-1).

Research Box 10-1

Elek SM, Hudson DB, Fleck MO: Expectant parents' experience with fatigue and sleep during pregnancy, *Birth* 24(1):49-54, 1997.

Background

Most research exploring fatigue and sleep disturbances in pregnancy have only looked at the woman's experience. Fathers also may experience decreased sleep because of interruption of sleep when the woman changes position or gets up to go to the bathroom. The completion of 90-minute sleep cycles, in addition to total hours of sleep, contributes to awakening feeling refreshed.

Research Questions

1. Do expectant mothers' and fathers' reported levels of morning and evening fatigue differ significantly during the last trimester of pregnancy?
2. Does the number of uninterrupted 90-minute sleep cycles or the total number of minutes of sleep differ significantly between mothers and fathers during the last trimester of pregnancy?
3. Is there a significant relationship between the number of mothers' and fathers' uninterrupted 90-minute sleep cycles or the total number of minutes of sleep and their reported level of morning and evening fatigue during the last trimester of pregnancy?

Methods

The authors used a longitudinal design to collect data concerning activity and sleep during 4 day periods of time each week during the last trimester. Data were collected from 9 AM Saturday through 9 PM Tuesday to sample working and nonworking days. The Visual Analog Scale for Fatigue (VAS-F) consisted of 13 items on a fatigue subscale and 5 items on an energy subscale. An activity diary consisted of 15-minute blocks of time in which the participants noted whether they were awake or asleep in each block. The totals of 90-minute uninterrupted sleep cycles and total numbers of minutes of sleep were calculated from the diary. A wrist actigraph was worn to assess validity and reliability of the diary. Parents were encouraged to keep the activity diary with them so that activity could be noted concurrently with events. Repeated measure analysis of variance was used to assess differences between groups, and Pearson product moment coefficients were used to determine relationships among variables.

Sample

A convenience sample of 28 couples agreed to participate in the study. Data from 24 couples were used, since four couples were unable to continue data collection under the study protocol. The mean age of fathers was 26.9 years; mean age of mothers was 25.3 years. All were white and married and had at least a high school education. Twenty expectant fathers were employed full time on day shifts, three were full-time students, and one worked part time and went to school part time. Twenty-three of the mothers were employed full time (days), and one part time. Most couples had incomes between $20,000 and $30,000.

Results

During each month of data collection, both mothers and fathers reported significantly lower levels of fatigue in the morning than in the evening. Levels of fatigue across groups increased from the seventh to the eighth month and from the eighth to the ninth month. Differences between fathers' and mothers' mean reports of fatigue both in the morning and evening increased as gestational age increased. Differences between mothers' morning and evening fatigue scores lessened as pregnancy progressed, but differences between the fathers' morning and evening scores remained constant. Mean number of total number of minutes of sleep did not differ across groups and across time. Mothers' reports of undisturbed 90-minute sleep cycles increased from the seventh to eighth month and decreased in the ninth month. Fathers' reports of uninterrupted 90-minute sleep cycles increased from the seventh to eighth and eighth to ninth months, but neither parents' changes reached statistical significance.

Clinical Application

The findings provide information that increases the clinician's understanding of sleep patterns in late pregnancy, thereby allowing discussion with couples of some of the changes they may experience. Clinicians may want to incorporate use of the VAS-F and/or activity diaries to assess parents' perceptions of fatigue and sleep patterns in order to develop individualized interventions to enhance sleep. Findings may be limited by the homogenicity of the sample; and the ability to be generalized to groups that differ in culture, employment, age, and other variables may be limited.

Data Collection

Subjective

Description of sleep habits, including bedtime, time necessary to get to sleep, sleep awakenings, total hours of sleep and naps
Identification of lifestyle behaviors that may increase fatigue
Identification of environmental factors that may increase fatigue
Description of exercise routine
Identification of depressive symptoms or history of depression

Objective

General appearance and affect
Current weight and any trend in weight gain or loss
Complete blood count if chronic or severe fatigue

Differential Diagnoses

Normal fatigue of pregnancy
Depression
Fatigue secondary to inadequate caloric intake or anemia

Interventions

The clinician should discuss the normal aspect of fatigue and the physiologic reasons for fatigue. Suggestions for enhancing sleep should be offered (see Sleep, Difficulty With). Counseling regarding the importance of proper nutrition and exercise, as well as treatment of anemia with diet and supplements, should be initiated.

Indications for Referral

Referral for pregnancy-related fatigue is rarely indicated. Fatigue secondary to anemia can be independently managed according to practice policies. When other pathology that predisposes to fatigue is suspected, appropriate consultation or referral should be initiated. Identification of depressive symptomatology requires referral for medical or psychologic evaluation.

FINGERS, NUMBNESS, OR TINGLING (CARPAL TUNNEL SYNDROME)

Cause

Carpal tunnel syndrome is the second most common muscular-skeletal discomfort reported in pregnancy. During the second and third trimesters, fluid retention in the wrists and hands may lead to compression of the median nerve. There can also be swelling of the carpal tunnel. This pressure results in numbness, tingling, and pain in the fingers and is usually bilateral. Signs and symptoms of carpal tunnel syndrome may be unilateral for women with previous symptoms, usually as a result of repetitive motion injury. In these cases the symptoms are exacerbated by the usual changes in pregnancy. The symptoms are most common in older primigravida who also are experiencing generalized edema (Heckman and Sassard, 1994). The symptoms are usually more pronounced at night. When there has not been repetitive motion injury before the pregnancy, the syndrome usually resolves spontaneously within days of delivery, although there are reports of onset or continuation during lactation.

Another reason for pain in the hands is de Quervain tenosynovitis which results from compression and inflammation of the tendons in the wrist. Fluid retention puts pressure on the tendons, and women will describe pain in the wrist and radial side of the hand. This type of tenosynovitis usually resolves after delivery but may continue with lactation (Heckman and Sassard, 1994).

Tingling of the fingers or numbness can also occur when the woman does not have good posture and the exaggerated lordosis of the upper back causes anterior flexion of the head. This position may compress the median and ulnar nerves of the arms.

Data Collection

Subjective

Description of the onset, frequency, duration, and character of the problem
Description of associated symptoms (swelling)
History of similar problem before pregnancy
Self-care interventions that have improved or worsened the problem

Objective

Inspection and palpation of the effected hand(s) to evaluate mobility, edema, and pain with manipulation
Observation of posture

Differential Diagnoses

Normal joint changes of pregnancy
Carpal tunnel syndrome

Intervention

Explanation of the cause of the problem and reassurance that the problem is usually self-limiting to pregnancy should be given. Severity requiring intervention is rare in healthy pregnant women (Stolp-Smith, Pascoe, and Ogburn, 1998). When intervention is necessary because of patient discomfort, splinting of the wrist using a removable soft plastic splint shaped to support the wrist in a neutral slight dorsiflexion is the most effective treatment (Courts, 1995; Heckman and Sassard, 1994). In severe cases, requests for change of work responsibilities may be needed, particularly in jobs that exacerbate the symptoms.

Indication for Referral

In severe cases, referral for medical evaluation and physical therapy may be indicated. Local steroid injections are occasionally used for severe inflammation. There is no research on the effectiveness of physical therapy alone when compared to other medical management. When generalized edema is present, dietary diuretics may help with elimination of excess fluid.

GAS, EXCESS (FLATULENCE)

Cause

Progesterone-induced relaxation of smooth muscles leads to decreased motility of intestines, resulting in increased occurrence of pockets of gas. This can cause bloating, gas pain, and flatulence.

Data Collection

Subjective

Description of onset, frequency, duration, and character of the problem
Identification of any food intake associated with the problem (e.g., milk intolerance)
24-hour diet recall
Identification of a history of similar problems before pregnancy

Objective

Inspection of abdomen for distention
Palpation of abdomen to confirm distention

Differential Diagnoses

Normal gastrointestinal changes of pregnancy
Other gastrointestinal problems, unknown etiology

Interventions

The intestinal changes in pregnancy should be explained. Avoiding problem foods such as onions, beans and lentils, collard greens, cauliflower, Brussels sprouts, cabbage, and turnips may help. Eating yogurt or drinking buttermilk may maintain normal intestinal flora.

Indication for Referral

Referral for medical intervention is rarely necessary.

GROIN PAIN/LOWER ABDOMINAL PAIN (ROUND LIGAMENT PAIN)

Cause

Rapid enlargement of the uterus in the early second trimester as the organ changes from being a pelvic organ to an abdominal organ leads to tension or stretching of the round ligaments. Women tend to notice the pain between 14 to 20 weeks' gestation, particularly with quick change of position. The round ligaments can be affected unilaterally or bilaterally. The pain is usually noted immediately above the level of the symphysis pubis in the right or left lower quadrants. Some women experience a return of the ligament discomfort in the third trimester secondary to the increasing weight of the uterus and its contents. The diagnosis is one of exclusion after all other reasons for lower abdominal pain have been ruled out.

Data Collection

Subjective

Description of onset, frequency, duration, and character of the pain
Description of any associated activity that triggers pain
Description of any associated symptoms such as back pain, uterine cramping, vaginal spotting, urinary burning, or urgency

Objective

Abdominal palpation for tenderness or masses
Palpation for identification of costovertebral angle tenderness
Cervical evaluation as indicated to rule out threatened abortion

Differential Diagnoses

Normal ligament pain of pregnancy
Threatened abortion/preterm labor

Urinary tract infection
Musculoskeletal discomfort, unknown etiology

Interventions

Education should include an explanation of the uterine and ligament changes in second trimester, reassurance of the fact that it is self-limiting, and instruction in slow position changes and guarding of the area with counterpressure of one's hand. Demonstration of proper body mechanics for bending and lifting may correct positions and activities that increase the risk of ligament strain. Heat may be used to alleviate symptoms.

Indication for Referral

Increased or severe pain requires further medical evaluation to rule out other organic causes.

GUMS, BLEEDING

Cause

Increased estrogen levels stimulate blood flow to the mouth and accelerate turnover of gum epithelial cells. The gums become more vascular than in the nonpregnant state. Increased numbers of small vessels, hyperplasia, edema, and decreased thickness of the gingival epithelial surface result in bleeding that can occur with chewing or brushing (Blackburn and Loper, 1992).

Data Collection

Subjective

Description of onset and amount of bleeding
Identification of history of bleeding gums before pregnancy
Description of usual dental hygiene routine
Identification of last dental evaluation and procedures

Objective

Observe teeth and gums for signs of decay or periodontal problems
Hematocrit/hemoglobin and platelets if history of chronic bleeding

Differential Diagnoses

Normal oral changes of pregnancy
Periodontal disease

Interventions

Explanation of the fact that bleeding gums are common in pregnancy can be offered. The clinician should recommend continued flossing and brushing with soft bristled brush, acknowledging that these dental hygiene measures may stimulate bleeding.

Indications for Referral

Since pregnancy offers an opportunity for women to obtain often neglected dental care, clinicians should be assertive in providing referrals for routine dental cleaning, evaluation, and treatment of problems. There are no contraindications to routine dental work, and women can be assured that local anesthetic is safe in pregnancy. Women should be counseled that, if the dentist prescribes antibiotic therapy, they should contact the midwife to determine whether the drug is safe in pregnancy.

HEADACHE

Cause

The most common cause of headache in pregnancy is muscle tension. The woman may describe the pain as persistent and viselike, extending from the base of the head to the forehead (Blackburn and Loper, 1992). Headaches can also be precipitated by stress, postural changes, eye strain, nasal or sinus congestion, fatigue, mild respiratory alkalosis, and altered cerebral fluid dynamics. Migraine headaches typically are described as throbbing and moderate to severe in intensity. They may be accompanied by nausea and vomiting, photophobia and/or phonophobia, and an aura. Women with a history of migraine headaches tend to experience remission or decreased frequency and severity during pregnancy (Chen and Leviton, 1994; Silberstein, 1997), although some studies have also found an increase in headaches in the third trimester (Scharff, Marcus, and Turk, 1997). A small proportion of women (4% to 8%) whose headaches worsen during pregnancy tend to experience migraines with aura (Aube, 1999).

Data Collection

Subjective

Description of onset, frequency, duration, location, and character of the headaches
Description of associated activities or behaviors
Description of self-care interventions that improve or worsen the pain

History of headaches before pregnancy
History of previous caffeine use, with cessation related to counseling to decrease use in pregnancy

Objective

General appearance (e.g., fatigued, acute distress)
Blood pressure
Weight
Palpation of extremities to identify edema
Palpation over sinuses to identify pain

Differential Diagnoses

Tension headache
Migraine headache
Sinusitis or sinus congestion
Hypertension

Interventions

If not associated with hypertension or other obvious medical disorder, reassurance that most headaches in pregnancy are benign may be offered. Interventions to decrease tension such as massage, warm compresses, and warm bath or shower may be beneficial. Rest in a darkened room and having a glass of juice have also been found helpful. Acetaminophen, 650 to 1000 mg PO every 6 hours, may be used in pregnancy, although some sources do not recommend its use in the first trimester unless absolutely necessary. Ibuprofen, 600 mg every 6 hours, can be used in early pregnancy. Acupuncture has been recommended as a nonpharmacologic approach to headache, but there has been little research done on its use in pregnancy. Women with a history of heavy caffeine use with abrupt cessation related to pregnancy concerns can be counseled regarding the headaches reflecting withdrawal from caffeine. Weaning oneself off caffeine using an increasing proportion of decaffeinated mixed with regular coffee or tea may decrease headache symptoms.

Indications for Referral

Severe headache that does not respond to comfort measures and analgesia is an indication for further medical evaluation. Severe headache accompanied by increased blood pressure, proteinuria, and/or edema requires immediate evaluation for preeclampsia. This evaluation can be done independently by the midwife or in collaboration with an obstetrician according to practice policies. Migraine headache requires consultation and collaborative care with an internal medicine physician.

HEARTBURN (GASTROESOPHAGEAL REFLUX)

Cause

Hormonal effects of estrogen and progesterone lead to relaxation of the cardiac sphincter, delayed emptying of the stomach, and pressure from the enlarging uterus that forces the acidic stomach contents into the lower esophagus late in pregnancy. It is estimated that as many as 85% of women experience heartburn during pregnancy (Broussard and Richter, 1998; Calhoun, 1992).

Data Collection

Subjective

Description of frequency and severity of symptoms
Identification of food intake associated with symptoms
Description of self-care interventions that have improved or worsened the discomfort

Objective

Diagnosis is usually by history alone, although, if the gastric reflux is inhibiting nutritional intake, the following data should be obtained:

- Weight, current and trend over time
- Urine ketones

Differential Diagnoses

Normal gastric reflux of pregnancy
Gastric reflux, unknown etiology

Interventions

Explanation of the probable cause and the probable self-limitation to pregnancy should be offered. Use of small, frequent meals or snacks should be encouraged. Avoidance of fatty or spicy food may help. Standing or sitting straight after eating may offer postural relief. Papaya tablets, 1 to 2 tablets after meals and before bedtime, or fresh papaya, may be beneficial. Anise or fennel seed tea after meals may assist digestion (Weed, 1985).

In moderate-to-severe cases of gastric reflux, nonsystemically absorbed medications, including antacids and sucralfate, are safe, with little risk to the fetus (Broussard and Richter, 1998) (Ching and Lam, 1994). Calcium carbonate is a commonly used ingredient in antacids (e.g., Tums), and these preparations are marketed in professional and lay literature as ideal sources of calcium for women. However, some women will experience a rebound gastric secretion, and there is the potential for development of hypercalcemia and decreased renal function with overuse (Brucker and Faucher, 1997). Aluminum hydroxide is a common ingredient in over-the-counter antacids; its most common side effect is constipation. Magnesium is also commonly used in antacids (e.g., Milk of Magnesia). The most common side effect for magnesium is diarrhea, and it should not be used with women who have compromised renal function. Combinations of aluminum and magnesium antacids have been developed to decrease the gastrointestinal side effects. Antacids containing sodium bicarbonate (e.g., Alka-Seltzer) should be avoided since they hinder absorption of B-complex vitamins and may aggravate edema.

Indication for Referral

Gastric reflux rarely requires referral for further medical evaluation and management.

HEMORRHOIDS

Cause

Progesterone-induced relaxation of smooth muscle contributes to the weakening of vessel walls. Pressure from the growing uterus on the veins around the rectum and anus further contributes to dilation of the vessels. Constipation with resultant straining with stools is also a factor in development of hemorrhoids.

Data Collection

Subjective

Description of the onset and character of the problem
Identification of any history of constipation or diarrhea
Identification of history of bleeding with bowel movements
Identification of self-care interventions that have improved or worsened the condition
24-hour diet recall

Objective

Inspection of hemorrhoids to identify size and signs of thrombosis

Differential Diagnosis

Hemorrhoids

Interventions

Explanation of the normal pregnancy changes that predispose women to hemorrhoids should be offered. Dietary and behavioral changes that will reduce the chance of constipation should be discussed. Sitz baths and witch hazel compresses offer symptomatic relief. Over-the-counter ointments or suppositories containing phenylephrine and/or hydrocortisone may provide relief.

"Natural" preparations for hemorrhoids include comfrey ointment, yellow dock root ointment, and plantain and yarrow ointment.

Indications for Referral

When venous thrombosis, anal fissure, or anal abscess is noted, medical referral for possible surgical intervention is recommended.

LEG CRAMPS

Cause

Up to 50% of pregnant women experience leg cramps, usually in the latter half of pregnancy (Hammar, Larsson, and Tegler, 1981; Sweet, 1997). The cramps are usually defined as "sudden tonic or clonic contractions of the gastrocnemius muscle, usually at night" (Pitkin, 1975). The cause is unknown, but they may be due to altered calcium/phosphorus ratio, magnesium deficiency, or buildup of lactic acid in the muscles. What little research has been done to explore this phenomenon has suggested that changes in calcium and magnesium levels in pregnancy may be contributing factors, but results of clinical trials are conflicting.

Data Collection

Subjective

Description of onset, frequency, duration, and character of the cramping
Identification of any precipitating activities
Identifications of self-care interventions that have improved or worsened the cramping

Objective

Inspection of legs

Differential Diagnoses

Leg cramps secondary to pregnancy
Leg cramps, unknown etiology

Interventions

Most sources suggest avoiding high-phosphorus/low-calcium foods such as soft drinks and processed snack foods. Studies that have analyzed the effect of calcium supplements on the frequency and severity of cramps are conflicting. There is some evidence that oral magnesium supplementation may decrease cramping (Dahle et al., 1995).

When cramping occurs, the woman should straighten the leg and pull the toes toward the body. Flexing the foot can also be done by a partner or friend. Daily exercise such as walking or swimming may decrease the episodes.

Indication for Referral

There is rarely the need for medical referral.

NASAL STUFFINESS/CONGESTION

Cause

Estrogen-induced nasal mucosal edema may lead the woman to think that she has a cold or allergies. Other factors, including allergy, infection, stress, and rebound rhinitis, may also influence the sensation of "stuffiness" (Mabry, 1986). Nasal congestion can lead to an increase in frequency and severity of snoring and may lead to sleep deprivation.

Data Collection

Subjective

Description of onset, frequency, duration, and character of the congestion
Identification of history of allergies
Identification of history of householders or acquaintances with upper respiratory infections (URIs)
Identification of current URI symptoms
Identification of self-care interventions that have improved or worsened condition

Objective

Inspection of nares

Differential Diagnoses

Nasal congestion secondary to hormonal changes of pregnancy
Allergic rhinitis
Upper respiratory infection
Deviated nasal septum

Interventions

Explanation of the physiologic changes in pregnancies that contribute to this condition should be offered. Increasing the humidity in the home through use of a cold steamer or humidifier is helpful. Normal saline nose drops may provide some symptomatic relief. The woman should be counseled to not use nose drops containing epinephrine-like drugs and to not use over-the-counter cold and flu remedies without consulting with the provider. Over-the-counter mechanical nasal dilators that are worn on the nose while sleeping have been found to improve the ease of breathing among patients with pregnancy-related nocturnal congestion (Turnbull et al, 1996).

Indication for Referral

There is rarely need for referral.

NAUSEA AND VOMITING

Cause

It is estimated that 50% to 80% of pregnant women experience nausea and vomiting and approximately 5% of pregnant women require treatment for fluid replacement and correction of electrolyte imbalance (Belluomini et al., 1994). Nausea and vomiting of pregnancy typically occur during the first trimester and are most likely caused by the elevated levels of human chorionic gonadotropin (hCG). Once the hCG levels begin to fall, nausea is relieved. This hormonal association is further supported by the fact that, in situations with higher than usual hCG levels (multiple gestation, trophoblastic disease), nausea and vomiting are increased. Nausea is also associated with the changes in smell and taste common in early pregnancy (Research Boxes 10-2 and 10-3).

There is some evidence that nausea may be associated with B-vitamin deficiencies, particularly B_6 (Vutyavanich, Wongtra-ngan, and Ruangsri, 1995). Although there is no relationship between the levels of pyridoxine and degree of morning sickness, evidence suggests that vitamin B_6 supplementation may relieve nausea and vomiting of pregnancy, particularly in cases of severe vomiting (Sahakian et al., 1991).

Data Collection

Subjective

Description of onset, frequency, and duration of the problem
Identification of associated environmental factors

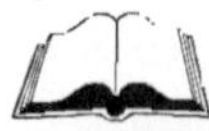

Research Box 10-2

O'Brien B, Zhou Q: Variables related to nausea and vomiting during pregnancy, *Birth* 22(2):95-100, 1995.

Background

Seventy to ninety percent of women experience nausea during pregnancy, and 50% experience at least one episode of vomiting. Although many theories are postulated as the underlying cause of the nausea and vomiting, precise causes are not well understood. Many women do not experience symptom relief with commonly recommended interventions to decrease the nausea and vomiting.

Research Question

What are the correlations between reported symptoms of nausea and vomiting with selected demographic, physiologic, and psychosocial variables identified in previous studies as associated with nausea and vomiting?

Methods

The authors used qualitative and quantitative methods to explore factors associated with nausea and vomiting in pregnancy. This report presented the associations among variables using the quantitative data. The Rhodes INV instrument was used to measure the duration, frequency, and distress associated with nausea and vomiting; the 16 personality factor (PF) questionnaire was used to evaluate 24 personality dimensions and traits. Data were collected at the initial prenatal visit, at 24 to 29 weeks' gestation, and at 4 to 6 weeks' postpartum.

Sample

One hundred forty-seven women who initiated prenatal care before 16 weeks' gestation and who were receiving care from three obstetric and nurse-midwifery practices volunteered to participate, and 126 completed the Rhodes INV. Participants were predominantly white, married, and employed outside the home. Almost two thirds of the sample attended or completed college. Twenty-eight percent were primiparas.

Results

No variables independently predicted or explained the presence or severity of nausea and vomiting. Younger age, nulliparity, female fetal gender, nonsmokers, and working outside the home were significantly associated with nausea and vomiting. When these variables were entered into the regression equations, it was found that they contributed to only 14% of variance that could be explained for overall symptoms. The sample size was not sufficient to interpret the personality data.

Clinical Application

Further research is necessary to develop more sensitive measures that can identify physiologic and psychosocial factors that explain the presence and severity of nausea and vomiting in pregnancy. Until these measures are developed, clinicians need to reassure women that the condition is usually self-limiting and that a variety of self-help measures may alleviate symptoms.

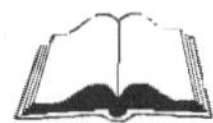

Research Box 10-3

Belluomini J et al: Acupressure for nausea and vomiting of pregnancy: a randomized, blinded study, *Obstet Gynecol* 84(2):245-248, 1994

Background

Fifty to eighty percent of pregnancies are complicated by nausea and vomiting. Pharmaceutic intervention is used only with the most severe cases. An effective, safe, self-care measure would improve the quality of life for women experiencing nausea and vomiting of pregnancy.

Research Question

Does the use of acupressure at the PC-6 point decrease the duration of nausea, amount of vomiting and level of distress caused by the condition?

Methods

Ninety women experiencing nausea and/or vomiting of pregnancy were randomly assigned into one of two acupressure groups. One group was instructed in use of the PC-6 pressure point, and the other was instructed to use a sham pressure point. The subjects and their providers were blinded to group assignment. Women were their own controls. For the first 3 days of study participation, women received no treatment; they then were instructed to use pressure point therapy for 10 minutes four times a day for 10 consecutive days. Data from the first 3 days were considered the pretreatment scores. Data for day 4 was discarded to allow time for treatment effect. The Rhodes Index of nausea and vomiting was used to collect data on the duration of nausea, the amount of vomiting, and the degree of distress from the condition. Student t test was used to compare differences between group means. Analysis of variance and analysis for variance for repeated measures were used to analyze treatment effects over time.

Sample

Thirty of the original 90 participants dropped out of the study, and the attrition by group assignment was similar. Participants were recruited from physician and midwife practices in a west-coast city.

Results

Nausea and vomiting improved in both groups over time, as would be expected from clinical experience. After controlling for condition improvement related to time, the investigators found a significant reduction of symptoms in the experimental group using the PC-6 point for acupressure.

Clinical Application

Although the use of pressure wrist band has resulted in similar improvement in nausea and vomiting in pregnancy, some women find the bands uncomfortable or conspicuous (particularly at a time when many women do not share knowledge of their pregnancies with friends, colleagues, or work supervisors). Acupressure can be easily taught in the office and requires no purchase of materials. Because the authors do not report characteristics of the sample, it is impossible to determine whether results are able to be generalized to other groups. Women with a previous knowledge of and experience with acupressure and other complementary approaches in health care may be more likely to experience positive results from the use of acupressure. The results may also be limited by the fairly high number of participants who dropped out of the study.

24-hour dietary recall
Identification of self-care interventions that have improved or worsened the condition

Objective

Palpation of skin turgor
Inspection of mucous membranes
Weight, current and trend over time
Urine ketones, specific gravity, color

Differential Diagnoses

Nausea and vomiting of pregnancy
Nausea and vomiting secondary to gastrointestinal infection

Interventions

Nausea and vomiting without signs of dehydration call for reassurance of the self-limiting nature of the problem, explanation of the probable cause, and discussion of self-help remedies that may be tried. Dietary approaches that seem to help include dry crackers or toast before getting out of bed, small frequent bland snacks, and sips of flat ginger ale or cola. Many women find that sour-tasting foods such as citrus fruit and pickles relieve the foul taste in the mouth. Likewise, strong mints (e.g., Altoids) may help both by changing the oral environment and altering the sense of smell. Dental hygiene helps eliminate the sour taste in the mouth and may relieve the symptoms. Avoidance of known triggers for nausea, such as smells associated with coffee and tobacco, may help.

There is evidence that vitamin B_6, 30 to 75 mg per day or 25 mg every 8 hours, may relieve nausea in some women (Murphy, 1998; Sahakian et al., 1991; Vutyavanich, Wongtra-ngan, and Ruangsri, 1995).

Several herbal remedies may decrease the nausea. Anise or fennel seed tea on awakening may be helpful. Eight ounces of water with one teaspoon of apple cider vinegar is also soothing on the stomach (Weed, 1985). Raspberry leaf tea eases nausea and cleanses the foul taste out of the mouth. Peppermint, spearmint, and chamomile tea are also commonly used to ease nausea and vomiting. Ginger in the form of root tea or crushed in capsules (250 mg four times per day) is especially effective for early morning nausea and motion sickness (Fisher-Rasmussen et al., 1990; Weed, 1985).

Homeopathic remedies commonly recommended for nausea include Ipecac 30x, Nux vomica 6x, and Cannabis 30x (Weed, 1985). No studies have explored the effectiveness of these interventions (Murphy, 1998).

A commonly available wristband that applies pressure on the P6 acupuncture point can be found in drug and marine supply stores. Several studies have found the acupressure can significantly reduce the frequency and severity of nausea and vomiting (Barsoum, Perry, and Fraser, 1990; Belluomini et al., 1994; Dundee et al., 1988; Evans et al., 1993; Hyde, 1989; Stannard, 1989). However, the effect may be associated with placebo rather than direct effect of the pressure (Murphy, 1998).

Indication for Referral

Nausea and vomiting accompanied by dehydration require referral for hydration, possible pharmacologic agents, and evaluation to rule out other causes of gastrointestinal distress.

NOSEBLEEDS (EPISTAXIS)

Cause

Increased vascularity of the nasal mucosa occurs under the influence of increased estrogen levels. Dry environment, such as that experienced in a centrally heated home with poor humidification or in a home heated by a wood stove, increases the friability of the vessels and the occurrence of bleeding. Factors associated with nosebleeds include upper respiratory infections, sinusitis, hypertension, vascular disease, ulcerative disease, trauma, and cocaine use.

Data Collection

Subjective

Description of onset, frequency, duration, and amount of bleeding
Identification of activities or behaviors associated with bleeding, including cocaine use
Identification of self-care interventions that increase or decrease the frequency or amount of bleeding

Objective

Inspection of nasal mucosa
Inspection of nasal septum
Inspection of skin color and other mucous membranes
Complete blood count with platelets if bleeding is severe or long-standing

Differential Diagnoses

Nosebleeds secondary to mucosal changes of pregnancy
Nasal polyps
Excoriation of nasal mucosa secondary to drug use

Interventions

Explanation of the vascular changes in pregnancy should be offered. Increasing the humidity in the environment through the use of a mister, humidifier, or boiling pots of water on the stove may be helpful. Normal saline drops may also decrease friability.

Indication for Referral

There is rarely reason for referral.

PERSPIRATION, INCREASED

Cause

Secretion from the apocrine glands, particularly in the axilla, decreases in pregnancy, but the physiologic cause is unclear. Conversely, secretion from the eccrine glands, located all over the skin surface, increases. This is possibly because of the increased thyroid activity during pregnancy. Increased dilation of the blood vessels in the skin enhances the body's ability to eliminate waste through this increase in perspiration and dissipate excess heat.

Data Collection

Subjective

Description of extent of discomfort experienced
Description of associated symptoms such as faintness, headache, chest pain, or shortness of breath

Objective

Inspection of skin
Temperature, if indicated from history

Interventions

Explanation of the physiologic reason for increased perspiration in pregnancy and reassurance that it is normal in pregnancy can be given. Counseling regarding bathing, wearing loose-fitting clothing of absorbent material, and controlling room temperatures in the home may assist in increasing comfort.

Indication for Referral

There is rarely need for referral for this problem.

PICA

Cause

Pica has been described as "the ingestion of nonfood substances and/or food staples in response to a craving" (Cooksey, 1995) and as "an eating disorder that is manifested by a craving for oral ingestion of a given substance that is unusual in kind or quantity" (Lacey, 1990). It has been estimated that as many as 68% of pregnant women in certain subgroups of the population of the United States experience pica. Some women are at higher risk of unusual ingestion of substances; those who are black, who live in rural or inner-city areas, and who have a family or childhood history of pica are more likely to demonstrate this behavior (Lacey, 1990). Pica has been associated with anemia, bowel obstruction, toxicity from certain heavy metals, poor nutrition, and parasites.

Data Collection

Subjective

Dietary recall
Identification of craving for food or nonfood items
Identification of family or personal history of pica
Identification of history of anemia or current anemia
Identification of faintness, weakness or lack of energy

Objective

General appearance
Weight, current and trend over time
Inspection of skin and mucous membrane color
Palpation of skin turgor
Inspection and palpation for identification of abdominal bloating, tenderness, or masses
Complete blood count
Stool for ova and parasites
Lead testing if lead toxicity is suspected

Differential Diagnoses

Pica
Anemia secondary to pica
Bowel obstruction secondary to anemia
Parasitic infection
Heavy metal toxicity secondary to pica

Interventions

Exploratory questions to identify pica should be included in every initial history. When women are in communities in which there is a high incidence of pica, follow-up assessment should be done each trimester. Education and counseling regarding the risks associated with the type of pica identified should be offered. When pica is associated with anemia, iron supplementation should be offered, along with nutritional education about iron-containing foods.

Indications for Referral

Severe anemia unresponsive to iron supplementation and signs of bowel obstruction or lead toxicity require referral for medical evaluation (Box 10-1).

Box 10-1 *Substances Identified As Consumed in Pica*

Nonfood	Food
Ashes	Carrots
Balloons	Celery
Burnt matches (cautopyreiophagia)	Croutons
Chalk	Licorice
Cigarette butts	Life Savers candy
Clay (geophagia)	Milk
Cloth	Parsley
Cotton balls	Potatoes, raw (geomelophagia)
Crayons	
Detergent	
Feces (coprophagia)	
Fuzz	
Grass	
Hair (tricophagia)	
Ice (pagophagia)	
Insects	
Lavatory fresheners	
Laundry starch (amylophagia)	
Lead paint chips (plumbophagia)	
Metal	
Newsprint	
Paper	
Pencil erasers	
Plant leaves	
Plastic	
Powder, baby	
Powder puffs	
Soap	
Stones (lithophagia)	
String, thread	
Toilet tissue	
Twigs	
Wood	

RASH OF PREGNANCY

Cause

Women commonly present with the complaint of a rash or itching in pregnancy. Common rashes, including varicella and other childhood diseases, insect bites, eczema, and contact dermatitis should be readily identified by the clinician. Four specific types of rashes are pregnancy related:

1. Papular dermatitis is characterized by discrete erythematous papules approximately 3 to 5 mm in diameter that do not occur in groups (Blackburn and Loper, 1992; Star et al., 1990). The lesions may occur anywhere on the body and usually heal within 10 days. Hyperpigmentation at the site of the lesion may occur. The condition may recur in future pregnancies.
2. Prurigo gestationis is characterized by small, excoriated pruritic papules on the abdomen, trunk, or extensor surface of the extremities (Star et al., 1990). The lesions usually appear in the late second trimester and may persist for several months following delivery.
3. Pruritic urticarial papules and plaques of pregnancy syndrome (PUPPPS) is characterized by discrete erythematous papules and urticarial plaques over the abdomen, thighs, buttocks, legs, and arms (Star et al., 1990). Excoriation is usually not present. PUPPPS usually develops in the third trimester and may persist for several weeks following delivery.
4. Pruritus gravidarum is characterized by abdominal pruritus without distinct lesions. The pruritus may spread to other areas of the body. Scratch marks may be present because of scratching. The itching typically occurs after the

twentieth week of gestation, and jaundice may develop 2 to 3 weeks after the initial outbreak. The condition resolves spontaneously within 4 weeks of delivery.

Pruritus gravidarum is the only pregnancy-related dermatologic condition for which the etiology is known. Intrahepatic cholestasis is diagnosed through the presenting complaint of pruritus without rash and the identification of elevated serum bile salts and transaminase and possible hyperbilirubinemia (McDonald, 1999; Reyes, 1997). The syndrome is associated with an increase in stillbirth, fetal distress in labor, and preterm labor (McDonald, 1999). Women who experience pruritus gravidarum face a 40% to 60% risk of recurrence with future pregnancies (Reyes, 1997).

Data Collection

Subjective

Identification of the history of the development and location of the rash
Identification of the degree of itching
Identification of history of similar condition in previous pregnancies
Identification of any history of jaundice

Objective

Inspection of skin to assess lesions and color
Serum liver panel, including serum alkaline phosphatase, serum glutamate oxaloacetate transaminase, and total bilirubin

Differential Diagnoses

Papular dermatitis
Prurigo gestationis
PUPPPS
Pruritis gravidarum
Other dermatologic lesions unrelated to pregnancy

Interventions

Education regarding the condition should be offered. Nonpharmacologic interventions include oatmeal baths and use of loose-fitting clothing. Calamine lotion may be applied to decrease itching. In severe cases topical corticosteroids and/or antihistamines may be used.

Indications for Referral

Consultation with a dermatologist or primary care physician for confirmation of diagnosis may be indicated. Consultation with an obstetrician is recommended for pruritus gravidarum because of the increased risk of preterm labor and fetal loss.

SALIVATION, EXCESSIVE

Cause

Whether ptyalism, or hypersalivation, actually occurs in pregnancy is controversial. It is unclear whether there actually is increased production of saliva or whether women do not swallow saliva because of nausea or changes in taste. Regardless, the need to spit out excess saliva can be an inconvenient problem. In addition, it can further contribute to nausea of pregnancy. In rare cases the condition can lead to electrolyte loss and dehydration. There appears to be a cultural component of this complaint, with some communities experiencing higher incidence.

Data Collection

Subjective

Description of onset, frequency, duration, and amount of spitting
24-hour dietary recall

Objective

Weight, current and trend over time
Assessment of skin turgor
Inspection of mucous membranes

Differential Diagnosis

Ptyalism

Interventions

The physiologic base for the increased saliva should be explained, with reassurance that it is rarely associated with pregnancy problems. Counseling regarding hygiene and nutrition should be offered.

Indication for Referral

Consultation or referral may be indicated if severe dehydration develops.

SHORTNESS OF BREATH (DYSPNEA)

Cause

Progesterone-induced respiratory changes and increased maternal metabolic rate and fetal oxygen consumption contribute to women feeling like they can't "catch their breath." This phenomenon often leads to the "sigh of pregnancy," a purposeful deep breath to try to increase respiratory reserve. The pressure of the enlarging uterus on the diaphragm further contributes to this problem.

Data Collection

Subjective

Description of onset, frequency, and duration of problem
Description of associated symptoms, including pain, palpitations, wheezing
Description of associated skin color changes, including paleness or cyanosis
Identification of history of respiratory problems before pregnancy, including asthma
Identification of history of upper respiratory infection symptoms
Identification of history of cardiac problems

Objective

Determination of respiratory rate and rhythm
Inspection of skin color
Auscultation of heart rate and lung fields

Differential Diagnoses

Normal respiratory changes of pregnancy
Asthma
Other respiratory or cardiac distress, not pregnancy related

Interventions

Client education should include the anatomic and physiologic causes of shortness of breath. Stretching the arms over the head and swinging the arms in a circular motion assist with respiratory expansion. Danger signs, including worsening of symptoms or chest pain, should be reported to the provider immediately.

Indications for Referral

Shortness of breath accompanied by elevated respiratory rate or chest pain requires referral to a physician immediately. Asthma symptoms exacerbated by pregnancy should be co-managed or referred for medical management, according to practice policies.

SKIN CHANGES

Cause

Pigmentation changes can occur because increased estrogen levels stimulate melanin. Stretch marks can occur anywhere on the body but most commonly are found on the abdomen, breasts, and thighs. They may become deep pink in color but usually fade to pale pink or silver following delivery.

Data Collection

Subjective

Description of skin changes

Objective

Inspection of affected areas

Differential Diagnoses

Chloasma
Linea nigra
Striae

Interventions

Explanation of the hormonal changes to skin pigmentation should be offered. The woman should be counseled that chloasma, linea nigra, and other pigmented areas of the skin may darken further in sunlight. Women should be encouraged to stay out of bright sun and apply PABA sunscreens liberally.

Keeping the abdomen well lubricated with an aloe- or vitamin E–based lotion may reduce the itching associated with the stretching of the skin. Women should be advised that there is no preparation that absolutely prevents stretch marks.

Indication for Referral

There is rarely need to refer for this problem.

SLEEP, DIFFICULTY WITH

Cause

Early in pregnancy sleep disturbances may be provoked by psychologic stressors, frequency of urination, and other first-trimester discomforts. Later in pregnancy physical discomforts, difficulty finding a position of comfort, fetal movements, and feelings of shortness of breath may also inhibit sleep.

Data Collection

Subjective

Description of sleep habits, including bedtime, time necessary to get to sleep, sleep awakenings, total hours sleep and naps
Identification of previous history of sleep disturbances
Identification of lifestyle behaviors that may increase fatigue
Identification of depressive symptomatology
Identification of environmental factors that may increase fatigue
Identification of self-care interventions that have improved or worsened condition

Objective

General appearance

Differential Diagnoses

Normal sleep disturbance of pregnancy
Sleep disturbance, preexisting

Interventions

Women can be reassured that sleep disturbances are common in pregnancy. Identification of factors that further inhibit sleep can direct counseling and education. Women can be encouraged to plan quiet time before going to bed; limit fluid intake several hours before bedtime; and use pillows to support the abdomen, back, and legs. A warm bath or shower and massage may further relax her. Meditation and visualization may further help calm her and prepare her for sleep.

Many awakenings are caused by dreams, particularly frightening dreams. The clinician can reassure the woman that dreams are common in pregnancy and that this experience is not unusual.

Warm milk may enhance falling asleep. Raspberry leaf tea may aid in relaxation, and skullcap tincture (30 drops of commercial tincture ½ hour before bedtime) enhances deep sleep (Weed, 1985).

Indication for Referral

There is rarely need for referral for this condition.

SWELLING (EDEMA)

Cause

Edema in the lower extremities is common in the latter half of pregnancy because of increased venous pressure caused by pressure of the enlarging. Edema of the hands is common in late pregnancy, particularly in the morning, and is most likely postural. Generalized edema may be a sign of preeclampsia.

Data Collection

Subjective

Description of onset, frequency, duration, and character of the swelling
Identification of associated danger signs such as headache, vision changes, chest pain, abdominal pain
24-hour dietary recall
Identification of self-care interventions that improve or worsen the condition

Objective

Inspection and palpation of site of edema
Blood pressure
Urine screen for protein
Weight, trend over time

Differential Diagnoses

Normal edema of pregnancy
Preeclampsia

Interventions

Education regarding the cause should be offered. Frequent elevation of the legs, use of a stool while sitting, and exercise help to mobilize the fluid. The woman should be reminded not to limit fluids but rather to maintain intake to enhance renal function. Support hose are often helpful, and the woman should be reminded to apply the hose before rising for best effect. Danger signs, including edema accompanied by headache, visual changes, and epigastric pain, should be reviewed.

Indications for Referral

Edema accompanied by the danger signs noted in the previous paragraph, elevation of baseline blood pressure, and/or proteinuria requires referral to a physician skilled in assessment of pregnancy-induced hypertension.

VAGINAL DISCHARGE

Cause

Increased vaginal discharge as the pregnancy progresses is caused by increased cervical mucus and transudate and increased vascularity of the cervix and vagina (Sweet, 1997). Normal pregnancy-related discharge is clear to whitish clear, with no associated symptoms of foul odor, itching, or burning. Microscopic examination demonstrates epithelial cells and gram-positive bacilli.

Data Collection

Subjective

Description of onset, trend, amount, color, and odor of discharge
Identification of associated symptoms, including itching, burning, or foul odor
Identification of signs of labor (rule out spontaneous rupture of membranes)
Identification of self-care interventions that have improved or worsened condition

Objective

Inspection of external pelvic structures for signs of irritation or inflammation
Speculum examination of vagina to assess discharge and vaginal walls
Microscopic examination of discharge

Differential Diagnoses

Normal vaginal discharge of pregnancy
Vulvovaginitis
Spontaneous rupture of membranes

Interventions

Once vaginitis and rupture of membranes have been ruled out, education regarding the normalcy of the discharge can be offered. Advice can include maintaining good hygiene and use of cotton panties to absorb secretions. Women can be reminded that the normal increase in secretions may influence the sexual practices used, as some partners may note changes in the smell and taste of the vaginal area.

Indications for Referral

There is no reason for consultation for normal discharge of pregnancy. Vaginitis can be independently managed according to practice policies.

VARICOSE VEINS

Cause

The relaxation of smooth muscle of vessel walls caused by progesterone and the anatomic pressure of the enlarging uterus lead to development or worsening of existing varicose veins. Heredity, obesity, constrictive clothing, and standing for long periods of time are all associated with varicosities. Pregnancy-related varicose veins are most pronounced in the legs and vulva.

Data Collection

Subjective

Description of onset, site, and character of the affected veins
Description of associated symptoms such as pain, redness, and tenderness
Identification of history of varicosities before present pregnancy
Identification of history of thrombophlebitis
Identification of self-care interventions that have improved or worsened the condition

Objective

Inspection of size and location of varicose veins
Identification of redness or tenderness over veins

Differential Diagnoses

Varicose veins, lower extremities
Vulvar varicosities

Interventions

Client education should include the anatomic and physiologic reasons for the problem. The woman should be encouraged to elevate the legs several times a day while in a side-lying position. Consistent use of maternity support hose should be encouraged, and proper application of the hose should be discussed. Support panty hose with additional reinforcement in the form of a porous peripad provide counterpressure for vulvar varicosities. Danger signs indicating possible venous thrombosis should be discussed.

Foods rich in vitamins A, C, E, and B complex are recommended for maintenance of vessel walls. Vitamin E, up to 600 IU daily, is considered safe in pregnancy and may contribute to maintaining vessel wall integrity and preventing thrombus formation.

Indications for Referral

Signs of venous thrombosis necessitate referral to a physician skilled in treatment. Women with a history of thrombophlebitis should be referred to a physician for consultation to determine whether prophylactic anticoagulant therapy is indicated in pregnancy.

WARMTH/FEELING UNCOMFORTABLY HOT

Cause

Progesterone can cause a thermogenic effect that includes vasodilation that increases skin temperature. In addition, maternal fatty stores may contribute to the sensation of warmth. During the latter part of pregnancy the placenta may contribute to the increased body temperature.

Data Collection

Subjective

Description of onset, frequency, duration, and extent of problem
Description of associated factors such as anxiety, activity, recent food intake

Objective

Temperature
Palpation of pulse
Inspection of skin for perspiration or obvious vasodilation

Differential Diagnoses

Normal thermogenic change of pregnancy
Fever

Interventions

When no fever is identified, education regarding the hormonally induced vascular changes in pregnancy can be offered. Reassurance regarding the normalcy of this condition in pregnancy should be given. The woman can be encouraged to wear light, layered clothes and to keep the thermostat at a lower setting than normal.

Indication for Referral

There is no reason for medical referral for this condition.

References

Aube M: Migraine in pregnancy, *Neurology* 53(4 suppl 1):S26-S28, 1999.

Barsoum G, Perry EP, Fraser IA: Postoperative nausea is relieved by acupressure, *J Royal Soc Med* 83(2):86-89, 1990.

Belluomini J et al: Acupressure for nausea and vomiting of pregnancy: a randomized, blinded study, *Obstet Gynecol* 84(2):245-248, 1994.

Blackburn ST, Loper DL: *Maternal, fetal, and neonatal physiology: a clinical perspective,* Philadelphia, 1992, WB Saunders.

Broussard CN, Richter JE: Treating gastro-oesophageal reflux disease during pregnancy and lactation: what are the safest therapy options? *Drug Safety* 19(4):325-337, 1998.

Brucker MC, Faucher MA: Pharmacologic management of common gastrointestinal health problems in women, *J Nurse Midwifery* 42(3):145-162, 1997.

Calhoun BC: Gastrointestinal disorders in pregnancy, *Obstet Gynecol Clin North Am* 19(4):733-744, 1992.

Chen TC, Leviton A: Headache recurrence in pregnant women with migraine, *Headache* 34(2):107-110, 1994.

Ching CK, Lam SK: Antacids. Indications and limitations, *Drugs* 47(2):305-317, 1994.

Cooksey NR: Pica and olfactory craving of pregnancy: how deep are the secrets? *Birth* 22(3):129-137, 1995.

Courts RB: Splinting for symptoms of carpal tunnel syndrome during pregnancy *J Hand Ther* 8(1):31-34, 1995.

Dahle LO et al: The effect of oral magnesium substitution on pregnancy-induced leg cramps, *Am J Obstet Gynecol* 173(1):175-180, 1995.

Dundee JW et al: P6 acupressure reduces morning sickness, *J Royal Soc Med* 81(8):456-457, 1988.

Evans AT et al: Suppression of pregnancy-induced nausea and vomiting with sensory afferent stimulation, *J Reprod Med* 38(8):603-606, 1993.

Fisher-Rasmussen W et al: Ginger treatment of hyperemesis gravidarum, *European J Obstet Gynecol Reprod Biol* 38:19-24, 1990.

Hammar M, Larsson L, Tegler L: Calcium treatment of leg cramps in pregnancy: effect of clinical symptoms and total serum and ionized serum calcium concentrations, *Acta Obstet Gynecol Scand* 60(4):345-347, 1981.

Heckman JD, Sassard R: Musculoskeletal considerations in pregnancy, *J Bone Joint Surg Am* 76(11):1720-1730, 1994.

Hyde E: Acupressure therapy for morning sickness, *J Nurse-Midwifery* 34(4):171-178, 1989.

Lacey EP: Broadening the perspective of pica: literature review, *Public Health Rep* 105(1):29-35, 1990.

Mabry RL: Rhinitis of pregnancy, *South Med J* 79(8):965-971, 1986.

McDonald JM: Cholestasis of pregnancy, *J Gastroenterol Hepatol* 14(6):515-518, 1999.

Murphy PA: Alternative therapies for nausea and vomiting of pregnancy, *Obstet Gynecol* 91(1):149-155, 1998.

Ostgaard HC, Andersson GB, Miller JA: Influence of some biomechanical factors of low back pain in pregnancy, *Spine* 18(1):61-65, 1993.

Pitkin RM: Calcium metabolism in pregnancy: a review, *Am J Obstet Gynecol* 121(5):724-737, 1975.

Pugh, LC, Milligan R: A framework for the study of childbearing fatigue, *Adv Nurs Sci* 15(4):60-70, 1993.

Reyes H: Review: Intrahepatic cholestasis: a puzzling disorder of pregnancy, *J Gastroenterol Hepatol* 12(3):211-216, 1997.

Sahakian V et al: Vitamin B_6 is effective therapy for nausea and vomiting of pregnancy: A randomized, double-blind placebo-controlled study, *Obstet Gynecol* 78(1):33-36, 1991.

Scharff L, Marcus DA, Turk DC: Headache during pregnancy and in the postpartum: A prospective study, *Headache* 37(4):203-210, 1997.

Silberstein SD: Migraine and pregnancy, *Neurol Clin* 15(1): 209-231, 1997.

Stannard D: Pressure prevents nausea, *Nurs Times* 85(4):33-34, 1989.

Star WL et al: *Ambulatory obstetrics: protocols for nurse practitioners and nurse-midwives,* ed 2, San Francisco, 1990, University of California, San Francisco.

Stolp-Smith KA, Pascoe MK, Ogburn PL: Carpal tunnel syndrome in pregnancy: frequency, severity and prognosis, *Arch Phys Med Rehabil* 79(10):1285-1287, 1998.

Sweet BR: *Mayes' midwifery: a textbook for midwives,* ed 12, London, 1997, Baillière Tindall.

Turnbull GL et al: Managing pregnancy-related nocturnal nasal congestion: the external nasal dilator, *J Reprod Med* 41(12):897-902, 1996.

Vutyavanich T, Wongtra-ngan S, Ruangsri R: Pyridoxine for nausea and vomiting of pregnancy: a randomized, double-blind, placebo-controlled study, *Am J Obstet Gynecol* 173(3):881-884, 1995.

Weed SS: *Wise woman herbal for the childbearing year,* Woodstock, NY, 1985, Ash Tree Publishers.

Chapter 11

Nutritional Needs and Counseling During Pregnancy

It is clear that the maternal adaptations in pregnancy and the fetal-placental demands require significant maternal energy expenditure. Recommendations for alterations in diet have always been culturally mediated in communities. Specific foods have been linked to infant growth, temperament, and physical appearance. Other foods have been linked to maternal health. This chapter explores the physiologic needs in pregnancy and the postpartum period, the influences of culture on nutrition, and nutritional recommendations for improving infant and maternal health status.

HISTORICAL ASPECTS OF NUTRITIONAL RECOMMENDATIONS IN PREGNANCY

It appears that, during the sixteenth, seventeenth, and eighteenth centuries, scholars in western Europe recognized that the fetus received its nutrients through the mother's system, and thus there was much emphasis put on the "proper" maternal diet in pregnancy (Food and Nutrition Board, 1990). However. in the mid-nineteenth century restriction in weight gain was suggested as a means to reduce birth weight and decrease the incidence of difficult births. The first published study of diet and pregnancy reported that the restricted maternal weight gain reduced birth weight by 400 to 500 g (Prochownick, 1901). Davis (1923) reported that mean birth weight increased with increasing maternal weight gain from 3100 g with a 7-kg maternal gain to 3600 g with a 13.6-kg gain. Excessive weight gain was attributed to edema; thus restricting weight gain seemed like a logical approach to decreasing the occurrence of toxemia. This theory led to the use of salt-restriction and diuretics to further reduce the occurrence of edema—a practice that continued in some areas of the United States into the 1950s. By the 1930s physicians were counseling women to restrict weight gain to 6.8 kg (15 pounds).

Early prenatal care initiatives in the 1920s document the public health nurse's role in giving advice about diet during pregnancy. Counseling usually occurred in the pregnant woman's home or at the health fairs supported by Shepard-Towner funding. As long as counseling occurred in the woman's own environment, culture and the woman's own belief system exerted strong influences on dietary choices. When physicians began providing instruction regarding weight gain in pregnancy, the context shifted to control of the woman's nutrition to address possible pathologic deviations in pregnancy. Historians have argued that the early inclusion of nutritional and weight-related care into medically defined prenatal care represents an example of social control of women in the medical system, rather than an example of inclusion of an intervention that was based on science (Wertz and Wertz, 1977). Relatively little research exploring the associations between nutrition and pregnancy outcome was generated until the second half of the twentieth century when researchers began to recognize the associations among quality of nutritional intake, weight gain, and infant outcome (Food and Nutrition Board, 1990; Worthington-Roberts and Klerman, 1990).

The emphasis on limiting weight gain in pregnancy was challenged as concern about the effects of less-than-optimal weight gain was raised. Retrospective studies using observational data during periods of hardship (e.g., war, famine, migration) suggested that severe nutritional deprivation is associated with lower birth weights, increases in fetal and neonatal mortality, and increase in congenital anomalies. Investigations of the association between maternal weight gain and birth weight have suggested that the additional variable of prepregnancy weight is also a major contributor to fetal nutrition. In contrast to previous physician counseling that women should not gain more than 18 to 20 pounds in pregnancy, recent findings suggest that women who gain less than 21 pounds during pregnancy are more than twice as likely to give birth to a low-birth-weight infant. Women who enter pregnancy underweight (80% of standard weight) are even more likely to deliver a low-birth-weight infant.

From 1970 to the present government panels and professional organizations have examined the issue of maternal nutrition and have promulgated numerous recommendations and guidelines. In 1970 the Committee on Maternal Nutrition of the Food and Nutrition Board (FNB) recommended an average maternal weight gain of 24 pounds, with a range of 20 to 25 pounds considered acceptable. The American College of Obstetricians and Gynecologists (ACOG) used the FNB recommendations in their own publications from 1972 through 1985. In 1981 the FNB revised their guidelines to consider pattern of weight gain as well as total amount. Inadequate weight gain was defined as a gain of 1 kg or less per month during the second and third trimesters, and excessive weight gain was defined as 3 kg or more per month (Food and Nutrition Board, 1990). Recommended caloric intakes have occasionally conflicted with professional guidelines. For example, the highest caloric recommendation for pregnancy ever published, 2700 kcal/day, was proposed in 1953 when weight gain was most restricted by physicians. The current recommendation for pregnancy is 2500 kcal/day.

The FNB has also published the recommended dietary allowances (RDAs) as standards for dietary intake since 1943. The RDA is defined as the average dietary intake necessary to meet the needs of 97% to 98% of healthy individuals in specific life-stage and gender groups (Food and Nutrition Board, 1999). Effective 1997 the FNB is publishing the estimated average requirement (EAR) for nutrients in its *Dietary Reference Intakes* (1999), a new format that provides extensive background information explaining the research that is considered when establishing nutritional standards. The EAR is the daily value that is estimated to meet the nutritional requirement in 50% of individuals in specific life-stage or gender groups (Food and Nutrition Board, 1999). When possible, the FNB also calculates the level for adequate intake (AI), which is the experimentally derived intake in a defined population that appears to sustain a defined nutritional state such as growth, and the upper limit (UL), which is the highest level of intake that is likely to pose no risk for toxicity.

A major contribution was made to the field when the Institute of Medicine issued *Nutrition During Pregnancy—Weight Gain and Nutritional Supplements* (1990). The major charge from the Bureau of Maternal and Child Health and Resources Development of DHHS to the National Academy of Sciences was to evaluate the scientific evidence and formulate recommendations for desirable weight gain and vitamin, mineral, and protein supplementation in pregnancy. The report summary recommendations are incorporated in the data collection and counseling sections of this chapter.

ENERGY REQUIREMENTS

The National Research Council's recommendation for increased caloric intake in pregnancy is an additional 300 kcal/day during the second and third trimesters, for a total daily intake of 2500 kcal/day. This recommendation is based on an expected weight gain of 12.5 kg during the pregnancy and doesn't consider the woman's prepregnant body mass index (BMI). While there have been no recent studies exploring the range of weight gain in healthy women, the 1980 National Natality Survey found that normal weight women who delivered 3- to 4-kg babies at term had a weight gain range of 16 to 40 pounds.

The IOM recommendations for weight gain in pregnancy are noted in Table 11-1. The higher end of the weight gain range is recommended for young adolescents and black women because of their higher risk

Table 11-1 *Institute of Medicine Recommended Weight Gains for Pregnant Women*

Weight-for-height category	Kilograms	Pounds
Low (BMI <19.8)	12.5-18	28-40
Normal (BMI 19.8-26.0)	11.5-6	25-35
High (BMI 26.0-29.0)	7-11.5	15-25

BMI, Body mass index.

of lower-birth-weight infants. The lower end of the weight gain range is recommended for short women (less than 62 inches). The recommended gain for obese women (BMI >29) is 6 kg (15 pounds). Parker and Abrams (1992) studied the associations among recommended IOM weight gains and the outcomes of small-for-gestational-age (SGA) infants, large-for-gestational-age (LGA) infants, and cesarean section and found that those women who experienced the recommended weight gains had decreased risk for SGA, LGA, and cesarean birth. Weight gains above the recommended levels were associated with increased risk of LGA infants and increase in cesarean birth. Weight gains below the recommended levels resulted in twice the risk of an SGA infant. Interestingly, their findings suggest that obese women who gain less than 6 kg have an increased risk of delivering an SGA infant, while there is only a nonsignificant trend ($p = 1\ 0.06$) of delivering an LGA infant when weight gain exceeds 17 kg. This conflicts with previous studies that have found no relationship between weight gain for obese women and birth weight. Two recent investigations (Caulfield, Stoltzfus, and Witter, 1998; Shieve, Cogswell, and Scanlon, 1998) found that the increased weight gain recommended for black women did not significantly reduce the risk of SGA infants, and investigators recommend more study to identify possible covariates that may influence the higher rate of SGA infants in black women.

Studies have consistently suggested that excess weight gain in pregnancy is associated with increased weight retention in the postpartum period. This is most likely because of the increase in maternal fatty stores, and there is a strong association between pregnancy weight gain and maternal fat gain. Studies have also suggested that postpartum weight retention is more likely after a first birth than after subsequent births. Women who breast-feed experience greater weight loss than those who do not breast-feed, and most of that loss is experienced during the third through sixth month after delivery.

The RDA recommendation for caloric intake during lactation is 2700 kcal/day, an additional 500 kcal/day when compared to nonpregnant recommendations. This calculation is based on the assumptions that average milk production is 750 ml/day during the first 6 months of lactation, average energy content of breast milk is 70 kcal/100 ml, efficiency of energy conversion into milk is 80%, and mobilization of fat for milk synthesis averages 100 to 150 kcal/day. Studies that have explored the actual intake of lactating women and their activity levels suggest that the recommended 2700 kcal/day may be an overestimate during the first months after delivery when the woman is more sedentary.

In addition to calories for energy, it is essential that adequate protein be ingested to meet the demands of rapid growth of the fetus and the uteroplacental unit and breasts, as well as increased plasma protein and blood cell production. The RDA for protein during pregnancy is 60 g/day and is usually exceeded in women with access to dietary sources and without cultural or religious restrictions in the diet.

VITAMIN AND MINERAL REQUIREMENTS

Maternal adaptations for pregnancy influence the levels of circulating and stored vitamin compounds. Water-soluble vitamins (vitamin C, the B vitamins, pantothenic acid, and biotin) commonly have decreased plasma levels in the second half of pregnancy as a result of hemodilution. Toxic effects of megadoses are rare since excess intake is excreted in urine in healthy women with normal renal function. Fat-soluble vitamins (vitamins A, D, E, and K) are stored in fatty tissue, and megadoses can lead to toxicity. The increased fatty stores that are deposited in pregnancy increase storage sites for the fat-soluble vitamins.

Vitamin A

The generic term vitamin A actually includes several compounds with similar biologic activities. Retinoids are found in animal tissue and include retinol, retinaldehyde, retinoic acid, and retinoic ester, which is the most commonly ingested retinoid. Carotinoids are found mainly in vegetable compounds. Both retinoids and carotinoids can be metabolized into vitamin A. Approximately 70% to 90% of ingested retinoid is absorbed, but absorption of carotinoids is less efficient with only 20% to 50% absorption.

The primary importance of vitamin A is its contribution of the photochemical reactions in the retina. It is also necessary in glycoprotein synthesis, promoting cell growth and differentiation, tooth bud formation, and bone growth. Vitamin A activity is expressed as international units (IU) or retinol equivalents (REs). IUs are determined by the growth-promoting activity of all retinoids or carotenoids. REs take into consideration the intestinal absorption of each compound. While confusing, both terms are used here, reflecting the units of measurement used in the studies or reports (Food and Nutrition Board, 1990). RDA for retinol equivalents is 800 μg/day, the same as for nonpregnant women. Since no vitamin A deficiency has been identified in the United States, routine supplementation has not been recommended.

Dietary sources for vitamin A include green leafy vegetables, dark yellow vegetables and fruits, chili peppers, beef liver, whole milk, and fortified margarine and butter.

High doses of retinoids can be toxic and teratogenic. The minimum dose associated with teratogenic effects is not known. Most sources suggest that doses of 20,000 to 30,000 IU are required for teratogenicity. Ingestion of large doses (15,000 RE for a sustained period of time) of retinoids is also associated with a syndrome that includes headache, vomiting, diplopia, alopecia, liver damage, and skin abnormalities. There have been only a few investigations on the effect of high doses of carotenoids in humans, and their findings suggest that they are neither teratogenic nor toxic. This is probably because of the poor absorption of these compounds so that little vitamin A is synthesized from them.

B Vitamins

Vitamin B_6 (pyridoxine) is a coenzyme necessary for amino acid and glycogen metabolism. Fetal uptake of vitamin B_6 and increased protein intake in pregnancy necessitate an increase in B_6 intake in pregnancy. Routine supplementation of vitamin B_6 does not appear to be necessary unless the pregnant woman is at risk for inadequate nutritional intake. Women at risk include those who abuse drugs and alcohol and smokers. When women are identified as at increased risk, a supplement of 2 mg/day is recommended. Dietary sources of vitamin B_6 include meat, poultry, eggs, organ meats, dark yellow vegetables, and whole grains and cereals.

Thiamine (vitamin B_1), riboflavin (vitamin B_2), and niacin (vitamin B_3) are necessary for energy metabolism. National surveys have found that American women typically exceed the RDA for these vitamins, primarily because of enriched and fortified grains and cereals. In addition, dietary sources of thiamine and niacin include pork, beef, and liver. Riboflavin is also found in milk products, eggs, organ meats, cheddar cheese, and green leafy vegetables. No supplementation is recommended in pregnancy.

Vitamin B_{12} is necessary for cell division, protein synthesis, maintenance of the myelin sheath of epithelial and nerve cells, and production of red and white blood cells. Vitamin B_{12} is found primarily in animal proteins and seaweed. The needs of pregnancy are met in the usual diet that includes meat, fish, eggs, and milk. Vegetarians who do not consume eggs, milk, and cheese should supplement their diets with 2 μg/day of vitamin B_{12}.

The RDAs and EARs for B vitamins in pregnancy are:

	RDA	EAR
Thiamine	1.4 mg	1.2 mg
Riboflavin	1.4 mg	1.2 mg
B_6	1.9 mg	1.6 mg
B_{12}	2.6 μg	2.2 μg
Niacin	18 mg	14 mg

Vitamin C

Vitamin C functions as an antioxidant and is essential in metabolism of tyrosine, folate, histamine, and some drugs. In addition, it is necessary for leukocyte function, immune responses, wound healing, and allergic reactions (Food and Nutrition Board, 1990). Vitamin C levels decrease somewhat in pregnancy, most likely as a result of blood volume expansion and hormone activity. The National Research Council estimates that an increase of 10 mg/day is necessary in pregnancy to meet the needs of the fetal and maternal systems. Drug use, smoking, alcohol use, long-term use of oral contraceptives, and multiple gestation increase the risk for deficiency; and a supplement of 50 mg/day is recommended for women with these risk factors.

The RDA for vitamin C is 70 mg in pregnancy. Dietary sources include citrus fruits, strawberries, melons, broccoli, tomatoes, peppers, potato skins, and raw dark green vegetables. Cooking destroys the available vitamin C.

Vitamin D

Vitamin D is necessary for absorption of calcium and phosphorous from the gastrointestinal tract and mineralization of maternal and fetal bones and teeth. Almost all vitamin D is synthesized from a precursor in the skin following exposure to ultraviolet light from the sun (Food and Nutrition Board, 1990). Because of this reliance on exposure to sun, there are seasonal and geographic differences in vitamin D synthesis in the United States. Vitamin D–fortified milk is the only major dietary source of this vitamin. International studies have identified cases of vitamin D deficiency in Britain and Western Europe, but this has not been the case in the United States, where most regions experienced greater numbers of days of sunshine. For this reason the Institute of Medicine does not recommend routine supplementation. Supplementation with 10 μg/day of vitamin D should be considered for vegetarians who do not include milk and eggs in their diets. In addition, pregnant women with low dietary intake who reside in northern climates may benefit from a 5-μg/day supplement of vitamin D during winter months. The RDA for pregnant women is 10 μg.

Vitamin E

Vitamin E is an important antioxidant in humans. It is necessary for maintenance of cell wall integrity and maintenance of red blood cells. Deficiency of this vitamin is associated with anemia, neuromuscular abnormalities, and reproductive failure (Food and Nutrition Board, 1990). Vitamin E is found in the polyunsaturated fatty acids (PUFA) of the cell membranes, and deficiency results in damage to the cells through the oxidation of PUFAs. Tocopherols and tocotrienols both include biologically active forms of vitamin E, with tocopherols being widely found in nature. Vegetable oils are the richest source of vitamin E in the American diet (e.g., margarine, shortening, wheat germ, whole grains, and nuts all contain large amounts of the vitamin). There have been no reports of toxicity, even in doses as large as 800 mg/day. Since there have been no reports of morbidity associated with intake below the RDA of 10 mg/day, routine supplementation is not recommended.

Folate

Folates, a generic descriptor of several compounds that have properties similar to folic acid, are necessary for metabolism of amino acids, synthesis of purine and thymidylate (essential in nucleic acid synthesis), production of hemes for hemoglobin, and completion of mitosis. Because of the necessary increase in cells in uterine enlargement, development of the fetal-placental unit, and increase in red blood cells, folate demands increase in pregnancy. Deficiency of folates has been associated with impaired cell growth and replication leading to spontaneous abortion, fetal and placental anomalies, and SGA infants. The role of folates in megaloblastic anemia has been well documented.

Folates are found in liver, fortified grains and cereals, dried peas and beans, leafy vegetables, and yeast. Effective January 1, 1998, all enriched cereal grains are required to be enriched with 1.4 mg of folic acid per kilogram of grain. Heat and ultraviolet light can destroy some forms of folates, so food preparation may diminish the available folates in a particular food. National surveys have identified that pregnant women in the United States tend to average 215 to 250 μg/day of folic acid, well below the RDA of 600 μg/day. However, since folates are readily available in leafy vegetables and fruits, the IOM recommends increased dietary folic acid rather than supplements.

Because of the apparent decreased risk of neural tube defects in women who have adequate folate intake, the Centers for Disease Control and Prevention recommends that all women of child-bearing age who are at risk of conceiving should have an intake of folic acid of at least 400 μg/day. There are no recommendations for additional supplements unless the women is identified as high risk for anemia, in which case a supplement of 400 μg is recommended.

Vitamin K

Vitamin K is required in the synthesis of prothrombin and clotting factors VII, IX, and X, as well as for the synthesis of proteins in the bone and kidney (Food and Nutrition Board, 1990). Vitamin K is absorbed in the small intestine. The effect of pregnancy on vitamin K activity is not understood. Placental transport of the vitamin to the fetus is likewise unclear.

Vitamin K is found in leafy vegetables, dairy products, meat, and egg yolks. Bacterial flora in the small intestine also contribute to vitamin K synthesis and absorption.

There has been no specific RDA established for pregnancy because of the lack of research available. The RDA for nonpregnant adults is 65 μg, which is well below the estimated daily intake of 300 to 500 μg found in a typical American diet (Food and Nutrition Board, 1990). Because of the availability of vitamin K from dietary and bacterial sources, no supplements are recommended in pregnancy.

Calcium

Calcium is necessary for increased maternal calcium needs and formation of fetal skeleton and teeth. There is an increase in both absorption and excretion of calcium in pregnancy, resulting in an overall positive calcium balance. Calcium is absorbed through active transport and passive diffusion in the intestine. Total serum calcium decreases, paralleling the decrease in serum proteins that occurs with expansion of intravascular fluid volume. When adjustments are made for this action, there is little or no change in total serum calcium.

Calcium is transferred to the fetus at a rate of 20 mg/day at 20 weeks' gestation, increasing to 330 mg/day at 35 weeks' gestation. It is theorized that this increased calcium is drawn from maternal bone, and it is believed that bone turnover begins in the first trimester and increases dramatically in the third trimester. Estimates of changes in bone mineral density in pregnancy have been conflicting. Dietary supplementation of calcium does not appear to have a relationship with changes in bone mineral density in pregnancy (Food and Nutrition Board, 1999). In addition, increased intestinal absorption begins early in pregnancy and continues until term.

The RDA for calcium in pregnancy is 1200 mg/day. Recent research has found that the median intake of calcium for pregnant American women is 1154 mg/day, with the twenty-fifth percentile at 939 mg/day and the seventy-fifth percentile at 1382 mg/day (Food and Nutrition Board, 1999). With these findings the Institute of Medicine now recommends supplementation only when it is clear that women who are between 14 and 18 years of age have an intake under 1300 mg/day and women who are 19 years of age or older have an intake under 1000 mg/day. Dietary sources include milk, yogurt, hard cheese, green leafy vegetables, nuts, dried beans, sardines or other fish with bones, and tofu.

Copper

Copper is necessary for the formation of many oxidative enzymes in the body, the synthesis of connective tissue and norepinephrine, and the transportation of iron. Animal studies have suggested that copper deficiency may be associated with infertility, abortion, and stillbirth, but these have not been replicated in humans. Copper deficiency has not been documented in pregnant women, and plasma levels usually increase as a result of changes in metabolism during gestation. Studies suggest that the estimated requirement for copper in pregnancy is 1.5 to 2 mg/day. Since there is no evidence that women in the United States experience insufficient intake of copper, there is no recommendation for supplementation in pregnancy. However, women who are taking iron supplements greater than 30 mg/day may benefit from supplementation of 2 mg of copper, since iron inhibits copper absorption.

Fluoride

Fluoride binds with hydrogen to form hydrogen fluoride, an acid that has been associated with decreased incidence of dental caries. Although it has been hypothesized that prenatal intake of fluoride offers preventive benefits through the uptake of fluoride by the enamel crystallites, the research on the effectiveness has been conflicting. Routine prenatal fluoride supplementation is not recommended by the American Dental Association or the American Academy of Pediatrics. There is no indication that pregnant women need more fluoride than nonpregnant women. The Institute of Medicine has determined that the AI for fluoride is 3 mg/day and the UL for fluoride in adult women is 10 mg/day. Intake higher than the UL increases the risk of skeletal and enamel fluorosis, with the related increased risk of skeletal fractures and fractures of dental enamel. The U. S. Public Health Service has set the optimal concentration of fluoride in drinking water at 0.7 to 1.2 mg/L, and the Environmental Protection Agency has set the maximum recommended concentration at 4 mg/L. Fluoride supplementation is also available in toothpaste and mouthwash.

Iodine

Iodine is necessary for synthesis of T_3 and T_4. Maternal iodine deficiency in pregnancy contributes to iodine deficiency disorders in the fetus, including endemic cretinism, profound deafness, spastic dysplasia, and a variety of neurologic impairments. Largely because of the availability of iodized salt in the United States, iodine intake is usually above the RDA of 150 μg/day in pregnancy.

Iron

Increased erythropoiesis in pregnancy results in an increased need for iron. In addition, many women enter pregnancy with depleted iron stores. Iron is present as heme (animal products) and nonheme (plant products) iron. Most of the iron in the diet is in the form of nonheme. The iron salts in nonheme vary in solubility, which affects the absorption in the upper part of the small intestine. Iron absorption is inhibited in meals that primarily consist of whole-grain cereals and legumes. Phytates in the cereals, calcium and phosphorous in milk, tannin in tea, and polyphenols in many vegetables inhibit iron absorption by decreasing iron salt solubility (Food and Nutrition Board, 1990). Inclusion of meat and ascorbic acid in meals increases absorption by facilitating solubility. Other iron-containing dietary sources are enriched breads and cereals, legumes, and dried fruits. Higher percentages of heme-iron are absorbed, and heme-iron absorption does not appear to be affected by the presence or absence of specific foods.

The current IOM recommendation for pregnant women who are not anemic is 30 mg of ferrous iron beginning at 12 weeks' gestation. Women with iron deficiency anemia should increase their iron intake to 60 to 120 mg/day elemental iron.

Phosphorus

Phosphorus is necessary for bone growth, and it appears that the absorption of phosphorus increases in pregnancy in a mechanism similar to the increased absorption of calcium. Because of the increased absorption, there is no indication for recommending increased intake in pregnancy. The RDA for pregnancy is 1250 mg/day for adolescents and 700 mg/day for women older than 18 years of age.

Zinc

Zinc is necessary for nucleic acid and protein metabolism and therefore essential in cell reproduction. With the rapid growth of fetal and maternal tissue in pregnancy, increased intake of zinc is necessary. Studies have shown that healthy adults in North America average 12 to 14 mg daily, which is probably sufficient in pregnancy, particularly if there are adaptations that increase zinc absorption. Dietary sources include liver, shellfish, meats, whole grains, and milk.

Women taking iron supplements of greater than 30 mg/day may benefit from a zinc supplement of 15 mg/day since iron inhibits zinc absorption. Vegetarians tend to have lower dietary intake of zinc and may benefit from supplementation. The RDA is 15 mg/day.

PHYSIOLOGIC CHANGES IN PREGNANCY THAT INFLUENCE NUTRITIONAL INTAKE

During pregnancy numerous maternal adaptations facilitate the growth of the maternal-fetal unit. Appetite increases, resulting in increased ingestion of food. Progesterone-induced relaxation of smooth muscles and inhibition of plasma motilin results in delayed transit time through the gastrointestinal system. Duodenal villi increase in size, leading to increased absorption of nutrients, including calcium, iron, lysine, valine, glycine, proline, glucose, sodium, chloride, and water (Blackburn and Loper, 1992). Alteration of enzyme transport systems decreases the absorption of niacin, riboflavin, and vitamin B_6. Absorption of calcium, sodium, and water also increases in the colon.

Hormonal influences of human placental lactogen, estrogen, and progesterone lead to metabolic changes that result in diabetogenic effects, altered lipid and protein metabolism, and increased glucose and amino acid availability for transfer to the fetus. Early in pregnancy lower glucose levels contribute to decreased insulin release. Later in pregnancy insulin resistance is associated with reduced maternal glucose use and increased production of insulin. The increased production of insulin is facilitated by hypertrophy of the beta-cells in the pancreas under the influence of estrogen. Protein metabolism is likewise affected. During the latter part of pregnancy, protein is used as an alternate energy source for fetal demands. Fat metabolism in the first two trimesters is altered in two ways: (1) increased triglyceride synthesis and fat storage, and (2) suppression of lipolysis. In late pregnancy lipolysis increases to meet maternal needs and spare glucose for fetal growth.

NUTRITIONAL INTERVENTION IN PREGNANCY

Studies evaluating the effectiveness of nutritional intervention programs are difficult to compare and contrast since they often suffer from lack of controls, poor definition of outcome variables, and poor identification of preexisting nutritional and health status variables. For that reason, two studies are presented to represent examples of the effectiveness of specific interventions.

Higgins Intervention Method for Nutritional Rehabilitation During Pregnancy

The Higgins Intervention Method was developed at the Montreal Diet Dispensary and is based on the determination of the calorie and protein needs of the individual woman during pregnancy. Following the establishment of the prepregnant caloric and protein requirements using ideal weight for height, 500 calories and 25 g of protein are added to the daily requirements after 20 weeks' gestation. Higher RDA requirements are used if the individual is an adolescent. Women who are underweight, under nutritional stress, or undernourished are given additional supplements of calories and protein. Throughout pregnancy 24-hour dietary recall and ongoing provider support lead to a greater proportion of women gaining an appropriate amount of weight during gestation. Programs that have used this approach have documented increased birth weight when the target intake has been met (Dubois et al., 1997; Dubois et al., 1991; Higgins, 1976; Higgins et al., 1989; Piechik and Corbett, 1985).

Special Supplemental Nutrition Program for Women, Infants, and Children

The Women, Infants, and Children (WIC) program is a federally regulated and funded program that has been available to pregnant women and children since 1974. The program is based on the assumption that poor women and children with nutritional risk will achieve better health status through food supplementation and health education and counseling. WIC goals include the improvement of fetal development and the reduction of the incidence of low birth weight, preterm deliveries, and incidence of anemia through intervention during the prenatal period (Food and Consumer Service, 1996). To qualify for services, women must demonstrate income below 185% of the poverty level and must be determined to be at nutritional risk by a physician, midwife, nurse, nutritionist, dietitian, or other qualified provider. The program provides services using a seven-level priority system to ensure that the most at-risk women and children receive services first when resources are limited. Examples of nutritional risk factors for pregnant and lactating women are noted in Table 11-2.

Numerous studies have found that participation in the WIC program is associated with decreases in the low-birth-weight and very low–birth weight rates. Because of the decreased morbidity associated with these outcomes, it has been estimated that the WIC program saves close to $2 billion annually, which more than offsets the costs of the program (Avruch and Cackley, 1995). Other studies have suggested that, for every dollar spent on the WIC program, there is a $2 to $3 savings on Medicaid costs during an infant's first 60 days of life (Devaney, Bilheimer, and Schore, 1992).

WIC programs are administered by local agencies under contract with the U. S. Department of Agriculture,

Table 11-2 *WIC Nutritional Risk Criteria*

Risk factor	Definition
Prepregnancy—underweight	BMI <19.8
Low maternal weight gain	<0.9 kg/month for nonobese women and <0.45 kg/month for obese women
Maternal weight loss in pregnancy	>2 kg in the first trimester and >1 kg in the second and third trimester
Prepregnancy—overweight	BMI >26
High gestational weight gain	>3 kg/month
Anemia	Institute of Medicine hemoglobin/hematocrit cut-offs
Medical conditions	Gastrointestinal disorders, diabetes, thyroid disorders, hypertension, human immunodeficiency virus infection
Closely spaced pregnancies	Interconceptional interval of 6 months (9 months if lactating)
History of preterm delivery	Delivery <37 weeks' gestation
Multiple gestation	More than one fetus
Dietary risks	Vegan, highly restrictive diets
Social problems	Homelessness, migrancy, battering

Adapted from Food and Nutrition Board, Institute of Medicine: *WIC nutrition risk criteria: a scientific assessment,* Washington, DC, 1996, National Academy Press.

and average monthly participation in fiscal year 1998 was 7 million individuals. In most states participants receive food vouchers that can be used to purchase specific foods. Foods provided under the program must be high in one or more of the following nutrients: protein, calcium, iron, and vitamins A and C. Examples of foods included in the supplementation program include milk, cheese, eggs, peanut butter, dried beans or peas, tuna fish, iron-fortified cereal, vitamin C–rich fruit and/or vegetable juices, and carrots. Research suggests that these foods may not be commonly used in many cultures, and it has been suggested that the WIC program expand coverage to ethnic foods, including tofu and dark green leafy vegetables (Horswill and Yap, 1999).

SCREENING AND DIAGNOSIS OF NUTRITIONAL PROBLEMS

Nutritional assessment using self-reported dietary intake can be completed by the health care provider, the nursing staff in the clinic or office, or a nutritionist working in the interdisciplinary team. The nutritional assessment should include an interview to identify the individual's and family's medical, social, and diet history and a physical examination that includes anthropometrics and laboratory tests to identify nutrition-related problems such as anemia and glucose intolerance in pregnancy. Even with the limitations of using weight gain as an indicator of nutrition, the measure of weight continues to be the most common screening measure when assessing for nutritional problems.

The initial prenatal nutrition interview should identify problems or potential problems associated with poor pregnancy outcome. Identification of usual caloric intake and source of the nutrients is essential to identify deficiencies in the diet. Food habits and attitudes reflect further influences on nutrition. Past or current medical conditions that may influence intake and absorption must be noted, as well as any medications that may affect nutritional status. Factors associated with high nutritional risk are noted in Box 11-1, and an example of an intake Nutrition Questionnaire is illustrated in Figure 11-1.

Anthropometric measurements of height and weight should be obtained using reliable equipment. Prepregnant weight for height and weight gain during pregnancy are important data obtained by the clinician. The use of other measures such as skin fold thickness have not been well examined for effectiveness. BMI (i.e., weight/height^2) is a better indicator of maternal nutritional status than weight alone (Food and Nutrition Board, 1990). Although no weight-for-height classification systems have been validated against pregnancy outcome, the committee made recommendations based on best clinical estimates.

All women should be screened for anemia at the initial visit and in late second trimester. Those with identified anemia should have follow-up laboratory studies to determine whether interventions are effective.

Box 11-1 *Factors Associated With High Nutrition Risk in Pregnancy*

Physical Factors

- Age under 15 or less than 2 years since menarche
- Obesity
- Low prepregnancy weight
- Insufficient weight gain in pregnancy
- Multiple pregnancy

Medical/Obstetric History Factors

- History of poor obstetric outcome, including habitual abortions, preterm deliveries, delivery of previous low-birth-weight infants
- Closely spaced pregnancies
- History of preeclampsia or preexisting hypertension
- Renal disease
- Diabetes
- Anemia
- Heart disease
- Liver disease
- Smoking
- Addictions to drugs or alcohol
- Pica
- Gastrointestinal disease
- Hyperthyroidism
- Hyperlipidemia
- Errors in metabolism (phenylketonuria, cystinuria)

Social/Cultural Factors

- Low income with limited food budget
- Unusual eating patterns (vegans, restrictive "health food" approach to nutrition)
- Religious beliefs that include special food proscriptions
- Inadequate knowledge or ability to make required food changes (handicapped individuals)
- Lack of access to food distribution programs when needed
- Poor social support

Adapted from Worthington-Roberts B, Klerman L: Maternal nutrition. In Merkatz IR, Thompson JE, editors: *New perspectives on prenatal care,* New York, 1990, Elsevier.

Nutrition Questionnaire

What you eat and some of the life-style choices you make can affect your nutrition and health now and in the future. Your nutrition can also have an important effect on your baby's health. Please answer these questions by circling the answers that apply to you.

1. Are you bothered by any of the following?
   Nausea Vomiting Heartburn Constipation Diarrhea
2. Do you skip meals at least 3 times per week? No Yes
3. Do you try to limit the food you eat to lose weight or limit weight gain? No Yes
4. Are you on a special diet now? No Yes
5. Do you avoid certain foods for religious or personal reasons? No Yes
6. Do you have a working stove? No Yes
7. Do you have a working refrigerator? No Yes
8. Do you ever run out of food before you are able to buy more? No Yes
9. Can you afford to eat the way you should? No Yes
10. Are you receiving any of the following food assistance?
    (Circle all that apply)
    Food Stamps WIC School Breakfast/Lunch Food from a pantry or food bank
11. Do you feel you need help obtaining food? No Yes
12. Which of the following did you drink yesterday?

Soda/soft drink	Coffee	Tea	Fruit drink
Orange juice	Other juice	Milk	Kool Aid
Water	Beer	Wine	Other alcohol

13. Which of the following did you eat yesterday?

Cheese	Pizza	Macaroni and cheese	
Yogurt	Cereal with milk		
Other food with cheese (for example, tacos, lasagna)			
Corn	Potatoes	Sweet potatoes	Green salad
Carrots	Collard greens	Spinach	Turnip greens
Broccoli	Green beans	Green peas	Other vegetables
Apple	Banana	Berries	Grapefruit
Melon	Orange	Peach	Other fruit
Meat	Fish	Chicken	Eggs
Peanut butter	Nuts	Seeds	Dried beans or lentils
Tofu			
Cold cuts	Hot dog	Bacon	Sausage
Cake	Cookies	Doughnut	Pastry
Chips	French fries		
Other deep fried foods			
Bread	Roll	Rice	Cereal
Noodles	Spaghetti	Tortilla	

Figure 11-1 Nutrition questionnaire. Adapted from Food and Nutrition Board, Institute of Medicine: *Nutrition during pregnancy and lactation: an implementation guide,* Washington, DC, 1992, National Academy Press.

The Food and Nutrition Board (1990, pp. 10-12) recommendations for data collection include:

1. Before conception use consistent and reliable procedures to accurately measure and record in the medical record the woman's weight and height without shoes.
2. Determine the woman's prepregnant BMI.
3. Measure height and weight at the first prenatal visit carefully by procedures that have been rigorously standardized at the site of prenatal care.
4. Use consistent, reliable procedures to measure weight at each subsequent visit.
5. Estimate the woman's gestational age from the best available dating parameters.
6. Record weight in a table and plot it on a chart included in the obstetric record.
7. Monitor the prenatal course to identify an abnormal pattern of gain that may indicate a need to intervene. Assess the pattern of gain at each visit relative to the established weight gain goal and the course leading to that goal.

Analysis of the data should yield the identification of problems or potential problems that will be addressed by specific intervention and counseling. Examples of commonly identified problems include prepregnant underweight status, obesity, anemia, restrictive diet, financial or environmental barriers to obtaining nutritious food. A plan to evaluate the effectiveness of each specific intervention should be developed using measurable outcomes.

NUTRITION COUNSELING FOR HEALTHY PREGNANT WOMEN

Nutritional counseling requires mutual exchange of information between the provider and the woman seeking care. Establishment of an environment that provides privacy and conveys the provider's supportive, nonjudgmental approach yields the most benefit for the client. Being honest about one's nutritional habits may be embarrassing, particularly in communities where there is much public discussion or media promotion of proper nutrition in pregnancy. It is important for the clinician to assume that a healthy woman wants to provide the best prenatal environment for her baby. Pregnancy is a time of great motivation for women, and it appears that women are more likely to make recommended changes in diet and lifestyle for the sake of the baby, even when it has been difficult to make changes in the past.

There are numerous instruments and client education materials available to assist the clinician with nutrition education. Most basic tools include the common "food groups" charts and sample diets. Table 11-3 illustrates a typical daily food plan appropriate for pregnancy.

Studies exploring the association between weight gain and pregnancy outcomes indicate the lowest incidence of low-birth-weight infants when women gain at least 26 to 35 pounds. Weight gain is influenced by the woman's body image and feelings about weight, race/ethnic variation, cultural attitudes about body im-

Table 11-3 *Daily Food Plan for Pregnancy*

Food	Nonpregnant woman	Pregnant woman
Dairy: Milk, cheese, yogurt, ice cream	2 cups	3-4 cups
Protein: Lean meat, fish, poultry, dried bean, lentils	1 serving (3-4 ounces)	2 servings (6-8 ounces)
Vegetables (dark green or yellow)	1 serving	1 serving
Vitamin-C rich foods: Citrus fruits, berries, cantaloupe, tomatoes, cabbage greens, potatoes with skins	1 good source or 2 fair sources	2 good sources or 1 good source and 1 fair source
Other vegetables and fruits	1 serving	2 servings
Bread and cereals: Enriched or whole grain	3 servings	4-5 servings
Fats: Butter/margarines	As desired or needed for calories	As desired or needed for calories

Adapted from Worthington-Roberts B, Klerman L: Maternal nutrition. In Merkatz IR, Thompson JE, editors, *New perspectives on prenatal care,* New York, 1990, Elsevier.

age and diet during pregnancy, and the guidance given by the health care provider (Caulfield, Witter, and Stoltzfus, 1996; Copper et al., 1995). Research suggests that health care professionals need to increase efforts to counsel women appropriately about target weight gain in pregnancy since about one fourth of women receive no counseling and one third of women receive advice that does not correlate with the Institute of Medicine recommendations for weight gain (Cogswell et al., 1996).

Vitamin and mineral supplementation became popular after World War II, in part because of the pharmaceutic industry's move to market prenatal vitamins. Trials involving supplementation of multiple vitamins or specific individual vitamins have resulted in conflicting findings (Keen and Zidenberg-Cherr, 1994). Data used to analyze nutritional status should provide rationale for recommendation for supplementation. To date there is no evidence to recommend universal vitamin and mineral supplementation.

Counseling recommendations published by the Institute of Medicine (1990, pp. 11-13) include:

1. Set a weight gain goal together with the pregnant woman, preferably beginning at the comprehensive initial prenatal examination, and explain to her why weight gain is important.
2. Base the recommended range of total weight gain and pattern of gain mainly on prepregnancy weight for height.
3. For women with a normal prepregnancy BMI, recommend gain at the rate of approximately 0.4 kg (1 pound)/week in the second and third trimesters of pregnancy.
4. When abnormal gain appears to be real rather than a result of an error in measurement or recording, try to determine the cause and then develop and implement corrective actions jointly with the woman.

CULTURAL INFLUENCES ON NUTRITION IN PREGNANCY

Food serves both a social and a nutritional purpose. Meals bring family and community members together; and rituals that tell about relationships, power, and beliefs are followed. The degree to which specific cultural beliefs and behaviors are incorporated into family life is related to the length of time the family has been in a community, the community composition, and the geographic and temporal distance from extended family and community of origin.

The pregnant woman's place in the family shapes her role in the rituals surrounding meals. A married woman in a nuclear family who is experiencing a second pregnancy may already be seen as the primary preparer of meals, whereas a young, newly married woman who has moved into her mother-in-law's home may have a role of helper to the family matriarch. The initial collection of social history data assists the provider in gaining understanding of the social, cultural, and economic factors that may influence the nutrition of the pregnant woman.

Eating patterns are influenced by community cultural patterns, religious proscriptions, personal preferences, and financial and community barriers to obtaining desired food. The clinician will sensitively explore all of these influences when completing a nutritional assessment and plan nutritional interventions collaboratively with the woman and any significant family members who participate in food planning and preparation. The following case studies illustrate ways that the health care professional and the client can mutually develop interventions to improve nutrition status.

Case Study 1

Annie Chen is a 24-year-old woman who came to the United States several years ago when her husband began graduate studies at a local university. She was unable to continue her studies here and is very unhappy with the lack of professional opportunities available for her. She shares that she is very lonely and doesn't usually feel like eating.

Her community has several stores that cater to the largely Chinese population, but the prices seem very high. Her family originates in the southern region of China, and her cooking reflects what is commonly referred to as Cantonese. She prepares seafood, occasional pork dishes, and numerous vegetarian dumplings (dim sum). She doesn't like to eat breakfast and only eats lunch if her husband comes home and expects lunch to be prepared.

Annie is 5'1" tall and weighed 102 pounds before pregnancy. Today, at 16 weeks' gestation, she weighs 95 pounds. She and her husband share an apartment with two other male graduate students who rarely eat with them. She feels money is "tight" and does not think that she can ask her parents for help.

Problems and interventions

Nutritional Problems

- Weight loss
- Diet inadequate in most nutrients and calories

Other Considerations

- Limited financial resources
- Possible depression
- Limited social support

Interventions

- Explore Annie's perception of the nutrition recommendations in her community in China.
- Explore student groups on campus that may provide support for international students and their families.
- In collaboration with the client, develop a meal plan that would increase calories and nutrients.
- Consider nutritional supplements, including iron, calcium, and multiple vitamins.
- Set target weight gain goals for each trimester and for total pregnancy.
- Discuss the importance of nutrition on fetal development, especially development of the brain and nervous system.
- Explore possible opportunities for volunteer work.
- Consider counseling if depression continues.

Evaluation of Effectiveness of Intervention and Counseling

- Annie gains a total of 25 to 35 pounds for a term pregnancy.
- Annie does not have any future weight loss.
- Annie maintains hemoglobin/hematocrit levels above the Institute of Medicine recommendations for each trimester.
- Annie reports dietary intake that provides adequate nutrients for her and her fetus.

Case Study 2

Latisha Johnson is an 18 year-old black woman who is 10 weeks' pregnant. She works in a local retail store 20 hours/week at minimum wage. While she works, her sister watches Latisha's 9-month-old son. Her boyfriend, the father of her son and this baby, comes around on weekends to play with his son and contributes about $25/week toward support. She lives with her mother, her sister, and her sister's two children (ages 4 and 6) in a three-bedroom home that her mother owns. Latisha gives "what she can" to help her mother out with bills. Her mother accompanies her at this visit and appears quite supportive, stating that she wants to do whatever is best for her grandbabies.

Latisha's mother does most of the shopping and cooking. Latisha tends to skip breakfast, taking a can of cola with her as she goes to work. When she is working, she has lunch at one of the nearby fast-food places and eats with co-workers. Her mother makes dinner, which usually consists of meat, potatoes, gravy, and greens. She drinks soda with her meals.

Latisha was upset that she gained 65 pounds with her last pregnancy and didn't lose much. She is 5′6″ tall and thinks she weighed around 210 pounds before conceiving. She currently weighs 225 pounds, and she attributes the weight gain to the fact that keeping something bland in her stomach decreases the nausea of pregnancy.

Problems and Interventions

Nutritional Problems

- Obesity
- Increased weight gain for gestational age
- Poor eating habits
- Diet low in dairy products, fresh fruits, and vegetables; many high-fat foods

Other Considerations

- Has little control over foods prepared in the home
- Limited income
- Closely spaced pregnancies
- History of excessive weight gain in last pregnancy

Interventions

- With Latisha's permission, include her mother in nutritional counseling.
- In collaboration with Latisha, identify foods that can be taken to work with her, decreasing the temptation to eat fast food.
- Set a target weight goal for a term pregnancy at 15 pounds.
- Consider vitamin and iron supplements because of closely spaced pregnancies and poor eating habits.
- Consult with a social worker to determine whether other publicly funded programs are available.
- Schedule frequent nutritional counseling sessions; provide positive reinforcement for appropriate nutritional changes.

Evaluation of Effectiveness of Intervention and Counseling

- Latisha gains 15 pounds during a term pregnancy.
- Latisha reports dietary intake that reflects appropriate calories and essential nutrients.
- Latisha reports adequate fluid intake of water and nutritious juices or milk.
- Latisha obtains nutritional support from WIC and food stamps.
- Latisha maintains hemoglobin/hematocrit levels above the Institute of Medicine recommendations for each trimester.

Case Study 3

Sunshine Abbott is a 22-year-old part-time college student who is 18 weeks' pregnant. She lives with her boyfriend, Jon, and they support themselves by working for a political group that lobbies for environmental reforms. She and Jon have a combined income of about $1200/month. She receives no assistance from her parents and is very firm that she would not approach them for help. They share an apartment with another couple who each work part-time jobs.

She is 5′5″ tall and weighs 115 pounds. Her prepregnant weight was about 110 pounds. Her pregnancy was planned and has been uneventful, except for nausea and vomiting during the first trimester and ongoing feelings of fatigue. Her hemoglobin is 9.2 g/dl. Sunshine is a vegetarian who eats no dairy or egg products. She does most of her shopping at a small natural food store in her neighborhood. She has obtained food stamps but doesn't have any other public support.

Problems and Interventions

Nutritional Problems

- Poor weight gain
- Low caloric intake
- Restrictive vegetarian diet, deficient in protein, iron, calcium, vitamin B_{12}, zinc, and iodine
- Anemia, probably iron deficiency

Other Considerations

- Low income
- No religious proscription
- Shops where food prices are most likely higher than larger markets
- Lack of extended family support
- Plans natural childbirth
- Plans to breast-feed

Interventions

- Mutually agree on the maternal and fetal need for certain nutrients.
- Provide nutritional counseling, individually or in groups.
- Suggest that Sunshine consider a lacto-vegetarian or lacto-ovo-vegetarian diet during the pregnancy and while breast-feeding.
- Consider vitamin and iron supplements.
- Recommend use of iodized salt.
- Discuss overpricing of organic foods in some markets; suggest larger stores where organic products may be available at more reasonable prices.
- Give positive reinforcement for positive dietary steps taken for herself and her baby.

Evaluation of Effectiveness of Intervention and Counseling

- Sunshine gains a total of 25 to 35 pounds during a term pregnancy.
- Sunshine increases the variety of food or uses supplements to ensure intake of essential nutrients.
- Sunshine maintains hemoglobin/hematocrit levels above the Institute of Medicine recommendations in the second and third trimesters.
- Sunshine obtains nutritional support from WIC.

Case Study 4

Jane Snyder-Johnson is 37 years old and experiencing her first pregnancy. She and her husband have been married for 9 years and have delayed planning a family until their careers were solid. Jane works as an attorney in a small law firm in town, and she is hoping to become a partner in the next year. She typically works 12- to 14-hour days and feels that she can't decrease her time because of the expectations of the firm. She is the first woman they have hired, and she feels little support from her colleagues. Because of her work schedule, she rarely exercises and tends to either eat "take-out" food at her desk or skip meals. Jane's husband is a physician in a group practice and, as the junior partner, covers a disproportionate share of nights and weekends. Although he would like to offer more help, he doesn't think he has the time. They have hired household help for cleaning and laundry and plan to have a live-in nanny when the baby is born.

Jane is 5′8″ tall; prepregnant weight was 120 pounds. She is currently 16 weeks' pregnant and has been experiencing a normal pregnancy. Her weight today is 128 pounds, and she is concerned about "gaining too much." Her hematocrit at her first visit (8 weeks' gestation) was 31%. Twenty-four hour diet recall is as follows:

Breakfast: Decaffeinated coffee, 8 ounces of orange juice, 1 piece whole wheat toast with jam

Lunch: Mixed salad brought in from a local deli, diet soda

Dinner: Snacks when she got home at 9 PM—cheese and crackers, celery, carbonated water

Other snacks: Popcorn at her desk, 2 cups of herbal tea at work

Problems and Interventions

Nutritional Problems

- Low caloric intake
- Inadequate protein, fruits and vegetables; inadequate iron, vitamin C, vitamin D, calcium, vitamin A
- Anemia, probably iron deficiency
- Entered pregnancy underweight

Other Considerations

- Demanding job; plans to work until she delivers, then 4 weeks leave
- No regular plan for meals
- Inadequate exercise
- Has adequate financial resources for meal planning
- Unrealistic expectations of impact of child on lifestyle
- Limited support from husband

Interventions

- Discuss deficiencies in diet, as well as nutritional needs for maternal and fetal health. Discuss the impact of inadequate nutrition on the developing fetus.
- Brainstorm ways that she could have five to six small meals throughout day and six to eight glasses of water or juice.
- Identify specific foods she likes and incorporate them into daily meal plan.
- Discuss expected weight gain and mutually plan a diet with sufficient calories to make that goal.
- Set target weight goals for each trimester and for a term pregnancy.
- Discuss realistic expectations of the demands of pregnancy and parenting.
- Brainstorm regarding work responsibilities and ways that some tasks can be delegated to others.
- Plan a way to exercise 3 days per week.
- Consider further counseling with the nutritionist.
- Encourage communication with mothers' groups or on-line list-serve that provide information and support regarding mothering.

Evaluation of Effectiveness of Intervention and Counseling

- Jane will gain 28 to 40 pounds during a term pregnancy.
- Jane will maintain hemoglobin and hematocrit levels above the Institute of Medicine recommendations for each trimester.
- Jane will report dietary intake that reflects adequate calories and all essential nutrients.
- Jane will report regular exercise three times per week.

CULTURAL, ETHNIC, AND RELIGIOUS PREFERENCES IN DIETS

Although it is important not to make broad, stereotypical assumptions about cultural, ethnic, and religious preferences in diets, the following common food preferences provide background for exploring the individual woman's nutritional pattern.

Black

- Meat: Beef; pork and ham; sausage, pig's feet, ears, etc.; bacon; luncheon meats; organ meats; scrapple; chitterlings; spareribs; hogshead; squirrel; opossum; rabbit; raccoon
- Poultry: Chicken, turkey
- Fish: Catfish, perch, red snapper, tuna, salmon, sardines, shrimp
- Eggs
- Legumes: Kidney beans, red beans, pinto beans, black-eyed peas
- Nuts: Peanuts, peanut butter
- Milk products: Little consumed, evaporated milk in coffee, buttermilk, cheddar cheese, cottage cheese, ice cream
- Grains: Rice, cornbread, hominy grits, biscuits, muffins, white bread, dry cereal, cooked cereal, macaroni, spaghetti, crackers
- Vegetables: Broccoli, cabbage, carrots, corn, green beans, greens, lima beans, okra, peas, potatoes, pumpkin, sweet potatoes, tomatoes, yams
- Fruits: Apples, bananas, grapefruit, grapes, nectarines, oranges, plums, tangerines, watermelon
- Other: Salt pork, carbonated beverages, fruit drinks, gravies

Chinese

- Meat: Pork, beef, organ meats
- Poultry: Chicken, duck
- Fish: White fish, shrimp, lobster, oysters, sardines
- Eggs
- Legumes: Soybeans, soybean curd, black beans
- Nuts: Peanuts, almonds, cashews
- Milk and milk products: Limited use of milk products, flavored milk, milk in cooking, ice cream
- Grains: Rice, noodles, white bread, barley, millet
- Vegetables: Bamboo shoots, beans (green and yellow), bean sprouts, bok choy, broccoli, cabbage, carrots, celery, Chinese cabbage, corn, cucumbers, eggplant, greens, leeks, lettuce, mushrooms, peppers, potatoes, scallions, snow peas, sweet potatoes, taro, tomatoes, water chestnuts, white radishes, white turnips, winter melon
- Fruits: Apples, bananas, figs, grapes, kumquats, loquats, mango, melons, oranges, peaches, pears, persimmons, pineapple, plums, tangerines
- Other: Soy sauce, sweet and sour sauce, mustard sauce, ginger, plum sauce, red bean paste, tea, coffee

Filipino

- Meat: Pork, beef, goat, deer, rabbit, variety meats
- Poultry: Chicken
- Fish: Sole, bonito, herring, tuna, mackerel, crab, mussels, shrimp, squid
- Eggs
- Legumes: Black beans, chick peas, black-eyed peas, lentils, mung beans, lima beans, white kidney beans
- Nuts: Cashews, peanuts, Pili nuts
- Milk and milk products: Limited use of any milk products, flavored milk, evaporated milk, Gouda cheese, cheddar cheese
- Grains: Rice, farina, oatmeal, dry cereals, pasta, rice noodles, wheat noodles, macaroni, spaghetti
- Vegetables: Bamboo shoots, beets, cabbage, carrots, cauliflower, celery, Chinese celery, eggplant, endive, green beans, leeks, lettuce, mushrooms, okra, onion, peppers, potatoes, pumpkin, radishes, snow peas, spinach, squash, sweet potatoes, tomatoes, water chestnuts, watercress, yams
- Fruits: Apple, bananas, grapes, guava, lemon, lime, mango, melons, oranges, papaya, pear, pineapples, plums, pomegranate, rhubarb, strawberries, tangerines
- Other: Soy sauce, coffee, tea

Mexican American

- Meat: Beef, pork, lamb, tripe, sausage, bologna, bacon
- Poultry: Chicken
- Eggs
- Legumes: Pinto beans, pink beans, garbonzo beans, lentils
- Nuts: Peanuts, peanut butter
- Milk and milk products: Milk, flavored milk, evaporated milk, condensed milk, American cheese, Monterey jack cheese, hoop, ice cream
- Grains: Rice, corn tortillas, flour tortillas, oatmeal, dry cereals, noodles, spaghetti, white bread, sweet bread

- Vegetables: Avocados, cabbage, carrots, chilies, corn, green beans, lettuce, onion, peas, potatoes, prickly pear, spinach, sweet potatoes, tomatoes, zucchini
- Fruits: Apples, apricots, bananas, guavas, lemons, mango, melons, oranges, peaches, pears, prickly pear cactus fruit, zapote
- Other: Salsa, chili sauce, guacamole, lard, park cracklongs, fruit drinks, Kool-aid, carbonated beverages, beer, coffee, excessive use of sugars, boil vegetables for long periods of time

Native American

- Meat: Pork, beef, lamb, rabbit
- Poultry: Chicken
- Fish: Depends on habitat
- Legumes
- Nuts: Walnuts, acorn, pine, peanut butter, sunflower seeds
- Milk and milk products: Milk, goat's milk, evaporated milk for cooking, ice cream, cream pies
- Grains: Refined white bread, whole wheat bread, cornmeal, rice, dry cereals, fry breads, tortillas
- Vegetables: Green beans, peas, beets, turnips, squash, peppers, lettuce
- Fruits: Few
- Other: Excessive use of sugar

References

Avruch S, Cackley AP: Savings achieved by giving WIC benefits to women prenatally, *Public Health Rep* 110(1):27-34, 1995.

Blackburn ST, Loper DL: *Maternal, fetal and neonatal physiology: a clinical perspective,* Philadelphia, 1992, WB Saunders.

Caulfield LE, Stoltzfus RJ, Witter FR: Implications of the Institute of Medicine weight gain recommendations for preventing adverse pregnancy outcomes in black and white women, *Am J Public Health* 88(8):1168-1174, 1998.

Caulfield LE, Witter FR, Stoltzfus RJ: Determinants of gestational weight gain outside the recommended ranges among black and white women, *Obstet Gynecol* 87(5 Pt 1):760-766, 1996.

Cogswell ME et al: Medically advised, mother's personal target, and actual weight gain during pregnancy, *Obstet Gynecol* 94(4):616-622, 1996.

Copper RL et al: The relationship of maternal attitude toward weight gain to weight gain during pregnancy and low birth weight, *Obstet Gynecol* 85(4):590-595, 1995.

Davis CH: Weight in pregnancy: its value as a routine test, *Am J Obstet Gynecol* 6:575-581, 1923.

Devaney B, Bilheimer L, Schore J: Medicaid costs and birth outcomes: the effects of prenatal WIC participation and the use of prenatal care, *J Policy Anal Manage* 11(4):573-592, 1992.

Dubois S et al: Ability of the Higgins Nutrition Intervention Program to improve adolescent pregnancy outcome, *J Am Diet Assoc* 97(8):871-878, 1997.

Dubois S et al: Twin pregnancy: the impact of the Higgins Nutrition Intervention Program on maternal and neonatal outcomes, *Am J Clin Nutr* 53(6):1397-1403, 1991.

Food and Consumer Service: *WIC program and participants' characteristics, April 1994,* Washington, DC, 1996, US Department of Agriculture.

Food and Nutrition Board, Institute of Medicine: *Nutrition during pregnancy. Part I, Weight gain. Part II: Nutrient supplements,* Washington, DC, 1990, National Academy Press.

Food and Nutrition Board, Institute of Medicine: *Dietary reference intakes for calcium, phosphorus, magnesium, vitamin D, and fluoride,* Washington, DC, 1999, National Academy Press.

Higgins AC: Nutritional status and outcome of pregnancy, *J Can Diet Assoc* 37:17, 1976.

Higgins AC et al: Impact of the Higgins Nutrition Intervention Program on birth weight: a within mother analysis, *J Am Diet Assoc* 89(8):1097-1103, 1989.

Horswill LJ, Yap C: Consumption of food from the WIC food packages of Chinese prenatal patients on the US west coast, *J Am Diet Assoc* 99(12):1549-1553, 1999.

Keen CL, Zidenberg-Cherr S: Should vitamin-mineral supplements be recommended for all women with childbearing potential? *Am J Clin Nutr* 59(suppl):532S-539S, 1994.

Parker JD, Abrams B: Prenatal weight gain advice: an examination of the recent prenatal weight gain recommendations of the Institute of Medicine, *Obstet Gynecol* 167:664-669, 1992.

Piechik SL, Corbett MA: Reducing low birth weight among socioeconomically high-risk adolescent pregnancies: successful intervention with certified nurse-midwife-managed care and a multidisciplinary team, *J Nurse Midwifery* 30(2):88-98, 1985.

Prochownick L: Ueber Ernihrumgscuiren in Schwangerschaft, *Ther Monatsh* 15:446-463, 1901.

Shieve LA, Cogswell ME, Scanlon KS: An empiric evaluation of the Institute of Medicine pregnancy weight gain guidelines by race, *Obstet Gynecol* 91(6):878-884, 1998.

Wertz RW, Wertz DC: *Lying in,* New York, 1977, The Free Press.

Worthington-Roberts B, Klerman L: Maternal nutrition. In Merkatz IR, Thompson JE, editors, *New perspectives on prenatal care,* New York, 1990, Elsevier.

Chapter 12

Psychologic, Emotional, and Social Aspects of Pregnancy

Jeanne F. DeJoseph, PhD, CNM, FAAN
and Linda Chapman, DNSc, RNC

INTRODUCTION

There are three components to prenatal care: ongoing risk screening, health promotion, and interventions for medical and other types of problems (Klerman, 1990). The developing maternal-fetal unit is the focus of much of the biophysiologic care during the prenatal period. Sociodemographic variables have also been considered for their relationship to pregnancy processes such as health status and timing of the onset of prenatal care (Enderlin et al., 1994). Yet the exclusive use of a biomedical perspective has been criticized for its narrowness of approach (Forde, 1996).

The purpose of this chapter is to provide an overview of equally important considerations in perinatal care such as the *s*ocial, *e*motional, *p*sychologic, *s*piritual, and *s*exual *a*spects of *p*regnancy (SEPSSAPs). Our intent is to raise questions for consideration by practitioners, and we expect that more questions will be generated than could be answered in any one book. Our goal is to support the practitioners who continue to move beyond the biomedical aspects of pregnancy toward a more integrated approach.

It is important to note at the outset that SEPSSAPs are not separate from the biophysiologic changes of pregnancy nor are they separate from each other (Bernazzani et al., 1997; Wadwah et al., 1996). The discussion will focus on the woman experiencing an uncomplicated pregnancy. SEPSSAPs will not be considered from the perspectives of women and men who adopt children nor for those who experience complications of pregnancy. As with the biophysical difficulties during pregnancy, complications of SEPSSAPs during the processes or outcomes of pregnancy add to the complexities of assessment and care. The references at the end of the chapter include information about some of the complications of pregnancy and SEPSSAPs (e.g., Parker et al., 1999).

To set the context for the discussion about SEPSSAPs, we present our view of the family and our beliefs about why it is important for perinatal clinicians to consider SEPSSAPs in their assessments during pregnancy.

WHO IS THE "FAMILY"?

In this chapter, as in the rest of the book, the "family" is defined by the woman herself. Some families are configured in a way that is often described as "traditional," with a woman, a man who is her husband and the father of the fetus, and possibly other siblings. This nuclear family configuration is still common in the United States at the turn of this century. However, in many cultures and/or geographic locations, the nuclear family is not the norm. For example, two generations besides the pregnant woman may live together or in close proximity. A pregnant woman also may have only one partner who is male or female or several partners. In addition, there is very little research to guide clinical practice about the experiences of other stakeholders such as grandparents in the pregnancy. In fact, most of the research about grandparents is related to adolescent mothers and their relationships with their grandmothers, with a special focus on family relations and depressive symptomatology (Caldwell, Antonucci, and Jackson, 1998; Kalil et al., 1998).

Support and acceptance of the woman's definition of her family by the practitioner is essential. Not every clinician is comfortable with all types of families. In some geographic areas or communities it is possible to refer to another practitioner; in some it is not. When it is not possible, the clinician must examine her or his own values and make a special effort to support the woman and the members of her support system.

In this chapter we have chosen to describe what information there is about SEPSSAPs among women and men during pregnancy. We include a section about lesbian parenting later in the chapter.

SEPSSAPS AND THE PRACTITIONER

A perspective is a set of lenses through which elements of pregnancy and birth can be viewed. SEPSSAPs may be described and evaluated differently, depending on the values and beliefs of an individual practitioner. For example, a person with a *developmental* perspective on pregnancy might focus on an individual's adaptation to pregnancy and childbirth, whereas one with a *community* perspective might focus on pregnancy and birth as they relate to the family or the community. In a *public health* perspective the focus is on pregnancy and childbirth within environments and the institutionalization of caring and oversight such as Women, Infants, and Children (WIC) programs. Someone with a *feminist* perspective views a woman's SEPSSAPs through the experiences and reports of the women themselves and attends to both differences and similarities based on individual women's situations. The feminist perspective has been used by researchers, educators, and clinicians (Doyal, 1995; Giarratano, Bustamante-Forest, and Pollock, 1999; Giele, 1997; McCool and McCool, 1989; Welles-Nystrom, 1997).

It is important for practitioners to assess their own perspectives on perinatal care, as well as their beliefs about SEPSSAPs (Grundstein-Amado, 1995). The personal practices of a clinician can lead to making assumptions about the pregnant woman's life (Zambrana and Scrimshaw, 1997). For example, a practitioner who organizes her or his world according to psychologic "types" may have a very different view of a woman and her family than someone who sees pregnancy and birth as a social event. For some women the emotions that are experienced during pregnancy are mainly positive; for others they are negative. For some women pregnancy is a time of emotional calm; for others a time of individual upheaval. It is important that each practitioner review her or his own experiences of the SEPSSAPs of pregnancy and parenting, whether as a child or as a parent. Clarifying values in this way can assist the clinician in providing woman-centered and family-focused care.

Descriptions of each of the elements of SEPSSAPs will also vary when specific questions are asked across categories. For example, one basic question is "Who is the identified 'patient'?" If a midwife is considering SEPSSAPs, the answer will depend on the whether that midwife defines the "patient" as the mother; the maternal-fetal unit; or the mother, fetus, and partner. Two other issues are also important: the *processes* and the *outcomes* of SEPSSAPs. What processes and outcomes are assessed and measured, what is done with the information, and what difference does it make? As each of the elements of SEPSSAPs is described, some of the research about SEPSSAPs during pregnancy will be presented.

In this chapter we are recommending that the *processes* of SEPSSAPs are important enough to be assessed by practitioners during each clinical visit. We also recommend that every clinician develop a list of questions or topics for the pregnant women in their specific practice rather than use standardized measures developed for those who do not represent a particular client population (Goldenberg et al., 1997). As we describe each aspect of SEPSSAPs we will suggest some questions/issues for assessment. We also recommend the use of such open-ended questions as, "Is there anything that you need now, like food, shelter, comfort, support, that I could help you arrange to get?" And, "Is there anything you want to talk about that I haven't mentioned?"

The research literature has a great deal of information about the *outcomes* of pregnancy and some of the elements of SEPSSAPs (Paarlberg et al., 1995; Wilson et al., 1996). Most of the research about pregnant women to date is quantitative in approach, with specific outcome variables measured. Thus, for example, we read of the contribution of social support, self-esteem, symptom distress, and stress severity to measurable perinatal outcomes such as birth weight (Hoffman and Hatch, 1996; Sheehan, 1996). Much of what we know about pregnancy has developed from early studies in which the participants were generally white, middle income, married, educated, and presumably heterosexual women. For the last three decades, numerous studies have been conducted to determine how other women experience pregnancy and what their outcomes were. In effect, the experiences of white married women have been the standard against which all other women's experiences and outcomes have been measured. The validity of assuming that all women everywhere are the same or even that all white married women are similar to each other in their experiences of pregnancy has been called into question by feminists (Morse, 1995), clinicians, researchers, and theorists (Curry, Burton, and Fields, 1998). Although it is important to have a broad knowledge of SEPSSAPs and biophysical research related to clinical practice, it is equally important to consider the relevance of each study to a specific clinical practice. This can be done by reading clinical and research literature carefully to determine if what is proposed fits for individual pregnant women in your specific practice. It can also be done by developing a short index to provide a practitioner with a woman's specific personalized responses about SEPSSAPs and her own experiences of pregnancy. Our approach to SEPSSAPs is to encourage the practitioner to pay attention to them throughout the woman's pregnancy and to develop and incorporate several questions about these important aspects of pregnancy for each woman into each visit. In the last section of this chapter we propose such a report.

The focus of care during pregnancy is usually directed toward the woman and her fetus. The woman's partner may be included in the care, but generally there has been little research about his experiences (Mayer et al., 1997). Expectant fathers report that they are often neglected (Chandler and Field, 1997). The changes that men experience during pregnancy may have a profound effect on their partners and their own transition to fatherhood. Expectant fathers experience pregnancy in a variety of ways. Some are emotionally attached, whereas others seem distant and detached from the pregnancy. Each man grapples with the meaning of fatherhood and how he will father this child. Pregnancy is a period of time when *partners* also prepare for birth.

Expectant fathers' responses to pregnancy and to their partners can affect the entire course of pregnancy, labor, birth, and transition to parenthood. Women who have a supportive partner and a strong couple relationship have been reported to have fewer problems during pregnancy, labor, and birth. Because of these relationships reported in research literature, it is imperative that practitioners who work with pregnant couples have a willingness to assess the partner's SEPSSAPs as well as those aspects for pregnant women.

WHAT DO WE CURRENTLY KNOW ABOUT SEPSSAPS?

In this chapter we consider aspects of SEPSSAPs separately. However, in clinical care, research, and education they are most often considered together and frequently are referred to as the "psychosocial" components of pregnancy. This characterization of anything other than "biophysical" as "psychosocial" can be limiting when specific components are not analyzed appropriately in the care process.

There are measures that have been used in research to determine the demographics of samples of pregnant women in relationship to the course and outcome of their pregnancies. For example, there is a clear connection between poverty and less favorable perinatal outcomes. Membership in a nondominant race (e.g., being of African descent, with or without financial resources, has also been noted to contribute to less favorable perinatal outcomes (Goldenberg et al., 1996). On the other hand, when a woman has emotional and tangible support from others in her social network, more favorable perinatal outcomes have been reported (e.g., Tilden, 1983). It is important to remember that the findings of most research studies support correlations between certain perinatal process and outcome variables. However, those findings seldom demonstrate linear, causal relationships.

SOCIAL ASPECTS OF PREGNANCY

When we discuss the "social" aspects of pregnancy, we mean those conditions and behaviors that are experienced outside of the self that may have an impact on the processes and outcomes of pregnancy. Social *conditions* would include social standings, economic situations, and other diverse experiences of regional, national ethnic, heritage, and cultural groups. Much of this information is gathered as demographic information. Social *behaviors* include nutritional habits; values about women, family, and childbirth; positive health behaviors such as education; and negative health behaviors such as smoking, the use of drugs, and violence against women (Faden, Hanna, Graubard, 1997; Parker et al., 1999; Richardson and Guttmacher, 1967). Other questions that arise include differences of opinion about the function and importance of women's health care itself to affect social change (Kassabian, 1995).

A pregnant woman can be seen as the center of a complex network of interlocking strands, something like a web. In a western perspective individuality is often stressed, and the nuclear family is still common. Elsewhere the woman may be part of a strong family system and an extended social network. Regardless of her network before conception, pregnancy brings new experiences and new opportunities to recast many of her relationships. Customs and practices for a pregnant woman, her family, and those in her social environment may be taught through storytelling by seasoned elders (Affonso et al., 1996; Richardson, 1990). The importance of the pregnant woman's social network has been confirmed in many studies (Langer et al., 1996; Schaffer and Lia-Hoagberg, 1997).

Another facet of the social milieu in which a woman carries a pregnancy has to do with economics and education. Since the turn of the last century, many epidemiologic studies have been conducted to determine the impact of mostly middle income women's employment on their perinatal outcomes (Saurel-Cubizolles and Kaminski, 1986). What those studies really demonstrate very clearly is the influence on research of prevailing social values and community beliefs and standards about the function and status of women. All women "work" throughout their pregnancies; however, only some women are employed and receive pay for their work. It is only in the last two decades that becoming pregnant did not signal an end to a married woman's paid employment (Northrup, 1998). Early studies found that, when a woman was employed during pregnancy, her perinatal outcomes were less optimal. In the last two decades researchers have reported more positive outcomes. Still there is only a small amount of recent research to guide clinicians to inform and support women with their activities in employment and nonemployment situations (Magann, Evans, and Newnham, 1996).

It is generally accepted among researchers and clinicians alike that women who have less education and less economic stability have less optimal pregnancy outcomes. Again, most attempts to change the relationships between poverty and pregnancy have centered around changing the woman and/or her social network. There has been little intervention research to alleviate poverty and then see if outcomes or processes of pregnancy improved.

Another facet in the social network is the woman's "culture." In every culture pregnancy and birth are significant rites of passage (Callister, 1995). Anthropologists have helped us to understand widespread differences in the perceptions about conception, pregnancy, and pregnancy care among different cultural groups (Helman, 1990; Sesia, 1996). Although the concept of culture is frequently explained in terms of ethnicity and heritage group membership (Burk, Wieser, and Keegan, 1995; Dempsey and Gesse, 1995; Facione, 1993; Fuentes-Afflick and Hessol, 1997; Sokoloski, 1995), these descriptions are not the only "culture" possible. There are also variations within cultures. For example, there are differences in SEPSSAPs between adolescents and mature gravidas (Stark, 1997). Membership in micro cultures (e.g., differences between and among people in various geographic, physical, and emotional situations) may affect clinical care. The best way to determine to what blend of cultures the women in their practice belong and what that belonging means to these women and their families is to ask them. The purpose of exploring cultures with a pregnant woman and her family is not to create a "cook book" that can train others to care for "that type of woman." Rather, it is to understand the processes, values, and meanings of pregnancy and childbirth within the context of the woman and her family.

For men, the social aspects of pregnancy are influenced by the relationship the man has with his partner, the relationship with his own parents, and his cultural beliefs. In contrast with the woman who is the center of the complex network of pregnancy relationships, the expectant father may be viewed as being on the edge of the network. The amount of support given to him is often minimal. Some men may feel jealous of all the attention their partners receive. Others may experience isolation because women can feel the baby move within their bodies. Expectant fathers may feel detached from their friends and may be less social. They may begin to move away from their friends who are childless and begin to form new relationships with men and couples who have children already or who are also expecting.

The man's primary support person is his partner; she is the person with whom he is most likely to share his thoughts and feelings. During pregnancy the woman's center of attention is focused toward the pregnancy and the developing child. As a result, she might have less energy to provide the type and amount of support needed by her partner. She may also be unaware of his needs for support during this life transition.

The relationship that the man has with his parents affects the type of support he seeks and receives from them. Men who were raised in a family that openly supported each other are more likely to have positive support during pregnancy. Men who were raised in an emotionally conservative or abusive family may not turn to their family of origin for support.

In general, men are less likely to share their personal concerns with other men. They may be hesitant to discuss their feelings and concerns about pregnancy and becoming a father. If men do not share their feelings with others, they are often left alone to deal with their feelings about and reactions toward the pregnancy.

Cultural beliefs can also influence the expectant father's involvement in pregnancy and the type of support he receives during the experience. In some cultures the expectant father is excluded from the experience. In others the man becomes the spokesperson for his pregnant partner. Culture also influences the role a man takes during labor, birth, and parenting. An assessment of the couples' cultural beliefs during the prenatal period can help the practitioner determine the type of involvement that both members of the couple are comfortable with across their childbearing experiences.

Some topics that may be useful to explore with the woman/partner/family about the social aspects of pregnancy include: "Among your friends, is becoming pregnant and bearing children what's expected of you?" "Some women have told me that most of their friends and family expect them to have a career before becoming pregnant." "What do you think about mothers who stay at home with their babies?—mothers who work outside the home?" "What did your mother do?" "What is a 'regular' day like for you?" "Who are you close to; who is going to be there for you?" "With whom do you live?" "What did the men in your life think about pregnant women?"

EMOTIONAL ASPECTS OF PREGNANCY

For the purposes of this chapter, an emotional aspect of pregnancy is considered to be that affective state of consciousness in which feelings are experienced. There is a range of feelings that is possible for all members of the family's network. "The perceptions of those involved, the coping mechanisms they possess, and the support systems to which they turn are components of emotional responses to pregnancy" (Jensen and Bobak, 1985, p. 293).

Most of the research has explored the relationship of a woman's feelings to the outcome of her pregnancy. For example, what effect does a negative mood state such as depression have on labor, birth, and neonatal outcome? Or, what is the relationship between pregnancy outcome and emotional conflict, anxiety, stress, or low self-esteem (Curry, Campbell and Christian, 1994). Recent research has also focused on women's expectations about pregnancy and birth and what connections they have to a woman's feelings of fulfillment, satisfaction, and emotional well-being (Green, Coupland, and Kitzinger, 1990).

It is commonly accepted that a woman has ambivalent feelings about being pregnant in the beginning of her pregnancy. In fact, there is little research information about how women perceive themselves and their feelings throughout their pregnancy (Hofmeyr, Marcos, and Butchart, 1990). Encouraging a woman to talk about her feelings can facilitate clinical care, and asking about feelings of others in her social network may also be helpful. Feelings of well-being and self-esteem, as well as of stress and/or anxiety, are connected to the biophysical and psychologic processes that the pregnant woman experiences. The most frequent mood changes during pregnancy have been reported to be anxiety and depression (Koltyn, 1994). Researchers generally report that these feelings fluctuate throughout gestation.

Men may experience mixed emotions about the pregnancy and impending fatherhood. Initially men who are experiencing a planned pregnancy may feel a sense of excitement and pride. Later they may experience an increase in anxiety and at times feel panicky about becoming a father and assuming increased responsibilities. They may be concerned about the increased financial obligations from their expanding family. They may have concerns about the health and safety of their pregnant partner and feel a need to protect and nurture her.

It is common for men to experience ambivalent feelings about the pregnancy even when it is a planned and desired event. The feelings usually decrease as the pregnancy advances. Men also need an opportunity to discuss their ambivalent feelings and to become aware that these are part of a normal process of role transition.

Questions that explore the emotional aspects of pregnancy include: "What's your energy level like these days?" "Some women have told me that their feelings are like a roller coaster when they are pregnant. What do you feel?" "Is there a difference between how you feel now and how you felt before you became pregnant?" "Do you dream?" "Some fathers have mixed feelings about the pregnancy, even when it is planned and wanted. How do you feel?"

PSYCHOLOGIC ASPECTS OF PREGNANCY

"Psychologic" aspects of pregnancy are considered to be the mental states and processes that women and families experience during pregnancy. Most of the studies about the psychologic aspects of pregnancy are related to their impact on outcomes (Westlander, 1991), although some researchers have studied pregnancy processes as well (Prince and Adams, 1990). Some of the psychologic changes of pregnancy are foundational to a woman's definition of herself and to preparation for her new activities as a mother. Particularly during a first pregnancy, she may use interpersonal and intrapersonal processes to expand her identity to include activities of "mothering" (Flagler and Nicoll, 1990). These processes are often referred to as "adaptation to pregnancy" (Lederman and Miller, 1998). Some of that psychologic work has been reported to be the work of transiting from woman-without-child to woman-and-child; reevaluating relationships with her partner and her own mother; and shifting patterns of dependence and nurturance (Grossman, Eichler, and Winikoff, 1980; Hees-Strauthamer, 1985; Lederman, 1984; Mercer, Ferketich, and Joseph, 1986; Tilden, 1983). In addition to the intrapsychic processes of identity reformation, some researchers have postulated that there are tasks specific to pregnancy that must be accomplished related to insurance of safe passage and social acceptance for the woman and her child; identification of the child and of self in relation to the child; and exploration of the meaning of giving/receiving (Rubin, 1970).

Psychologic aspects of pregnancy have also been studied relative to specific groups of women (e.g., women in the armed forces [Lombardi, Wilson, and Peniston, 1999; Tam, 1998]) or among women who use illegal substances during pregnancy (Hutchins and DiPietro, 1997). These studies are often focused on pregnancy outcomes within a particular group. Psychologic variables such as anxiety and depression may also be considered as they are related to potential adverse effects on pregnancy processes and outcomes (Dragonas and Christodoulou, 1998).

Very little research has been conducted about the psychologic aspects of pregnancy for men. One reflection of a man's psychologic processes may be the involvement he exhibits with the pregnancy. May (1980) reported that there are three styles of involvement that men adopt during pregnancy. These styles range from being very involved to extremely detached. The styles she described are expressive, instrumental, and observer. The expressive father is the man who is outwardly very emotionally involved in the pregnancy. He feels that "we" are pregnant and he is a full partner in the pregnancy. He is eager to learn as much as he can about the pregnancy and to be as much a part of the pregnancy as he can. He will often attend as many of the prenatal appointments as he can. He can freely express his emotions and excitement and thus generally receives a great deal of support from family, friends, co-workers, and health care providers.

Men who take on the instrumental style view themselves as the managers of the pregnancy and generally have a more businesslike involvement. They do not freely share their emotional feelings about the pregnancy, and they frequently maintain a degree of emotional distance from the pregnancy. These men can seem to be very controlling as they "manage" their partner's pregnancy. They may ask numerous questions of the provider, since they think they are responsible for the care provided to their partner.

The third style is that of observer. Men who adopt this style appear to be extremely detached from the pregnancy. Their partners may report that they are not interested in the pregnancy. These men place an emotional distance between themselves and the pregnancy as they work through what it means to be a father. They can be encouraged to attend prenatal appointments and expectant parent's classes.

When providing care for a pregnant family, practitioners can include an assessment of the style the expectant father has adopted. For example, the practitioner may more easily develop a rapport with the instrumental father by anticipating his need to receive in-depth information and to feel a part of the decision-making during the pregnancy. Because he is so emotionally attached to the pregnancy and the unborn child, an expressive father may need more support if a complication occurs. The observer might need encouragement to participate in the pregnancy and to demonstrate that he is interested in his partner and the pregnancy. In addition, explaining to the expectant mother that there are different styles and that each man is interested in the pregnancy but has different ways of expressing it might decrease any concerns she might have.

Again, many psychologic processes that occur during pregnancy are evaluated by clinicians against their own set of beliefs and values. For example, a clinician may assess that a particular woman's motivation for becoming pregnant may be "healthy" if the woman is in a stable relationship, is financially secure, and chooses to become pregnant. There are other motivations for becoming pregnant that a clinician may judge to be "less healthy"; for example, hoping to replace a child lost by miscarriage or to shore up a weak relationship. The clinician may also consider that the responses of the woman's family may not be optimal (e.g., if the partner does not plan to participate in any part of the pregnancy, labor, or delivery). Again, knowledge of one's own beliefs and values is an important part of preparing to give clinical care.

Pregnancy may be potentially beneficial or detrimental to a woman's psychologic growth and health, but we believe that it is rarely neutral. Psychologic elements of a SEPSSAPs assessment could include the following sample issues: "How do you know you're doing a good job?" "What are your strengths?" "What makes you happy, sad, or mad?" "What do you do when you are mad, or sad, or happy?" "What do you think about the changes in your body?"

SPIRITUAL ASPECTS OF PREGNANCY

The definition of *spiritual* and *religious* are contested. The meaning frequently depends on those who are discussing it. Hall (1998) deconstructs two assumptions that have been problematic in the study of spirituality. "First, the presumed fusion of spirituality with religion has guided attention to religiosity and religious practices . . . and second, [there has been] a professional reification of concepts, including those that arise from the field of human development and their attendant measurements. Many concepts have been put forth to stand for spirituality, such as harmonious interconnectedness, inner strength, being, knowing, doing, [and others]" (p. 144). There is also a body of literature about various forms of directed and nondirected energy or intent such as prayer, spiritual, and/or psychic healing (Levin, 1996). In this chapter we define "spiritual" very broadly as a relationship that the individual constructs outside of herself/himself that supports that person's search for meaning and purpose. The manifestations differ among women and may include ceremonies and blessings, as well as rituals such as baby showers. We agree with Dyson, Cobb, and Forman (1997) that "religion" is more about systems of practices and beliefs within which a social group engage.

Lukoff and his colleagues (1999) reviewed four million abstracts of general case reports indexed on Medline between 1980 and 1996 and found only 364 abstracts related to spiritual and/or religious issues. Others have described the importance of an individual's world view in constructing the interactions between spiritual and cultural practices (Engebretson, 1996). This aspect of human life has not received much study because it is a very personal and intangible issue (Long, 1997). There is some literature about religiosity and birth outcomes (Magana and Clark, 1995); but in medical, midwifery, nursing, and other clinical literature, there is relatively little written about spiritual aspects of pregnancy. And there is no research literature that links spirituality with processes and/or outcomes of pregnancy for the woman or any members of her family. However, we believe that pregnancy offers women and their partners an opportunity to explore their systems for determining meaning in their lives and ways of looking beyond day-to-day experiences. Because spirituality is an important reality in *some* women's lives, we believe that clinicians can include questions related to spirituality in at least some of their assessments during pregnancy. Again, it is an *invitation,* an opening for women to talk about their spirituality *if they choose.* The purpose is to determine if she has any needs or wishes that may change our clinical practice related to her or her family.

Some topics that might be useful for assessment include: "Do you have any spiritual beliefs that will help me care for you during your pregnancy?" "Do you have any religious practices that might change the way we give you prenatal care?" "Do you have any special events (rituals) such as baby showers to celebrate your pregnancy or any special ceremonies you observe around birth?"

SEXUAL ASPECTS OF PREGNANCY

Sexuality is another term that is described differently when considered from various perspectives. Physical, psychologic, and interactional components of sexuality have been described within a sociocultural context (MacLaren, 1995; Warner, Rowe, and Whipple, 1999). In this chapter "sexuality" is defined as an individual's identity that is a socially constructed set of biologic components, beliefs, values, interests, attractions, expectations, and behaviors. During any type of transition there may be an opportunity to create or experience changes in some aspects of sexuality. Pregnancy is one such transition and has been described as "a potent influence on sexuality irrespective of an individual's conditioning" (Oruc et al., 1999, p 48).

One difficulty in basing clinical care on the research about sexuality during pregnancy is that many of the studies are descriptive and also have conflicting results

(Byrd et al., 1998). There are no published intervention studies that could provide a clinician with information to help couples improve sexual satisfaction during pregnancy, if that is something they wish to do. Clinicians have reported that both sexuality and spirituality are very difficult subjects to discuss (Warner, Rowe and Whipple, 1999). Some even consider that neither of these topics is appropriate for discussion with pregnant women and their families.

There are several reasons why it is important to incorporate assessments of a woman's sexuality during her pregnancy. First, conception is most often the result of a sexual act. Although technology exists to help a woman conceive separately from her sexual expressions, most babies are conceived through heterosexual intercourse. When pregnancy occurs as a consensual experience, regardless of how the fetus was conceived, it takes place within a context of specific beliefs about the nature of men and women and values about families, children, and the purposes of sexuality (Doyal, 1995).

Pregnancy may offer the woman and her partner an opportunity to explore different expressions of their sexuality. For some this opportunity may be welcome; for others it may be distressing. Difficulty within the couples' sexual expressions is common during pregnancy. The women's interest during the early weeks and months of pregnancy may decrease, while her male partner's remains the same as it was before pregnancy (Byrd et al., 1998). The women's increasing body size during the last months of pregnancy may interfere with the couple's usual sexual positions and activities. Some men think that their partner's pregnant body is sexually attractive; others do not.

Some expectant fathers may experience an overall decrease in their interest in sex. It is not uncommon for men to abstain from sex throughout the pregnancy. These men may feel that they might injure their unborn child or cause a miscarriage. Some men find that feeling the baby kicking them during sexual activity is very disconcerting. They may feel that they are no longer alone with their partner and that the unborn child is aware of what they are doing.

We recommend that clinicians use the PLISSIT model (Alteneder and Hartzell, 1997) when working with pregnant families. Briefly, this model of approaches to sexual concerns includes: permission *(P);* limited information *(LI);* specific suggestions *(SS);* and intensive therapy *(IT)* (Annon, 1976). By introducing the topic of sexuality and providing basic simple facts, the practitioner legitimates the topic for the pregnant woman. Making specific suggestions with pictures can also be useful. We believe that it is important to *invite* women to share information about their sexuality if they wish and not impose on them the responsibility to give us their intimate details. If the provider assesses that the family needs more help than can be available during clinical visits, referrals to therapists may be indicated.

Some background information might include: Within the context of a particular woman's community, what are the beliefs about sexuality? For example, in a given group, who controls women's sexuality and reproduction? What is expected of women regarding the number and spacing of children? What are the partner's sexual responsibilities before, during, and after pregnancy? What are the social and economic realities of the community into which this new member will be born, and does that affect sexual behaviors? Some sexual issues to explore with the woman/partner/family include: "Some women have told me that their sex life changes a lot when they get pregnant. Have you noticed any changes in yours?" "What was it before? What is it like now?" "Are you and your partner having any struggles about your sex life?" "Sometimes when women are pregnant, they may have strong feelings about having or not having sex. What's that been like for you?" "Besides sex, are there any changes in your relationship with you husband/partner/family that you'd like to talk about?"

LESBIAN PARENTING

The definition of who is a "lesbian" is contested, and even the term *lesbian* itself may be defined differently among various generations of lesbians (Gruskin, 1999). In this chapter we consider that it is the woman herself who defines her sexual orientation/identity. If a woman says she is a lesbian, she is.

There have always been lesbian mothers: women who had children while in heterosexual relationships; lesbians who chose to marry so that they could have children; and sisters, aunts, grandmothers, and family friends who were lesbians and who also provided maternal support and caring to children. Since the 1970s in the United States, there are more options for lesbians. As Pies noted (1985, p. xvi), "There are lesbians all over the world having children, adopting, and raising children as 'out' lesbians." However, both lesbians and bisexual women may face certain decisions not generally shared by women who define themselves as heterosexual (Kenney and Tash, 1992).

Many lesbians give birth to or adopt a child or children within the context of a committed relationship. It is their intention to create a family. There is no research that compares lesbian and heterosexual women with regard to intentionality of pregnancy. Nor is there research to compare or contrast lesbian and heterosexual women who adopt children. Gruskin (1999) discussed many of the questions around birth and/or adoption (e.g., if the woman is in a committed relationship, who will be the biologic mother?). Who will be the father/sperm donor, and will he have a role in the child's life? If she or they are adopting, will it be the adoption be domestic or international?

There is relatively little specific research about lesbians and pregnancy. The literature contains a bit of information about lesbian families (Levy, 1996), lesbian mothers (Kirkpatrick, 1987), general health care for lesbians (Rankow, 1995) and pregnancy care (Carroll, 1999; Tash and Kenney, 1993; Zeidenstein, 1990). Another group of studies focuses on issues surrounding donor insemination among both lesbian and heterosexual women (Fasouliotis and Schenker, 1999; Leiblum, Palmer, and Spector, 1995; Wendland, Burn, and Hill, 1996). Psychologic issues in lesbian parenting from the planning of pregnancy through the first 2 years of parenthood were explored by Rohrbaugh (1988) and involved interactions among identity, relationships, homophobia, and the definition of parenting roles. Contemporary issues about disclosure and parenting, as well as those related to the legal system, are complex, and yet in the 1990s more and more lesbians chose to become parents. Questions that assist in exploring the lesbian mother's experience in pregnancy include: "Who in your family/community is an important support person for you? Will that person continue to be involved in the child's life?" "Have you planned any legal actions to ensure that your partner's parental rights are protected?"

A FRAMEWORK FOR INTEGRATING SEPSSAPS INTO PRENATAL CARE

In each of the preceding sections we have described some issues and some potential questions to use to develop a SEPSSAPs index that is appropriate and relevant for your practice. You can use the information to chart and report to other clinicians in your practice about SEPSSAPs for a specific woman. The following is an example of such a report.

SEPSSAPs Report

This is Ms. X....

(S) 1. The following people will support her during her pregnancy:

____

____

____

{plus demographic information}.

(E) 2. Currently she is feeling ______________

____

____

______________ *re: her pregnancy.*

(P) 3. She identifies her psychologic strengths as

____

______________________________.

(S) 4. Her spirituality involves ______________,

____

and she would like us to do x, y, and z to support her.

(S) 5. Her primary relationship is with (FOB/other)–current issues for them include:

____

______________________________.

6. She identifies her current SEPSSAPs needs as:

____

______________________________.

PLAN

____

____

____

(e.g., "referred to WIC")

SUMMARY

The inclusion of a SEPSSAPs index into a clinical practice can be an opportunity to obtain and share important information about the pregnant woman and her family. The base for assessment as social, emotional, psychologic, spiritual, and sexual aspects of pregnancy has been presented. Because sexuality and spirituality may be difficult for some clinicians to discuss, we have highlighted their potential impact on clinical care. Finally, an example of how the clinician might construct a SEPSSAPs report in practice is presented.

We would like to thank the students from the UCSF/SFGH Interdepartmental Nurse-Midwifery Education Program who participated in the development of several versions of the SEPSSAPs index questions and reports.

References

Affonso DD et al: Hawaiian-style "talkstory": psychosocial assessment and intervention during and after pregnancy, *J Obstet Gynecol Neonatal Nurs* 25(9):737-742, 1996.

Alteneder RR, Hartzell D: Addressing couples' sexuality concerns during the childbearing period: use of the PLISSIT model, *J Obstet Gynecol Neonatal Nurs* 26:651-658, 1997.

Annon J: *Behavioral treatment of sexual problems: brief therapy,* vol I, New York, 1976, Harper & Row.

Bernazzani O et al: Psychosocial factors related to emotional disturbances during pregnancy, *J Psychosom Res* 42(4):391-402, 1997.

Burk ME, Wieser PC, Keegan L: Cultural beliefs and health behaviors of pregnant Mexican-American women: implications for primary care, *Adv Nurs Sci* 17(4):37-52, 1995.

Byrd JE et al: Sexuality during pregnancy and the year postpartum, *J Fam Pract* 47(4):305-308, 1998.

Caldwell CH, Antonucci TC, Jackson JS: Supportive/conflictual family relations and depressive symptomatology: teenage mother and grandmother perspectives, *Fam Relations: Interdis J Appl Fam Studies* 47(4):395-402, 1998.

Callister LC: Cultural meanings of childbirth, *J Obstet Gynecol Neonatal Nurs* 24(4):327-342, 1995.

Carroll NM: Optimal gynecologic and obstetric care for lesbians, *Obstet Gynecol* 93(4):611-613, 1999.

Chandler S, Field PA: Becoming a father: first-time fathers' experience of labor and delivery, *J Nurse Midwifery* 42(1):17-24, 1997.

Curry MA, Burton D, Fields J: The prenatal psychosocial profile: a research and clinical tool, *Res Nurs Health* 21:211-219, 1998.

Curry MA, Campbell RA, Christian M: Validity and reliability testing of the prenatal psychosocial profile, *Res Nurs Health* 17(2):127-135, 1994.

Dempsey P, Gesse T: Beliefs, values and practices of Navajo childbearing women, *West J Nurs Res* 17(6):591-604, 1995.

Doyal L: Regulating reproduction. In Doyal L: *What makes women sick: gender and the political economy of health,* New Brunswick, NJ, 1995, Rutgers University Press.

Dragonas T, Christodoulou GN: Prenatal care, *Clin Psychol Rev* 18(2):127-142, 1998.

Dyson J, Cobb M, Forman D: The meaning of spirituality: a literature review, *J Adv Nurs* 26:1183-1188, 1997.

Enderlin MC et al: Health status and timing of onset of prenatal care: is there an association among low-income women? *Birth* 21(1):71-76, 1994.

Engebretson J: Considerations in diagnosing in the spiritual domain, *Nurs Diag* 7(3):100-107, 1996.

Facione N: The Triandis model for the study of health and illness behavior: a social behavior theory with sensitivity to diversity, *Adv Nurs Sci* 15(3):49-58, 1993.

Faden VB, Hanna E, Graubard BI: The effect of positive and negative health behavior during gestation on pregnancy outcome, *J Subst Abuse* 9:63-76, 1997.

Fasouliotis SJ, Schenker JG: Social aspects in assisted reproduction, *Hum Reprod Update* 5(1):26-39, 1999.

Flagler S, Nicoll L: A framework for the psychological aspects of pregnancy, *NAACOG's Clin Iss Perinatal Women Health Nurs* 1(3):267-278, 1990.

Forde R: Inclusion of psychosocial conditions in clinical practice and the problem of medicalization, *Theoret Med* 2(17):151-161, 1996.

Fuentes-Afflick E, Hessol NA: Impact of Asian ethnicity and national origin on infant birth weight, *Am J Epidemiol* 145(2):148-155, 1997.

Giarratano G, Bustamante-Forest R, Pollock C: New pedagogy for maternity nursing education, *J Obstet Gynecol Neonatal Nurs* 28(2):127-134, 1999.

Giele JZ: Windows on new family forms: Insights from feminist and familist perspectives, *Qual Soc* 20(2):143-152, 1997.

Goldenberg RL et al: Medical, psychosocial, and behavioral risk factors do not explain the increased risk for low birth weight among black women, *Am J Obstet Gynecol* 175(5):1317-1324, 1996.

Goldenberg RL et al: Abbreviated scale for the assessment of psychosocial status in pregnancy: development and evaluation, *Acta Obstet Gynecol Scand* 165(suppl):19-29, 1997.

Green JM, Coupland VA, Kitzinger JV:. Expectations, experiences and psychological outcomes of childbirth: a prospective study of 825 women, *Birth* (17(1):15-24, 1990.

Grossman FK, Eichler LS, Winikoff SA: *Pregnancy, birth, and parenthood,* San Francisco, 1980, Josey-Bass.

Grundstein-Amado R: Values education: a new direction for medical education, *J Med Ethics* 21:174-178, 1995.

Gruskin EP: *Treating lesbians and bisexual women: challenges and strategies for health professionals,* Thousand Oaks, Calif, 1999, Sage Publications.

Hall B: Patterns of spirituality in persons with advanced HIV disease, *Res Nurs Health* 21:143-153, 1998.

Helman CG: Reproduction and childbirth. In Helman CG, editor: *Culture, health and illness,* London, 1990, Wright.

Hees-Strauthamer JC: *The first pregnancy: an integrating principle in female psychology,* Ann Arbor, 1985, University of Michigan Research Press.

Hoffman S, Hatch MC: Stress, social support and pregnancy outcome: a reassessment based on recent research, *Paediatr Perinatal Epidemiol* 19(4):380-405, 1996.

Hofmeyr GJ, Marcos EF, Butchart AM: Pregnant women's perceptions of themselves: a survey, *Birth* 74(4):205-206, 1990.

Hutchins E, DiPietro J: Psychosocial risk factors associated with cocaine use during pregnancy: a case-control study, *Obstet Gynecol* 90(1):142-147, 1997.

Jensen MD, Bobak IM: *Maternity and gynecologic care: the nurse and the family,* St Louis, 1985, Mosby.

Kalil A et al: Effects of grandmother co-residence and quality of family relationships on depressive symptoms in adolescent mothers. *Fam Relations: Interdis J Appl Fam Studies* 47(4):433-441, 1998.

Kassabian L, editor: *Prelude to action II: reforming maternity care,* New York, 1995, Maternity Center Association.

Kenney JW, Tash DT Lesbian childbearing couples' dilemmas and decisions, *Health Care Women Int* 13(2):209-219, 1992.

Kirkpatrick M: Clinical implications of lesbian mother studies, *J Homosexuality* 14(1-2):201-211, 1987.

Klerman LV: The need for a new perspective on prenatal care. In Merkatz I, Thompson J, editors: *New perspectives on prenatal care,* New York, 1990, Elsiever.

Koltyn KF: Mood changes in pregnant women following an exercise session and a prenatal informational session, *Women Health Iss* 4(4):191-195, 1994.

Langer A et al: The Latin American trial of psychosocial support during pregnancy: effects on mother's well-being and satisfaction. *Soc Sci Med* 42(11):1589-1597, 1996.

Lederman RP: *Psychosocial adaptation in pregnancy,* Englewood Cliffs, NJ, 1984, Prentice Hall.

Lederman RP, Miller DS: Adaptation to pregnancy in three different ethnic groups: Latin-American, African-American, and Anglo-American, *Can J Nurs Res* 30(3):37-51, 1998.

Leiblum SR, Palmer MG, Spector IP: Non-traditional mothers: single heterosexual/lesbian women and lesbian couples electing motherhood via donor insemination, *J Psychosom Obstet Gynaecol* 16(1):11-20, 1995.

Levin J: How prayer heals: a theoretical model. *Altern Ther Health Med* 2(1):66-73, 1996.

Levy EF: Reproductive issues for lesbians. In Peterson KJ, editor: *Health care for lesbians and gay men: confronting homophobia and heterosexism,* New York, 1996, Harrington Park Press/Haworth Press.

Lombardi W, Wilson S, Peniston PB: Wellness intervention with pregnant soldiers, *Mil Med* 164(1):22-29, 1999.

Long A: Nursing: a spiritual perspective, *Nurs Ethics* 4(6):496-510, 1997.

Lukoff D et al: Religious and spiritual case reports on Medline: a systematic analysis of records from 1980 to 1996. *Altern Ther* 5(1):64-70, 1999.

MacLaren A: Primary care for women: comprehensive sexual health assessment, *J Nurse Midwifery* 40(2):104-119, 1995.

Magana A, Clark NM: Examining a paradox: Does religiosity contribute to positive birth outcomes in Mexican American populations? *Health Educ Q* 22(1):96-109, 1995.

Magann EF, Evans SF, Newnham JP: Employment, exertion, and pregnancy outcome, assessment by kilocalories expended each day, *Am J Obstet Gynecol* 175(1):182-187, 1996.

May K: A typology of detachment/involvement styles adopted during pregnancy by first time expectant fathers, *West J Nurs Res* 2:445-461, 1980.

Mayer BA et al: Health assessment for partners of pregnant women: a pilot study of four survey methods, *J Am Board Fam Pract* 10(3):192-198, 1997.

McCool WF, McCool SJ: Feminism and nurse-midwifery: historical overview and current issues, *J Nurse Midwifery* 34(6):323-334, 1989.

Mercer RT, Ferketich S, De Joseph J: Theoretical models for studying the effect of antepartum stress on the family, *Nurs Res* 35(6):339-346, 1986.

Morse GG: Reframing women's health in nursing education: a feminist approach, *Nurs Outlook* 43(6):273-277, 1995.

Northrup C: *Women's bodies, women's wisdom,* New York, 1998, Bantam.

Oruc S et al: Sexual behavior during pregnancy, *Aust NZ J Obstet Gynaecol* 39(1):48-50, 1999.

Paarlberg KM et al: Psychosocial factors and pregnancy outcome: a review with emphasis on methodological issues, *J Psychosom Res* 39(5):563-595, 1995.

Parker B et al: Testing and intervention to prevent further abuse to pregnant women, *Res Nurs Health* 22:59-66, 1999.

Pies CA: *Considering parenthood: a workbook for lesbians,* San Francisco, 1985, Spinsters Ink.

Prince J, Adams M: The psychology of pregnancy. In Alexander J, Levy V, Roche S, editors: *Antenatal care: a research-based approach,* Toronto, 1990, University of Toronto Press.

Rankow EJ: Lesbian health issues for the primary care provider, *J Fam Pract* 40(5):486-496, 1995.

Richardson L: Narrative and sociology, *J Contemp Ethnog* 19(1):116-135, 1990.

Richardson SA, Guttmacher AF: *Childbearing—its social and psychological aspects,* Philadelphia, 1967, Williams & Wilkins.

Rohrbaugh JB: Choosing children: psychological issues in lesbian parenting. *Women Ther* 8(1-2):51-64, 1988.

Rubin R: Cognitive style in pregnancy, *Am J Nurse* 70(3):502-508, 1970.

Saurel-Cubizolles MJ, Kaminski M: 1986 Work in pregnancy: its evolving relationship with perinatal outcomes: a review, *Soc Sci Med* 22(4):431-441.

Schaffer MA, Lia-Hoagberg B: Effects of social support on prenatal care and health behaviors of low-income women, *J Obstet Gynecol Neonatal Nurs* 26(4):433-440, 1997.

Sesia PM: "Women come here on their own when they need to": prenatal maternal health in Oaxaca, *Med Anthropol Q* 10(2):121-140, 1996.

Sheehan TJ: Creating a psychosocial measurement model from stressful life events, *Soc Sci Med* 43(2):265-271, 1996.

Sokoloski EH: Canadian First Nations women's beliefs about pregnancy and prenatal care, *Can J Nurs Res* 27(1):89-100, 1995.

Stark MA: Psychosocial adjustment during pregnancy: the experience of mature gravidas, *J Obstet Gynecol Neonatal Nurs* 26(2):206-211, 1997.

Tam LW: Psychological aspects of pregnancy in the military: a review, *Mil Med* 163(6):408-412, 1998.

Tash DT, Kenney JW: The lesbian childbearing couple: a case report, *Birth* 20(1):36-40, 1993.

Tilden VP: The relation of life stress and social support to emotional disequilibrium during pregnancy, *Res Nurs Health* 6:176-184, 1983.

Wadwah PD et al: Prenatal psychosocial factors and the neuroendocrine axis in human pregnancy, *Psychosom Med* 58(5):432-446, 1996.

Warner PH, Rowe T, Whipple B: Shedding light on the sexual history, *Am J Nurs* 99(6):34-40, 1999.

Welles-Nystrom B: The meaning of postponed motherhood for women in the United States and Sweden: aspects of feminism and radical timing strategies, *Health Care Women Int* 18(3):279-299, 1997.

Wendland CL, Burn F, Hill C: Donor insemination: a comparison of lesbian couples, heterosexual couples and single women, *Fertil Steril* 65(4):764-770, 1996.

Westlander G: The psychological background of pregnancy outcome: a critical evaluation of research, *Women Health* 17(3):79-99, 1991.

Wilson LM et al.: Antenatal psychosocial risk factors associated with adverse postpartum family outcomes. *Can Med Assoc J* 154(6):785-799, 1996.

Zambrana RE, Scrimshaw SC: Maternal psychosocial factors associated with substance use in Mexican-origin and African American low-income pregnant women, *Pediatr Nurs* 23(3):253-259, 1997.

Zeidenstein L: Gynecological and childbearing needs of lesbians, *J Nurse Midwifery* 35(1):10-18, 1990.

Chapter 13

Screening for Fetal Health

Specific strategies to assess fetal status have been proposed as a way to (1) confirm the well-being of the normal fetus, thereby preventing unnecessary intervention, and (2) improve perinatal outcome through timely diagnosis and treatment of fetal compromise (Miller,Rabello, and Paul, 1996). In addition, fetal assessment should provide information that is useful in making clinical decisions regarding whether pregnancy should continue or further intervention is justifiable (Ware and Devoe, 1994). Fetal assessment is an important part of the broader, ongoing risk assessment that occurs from the preconceptual period until delivery of the infant.

The types of fetal assessment strategies vary from country to country and from community to community. For example, women from many of the European countries expect multiple ultrasound examinations throughout the pregnancy and are often surprised when they find themselves in a community where ultrasound screening may be done for medical indications only. The strategies used for fetal assessment are influenced by the providers' beliefs about the predictive value of the testing, the availability of the technology, and the source of payment for the procedures. Providers practicing with a midwifery philosophy of care need to continually balance the woman's knowledge of her fetus' health and the information that can be gained from technology.

HISTORY

Although there is historic evidence that women have recognized the importance of perception of movement of their fetuses, procedures done by a third party to establish fetal status are fairly recent. Early nineteenth-century writings document interest in listening to the fetal heart with a rudimentary fetoscope. However, it was not until the mid-twentieth century with the development of biochemical assays (plasma and urinary estriols) followed by the development of technology to continuously monitor fetal heart rates (FHRs) that researchers recognized the possibility of preventing fetal and neonatal mortality and morbidity through active fetal assessment.

Investigation into the identification of fetuses at risk during labor led to the development of continuous FHR monitoring for women experiencing high risk pregnancies. The association between late decelerations of the FHR during labor with fetal asphyxia provided the basis for the idea that similar changes may predict those fetuses who will not adapt well to labor. This concept of providing transient stress to the fetus to identify uteroplacental insufficiency led to the introduction of the oxytocin challenge test (OCT). The rationale for the testing was the belief that that late FHR decelerations were a reflection of relative myocardial hypoxia in a compromised fetus (Ware and Devoe, 1994). As it became clear that any contraction activity—not just that induced by administration of oxytocin—could be used in the testing, the terminology was changed to contraction stress test (CST).

The OCT/CST quickly became a standard antepartum means of assessing whether the fetus would benefit from continued intrauterine life or be better off delivered. However, the OCT/CST had several drawbacks, including the need for use of interventions that would induce naturally produced oxytocin (nipple stimulation) or exogenous oxytocin (intravenous induction), the fact that it was time consuming, and the fact that the intervention was contraindicated in many high-risk cases (e.g., preterm labor). It was during the investigations and use of the OCT/CST that it was noted the FHR accelerations were associated with a decrease in abnormal CSTs (Lee, DiLoeto, and Logrand, 1976; Lee and Drukker, 1979). These findings led to the development of the nonstress test (NST). Advantages of the NST were quickly noted. It was easier to perform, took less time, and had no contraindications.

Although it became clear that both the CST and NST have low false-negative rates (accurate in identifying healthy fetuses), they both have rather high false-positive rates (incorrect prediction of a problem in a healthy fetus). The development of ultrasound technology that allowed imaging of the intrauterine environment allowed other fetal biophysical activities to be documented. The research of Manning, Platt, and Sipos' suggested that assessing fetal breathing movements, fetal movements, fetal tone, and amniotic fluid volume in addition to the NST would decrease the false-positive rate of the single NST (Manning, Platt, and Sipos, 1980). These three tests—the NST, CST, and biophysical profile (BPP)—continue to be used in practice, although there is controversy regarding whether there is an ideal sequencing of testing. In addition to these tests, use of Doppler effect to document umbilical vessel flow and fetal movement has also been introduced into practice for screening and diagnosis. Ultrasound visualization continues to develop as a means to identify anomalies and deviations in growth.

INDICATIONS FOR FETAL ASSESSMENT

Ideally fetal assessment is done at every prenatal visit. Uterine growth, FHR and rhythm, and fetal movement are all criteria that are assessed by the clinician during the abdominal and pelvic examinations. Specialized fetal testing, often requiring specially trained personnel and equipment not always immediately available in the office or clinic setting, continues to be used primarily for fetuses at increased risk for poor outcome. Since research has not identified any one particular screening test that can be used to effectively screen all pregnant women for potential fetal problems, the need for fetal testing is determined by indications or risk factors. Box 13-1 identifies commonly accepted indications for antepartum testing.

When determining whether a screening test will be effective in obstetric care, one needs to understand the sensitivity, specificity, and positive and negative predic-

Box 13-1 *Indications for Fetal Antepartum Testing*

- Abnormal heart rate or rhythm by auscultation or doptone
- Asthma
- Cardiac disease—Stage III-IV
- Cholestasis of pregnancy
- Chronic hypertension
- Collagen vascular disease
- Congenital anomalies in the fetus
- Decreased fetal movement
- Diabetes
- Intrauterine procedures—percutaneous umbilical blood sampling or intravascular intrauterine transfusion
- Multiple gestation
- Oligohydramnios
- Placenta previa
- Polyhydramnios
- Poor obstetric history (history of repeated losses or previous preterm births)
- Poor fetal growth (suspected or documented intrauterine growth restriction)
- Postterm pregnancy
- Preeclampsia
- Premature labor
- Premature rupture of membranes
- Previous stillbirth
- Renal disease
- Rh disease
- Sickle cell disease
- Substance abuse
- Third trimester bleeding
- Thyroid disease

tive values (see Chapter 2). In healthy women at low risk for perinatal problems, the predictive values may not appear adequate and may result in high false-positive rates. However, if the abnormality is one that represents a very real threat to the life or quality of life of the infant and if intervention is available to decrease the effects of the abnormality, it would seem reasonable to accept an otherwise high false-positive rate.

When counseling women and their partners about fetal assessment strategies, it is important to explain the rationale for the testing and what the testing can and cannot determine. Parents should be encouraged to actively participate in the decision making surrounding the assessment of their child's status, and their beliefs and decisions should be honored. Investigators have argued that women are often faced with "options" that they think they can't refuse. Wertz and Fletcher (1993, p. 175) note, "(I)t is extremely difficult, if not impossible, for women to choose to reject technologies approved by the obstetric profession. Once tests are offered, to reject them is a rejection of modern faith in science and also a rejection of modern beliefs that women should do everything possible for the health of the future child." When a woman rejects the use of a screening test, she is usually reframing the concept of "risk" from the expert's perception of risk to her own perception—a perception shaped by her knowledge, beliefs, values, and previous experiences. For example, a woman may be concerned that the "risk" of NST/amniotic fluid index (AFI) screening for her postdates pregnancy leading into an unwanted induction may be greater than the risk that the baby may be compromised (Research Box 13-1).

FETAL MOVEMENT COUNTS

Documenting the woman's perception of fetal movement is the oldest and simplest method of monitoring fetal well-being in the late-second and third trimesters. Since the 1970s a variety of counting techniques have been described in the literature, yet few have been evaluated for predictive values.

Physiology Considerations

During the third trimester the fetus spends about 10% of its time making gross body movements, with the most activity occurring between 9 PM and 1 AM (Patrick et al., 1982). Periods without activity generally last about 20 minutes, although they can last up to 75 minutes in normal pregnancies. Gross body movements are usually described as movement of the trunk (stretching) with associated coordinated movements of the limbs. Women tend to feel 85% to 90% of these gross movements, and studies suggest that maternal perception of movement is a reliable measure (Rayburn et al., 1980; Sadovsky, Yaffe, and Polishuk, 1974). Women also feel movement that is a result of hiccups—repetitive, regular movement of the trunk that may last for several minutes. Occasionally movement of the fetal arms and legs will be present during the hiccups. Women tend not to feel finer fetal movement such as hand grasp or finger sucking, nor do they tend to note passive fetal movement. Passive movement includes the longitudinal movement that occurs as the maternal diaphragm moves with respiration or the front-to-back movement that occurs with aortic pulsing.

Decreased fetal movements may be associated with fetal anoxia; a decrease in movements usually occurs over 2 to 3 days before complete cessation of movement. Decreased movement has been found to be associated with conditions that involve uteroplacental insufficiency, including preeclampsia, chronic hypertension, and diabetes. Cessation of movement may precede intrauterine death by 24 hours or more (Sadovsky, Yaffe, and Polishuk, 1974). The decrease in movements has been referred to as an "alarm signal," but the degree of decrease and the time frames have differed among studies. Lack of three movements per hour or no movement in 12 hours, lack of ten movements in 12 hours, lack of ten movements in 2 hours, and a serial increase in the amount of timeit takes the woman to count ten movements all have been proposed as alarm signals (Liston et al., 1982; Rayburn et al., 1980; Sadovsky, Yaffe, and Polishuk, 1974).

Procedure for Documenting Fetal Activity

Since there appears to be a strong relationship between decreased fetal movement and fetal death, teaching women to monitor fetal movement should be included in all third-trimester patient education. Documenting maternal perception of fetal activity provides a means for the woman to actively participate in her care, and the teaching may also enhance maternal-fetal attachment. Although some clinicians have expressed concern that maternal monitoring may increase stress during pregnancy, research suggests that self-monitoring does not significantly increase psychologic distress.

Perhaps the easiest mode of maternal monitoring is counseling the woman to rest on her left side for 30 to 60 minutes and count each fetal movement. If less than

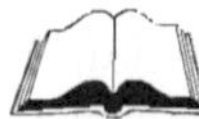

Research Box 13-1

Markens S, Browner CH, Press N: Because of the risks: how U. S. pregnant women account for refusing prenatal screening, *Social Sci Med* 49:359-369, 1999.

Background

Prenatal screening has become a routine intervention in the United States, and maternal serum alphafetoprotein (AFP) screening has become a community standard of care. Most research on prenatal fetal testing has focused on the women who accept prenatal diagnosis, and the few studies that have explored the decision to decline testing have sought associations among sociodemographic factors and the decision to accept or reject screening and/or diagnosis. A common assumption is that women who refuse AFP screening do so because of their opposition to abortion since abortion is often the only intervention that medicine can offer when fetal anomalies are detected. Other investigators have assumed that rejection of screening is associated with the perception that pregnancy and childbirth have been overly medicalized.

Research Questions

(1) How do a group of U. S. women who refuse AFP screening account for their decision? (2) How do their explanations compare with those explanations given by women who accept the screening?

Methods

Women who refused AFP screening were recruited from a southern California HMO. Face-to-face interviews were conducted, and content included women's understandings about, attitudes toward, and experiences with prenatal diagnosis; self-care practices during pregnancy; attitudes toward prenatal care, motherhood, and childbearing; and experiences with and attitudes toward disability. Interviews were tape recorded and transcribed, and content was analyzed for themes. Stratification by ethnicity and social class was done to identify potential differences between groups.

Sample

One hundred and thirty-eight women were interviewed; 25 of those interviewed had refused AFP screening. Women recruited into the study were assumed to represent a "low-risk" population as defined by the inclusion criteria: age between 18 and 35 years and no known risk for bearing a child with an anomaly. The mean age of the sample was 26.6 years, mean number of children was 1.3 (range 0-6), and mean parity was 2.2 (range 0-9). Sixty-eight percent were European-American, and 32% were Mexican-American. Median family income was $30,000 to $35,000, with 24% having annual incomes below $15,000. Nineteen percent had not finished high school, and 14% had more than a high school education.

Results

Women who accepted and those who refused AFP screening did not form two distinct groups in terms of factors affecting decision making. The findings suggest that women in the two groups shared many of the same beliefs in and attitudes toward medical management of pregnancy. Women who refused screening incorporated and used biomedical categories to provide rationale for their decisions, and these categories went beyond the expected categories of religious concerns and attitudes about abortion. Women who refused the screening tended not to accept the test as an integral part of prenatal care both because of the voluntary nature of the screening and the understanding that there is a significant false-positive rate. Women in both groups considered the concept of "risk" in making their decision to accept or reject screening, with those who refused believing that they were protecting their fetuses/babies from the risks of further interventions.

Clinical Application

Clinicians can use the findings of this study to increase understanding of the factors affecting the decision to accept or reject fetal screening or diagnostic tests. Although it is easy to assume that opposition to abortion is the primary reason for rejecting fetal diagnosis, findings suggest a much more complex decision-making model. Women who refuse screening do not articulate rejection of other biomedical interventions in pregnancy or childbirth but frame their rejection of screening in terms of their own interpretation of risk. The primary limitation of the study is the homogeneity of the sample, since the Mexican-American group was highly acculturated and similar to the European American group in all sociodemographic factors.

three movements are felt in 60 minutes, she should contact her health care provider. Most women find the Cardiff Count-to-Ten chart easy to use for monitoring (Figure 13-1). Completion of the record takes an average of 20 minutes, as opposed to 1 or more hours used in other screening methods (Smith, Davis, and Rayburn, 1992). Women are counseled to select a time of day to record the movement. Immediately on arising or following a meal is typically recommended as an appropriate time. Fetal movements should be counted until the tenth movement. The woman then notes how many minutes (sometimes rounded to 10- or 15-minute increments) pass until the tenth movement.

Although some clinicians suggest that fetal movement can be stimulated by an increase in maternal glucose levels, assessment of fetal movement in experimental conditions has not shown any association between increased glucose levels and fetal activity (Bocking et al., 1982; Druzin and Foodim, 1986). However, glucose administration has been associated with an increase in fetal breathing movements (Bocking et al., 1982).

Findings that would be considered alarm signals include fewer than ten movements in 12 hours, no perception of movement for 8 hours, a change in the usual pattern of fetal movement, and a sudden increase in violent

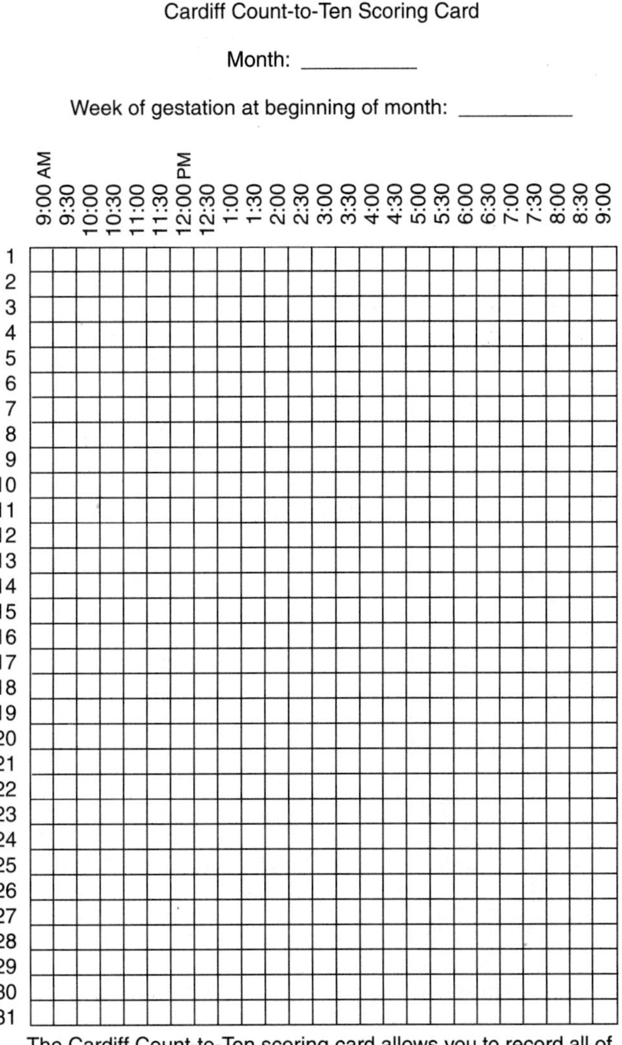

Figure 13-1 Cardiff count-to-ten chart.

fetal movements followed by complete cessation of movement (Lehman and Estok, 1987). When an alarm signal is noted by the woman, she should contact her health care provider, and a plan should be made for further evaluation of the fetal status.

ASSESSMENT OF FETAL HEART RATES

Physiology Considerations

FHR patterns are influenced by anatomic, biochemical, and pharmacologic factors. Intact peripheral receptors, spinal column, brain, autonomic nervous system, and myocardium are necessary for reactivity of the FHR. The autonomic nervous system, balancing sympathetic and parasympathetic effects, leads to the changes in FHR known as "beat to beat" variability. Research suggests that vagal stimulation—cardiodecelerator action—demonstrates a more rapid effect than the sympathetic, or cardioaccelerator, effect (Warner and Cox, 1962). During the first and second trimesters baseline heart rate is relatively elevated, most likely reflecting dominance of the sympathetic system. As pregnancy progresses and the fetal systems mature, there is an increase in parasympathetic influence, resulting in a decrease in baseline FHR. Baseline FHR is also influenced by chemoreceptors in the carotid arteries and aortic arch. Sudden decrease in arterial oxygen tension may stimulate these receptors, leading to acute slowing and increased variability of heart rate. Chronic hypoxia is associated with decreased variability in FHR (Ware and Devoe, 1994). FHR and variability can also be affected by maternal factors. Maternal fever, thyrotoxicosis, and other factors that increase sympathetic stimulation increase rate; maternal hypotension decreases rate. Drugs such as atropine and β-adrenergic agents increase rate; β-adrenergic blockers decrease rate. Chronic placental insufficiency is associated with a decrease in variability, as are drugs such as narcotics, barbiturates, tranquilizers, and atropine (Ware and Devoe, 1994).

When the fetus moves, there is an increased demand for oxygen. This in turn stimulates the FHR accelerations to meet demand. Therefore demonstration of the increase in heart rate is associated with a healthy fetus/newborn. This reactivity of the FHR is influenced by gestational age of the fetus. From 24 through 28 weeks approximately 50% of NSTs will be nonreactive, and by 32 weeks 15% of NSTs remain nonreactive (Druzin and Gabbe, 1996). The effect of gestational age on decelerations of the FHR is not as clear. Some investigators have found that decelerations not associated with accelerations decrease as gestational age increases (Ware and Devoe, 1994). The occurrence of variable decelerations is more dependent on factors such as amount of amniotic fluid, length of umbilical cord, and condition of the cord than gestational age. Likewise, development of late decelerations is associated more with the acid-base balance of the fetus than with gestational age.

Research suggests that there may be population differences in the sensitivity, specificity, and predictive values of testing based on FHR patterns. It has been reported that black women have a higher rate of nonreactive NSTs than white women (Paine et al., 1991). This finding may be influenced by the associated finding that black fetuses demonstrate a higher mean baseline than white fetuses and the finding that there are fewer accelerations of 15 beats/min when the FHR is greater than 140 beats/min (Johnson et al., 1992). Therefore the NST may be less reliable in predicting good perinatal outcomes among blacks, and it may have a lower false-negative rate when compared with white women (Johnson et al., 1998). These differences may be physiologic, or they may be associated with variables that were not controlled in the studies. The fact that the prevalence of certain diseases varies among population also may contribute to the observed differences. Further studies are needed to understand the population differences in each fetal testing approach (Research Box 13-2).

Decelerations in FHR are associated with transient fetal hypoxia. This can be caused by mechanical obstruction (cord compression) or uteroplacental insufficiency. A healthy infant with a normally functioning uteroplacental unit tolerates the decreased intervillous blood flow during contractions well. Poor placental reserves as found in a compromised uteroplacental unit will lead to FHR heart rate decelerations in response to contractions. These late decelerations can be intermittent or repetitive.

Procedures for Using Fetal Heart Rate Changes for Screening

Auscultation of fetal heart rate. Auscultation of the FHR was introduced into obstetric practice in the nineteenth century, but little research was done to evaluate the association with fetal outcome until the mid-twentieth century. Several investigators have found that obstetric personnel are not consistent in their technique of counting FHR, and many are inaccurate in their calculations, especially when the FHR is outside the normal range (Schifrin, Amsel, and Burdorf, 1992). Accuracy is maxi-

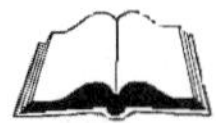

Research Box 13-2

Johnson M J et al: Population differences of fetal biophysical and behavioral characteristics, *Am J Obstet Gynecol* 166(1 pt 1):138-142, 1992.

Background

The nonstress test (NST) is a common screening test used to assess fetal status before labor. Previous research findings suggested that maternal race may influence NST results, with black women noted to have nonreassuring tests three times more often than white women. One theory to explain those findings is that black fetuses spent more time than white fetuses in states associated with nonreactivity.

Research Question

Can the difference in reactivity be attributed to differences in time spent by black and white fetuses in the four fetal behavioral states?

Methods

Women between 38 and 41 weeks' gestation were recruited from the low-risk obstetric clinic and the faculty practice of a large teaching hospital. After eating lunch, women were placed in the left lateral supine position and monitored for 2 hours using an electronic fetal monitor that records both FHR and fetal movement. An ultrasound transducer was also placed to observe fetal lens movement. Two observers interpreted the fetal monitoring strips. Percent time in each fetal state and mean baselines during each state were computed. Chi-square, Fisher's exact test, and independent t-tests were used to identify differences between the groups.

Sample

Fifteen white and 14 black women participated in the study. All of the black women were clinic patients and 13 of the 15 white women were private patients. Parity was similar in both groups, but the black women had a mean age of 20.4 years, and the white women had a mean age of 30.7 years ($p<0.05$).

Results

Fetal outcome, APGAR scores, and birth weight were similar in both groups. No significant differences in fetal state were found between the two groups. When overall mean FHRs were analyzed, black fetuses were found to have a statistically significant higher mean FHT by 9.5 beats/min. The higher baseline persisted in all four behavioral states. When the groups were controlled for fetal sex, there was no difference in mean FHR. These findings are limited by small sample size.

Clinical Application

When the FHR is greater than 140 beats/min, there are less accelerations of 15 beats/min. Therefore race may be an important variable when assessing the sensitivity and specificity of the NST and other screenings tests that use FHR as an indicator. Further study is needed using larger sample sizes to confirm the impact of race on fetal assessment screening.

mized by using several short periods of time (e.g., 5- to 15-second increments) rather than counting for a full minute. Auscultation can be done using a standard fetoscope or a handheld Doppler.

Traditionally auscultation has been used to establish FHR without consideration of the periodic changes that occur. Paine and colleagues (1992) proposed using auscultation of accelerations in the office or clinic setting as an alternative to the conventional NST. Advantages of the auscultated acceleration test (AAT) include decreased testing time, decreased inconvenience for the patient (since in many settings she would need to go to a different site for the NST), and the ability to offer a "low-tech" technique for screening. Sensitivity of the AAT is 75% to 100%, and specificity is 85% to 98%. Positive predictive value is 28% to 33%, and negative predictive value is 100% (Daniels and Boehm, 1991) (Research Box 13-3).

Women should be positioned in a semi-Fowler position with a left or right tilt. FHR should be located using the fetoscope or Doppler, and the clinician then counts the number of beats heard every other 5-second period. The 5-second counts are recorded on a graph. An acceptable acceleration is considered when there is an increase in any given 5-second interval of two or more beats above baseline (Daniels and Boehm, 1991). This increase is equivalent to an increase of 24 beats/min, exceeding the criteria for an NST. Fetal movement is noted when either the mother perceives the movement or the examiner palpates movement. If no accelerations are

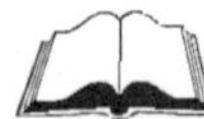

Research Box 13-3

Paine LL et al: A comparison of the auscultated acceleration test and the nonstress test as predictors of perinatal outcomes, *Nurs Res* 41(2):87-91, 1992.

Background

The nonstress test (NST) is the most widely used electronic fetal monitoring technique for fetal assessment. However, it requires the use of fetal monitors and specially trained personnel. It also is inconvenient for women in many sites because the testing requires them to go to a different site than their usual site of care. The auscultated acceleration test (AAT) is a 6-minute test that can easily be administered by nurses, midwives, and physicians using a fetoscope or Doptone device. Previous research has indicated that the AAT has a sensitivity of 75% and specificity of 93% to 98%. However, previous assessment of the AAT has not evaluated its predictive ability for perinatal outcome.

Research Question

What is the validity of the NST and AAT as screening tests in predicting selected perinatal outcomes in a sample of women with high-risk pregnancies?

Methods

Four data collectors performed the AATs and gathered demographic and clinical data on participants. They were blinded to the results of the NST. The NST was interpreted by the faculty physician and the most experienced data collector. Measures of perinatal outcomes included identification of the following as noted in the delivery record: small for gestational age, late decelerations, fetal distress, operative delivery for fetal distress, thick meconium, neonatal resuscitation, and admission to the neonatal intensive care unit. Sensitivity, specificity, positive and negative predictive ability, and false-positive and false-negative rates were calculated. Z-scores were used to detect significant differences in estimates of each validity measure.

Sample

Two hundred and five women referred to a fetal assessment center met the study criteria and agreed to participate. The mean age of the sample was 24.7 years, and mean completed years of education was 12.3 years. Most were black and unmarried. More than half were receiving medical assistance.

Results

Sensitivity was very low for all outcomes for the NST. The sensitivity of the AAT was somewhat higher than that of the NST, but only presence of thick meconium and neonatal resuscitation had significant differences in sensitivity between groups. Specificity exceeded 90% for all outcomes for the NST; it ranged from 70% to 75% for the AAT. All differences in specificity between groups were not significant. Outcomes were also examined by creating two groups: fetal distress and neonatal morbidity. The sensitivity of the AAT in predicting fetal distress was significantly higher than that of the NST, but the specificity of the AAT was lower. The sensitivity of the AAT in predicting neonatal morbidity was higher than that of the NST but not statistically significant. Specificity of the AAT was lower than that of the NST at a significant level.

Clinical Application

Results suggest that the AAT may be a better predictor of poor perinatal outcome than the NST, whereas the NST may be a better predictor of favorable outcome. Specificity for the AAT may be improved by repeating the test in 20 to 30 minutes or by adding maternal perception of fetal movement counts into the assessment. The study findings are limited by the low incidence of nonreactive NSTs and poor perinatal outcomes. Also, the criteria for referral to the fetal testing center in this particular center may not be representative of other clinical sites, so that the sample may differ in high-risk characteristics. Findings support the use of the AAT in clinical practice, with follow-up NST for nonreactive tests.

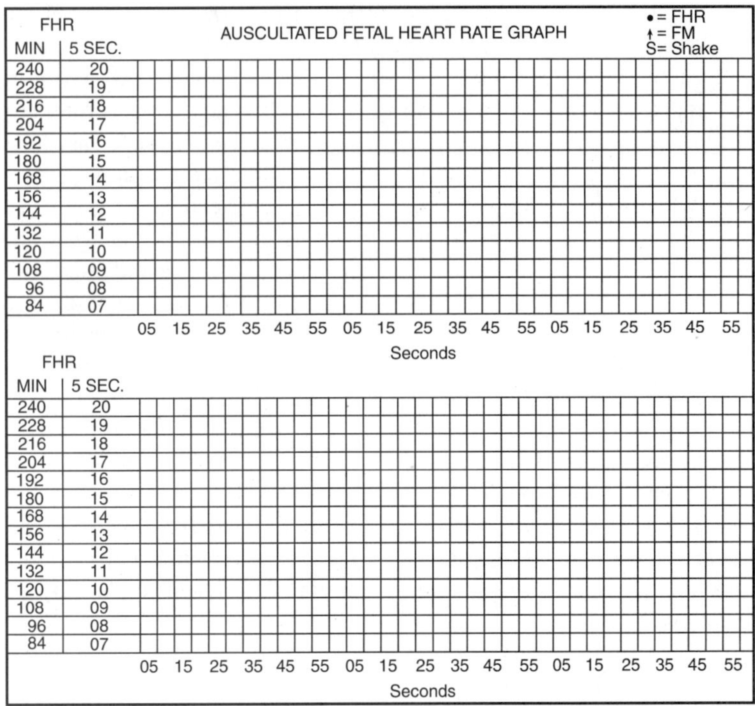

Figure 13-2 Auscultated acceleration test

noted over 3 minutes, the baby is stimulated by shaking or by exposure to vibroacoustic stimulation (VAS). If no accelerations are noted over an additional 2 minutes, the test is considered nonreactive. An NST should be performed when the AAT is nonreactive (Figure 13-2).

There are no contraindications to auscultated acceleration testing.

Nonstress test. The woman should be positioned in a way that decreases aortocaval compression. Left lateral recumbent or semi-Fowler position with a wedge under one hip is most often used. It appears that left- and right-tilt are comparable when assessing FHR (Moffatt and Van den Hof, 1997). The best positioning for the ultrasound transducer is determined using Leopold maneuvers, and the transducer is applied with the appropriate belts. Fetal movement can be noted with an "event marker" that the mother presses when she perceives movement. A distinctive mark is then documented on the fetal monitoring paper, allowing comparison of the FHR with the mother's perception of movement. Uterine activity can be assessed through palpation by the examiner and/or use of the tocodynamometer strapped to the abdomen. External monitoring of the contractions indicates frequency and to a lesser degree, duration. Accuracy of the monitoring of uterine activity is influenced by maternal body type and fetal position.

An NST is considered reactive when two FHR accelerations of at least 15 beats/min for at least 15 seconds in a 20-minute cycle are observed. When the test is nonreactive in the first 20 minutes, it is usually extended for another 20 minutes. The most common reason for a nonreactive test is a fetal sleep cycle. VAS may be used if the test is nonreactive in the first 20 minutes. An NST is considered equivocal or inconclusive when there is an acceleration above baseline that is less than 15 beats/min or lasts less than 15 seconds, if variability is less than 6 beats/min, or if the quality of the fetal monitoring strip is not adequate for interpretation (Tucker, 1996).

Women with reactive NSTs usually are scheduled for repeat testing twice weekly when conditions associated with increased risk of sudden deterioration of the uteroplacental unit (e.g., diabetes, IUGR, postdates gestation) are present. Equivocal NSTs should be repeated within 24 hours.

When the NST is nonreactive, additional testing is indicated. Most clinicians use a BPP as the next level of testing. Others use the CST. Ideally further testing can be done immediately following the NST. A nonreactive NST followed by a negative (normal) CST is considered equivocal and requires repeat testing within 24 hours.

Sensitivity of the NST appears to range from 45% to 55%, with specificity ranging from 85% to 100% (Ware and Devoe, 1994). As expected, the test is less sensitive and specific in populations with low morbidity and mortality rates. There are no contraindications to nonstress testing.

Vibroacoustic stimulation. Fetal response to acoustic stimulation was first described in 1925 when Peiper reported an increase in fetal movement with the stimulation (Marden et al., 1997). Fetal activity response to acoustic stimulation increases with gestational age, and after 31 weeks 70% to 96% of fetuses respond (Crade and Lovett, 1988; Inglis et al., 1993). Vibroacoustic stimulation appears to have no effect on fetal state changes, long-term hearing loss, or fetal compromise (Marden et al., 1997). Fetal movement following exposure to VAS has been associated with BPP scores of 8 or more, and use of VAS to improve BPP scores is not associated with any increase in false-negative rates (Inglis et al., 1993). Palpation of fetal movement following VAS is almost always associated with reactive NSTs. Fetal tachycardia has been noted in some studies evaluating the use of VAS. The FHR usually returns to normal within 5 minutes but may remain elevated for up to 1 hour.

VAS is usually used when an NST is nonreactive. Some clinicians support routinely using VAS as a way to shorten the time necessary for fetal assessment. After determining the position of the fetus, the clinician applies an artificial larynx or fetal acoustic stimulation device firmly on the maternal abdomen over the fetal head. A 1- to 3-second exposure is administered, with repeat exposure at 1-minute intervals up to three times. The test is considered reactive when two FHR accelerations of at least 15 beats/min for at least 15 seconds are observed.

Further research is needed to determine whether there are contraindications to VAS.

Contraction stress test. Contractions can be stimulated by endogenously produced oxytocin using nipple stimulation. When nipple stimulation is not feasible, exogenous oxytocin can be used.

Nipple stimulation is commonly used before using exogenous oxytocin. The woman should be positioned in semi-Fowler position with a lateral tilt. The tocodynamometer and ultrasound transducer should be positioned on the maternal abdomen. FHR and uterine activity should be monitored for at least 10 minutes to

Box 13-2 *Interpretation of Contraction Stress Test*

Interpretation According to Contraction Pattern and Fetal Heart Rate Decelerations

Positive (abnormal)	Late decelerations occur with >50% of contractions; indicates fetal compromise secondary to uteroplacental insufficiency
Negative (normal)	No late decelerations noted with contractions that are at least 40 seconds in duration, with a frequency of three per 10 minutes; indicates fetal well-being and normal uteroplacental function
Suspicious (equivocal)	Inconsistent late decelerations with contractions
Unsatisfactory	Inability to stimulate contractions with a frequency of three per 10 minutes; unsatisfactory tracings secondary to maternal habitus

Interpretation according to Presence or Absence of Fetal Heart Rate Accelerations

Reactive negative	Accelerations of at least 15 beats/min for at least 15 seconds following fetal movement and no late decelerations associated with contractions
Nonreactive negative	Absence of accelerations following fetal movement and no late decelerations with contractions
Reactive positive	Accelerations of at least 15 beats/min for at least 15 seconds following fetal movement and the presence of late decelerations with some of the uterine contractions
Nonreactive positive	No accelerations noted and persistent late decelerations associated with contractions

establish baseline parameters. If three spontaneous contractions of at least 40 seconds are noted over a 10-minute period of time, no further stimulation should be attempted.

Nipple stimulation can be done by having the woman either stroke the nipple with the palmar surface of her fingers or by gentle nipple rolling. Some sites use a breast pump for stimulation. Typically women are instructed to stimulate the nipple on one breast for 2 minutes or until a contraction begins, then rest for 2 to 5 minutes. The stimulation is repeated for up to 20 minutes or until contractions occur every 3 minutes.

When spontaneous contractions are not observed, oxytocin can be administered intravenously using a controlled-rate infusion pump. Dosage of 0.5 mU/min is used to begin the infusion, and the rate is increased 1 to 2 mU every 15 to 20 minutes until contractions with a frequency of three per 10 minutes are achieved. Once the contractions are adequate for evaluating fetal response, the infusion is discontinued. The infusion is discontinued immediately if hyperstimulation or tetany occur. Interpretation of CSTs is summarized in Box 13-2.

When the CST is negative, testing is repeated on a weekly basis. When the CST is equivocal, repeat testing should be scheduled within 24 hours. A positive CST requires consultation with the obstetrician and consideration for delivery.

CST is contraindicated in women at increased risk for preterm labor, premature multiple gestation, incompetent cervix, previous vertical uterine incision, placenta previa, preterm premature rupture of membranes, polyhydramnios, and third trimester bleeding.

AMNIOTIC FLUID VOLUME

Physiology Considerations

Extremes in volume of amniotic fluid are associated with adverse fetal outcomes. Decreased volume is associated with fetal growth restriction, postural deformities, stillbirth, pulmonary hypoplasia, meconium-stained fluid, and abnormal FHR patterns in labor. Increased volume is associated with fetal anomalies, aneuploidy, macrosomia, and stillbirth. Dye-dilution techniques are the most accurate means of estimating volume, but they are invasive, carrying risk to the pregnancy. The development of ultrasound imaging has provided an indirect means of measuring fluid level, but there is evidence that the most common techniques for measuring fluid may not provide adequate ability to predict adverse pregnancy outcome (Chauhan et al., 1997; Magann et al., 1999a; Magann et al., 1999b). The prediction of oligohydramnios is especially problematic, with unacceptably high false-positive rates.

The ability to correctly identify fetuses with abnormal low volumes of fluid is important in planning management for a potentially compromised fetus. A fetus who experiences hypoxemia experiences decreased renal and pulmonary perfusion secondary to the shunting of fluid to the heart and brain. When this process is chronic, it can lead to decreased production of amniotic fluid, resulting in oligohydramnios. Thus the amount of fluid can be used as a marker for chronic fetal compromise.

Procedures for Estimating Amniotic Fluid Volume

Amniotic fluid index. The woman is positioned in a semi-Fowler or recumbent position with a lateral tilt. The uterus is divided into four quadrants, with the umbilicus as the landmark for dividing the upper and lower segments and the linea nigra for dividing the left and right segments. The maximum vertical diameter of a pocket of fluid without loops of cord or extremities is determined in centimeters. The maximum vertical diameters for the largest pockets in each quadrant are added to obtain the AFI. A sum of 0 to 5 cm is considered oligohydramnios; 5.1 to 8 cm indicates low normal (borderline); 8.1 to 18 cm indicates normal volume; and greater than 18 cm indicates high volume.

Two-diameter pocket measurement. Positioning is similar to that for determining AFI, and the uterus is divided into four quadrants using the same landmarks. The largest pocket of fluid for each quadrant is identified, and the vertical diameter is multiplied by the horizontal diameter for each. The largest pocket provides the final two-diameter pocket measurement. A measurement of 0 to 15 cm^2 indicates oligohydramnios; 15.1 cm^2 to 50 cm^2 indicates normal fluid volume; greater than 50 cm^2 indicates increased fluid volume.

When fluid volume is normal, rescreening is recommended weekly for women less than 41 weeks' gestation (Lagrew et al., 1992). Women who are greater than 41 weeks' gestation and those with low normal estimates should be evaluated twice weekly. When polyhydramnios is identified, rescanning twice weekly is indicated to document worsening of the condition. When fluid estimates suggest oligohydramnios or polyhydramnios, a full anatomic screen of the fetus for anomalies should be done.

When oligohydramnios or low normal volume is identified, the scan can be repeated in 24 hours, with the woman being instructed to increase oral fluid intake and maintain bed rest in the lateral position. Traditionally physicians have induced labor in women with low fluid volume at 36 weeks' gestational age or greater. Recent research suggests that this interventive approach may not be necessary for fetuses with appropriate growth and/or those with reactive NSTs.

BIOPHYSICAL PROFILE

Physiology Considerations

Fetal response to hypoxemia reflects the sensitivity of the central nervous system (CNS) to decreases in oxygen levels. It is recognized that CNS tissue is highly sensitive to decreases in oxygen, and the development of hypoxemia rapidly affects CNS-mediated system functions. Since FHR reactivity, breathing, movement, and tone are mediated by the CNS, changes in these activities can be used as an indirect measure of CNS status. Fetal movement and fetal breathing are coordinated, complex biophysical activities, and, when they are observed, one can assume that the CNS is not hypoxemic (Manning, Platt, and Sipos, 1980). When these complex activities are not observed, the fetus may simply be in a quiet sleep. Lack of fetal breathing and movement may also be associated with true fetal compromise. Manning, Platt, and Sipos (1980) provided strong evidence that using several biophysical fetal tests in combination decreases both the false-positive and false-negative rates inherent in a single test alone.

Fetal responses to CNS hypoxemia can be divided into two categories: acute and chronic responses. Acute responses represent changes in CNS-regulated activities such as fetal movement, tone, breathing movements, and heart rate. Acute hypoxemia in an otherwise healthy fetus results in changes in the CNS-regulated activities but does not affect the chronic markers. Research suggests that the biophysical indicators that present earliest in fetal life are the last to be affected by hypoxemia (Vintzileos et al., 1983). Control of fetal tone in the cortex begins at 7.5 to 8.5 weeks' gestation and is the last indicator to be lost in fetal compromise. Cortex control of fetal movement begins around 9 weeks' gestation and is therefore more sensitive to hypoxemia-influenced changes. Fetal breathing movements and FHR control occurs later in the second trimester, and loss of each of those indicators is an early sign of fetal compromise. Repetitive acute episodes have the potential to lead to chronic responses to hypoxemia.

Chronic responses represent decreased amniotic fluid production and impaired fetal growth. Chronic hypoxemia, such as that seen with a compromised uteroplacental unit, leads to a loss of both acute and chronic response markers.

More recently a modified BPP using only the NST and AFI as variables has been proposed to decrease time and cost while maintaining adequate predictability. Results of studies demonstrate conflicting findings regarding the effectiveness of the modified BPP. Some investigators have found that it has an intermediate false-positive rate of 60% and a low false-negative rate of 0.8%, which compares favorably to the CST and complete BPP (Miller, Rabello, and Paul, 1996). Others have not found this to be true (Manning et al., 1990). Clearly the incidence of perinatal morbidity and mortality in a given patient population needs to be considered when assessing the effectiveness of the testing scheme.

The BPP combines markers for both acute and chronic hypoxemia, and the findings can be evaluated to estimate the severity, repetitive frequency, and chronicity of the hypoxemic state. Advantages of the BPP over other single tests include greater accuracy of fetal compromise and improved ability to follow the progressive effects of fetal pathophysiology, leading to the option of conservative management when warranted. To date there have been no population-based differences found in fetal state as determined by fetal movement (Johnson et al., 1992).

Procedure for Obtaining a Biophysical Profile Score

The patient is positioned in a semirecumbent position with a lateral tilt. The fetus is scanned until the transducer is positioned so that the fetal thorax and hand can be observed. The time is noted and observation for fetal breathing movements begins. When at least 30 seconds of breathing activity has been observed, identification of fetal movements and tone is accomplished. Fetal tone is considered normal when the trunk or an extremity extends and returns to flexion or if the clinician observes the opening and closing of a hand. Assessment of amniotic fluid volume is then completed. Recent research suggests that, when all fetal biophysical properties identified visually by ultrasound are normal, the NST can be eliminated without altering the negative predictive accuracy of the testing (Druzin and Gabbe, 1996).

A BPP score of 8 to 10 represents a fetus that is at low risk for chronic asphyxia. Testing is usually repeated

Table 13-1 *Variables in the Biophysical Profile*

Variable	Normal (2 points)	Abnormal (0 points)
Fetal breathing movements	At least one episode of fetal breathing movement lasting at least 30 seconds during a 30-minute observation	Absent fetal breathing movements or fetal breathing movement less than 30 seconds' duration
Gross body movements	At least three distinct body/limb movements in a 30-minute observation	Two or less gross body/limb movements
Fetal tone	At least one episode of active extension and return to flexion of the limbs or trunk, or one episode of opening and closing of the hand	Either slow extension with return to partial flexion or movement of limb in full extension; no fetal movement
Amniotic fluid index	One pocket of fluid that measures at least 2 cm in two perpendicular planes	No pockets of fluid or pocket less than 2-cm diameter in two perpendicular planes
Nonstress test	Reactive	Nonreactive

weekly, except in cases in which rapid deterioration may be expected (e.g., diabetes, postmaturity). A score of 4 to 6 represents suspected chronic asphyxia, warranting consultation with the obstetrician. If there is oligohydramnios or if the gestational age is greater than 36 weeks with a favorable cervix, immediate delivery may be considered. In other cases repeat testing in 24 hours is expected.

Scores of 0 to 2 require immediate referral to the obstetrician, preferably to a perinatologist. Immediate delivery may be considered (Table 13-1).

DOPPLER FLOW STUDIES

Physiology Considerations

Doppler flow studies are used to measure velocity of blood flow through a vessel. Normal flow through the umbilical arteries indicates normal decreased placental resistance. When placental resistance is increased (e.g., when maternal hypertension is present), flow velocity is altered. Therefore alterations in Doppler flow waveforms can be an indirect measure of risk for impaired fetal growth and chronic hypoxemia. Abnormal uterine and umbilical artery velocity waveforms are associated with shorter gestational age, lower birth weight, increased cesarean section rate, and increased neonatal intensive care unit admissions (van Asselt et al., 1998).

Doppler waveform patterns are influenced by gestational age. Pulsatility decreases and diastolic flow increases as gestation progresses. Development of decreased end-diastolic flow or absent or reversed end-diastolic flow is an abnormal finding and may represent true extreme fetal compromise.

Several indices have been proposed to describe the flow velocity waveforms. The peak systolic/diastolic ratio (S/D ratio, or A/B ratio) is most commonly used. The greater the diastolic flow (normal flow), the lower the ratio. When the diastolic flow decreases, as with increased resistance, the ratio increases. The S/D ratio is considered abnormal when it is elevated above the 95 percentile for gestational age or if diastolic flow is absent or reversed after 18 to 20 weeks' gestation (ACOG, 1997a). Another common index is the pulsatility index, which is the systolic-minus-diastolic values divided by the mean of the velocity waveform profile (S–D/mean) (Druzin and Gabbe, 1996). The resistance index is the systolic minus diastolic divided by the systolic.

An elevation of the umbilical artery S/D ratio may precede restriction in fetal growth, and once fetal growth restriction is identified, velocity flow indices can be used to assess the degree of compromise.

Umbilical artery velocimetry provides the most benefit in pregnancies with a presumptive diagnosis of intrauterine growth restriction (ACOG, 1997a). The use of umbilical artery Doppler velocimetry is not indicated for screening in a low-risk population because of its low sensitivity and extremely low positive predictive values for fetal growth restriction and preeclampsia (ACOG, 1997a; Atkinson et al., 1994).

Procedure for Obtaining Doppler Waveform Indices

When the need for Doppler waveform studies is identified, the woman should be referred to a perinatal diagnostic centered skilled in fetal screening and diagnosis.

ROUTINE ULTRASOUND SCREENING

Ultrasound technology has been accepted as a reliable means of documenting fetal viability, gestational age, fetal growth patterns, and selected anomalies. Although the technology was developed to provide data that would be useful in managing pregnancies at increased risk for perinatal problems, it was rapidly incorporated into general prenatal care. Routine screening of healthy, low-risk women is included in the prenatal care in many countries, but its use has provoked controversy in the United States. To date no American professional organization or national panel has recommended routine ultrasound screening of all pregnant women, but most obstetricians are currently recommending at least one routine scan, usually at 18 to 20 weeks' gestation.

Ultrasound screening is commonly thought to improve the outcome of perinatal care by improving gestational dating and identifying fetuses for whom intervention was indicated. The results of most randomized control studies have not supported this assumption (Crane et al., 1994; Ewigman, LeFevre, and Hesser, 1990; LeFevre et al., 1993; Neilson, Munjanja, and Whitfield, 1984; Saari-Kemppainen et al., 1990; Waldenstrom et al., 1988). Only one controlled study has shown an improvement in perinatal mortality rate, and that was primarily because of the termination of pregnancies in which anomalies were detected (Saari-Kemppainen et al., 1990). The largest trial conducted in the United States found no differences in perinatal mortality, severe perinatal morbidity, and moderate perinatal morbidity when comparing the experimental group that received ultrasound screening at 18 to 20 weeks' gestation and 31 to 35 weeks gestation to the control group that received screening only for clinical indications (Ewigman et al., 1993). The sensitivity to detection of fetal anomalies in routine screening in low-risk pregnancies ranges from 17% to 74%, with higher rates of detection found in tertiary hospital-based practices and lower rates in community obstetric practices. It appears that the skill of the individual is highly influential in the accuracy in scanning.

The American College of Obstetricians and Gynecologists notes, "In a population of women with low-risk pregnancy, neither a reduction in perinatal morbidity and mortality, nor a lower rate of unnecessary interventions can be expected from routine diagnostic ultrasound. Thus, ultrasound should be performed for specific indications in low-risk pregnancy" (ACOG, 1997b). The indications identified by the Consensus Development Conference sponsored by the National Institute of Child Health and Human Development are listed in Box 13-3.

Even though research has not supported the routine ultrasound screening of healthy pregnant women, women themselves have increasingly sought screening to "see" their babies. Midwives and physicians are often faced with the fact that there may be no medical indication for ultrasound screening, yet there is patient demand. Most third-party reimbursers cover the cost of one screening ultrasound, further encouraging the use of ultrasound for nonmedical purposes. Excessive use of ultrasound screening adds to the cost of routine prenatal care, with one study estimating that this cost may exceed $500 million dollars annually (Ewigman et al., 1993). Using a decision analysis model, Berwick and Weinstein (1985) found that women demonstrated their desire for ultrasound examination by indicating that they would pay out-of-pocket for the information obtained on an ultrasound scan, even when almost half of the expected information would not be used for medical decision-making. One can imagine that, with the improvement in clarity and the introduction of three-dimensional imaging, patient demand most likely has increased since their study was done.

The routine use of ultrasound screening in healthy pregnancies raises numerous philosophic and ethical issues. American society has become technology dependent, and it is no surprise that belief in the power of technology has permeated medical care. The clinician providing the midwifery model of care needs to carefully balance the philosophic beliefs underlying the use of technology and interventions in care, the beliefs held by the client, and the assessment of the rational use of limited resources. When that is done, it may be difficult to accept routine ultrasound screening of healthy pregnant women for medical reasons. As the

Box 13-3 *Indications for Prenatal Diagnostic Ultrasound*

Estimation of gestational age for patients with uncertain clinical dates
Verification of dates for patients who are to undergo scheduled elective repeat cesarean, delivery, indicated induction of labor, or other elective termination of pregnancy
Evaluation of fetal growth
Vaginal bleeding of undetermined etiology in pregnancy
Determination of fetal presentation
Suspected multiple gestation
Adjunct to amniocentesis
Significant uterine size/clinical dates discrepancy
Pelvic mass
Suspected hydatidiform mole
Adjunct to cervical cerclage placement
Suspected ectopic pregnancy
Adjunct to special procedures
Suspected fetal death
Suspected uterine abnormality
Intrauterine contraceptive device localization
Ovarian follicle development surveillance
Biophysical evaluation of fetal well-being
Observation of intrapartum events (e.g. version/extraction of second twin)
Suspected polyhydramnios or oligohydramnios
Suspected abruptio placenta
Adjunct to external version from breech to vertex presentation
Estimation of fetal weight and/or presentation in premature rupture of membranes and/or premature labor
Abnormal serum alpha-fetoprotein value
Follow-up observation of identified fetal anomaly
Follow-up evaluation of placenta location for identified placenta previa
History of previous congenital anomaly
Serial evaluation of fetal growth in multiple gestation
Evaluation of fetal condition in late registrants for prenatal care

U.S. Department of Health and Human Services: *Diagnostic ultrasound imaging in pregnancy,* Washington, DC, 1984, National Institute of Child Health and Human Development, pp. 7-9.

technology becomes more consumer friendly and better able to clearly image the fetus, professionals in the health care system may have to identify whether there are social, nonmedical indications for routine ultrasound imaging.

References

ACOG, Committee on Clinical Practice: *Utility of antepartum umbilical artery Doppler velocimetry in intrauterine growth restriction,* No. 188, Washington, DC, 1997a, American College of Obstetricians and Gynecologists.

ACOG: *Practice patterns—evidence-based guidelines for clinical issues in obstetrics and gynecology: routine ultrasound in low-risk pregnancy,* Washington, DC, 1997b, American College of Obstetricians and Gynecologists, p 5.

Atkinson MW et al: The predictive value of umbilical artery Doppler studies for preeclampsia or fetal growth retardation in a preeclampsia prevention trial, *Obstet Gynecol* 83(4):609-612, 1994.

Berwick DM, Weinstein MC: What do patients value? Willingness to pay for ultrasound in normal pregnancy, *Med Care* 23(7):881-893, 1985.

Bocking A et al: Effects of intravenous glucose injections on human fetal breathing movements and gross fetal body movements at 38 to 40 weeks' gestational age, *Am J Obstet Gynecol* 142(6):606-611, 1982.

Chauhan SP et al: Intrapartum oligohydramnios does not predict adverse peripartum outcome among high-risk parturients, *Am J Obstet Gynecol* 176:1130-1138, 1997.

Crade M, Lovett S: Fetal response to sound stimulation: preliminary report exploring use of sound stimulation in routine obstetrical ultrasound examinations, *J Ultrasound Med* 7:499-503, 1988.

Crane JP et al: A randomized trial of prenatal ultrasonographic screening: impact on the detection, management, and outcome of anomalous fetuses, *Am J Obstet Gynecol* 171(2):392-399, 1994.

Daniels SM, Boehm N: Auscultated fetal heart rate accelerations—an alternative to the nonstress test, *J Nurse Midwifery* 36(2):88-94, 1991.

Druzin ML, Foodim J: Effect of maternal glucose ingestion compared with maternal water ingestion on the nonstress test, *Obstet Gynecol* 67:425, 1986.

Druzin ML, Gabbe SG: Antepartum fetal evaluation. In Gabbe SG, Niebyl JR, Simpson JL, editors: *Obstetrics—normal and problem pregnancies,* New York, 1996, Churchill Livingston, pp 327-367.

Ewigman B, LeFevre M, Hesser J: A randomized trial of routine prenatal ultrasound. *Obstet Gynecol* 76(2):189-193, 1990.

Ewigman BG et al: Effect of prenatal ultrasound screening on perinatal outcome, *N Engl J Med* 329(12):821-827, 1993.

Inglis SR et al: The use of vibroacoustic stimulation during the abnormal or equivocal biophysical profile, *Am J Obstet Gynecol* 82(3):371-374, 1993.

Johnson MJ et al: Population differences of fetal biophysical and behavioral characteristics, *Am J Obstet Gynecol* 166(1):138-142, 1992.

Johnson TRB et al: Population differences affect the interpretation of fetal nonstress test results, *Am J Obstet Gynecol* 179:779-783, 1998.

Lagrew DC et al: How frequently should the amniotic fluid index be repeated? *Am J Obstet Gynecol* 167(4 Pt 1):1129-1133, 1997.

Lee CY, Drukker B: The nonstress test for the antepartum assessment of fetal reserve. *Am J Obstet Gynecol* 134:460-466, 1979.

Lee CY, DiLoeto PC, Logrand B: Fetal activity acceleration determination for the evaluation of fetal reserve, *Obstet Gynecol* 48:19-24, 1976.

LeFevre ML et al: A randomized trial of prenatal ultrasonographic screening: impact on maternal management and outcome, *Am J Obstet Gynecol* 169(3):483-489, 1993.

Lehman AE, Estok PJ: Screening tool for daily fetal movement, *Nurse Pract* 12(1):40-42, 44, 1987.

Liston R et al: Antepartum fetal evaluation by maternal perception of fetal movement, *Obstet Gynecol* 60:424-428, 1982.

Magann EF et al: Does an amniotic fluid index of </= 5 cm necessitate delivery in high-risk pregnancies? A case control study, *Am J Obstet Gynecol* 108(6 Pt 1):1354-1359, 1999.

Magann EF et al: Antenatal testing among 1001 patients at high risk: the role of ultrasonic estimate of amniotic fluid volume, *Am J Obstet Gynecol* 108(6 Pt 1)1330-1336, 1999.

Manning FA, Platt LD, Sipos L: Antepartum fetal evaluation: development of a fetal biophysical profile, *Am J Obstet Gynecol* 136(6):787-795, 1980.

Manning FA et al: The abnormal fetal biophysical profile score: V. Predictive accuracy according to score composition, *Am J Obstet Gynecol* 162(4):918-927, 1990.

Marden D et al: Randomized controlled trial of a new fetal acoustic stimulation test for fetal well-being, *Am J Obstet Gynecol* 176(6):1386-1388, 1997.

Miller DA, Rabello YA, Paul RH: The modified biophysical profile: antepartum testing in the 1990s, *Am J Obstet Gynecol* 174(3):812-817, 1996.

Moffatt FW, Van den Hof M: Semi-Fowler's positioning, lateral tilts, and their effects on nonstress tests, *JOGNN* 26(5):551-557, 1997.

Neilson JP, Munjanja SP, Whitfield CR: Screening for small-for-dates fetuses, *Br J Med* 289:1179-1184, 1984.

Paine LL et al: Population differences affect nonstress test reactivity, *J Perinatol* 11:41-45, 1991.

Paine LL et al: A comparison of the auscultated acceleration test and the nonstress test as predictors of perinatal outcomes, *Nurs Res* 41(2):87-91, 1992.

Patrick J et al: Patterns of gross fetal body movements over 24-hour observation intervals during the last 10 weeks of pregnancy, *Am J Obstet Gynecol* 142(4):363-371, 1982.

Rayburn W et al: An alternative to antepartum fetal heart rate testing, *Am J Obstet Gynecol* 138(2):223-226, 1980.

Saari-Kemppainen A et al: Ultrasound screening and perinatal mortality: Controlled trial of systematic one-stage screening in pregnancy, *Lancet* 336:387-391, 1990.

Sadovsky E, Yaffe H, Polishuk WZ: Fetal movement monitoring in normal and pathologic pregnancy, *Int J Gynaecol Obstet* 12(3):75-79, 1974.

Schifrin BS, Amsel J, Burdorf G: The accuracy of auscultatory detection of fetal cardiac decelerations: a computer simulation, *Am J Obstet Gynecol* 166(2):566-576, 1992.

Smith CV, Davis SA, Rayburn WF: Patients' acceptance of monitoring fetal movement: a randomized comparison of charting techniques, *J Reprod Med* 37(2):144-146, 1992.

Tucker S: *Fetal monitoring and assessment,* ed 3, St Louis, 1996, Mosby.

van Asselt K et al: Uterine and umbilical artery velocimetry in pre-eclampsia, *Acta Obstet Gynecol Scand* 77(6):614-619, 1998.

Vintzileos A et al: The fetal biophysical profile and its predictive value, *Obstet Gynecol* 62:271-275, 1983.

Waldenstrom U et al: Effects of routine one-stage ultrasound screening in pregnancy: a randomised controlled trial, *Lancet* 2:582-588, 1988.

Ware DJ, Devoe LD: The non-stress test: reassessment of the "gold standard," *Clin Perinatol* 21(4):779-796, 1994.

Warner HR, Cox A: A mathematical model of heart rate control by sympathetic and vagus efferent information, *J Appl Physiol* 17:349, 1962.

Wertz DC, Fletcher JC: A critique of some feminist challenges to prenatal diagnosis, *J Women Health* 2:173-188, 1993.

Chapter 14

Midwives As Teachers: the 5-Minute Curriculum

Pam England, CNM, MA,
and Rob Horowitz, PhD

Every midwife is a childbirth teacher. Every prenatal appointment is a class. Midwives underestimate the power and depth of their influence on the pregnant women and fathers in their care. They think childbirth preparation is what happens on Tuesday nights down the hall with the childbirth "teacher." This view is understandable when one considers how fragmented health care has become.

Many nurse-midwives are experiencing increased stress from the intensifying demands of managed care. This trend has narrowed the focus of prenatal care and restricted the time midwives can spend with expectant parents. Intense time pressure to meet clinical responsibilities and stay on top of paper work often leads midwives to believe there is no time for the creative or emotionally engaging aspects of midwifery care.

These circumstances threaten the heart and soul of midwifery and often result in professional burnout. We hope this chapter inspires new midwives to keep alive the tradition of holistic midwifery.

Even when a midwife has only 15 minutes for a prenatal visit, she can still make a difference with parents by offering *5-minute teaching modules*. Creative 5-minute "classes" over a course of six, eight, or ten prenatal visits can have a profound cumulative impact on parents (and the midwife as well). They create a mindset of self-reliance and empowerment within the couple, which serves as an antidote to the increasingly prevalent attitude that all parents need to do is "show up for the birth" (especially if they've written a birth plan).

Each 5-minute teaching module becomes a small "gift" to parents' initiation into parenthood. As prenatal visits come alive, mothers and fathers more eagerly anticipate their next visit. Most important, by teaching labor-coping skills, the midwife is increasing their self-confidence and deepening their relationship with her or him. These 5-minute modules become interventions into the anxiety that otherwise could undermine the natural physiology of labor (Box 14-1). This chapter presents six mini-modules; we hope you'll enjoy developing some of your own.

Pam England and Rob Horowitz are the authors of *Birthing From Within: an Extra-Ordinary Guide to Childbirth Preparation*, Albuquerque, NM, 1998, Partera Press; www. birthpower.com. The book provides more about the Birthing From Within philosophy, birth art, pain-coping techniques and certification. Pam England—midwife, mother, artist, and lecturer—graduated from Frontier Nursing Service and is the founder of the Art of Birthing Center in Albuquerque, New Mexico. Rob Horowitz—psychologist, father, and writer—received his doctorate in clinical psychology from Peabody College of Vanderbilt University. He has specialized in working with families for 25 years.

Box 14-1 *Suggested Topics for Your 5-Minute Curriculum*

- Pain-coping techniques*
- Building a pain-coping mindset*
- Labor "theatrics"*
- Foot massage*
- Birth art*
- Assessing your clients' experience in childbirth class*
- Pushing effectively while avoiding tearing
- Doula referral
- Breast-feeding basics
- How to swaddle a baby

* These topics are discussed in this chapter.

BUILDING A PAIN-COPING MINDSET

Nowadays many women either are not interested in or lack the confidence to birth through pain; they *assume* that drugs and epidurals will be part of their birth. Unfortunately, because of this social trend, nurse-midwives find themselves in a dilemma.

On the one hand, those following the midwifery tradition of encouraging and supporting women to birth through normal pain sometimes are surprised and hurt when their efforts are unappreciated or even criticized by parents and colleagues. On the other hand, after a medicated birth, they may be attacked for having cooperated too readily with a parent's request for drugs. As a result of this dilemma, many nurse-midwives have abdicated their responsibility to encourage and prepare mothers to cope with pain; parents are left to make "decisions" about drugs out of fear and ignorance, not experience.

Initially not all parents are receptive to learning pain-coping techniques. You may need to inspire a "pain-coping mindset." As a first step, teach mothers the difference between pain and *suffering*. They need to know that although pain is an inevitable part of normal labor, a great deal of the suffering comes from people feeling helpless and frightened by it. In general, the Birthing From Within approach to coping with pain emphasizes *immersion* into it rather than trying to deny, control, or escape it.

Midwives can continue to build a pain-coping mindset in parents by teaching them how pain can be an ally in normal labor and by guiding the mothers *and* fathers to explore their attitudes, beliefs, and expectations about labor pain.

Teaching new parents pain-coping techniques during prenatal care communicates confidence in parents' ability to cope with pain. It is important to begin by telling a mother the truth: that labor *is* painful, *and* that she can do it!

Even when mothers are committed to getting an epidural, you can still encourage them to learn a few pain-coping techniques to use while waiting for it. Pain-coping techniques can be taught in 5 minutes in the prenatal clinic or at the bedside during labor. One basic technique follows.

BREATH AWARENESS: A PAIN-COPING TECHNIQUE YOU CAN TEACH IN 5 MINUTES

Materials and Instructions

You will need ice cubes and paper towels. Ice cubes provide expectant parents with a simulated pain experience. If you teach a pain-coping technique *without* a contrasting sensation of pain, your clients will probably find it deeply relaxing but will not grasp its effectiveness with pain.

Begin by explaining how breath awareness works.

1. Emphasize that women's bodies instinctively know how to breathe through each contraction. Suggest that both mother and birth companion become *curious witnesses* of labor's perfect breathing and contracting patterns. (Superimposing rigid or stylized breathing patterns is rarely helpful.)
2. It is important for parents to know that much of the tension and suffering in labor arises from anxiety-producing mental chatter, not from the pain itself. When a woman focuses *intensely* on her outward breath during contractions, there is no room for desperate or panicky thoughts or looking for a way out.

Guide parents through breath awareness.

1. Before giving instruction in breath awareness, establish parents' baseline for ice-cube pain by having them hold an ice cube in their hands for a full minute; ask them to rate the intensity of pain on a scale of 0 to 10.
2. Prepare the parents to practice breath awareness by instructing them to, "Bring your *full* attention to

each outward breath. Notice exactly when your exhalation begins . . . and ends. Make no effort to change, improve, or slow down your natural breathing pattern. Even in early labor, a mother breathes out through her mouth, so it will help if you do the same during practice sessions."

3. Tell the parents to practice breath awareness while holding an ice cube in their hand or against their wrist for a minute-long "contraction" (time it for them).
4. Ask the parents to rate their experience of pain this time (0 to 10) and contrast it with their baseline rating.

Variations to Increase Mastery of Breath Awareness

1. After the mother learns the basic technique, challenge her by placing an ice cube in both hands or behind her ears. This dual locus of pain makes it more difficult to isolate, ignore, or escape.
2. Demonstrate how "losing control" is in their control
   a. Instruct parents to practice breath awareness for a 1-minute "contraction." Have them put down the ice, and continue breath awareness for another half-minute between "contractions."
   b. Instruct the parents to pick up the ice cube in the *opposite* hand (so the original hand doesn't become numb) and continue practicing breath awareness. About 15 seconds into the "contraction," without warning, instruct the mother/parents to shake their head and whine, "No, I can't do this any more!" After about 20 seconds, instruct them, "Stop fighting it," and calmly encourage them to, "Bring your full attention to your next outward breath . . . from beginning to end . . . continue practicing your breath awareness. . . ." After approximately another 15 seconds, tell them the "contraction" is over and ask them what they noticed.
   c. Reinforce their typical observation that, when they began *thinking* that they couldn't do it, they began to "suffer." Their suffering resulted from the change in their mental focus, not a change in the intensity of the pain stimulus. Parents are empowered when they learn that what they tell themselves in labor will have a huge impact on how they experience pain.
   d. This is more than an exercise; it is a revelation. Parents are excited and encouraged to discover that, if they're losing confidence or looking for a way out (even though labor is progressing normally), they can get on track again by bringing their attention back to breath awareness.

5-MINUTE LABOR "THEATRICS"

New mothers and fathers benefit from getting a preview of the gritty, sometimes sexual, aspects of hard labor. Admittedly this module will be a "stretch" for the shy midwife, but it becomes rewarding as you observe its positive impact on clients.

Many mothers, failing in their efforts to appear "strong" during labor, wind up turning to drugs to achieve that "in-control" look. A midwife becomes a powerful teacher and myth-breaker when she challenges parents' unrealistic images of relaxation and staying-in-control by *showing* them what strong women often look and sound like in labor. As an authority figure, she also implicitly gives women permission to do *whatever* may be natural for them to get their baby out.

A midwife's theatrical, even startling role-play alerts the father to the possibility of "wild" behavior from his laboring wife. Seeing what the mother might look and sound like helps prepare him to stay calm during labor, rather than to think that *he* needs to calm *her.* Mothers who know they don't *have* to be calm and relaxed through labor pain are, paradoxically, more able to relax.

Here are a few ways to desensitize parents to the loud, active, and sensual quality of labor:

- Demonstrate a range of vocalizations, including moaning, groaning, and chanting phrases such as "open" or "baby get o o o u u t," mixed with loud, forceful breathing.
- Hang over a chair or examination table and rhythmically rock your hips while exhaling forcefully . . . even moan a little.
- Get on your hands and knees and sway back and forth while exhaling forcefully.

TEACHING FOOT MASSAGE IN 5 MINUTES

Dona Juana was an old *partera empirica* (midwife) and mother who lived in Mexico's Yucatan peninsula. During the winter of 1972, anthropologists Bridgette Jordan and Nancy Fuller followed Dona Juana to learn about the Yucatan's prenatal rituals (which are described in *Birth in Four Cultures* [Jordan, 1980]).

In the Yucatan a pregnant woman visits her *partera* several times in pregnancy. During prenatal visits Dona Juana and the mother get acquainted (if they have not already met at previous family births). Dona Juana asks about the mother's reproductive history, her family relationship, and who will be the 'helpers' at her birth. Getting to know the pregnant woman helps a *partera* predict how she will labor and withstand pain.

During the typical prenatal visit the mother lies on the floor, and Dona Juana sits on a low stool or squats beside her. While Dona Juana gives a *sobada* (massage), she asks how the mother is feeling and prepares her for childbirth by telling birth stories. Not all talk is focused on pregnancy; the women also gossip and discuss local events, which brings birth into the normal routine of living.

The prenatal *sobada,* one of the midwife's most valuable skills, allows her to assess the position and growth of the baby, and also how the mother responds to touch and relaxation. If the baby is in the breech position, Dona Juana gently changes the baby's position so it will be born head first, which is safer for the baby. After the *sobada,* the mother is encouraged to rest a while in a hammock.

Many western midwives, inspired by Dona Juana, experience flickers of guilt or frustration because their busy appointment schedule and clinical environment are not conducive to giving a complete prenatal massage. This doesn't mean that *nothing* can be done! Even busy midwives can sprinkle Dona Juana's care and nurturing into prenatal visits by giving or teaching the 5-minute foot massage and reflexology module.

Don't underestimate the power of this intervention! When asked about what was most helpful in their Birthing From Within childbirth classes, couples frequently mention the footbath ritual and massage (described in *Birthing From Within*). They say that experiencing the foot massage (instead of just reading or being told about it) taught the fathers *how* to touch and nurture their wives during labor. It also helped some women become more comfortable receiving nurturing from their husband/birth companion. The positive feelings during this process bring couples closer together.

Sadly, many pregnant women are touched only in the course of clinical assessment: to measure the baby's growth and check for swelling and cervical changes. During the foot massage the woman is touched as a person, not a patient.

Materials and Instructions

1. All you need is a small bottle of oil or lotion and a willingness to expand your professional skills and identity.

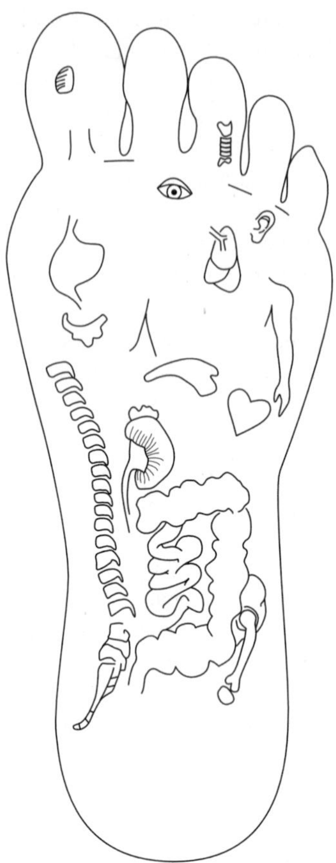

Figure 14-1 Sole of foot. "The foot is a 'map' of the entire body. No muscle, no gland, no organ, whether internal or external, is without a set of nerves whose opposite ends are anchored in the foot." — George Downing, *The Massage Book,* 1998, Random House.

2. Oil and rub your hands together to generate some warmth. Massage the sole of the foot with the thumbs, working both thumbs in small circles. *Massaging* slowly and rhythmically helps the mother *breathe* slowly and rhythmically. As you cover every inch of the sole, imagine you're touching every one of the thousands of nerve endings connected to her entire body (Figure 14-1).
3. Then, using your thumbs in the same way, work the top of the foot, beginning near the toes. As you approach the ankle, massage with your fingertips. Simultaneously make smooth circles around both sides of the ankle bone (Figure 14-2).
4. Another nice touch is to squeeze the foot by placing the heels of the hands against the top of the foot with fingertips pressing into the middle of the sole. Simultaneously press very hard downward onto the top of the foot while pressing upwards into the sole with your fingertips. Very slowly let the heels of

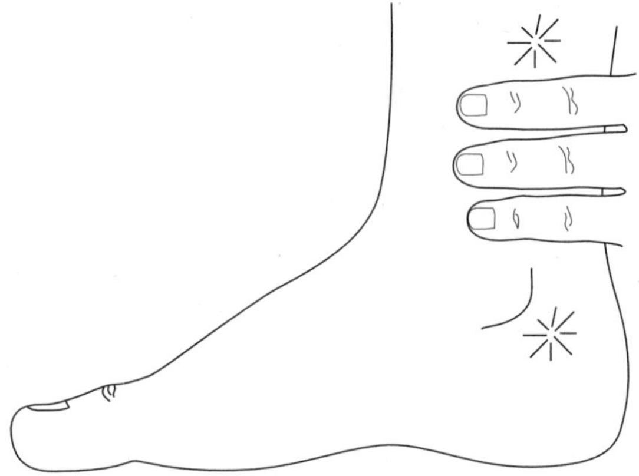

Figure 14-2 Uterine reflexology points on ankle.

your hands slide from the middle of the top of the foot down the sides. Do this several times.

Making Foot Massage a Pain-Coping Resource

1. If ice cubes are available, help the mom experience the power of relaxation-through-massage by having her hold an ice cube against her wrist while you or her birth partner massage her foot.
2. Suggest to the mother/partner that they use pain-coping techniques such as Breath Awareness or Nonfocused Awareness (described in *Birthing From Within*) during the massage. Combining mental concentration techniques with soothing touch works especially well in labor.

DISCOVERY THROUGH BIRTH ART: THE 5-MINUTE UNIT

Mothers love learning from their birth art! Over and over I hear mothers report that before making birth art, they had never thought about how they envisioned their own pregnancy or birth. Here's what pregnant women who participated in my master's thesis research (England, 1989) said about their experience:

- "Incredible, made me think of things I never thought of before. I got in touch with what was going on inside of me."
- "Making birth art forced me to sit down and let me *see,* which I would not have done without the drawing sessions."
- "I was anxious about labor and didn't know it—using my head and hands got me in touch with it."
- "Gave me insight into how I anticipated medical intervention."
- "Talking about being pregnant during the drawing sessions acknowledged my pregnancy as important . . . very affirming."

Waiting Rooms Can Be "Classrooms"

Clinic waiting rooms often provide health education materials (e.g., magazines, posters, pamphlets, and videos). Although parents may enjoy or glean information from these materials, this kind of learning is *passive.* The mother is a receptacle for information from the outside, from the experts.

Passive learning is different from the learning that can take place when the mother is *actively* involved, as she is when making birth art. In our culture there is a pervasive message that health care and education are passive processes. Thus initially you may face resistance from some clients if you ask them to become more actively involved in their childbirth preparation. Be patient: mothers need to *learn* how to be active in learning. Their body-mind is already rich with primordial knowing—they just don't *know* it!

Women tend to adopt the images of either the medical or the advertising culture, without ever exploring their own images. Yet it is their *own* images (whether ignored or acknowledged) that determine how they prepare for and experience their spiritual and physiologic journey through birth.

For some mothers the wait to see their midwife or doctor is a relaxing break in a busy day. For others waiting is stressful. Either way, it's possible, given the opportunity and encouragement, that most mothers (and fathers) would enjoy spending 15 to 30 minutes making birth art. Exploring their birth art could be a highlight of the prenatal visit; it can be done in a 5-minute teaching module.

Materials and Instructions

Art supplies: pastels, crayons, magic markers, paper and a drawing surface Although pastels can be messy, they have proven to be the best medium for mothers' self-expression. (All you need is a box of eight to twelve student-grade sticks.) If you're concerned about pastel dust getting on your office furniture or carpet, use crayons or markers.

Typing paper will do, but larger sheets of paper get better results. Newsprint is inexpensive, especially when you buy end rolls at your local newspaper. You will also need a hard surface such as a small table or drawing board on which parents can draw.

Favorite drawing assignments Certain drawings in early pregnancy, such as "Pregnant Woman," "Womb With a View," or "Drawing On Your Animal Nature" increase parents' awareness of their unborn and heighten protective feelings toward their baby. Enhanced early bonding motivates a mother to eat well, avoid habits that could be harmful to her unborn, and generally participate more fully in her prenatal care.

Later in pregnancy exploring drawings of "Fantasy of Birth," "Birth in Our Culture," or "Opening" often brings to the surface previously unacknowledged questions and concerns. A little attention paid to these deeper issues can relieve anxiety and help the parents tap personal strengths and resources, thus moving a mother's mind-body toward harmony. Unresolved fears produce adrenalin and tension throughout the body, disrupting the normal physiology of pregnancy and labor.

Here are several drawing assignments you can suggest that a mother do while waiting in the waiting room, or at home:

- Pregnant woman: "How do you see yourself as a pregnant woman/mother?"
- Tree mother: "Draw a tree that represents how you see yourself as mother."
- Drawing on your animal nature: "Draw the animal you associate with easy birthing or good mothering."
- Womb with a view: "Imagine you could peek through a window into your womb. What is your baby doing in her or his womb all day? What does she or he look like?"
- Opening: "The primary activity in labor is opening: opening your body, heart, and mind to let the baby out. Draw your strongest image of *opening* in labor."
- Fantasy of birth: "Everybody has a fantasy of how they would like their birth to go. What is your fantasy of labor and birth? It can be realistic or symbolic. Depict the physical or emotional aspects. Include details!"
- Birth in our culture: "Make a drawing that shows someone from another planet or culture what birth in our culture is like. Draw the birthplace and illustrate our current customs. If people are present, show what they are doing."

5-Minute exploration of parents' birth art

1. Describe what is happening in your drawing.
2. What did you learn from making this drawing?
3. What surprised you about your drawing?
4. What might be missing? How might that be significant for you?

Seizing teachable moments As a midwife, you are *not* functioning as an art therapist. You *are* creating a space for parents' self-expression and introspection through birth art.

For parents, drawing a birth image, no matter what it looks like, has healing power in itself. Try to keep in mind that, when making birth art, parents often express their unconscious images or beliefs about birth. The art isn't always positive or pretty; there are no "good" or "bad" images. Parents do not need to "heal" their image (i.e., make it match their [or your] idea of what a good birth [image] should look like).

Some parents will be shy or inhibited, and say, "I can't draw." Help them understand that making birth art has nothing to do with art talent but is an act of self-expression (and acceptance), just as giving birth will be. If "doing it right" becomes an issue, gently point out how that attitude might also become an obstacle in birth. Overcoming her inhibition about making birth art may set the stage for her being more spontaneous and expressive in labor. If a mother seems stuck, ask her to take the paper home and, "Draw anything, any way you can, that connects with the feelings you are having about birth."

Sometimes you may notice a potential problem depicted in a drawing. For example, a woman draws a birth room filled with ten friends and family members and a video camera. Use this opportunity to talk to her about the importance of privacy in the physiology of birth. When you see a drawing that expresses parents' intuitive understanding about what will help them birth more easily (e.g., such as a drawing showing pushing in an upright position), reinforce her intuitive wisdom. Teach her more about why pushing in an upright position is effective.

When asked to draw his "Strongest Image of Birth," Daniel, a first-time father, drew Figure 14-3. He described his idea of being supportive in labor as keeping his wife calm and relaxed. In his drawing his wife is lying down and relaxing while he massages her. Using his drawing as a critical teaching moment, I taught him how to massage her in labor. We also talked about how to be supportive even when the intensity of labor makes her wild and not want to be touched.

In this drawing, when asked to draw her strongest image of being in birth, a first-time mother drew a picture of herself holding her baby under a tree (Figure 14-4). While exploring her drawing, she realized that she had been wishfully thinking her birth would be natural (and would not require preparation or hard work). With deeper exploration she discovered she could not imagine giving birth at all, and her fears of being in the hospital surfaced. This drawing opened the way to more active and personal preparation for the birth (Box 14-2).

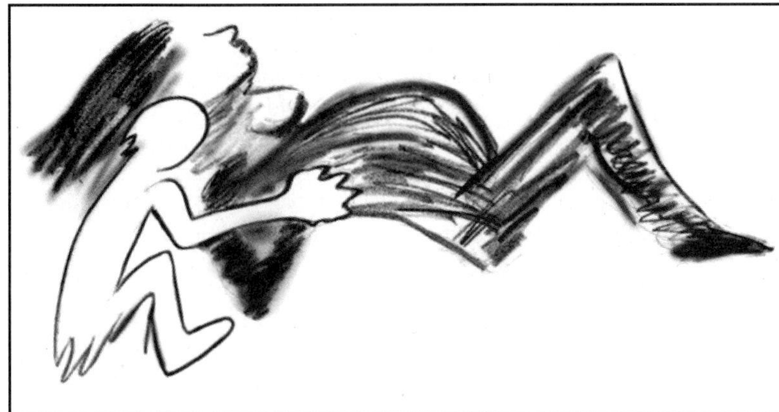

Figure 14-3 Father's drawing.

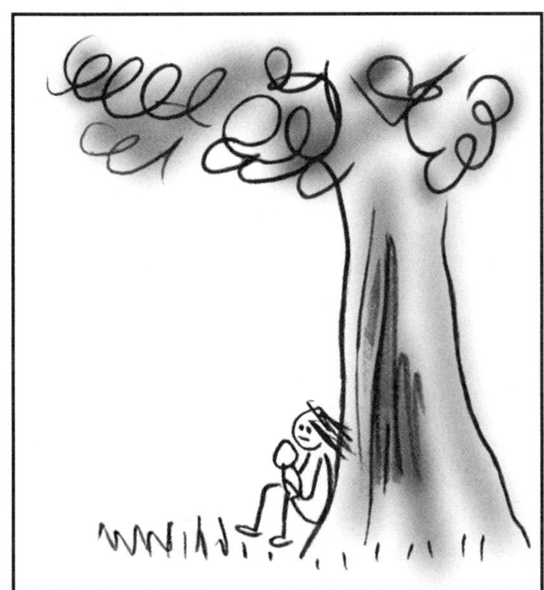

Figure 14-4 Mother's drawing.

Box 14-2 *Belly Birth Art*

Another way birth art can fit into midwifery practice is exemplified by a story from midwife Candace Fields Whitridge (1987). Notice how a moment of her time, used creatively, had a profound and lasting impact on both the mother and Candace:

"I remember one mom who lived tucked away in the hills and who had suffered a life of terrible abuse. Basic amenities like adequate food, kindness, and friendship did not readily come her way. Her first child was born with a neurological impairment after a difficult pregnancy.

"I drew a picture of a twelve-week fetus on her tummy one day. She looked and looked at it, saying not a word. Then big tears flooded her caricature, saying, 'Oh, you sweet little baby, my sweet little child. What ever do you do inside of that big house all day alone?' And then she began to laugh with delight. Her pinched face softened as she continued to talk to the baby, seemingly oblivious to my presence.

"From that day on that little unborn child became her friend. She nourished and cared for him with diligence, and went on to deliver a perfectly healthy baby boy who continues to thrive."

ASSESSING WHAT PARENTS ARE LEARNING FROM THEIR CHILDBIRTH CLASSES AND BOOKS

Childbirth classes have become a significant birth ritual. Whatever the content of classes, their message profoundly affects how a woman negotiates birth. Midwives and teachers who understand the power of childbirth classes can make them an *initiation* into motherhood rather than an obstacle to a woman's personal growth and self-discovery.

Birth is a universal rite of passage. However, the rituals surrounding it are remarkably diverse across cultures and over time. Traditional birth rituals offer inspiration, illumination, and group support. In western cultures few women experience these kinds of spiritual, communal birth rituals. Nevertheless, birth rituals do exist in our culture. Childbirth classes are one of our key birth rituals and wield great power to influence expectant parents.

What is a ritual? A ritual repetitively and nonverbally communicates a message. Its intent is to bring the behaviors and values of its recipient into alignment with those of the sender. When I learned how elders and shamans traditionally have used rituals to celebrate major life transitions, I became excited thinking about what the "ritual" of childbirth classes could offer women.

Before referring your clients to childbirth classes, know the messages and philosophy of the childbirth teachers in your birthing community. For example, most childbirth teachers, as employees of hospitals, understandably reflect the policies, protocols, and concerns of those institutions. Therefore many hospital-based classes are embued with medical/institutional birth rituals rather than those that emphasize self-discovery or birthing through the pain of normal labor.

A medical birth initiation can happen in many ways. One distraught mother dropped out of hospital classes and transferred to Birthing From Within classes after experiencing a panic attack and bolting from her third class. She described how the teacher, a hospital nurse (intending to put parents at ease with hospital procedures), pulled from a black bag, one-by-one, a wide array of instruments and equipment used in medical birth (e.g., oxygen mask, intravenous needles, vacuum suction, internal fetal monitor electrode, urinary catheters). The teacher asked the parents to guess the purpose of each item . . . then told them. As the mother absorbed the message that birth was *dangerous* and that she would be helpless to protect herself and her baby, her anxiety soared, and she left the class in tears.

When class after class focuses on birth complications, medical management, and anesthesia options, a mother's confidence to protect and safely deliver her baby erodes. Too much of this kind of "information" inadvertently communicates to a woman that she is a weak, helpless, *patient* who needs coaching, drugs, and advanced technology to have a baby. Because of the mind-body connection in birth physiology, such a message may become a self-fulfilling prophecy.

Questions for Your 5-Minute Parent Education Assessment

1. Find out what the mother is reading:
   a. What is your favorite book on childbirth?
   b. What is the most important thing you've learned from it?
   c. What effect has the book had on your confidence to give birth?
2. If the parents are already taking childbirth classes, find out:
   a. What do your classes emphasize?
   b. What are you learning from the classes about what *you* can do to give birth as easily as possible?
   c. Do the classes validate that you instinctively already know something about how to give birth?
   d. Are you becoming more, or less, afraid of giving birth?
   e. What pain-coping techniques are you learning? Are you learning how to birth through pain? Or are you learning to see drugs and epidurals as the primary ways to cope with pain?
   f. Are your classes interactive (with the teacher *and* other parents), or do you just sit there, listening to the teacher?

BEDSIDE TEACHING IN LABOR

Endless teaching opportunities occur not only during pregnancy but during labor as well. Even if a mother has taken classes and is well informed, she really learns about being in labor when she is *in* labor. From time to time in labor, a mother needs a kind, experienced guide to show her (and her inexperienced partner) the way.

During hospital admission the midwife's greeting of parents in the first 5 minutes is a teaching in itself. When her first sentence focuses on medical assessment or admission procedures, a message is sent to the parents that they are, above all, *patients.* But, if her first words communicate warmth and encouragement, a different psychologic space for the labor, and their relationship, is created.

As labor progresses, if a woman and her husband/birth companion seem like they are doing well, nurses or nurse-midwives often leave them alone. Sometimes this reflects the fact that the staff is too busy to sit with a laboring couple; sometimes their absence is because of a well-intentioned respect for the couple's privacy.

However, many women describe the loneliness and anxiety they felt when they were left alone in labor, didn't really know what they were doing, and couldn't quite trust their equally inexperienced or nervous partner. These same women describe the profound internal relaxation and confidence they felt when the nurse or midwife sat with them for a few minutes and offered encouragement. (One frequently overlooked option is to encourage couples to have a doula who can offer continuous support in labor.)

Penny Simkin, well-known birth author, lecturer, and founder of Doulas of North America, teaches doulas and nurses to assess how mothers are doing *within* by asking them, "During that last contraction, what were you thinking about?" Even if the mother is thrashing and hollering, if she answers, "I was thinking about how much you are helping me and that my baby is coming soon,"—she's okay. On the other hand, if a mother (even when she appears calm and relaxed on the outside) answers, "I'm thinking I can't do this, I need drugs," it's time to give more support and encouragement and, of course, to assess whether or not drugs would be right for her.

Ideally midwives and nurses, as well as childbirth educators, are in a position to empower a pregnant woman, and as Gayle Peterson (1981) points out, to "teach her that she can give birth and that only she can do it. No one else can push her baby out, except by intervention." A first-time mother remembers the impact of just this kind of firm support from her nurse-midwife during a turning point in her long labor:

> I remember giving up, feeling too tired to go on and saying, "I can't do this anymore." My midwife, standing nearby me, said matter-of-factly, "Well, Lois, if you don't birth your baby, who do you think will?" I remember getting so angry, thinking, "I'll just show her." And soon after, I gave birth to my son.

Bedside teaching doesn't just involve techniques. One of the gifts you can give a mother is your confidence in her strength and her body's wisdom to get her baby out.

SUMMARY

We hope this chapter will inspire and guide you to take advantage of brief teaching opportunities, even when working in demanding clinical settings. Five-minute teaching modules are not a prescription for *every* prenatal visit or *every* prenatal client. Do what you can, when you can, and have fun keeping the art of midwifery alive.

References

England, Pam: *Childbirth images of modern and ancient women,* Unpublished masters thesis, Yellow Springs, Ohio, 1989, Antioch University.

Jordan B: *Birth in four cultures,* Montreal, 1980, Eden Press, Women's Publication. pp 11-20.

Peterson G: *Birthing normally,* Berkeley, Calif, 1981, Mind-Body Press, p 17.

Whitridge CF: The power of joy: pre-and peri-natal psychology as applied by a mountain midwife, *Prenat Perinat Psychol* 2(3):188, 1987.

Chapter 15

Perinatal Care Among Diverse Populations of Women

Catherine A. Carr, CNM, Dr.P.H.
and Jeanne F. DeJoseph Ph.D., CNM, FAAN

INTRODUCTION

This chapter provides an overview of some of the most interesting challenges for perinatal clinical practice in the late twentieth century. Communities are increasingly multicultural and multiethnic. The "childbearing years" have been extended beyond their historical limits. The "traditional family," in which the husband is employed outside the home, the wife is a homemaker and there are two children, one of each gender, has nearly vanished, representing less than 10% of the families in the United States. In its place there is a "new family" primarily defined by those who live within it. Providing care to the childbearing family within such a shifting context requires new skills of perinatal practitioners.

Certain definitions are used throughout the chapter in the discussion of midwifery care in an increasingly diverse population. The first is *culture,* which is a pattern of learned behavior, attitudes, beliefs, and values exhibited by a group that shares a common history and usually geographic proximity (Spector, 1991). Culture is the result of the processes of socialization. Young people and newcomers to a particular culture are socialized to assume the norms and/or roles sanctioned as appropriate, including sex, gender, behavioral, and economic roles. Culture also prepares individuals to exhibit attitudes, behaviors, and feelings in relation to health and illness events. Appropriate behaviors are ascribed to both the provider of health care and the recipient.

A second definition is *race/racial group.* Originally this term was used to refer to kinship groups in sixteenth century Europe. Since the eighteenth century the term race has been used to define a group by primarily physical characteristics. Although by no means biologically useful, race and racial group have been and are currently politically and socially important terms. Historically, oppression of particular cultural and ethnic groups has been justified on the basis of the importance of racial characteristics (Hannaford, 1996). *Ethnicity* is a term determined by a specific group of people to refer to those who share cultural, social, and political ties. Ethnic groups may also share language, history, religion, economic interdependence and a set of social values. Ethnicity represents a sense of identity and a way to allocate limited resources. It may provide particular structures to marriage, childrearing practices, economic ties, and place of residence (Adams, 1995; Lipson, Dibble, and Minarik, 1996).

Although the recipients of midwifery care have traditionally been heterosexual women, increasing numbers of lesbians are seeking the care of midwives for their childbearing and gynecologic needs. *Lesbian* may be defined either behaviorally or as an identity affiliation. Behavior refers to a woman whose sexual practices are with other women, although she may also have heterosexual relationships. Although sexual behavior is a plausible construct to use for contraception provision or to ascertain risk of sexually transmitted infections, it omits the social context within which the lesbian exists. In this chapter lesbian refers to a woman whose identity is as a lesbian, whether or not she is currently in a sexual relationship with another woman. Lesbian health care is rarely included in literature on minority health, nor is it commonly discussed in texts addressing the health care of women. This may be because of the invisibility of many lesbians in society. Others have proposed that the omission is the result of systematic homophobia (Stevens and Hall, 1991). Demographically lesbians are a very diverse group and also share commonalties with women who are not lesbian. However, their oppression needs to be recognized as a potential threat to their health and well-being.

HOW DO PRACTITIONERS DETERMINE THE USUAL EXPERIENCES OF PREGNANCY?

To provide perinatal care, practitioners must know what can be expected during the usual pregnancy to assess how a particular pregnancy in an individual woman is progressing. Over time, through direct observation and other forms of research, knowledge about normal pregnancy has increased. A range of experiences has been noted within which optimal results are seen. Within a range, there is an average that represents the most common experience.

An average (e.g., the arithmetic mean of a set of numbers) can be useful for certain types of perinatal calculations. Often decisions for individual childbearing women are made on the basis of averages. For example, care decisions are regularly made regarding the appropriate length of gestation or how long labor should last on the basis of observations that, on the average, women who have a 40 weeks' gestation generally have better outcomes than those who give birth at 26 weeks, and women who have about a 2-hour second stage of labor have better outcomes than those who labor in second stage for 10 to 15 hours. Averages, then, can be used to construct a range of care practices for optimal results.

In a complex world, using the concept of averages about people is convenient. It is helpful for a solicitous midwife who wants to provide appropriate care to seek information about childbirth from the perspective of many women. Some of these women might be from many cultures and of diverse age, marital status, and sexual orientation. Early attempts to assist practitioners in developing their knowledge base often highlighted group characteristics believed to represent all individuals within that group. Articles in professional journals in the 1970s and 1980s often provided helpful information for clinicians and others in increasingly multicultural practices, although most authors did acknowledge that the characteristics, traits, or practices that they highlighted were not absolute or stereotypical among women who belong to a particular group and that there was a wide range of variation. For example, most would agree that all adolescents who were pregnant were not irresponsible, drug-using high school dropouts or that machismo was not something experienced by every Latina in her daily life. However, care and education were frequently arranged around assumptions of what was common to a culture, an age group, and/or women of certain economic circumstances.

Averages are appealing because they are so useful. A set of numbers may easily yield an average, but the "average" experience of a set of people depends on the sample that is studied. Convenience samples predominate in the published research about perinatal populations. Knowledge about women's childbirth practices is frequently obtained from women who were available and willing to volunteer for research studies. This may mean that the "average" experience is that of the white, eurocentric, middle class, educated, conservative married woman in her late 20s. Her experiences become the central point from which all other women's experiences are measured. Others who are outside of that experience are labeled "different" and are the object of study, but they are not the "norm." Childbirth practices that are not reflected in the center are considered to be marginal and can be possible objects of interest and speculation, but they are not the material out of which foundational texts about childbirth are written. Projecting the eurocentric perspective as the norm is pervasive in law, politics, policy, art, education, and most types of clinical care. It is so present that it is often taken for granted, and its effect is that all whose experiences are not seen as the norm are defined as "other."

Political and economic power have traditionally provided the power-owning group the privilege of defining "otherness." When a group or population is defined as "other," it can be looked at as a problem to be fixed, eradicated, or otherwise changed. Historically otherness has included ethnicity (the Irish, Italian, Jewish, Eastern European "problems" as immigrant waves moved across the Atlantic), race (the enslavement of African and Native populations, the "Yellow Peril" of Asian immigrants), disability, and often poverty, lifestyle, and age. All of these groups have been and some continue to be "other" as defined by groups with economic and political power. Solutions have included cultural destruction in the form of family disruption, institutionalization, removal of children from their homes, and restrictions on land ownership, jobs, marriage, and location.

Health policy development and implementation follow the definitions of what is a problem. In a relatively contemporary example the "welfare problem" is a leading concern of policy makers. In a policy speech in January 1997, the governor of California, Pete Wilson, suggested that adolescent mothers be "strongly advised and counseled" to release their children for adoption. He also included poor families in the group that should relinquish their children. Inability to find work or pay the electric bill (his examples) should result in the parents being encouraged to give up their children (1997). The definition of problem and subsequent policy development are often not based on current research.

The definition of a problem in health care tends to be somewhat consistent across groups. For example, hypertension within a certain range is recognized as a potentially life-threatening problem in any population and one that needs to be followed and treated. But the politics of problems and policy are rarely consistent. The problem of pregnancy in certain groups, particularly drug-using and adolescent women, has resulted in free, if not mandatory family planning. But free family planning services have not been extended to nonsubstance abusing women and women who are over 19 years of age. It can be argued that unwanted pregnancy is no less devastating in a 23-year-old woman than it is in a 19-year-old woman. Similarly, prenatal care is mandated for teenage mothers but is increasingly less available for undocumented immigrants (Chapin and Pereles, 1995). Although health care needs may vary for these two groups, the need for prenatal care is undeniable. The possibility of access is determined by the policy decisions of those who decide who, and what, is the problem.

THE NORM VS. THE "OTHER?"

Definition of otherness can preclude research into actual health problems. Investigation is often done on the "standard" or "norm," and, when the standard does not fit, incorrect information may be the result. A classic example is the study of heart disease. Men were the norm for the study, and for decades all the participants in the research were men. Results were generalized to women, who are at the very least theoretically different in a biologic sense, particularly in a condition affected by hormone levels. Another example is that of eating disorders. Nonwhites are far less frequently referred for treatment of eating disorders, making the research participant pool largely white. Because of this research bias, the incidence of eating disorders in nonwhites is unknown. The most effective treatment of this and many other conditions may vary significantly with different cultures, economic situations, and levels of education.

It is important to note that all pregnant women have needs related to the fact that they are pregnant, but many women have further needs related to their economic, social, and ethnic circumstances and to their physical abilities, age, and sexual orientation. Practitioners must develop attitudes and skills that will help them behave in culturally appropriate ways. Culturally competent practice demonstrates sensitivity to cultural differences and similarities through the effective use of cultural symbols in interactions and effective communication (Adams, 1995). Green (1982) refers to the culturally competent worker as one "who knows, appreciates and can use the culture of another group in assisting with the resolution of a problem." The culturally competent midwife accepts and works with cultural differences in an open, sincere manner without condescension or patronization. Culturally competent care is sensitive to issues related to culture, race, gender, sexual orientation, social class, and economic situation (Meleis et al., 1995). According to Lipson, Dibble, and Minarik (1995), although cultural competency does not require language or cultural fluency, it does require awareness and the ability to intervene effectively.

CONTEMPORARY PRENATAL PRACTICES

Across the world, women are generally responsible for the health of their families. In most places health care providers are from the upper classes and are trained to be responsible for their "patients." This creates a situation in which careful communication is essential. When the provider and client come from different cultures and/or points of view, there is an added variable. There must be negotiation for appropriate care to occur. The "clash of cultures" that occurs when incongruent understandings of health care collide can lead to poor care and unhappy clients and providers. This ineffective care not only affects the prenatal period in question but may result in alienation of the woman and her family from the health care system. Therefore learning how to assess a woman *within her own context* and learning to negotiate within the health care setting are important skills for the prenatal provider of the 21st century.

Although there are differences among childbearing women, some of which are apparent and some that are hidden, there are also commonalties among women. Almost all women are concerned about the well-being of their families. Whatever their cultural background, women must cope with the challenges of childrearing and attempt to balance the needs of work and home. Culture, race, sexual orientation, social class, and economic situation affect the ways women adapt to these common concerns. Although childrearing may look drastically different in two population groups, women in each one are working to rear children who are successful group members and citizens of society as they see it.

In a decade that is increasingly marked by multiple mixtures of cultures, ethnicities, economics, races, ages, and sexual orientations, practitioners may experience a need for additional knowledge to provide competent clinical care. There is no single protocol that can be devised to meet all needs of all pregnant women in their practices at all times.

CRITICAL QUESTIONS

Certain information gathered during the course of a pregnancy can be extremely useful to provide culturally competent care. As communities become more culturally diverse, these data are essential, whether the woman is from across town or across national borders. These issues are not meant to be considered in isolation of each other but rather to be used to develop a tapestry of information about a particular woman. The list does not include all areas that could be considered. It is meant to be a guide that practitioners can adapt to their own clinical settings.

What are her goals for herself?

Pregnant women are more than containers to incubate a fetus, and most practitioners acknowledge this. However, the focus of prenatal visits is often on the health of the developing maternal-fetal unit. Beyond the spotlight on that unit, it is important to understand how this pregnancy fits into her life, her personal goals, and her family. In an approach to prenatal care that is based on public health goals, the community has a stake in the aggregate of each woman's health and in the outcome of each pregnancy.

What is the place of women in the family/community in which she was raised?

In the women's congress in Beijing, one of the most critical areas to be noted in women's health was the status of women (Morgan, 1996). The women at that conference discussed the differences in the status of women from one community to another. Lessor status in the community is a significant health concern because it is directly related to the amount and kind of food a woman gets to eat, the amount of resources she can accumulate, and where her sphere of influence can extend. Control of the number and spacing of pregnancies is also related to the amount of self-determination that is extended to women of a given group. There are also differences related to the age of the woman, her physical abilities, her economic status, and her sexual orientation. Although it is relatively easy to consider these differences when the culture, ethnicity, and/or racial characteristics of the practitioner are different from those of the pregnant woman, they may be missed entirely and thus not considered in developing a competent assessment of the woman when culture/ethnicity/race/class are similar.

Where/what signifies home?

Geographically and culturally the woman may be living in a place now that is different from the place in which she was raised. The current "home" may be vastly different from that which she knows from her family of origin. It is important to gain an understanding of the life experiences that occurred during the transition to the new community. For example, some Southeast Asian refugees spent years in resettlement camps before finally moving to a host country. Children who grew up in refugee camps may be less likely to have had basic education or job training. Currently Vietnamese refugees of Chinese ancestry are being refused repatriation to their country of origin even as they are being turned away by host countries. Some Navajo women may reside in one place for 95% of the year, but "home" is where their sheep are. A woman raised in the northeast United States might experience some cultural differences in a move to the southeast. Changes in the geographic and cultural home will influence how a woman relates to her community and those with whom she interacts.

Is the woman safe in her home and community?

Violence against women must also be considered in any public health approach to prenatal care. It is mentioned here because the competent practitioner must be aware of the community in which women and families dwell. For example, it is useless to suggest that a woman walk for exercise during pregnancy if her neighborhood is not a safe place to walk. If the woman is employed in the formal or informal labor market, it is also important to consider the occupational hazards to which she is exposed, including sound, motion, chemicals, and long hours without breaks. Intimate partner abuse has a prevalence of 10% to 20%, and abuse during pregnancy is associated with less than optimum outcomes. All women should be screened for current or past incidents of abuse.

When immigration has occurred, what is known about the group's history and current status?

Immigration by choice is significantly different from immigration by force. Those who have immigrated by choice usually have planned their moves, thereby easing the transition into the new culture. Those who immigrate because of force usually face major challenges. Political refugees may have fled with minimal notice, leaving land, money, and family behind. Refugees who were on the losing side may rightfully fear for their own health and safety or that of family and friends who remained in the country of origin. Refugees dislocated by war or famine may find themselves in completely different circumstances compared to those experienced in the home community. The Vietnamese war displaced a large urban, middle-class, professional population as well as rural farming populations without educational or monetary resources. The war and geopolitical region are the same, but the immigrant experiences are vastly different.

What is the history of inclusion or exclusion of the group in the power structure of the United States?

Some groups were initially excluded from participation in the economy and culture of the United States (e.g., Irish, Italian, and Jewish immigrants) but have become acculturated and accepted in many areas of American society. Other groups, including blacks and American Indian populations, have remained marginalized. How the group is accepted or rejected by mainstream American society will influence the resources available for the woman and her family, as well as the interactions between the woman and health and human service professionals.

How long has it been since the family was "home"?

Typically school-age children are the first to learn a new language and may end up in the awkward position of interpreting the new culture to their parents. Working male members in the family usually learn English next, followed last by women, particularly those who do not work outside the home. Women may be the last to learn English, but they are still expected to maintain their duties and attend to the family's well-being, negotiate with the educational system for the children, and provide a cultural home. Immigrant or refugee families may be facing the tasks of childrearing without the support of an extended community and family, a daunting task for those from cultures that depend on a large and supportive kinship network. The U. S. norm of the small family living without extended members can be quite shocking to a family from a community where extended families are the norm.

Who will be there for her during the pregnancy, the birth, and the rearing of the child?

The answers to these questions may provide another view of the woman's support system. That information is important because, although pregnancy is a biologic experience, it is also a social experience, and support is generally a very necessary part of the experience. Early identification of what comprises the woman's support system may help the practitioner suggest focused, individualized care suggestions.

Who is the authority in health care matters? Who is the family decision maker?

If the community leader must be consulted for all important health decisions, it is important to allow time for consultation rather than to expect the client to make decisions at the time of the office or clinic visit. Older relatives may need to be notified of health questions or pending decisions and may wish to negotiate directly with the provider.

What are the woman's plans for the pregnancy? What does she want from the care provider and the health care system?

Some women look to their provider to confirm the normalcy of their pregnancy and to tell them how to manage during pregnancy. Other women wish to be full partners with the practitioner, sharing in the decision-making about their care. Still others wish to use their practitioner as a consultant and manage their own pregnancy. The clinician should explore whether the woman plans to continue the pregnancy, whether she believes in ongoing prenatal visits with the provider, and whether she plans to seek other health care guidance during the pregnancy (e.g., from a traditional healer). The interview should also establish what the woman's priorities are for the pregnancy. If she is a healthy multipara, she may be more concerned about being at home to care for other children than keeping prenatal appointments.

To identify barriers or conflicts, practitioners should also explore what the woman expects from the health care system. For example, a woman may expect a female provider because of religious beliefs. If a particular clinical service cannot meet that expectation, alternative clinical practices may have to be explored.

THE COMPETENT PRACTITIONER

To practice midwifery within complex systems, it is necessary that each practitioner prepare herself or himself to effectively care for diverse communities of families. This preparation certainly includes acquiring academic knowledge and skills about women's health, families, communities, and childbirth. It also includes some personal preparation to recognize and acknowledge biases, assumptions, strengths, and personal weaknesses. We believe that that preparation begins with collecting information about ourselves—how we choose, what we choose, how we feel about what we choose, and how we act on our choices (Simon, Howe, and Kirschenbaum, 1978, p. 169). Those processes have come to be known collectively as values clarification and can be useful in understanding the relation between a person's own opinions and stereotypes (Sheffield and Sheffield, 1975). In addition, values clarification can help individuals understand their own values and the choices they make (Sheffield and Sheffield, 1975). These processes can also be an important component of determining public values for complex policy decisions (Keeney, Von Winterfeldt, and Eppel, 1990).

In women's health care the practitioner's beliefs and assumptions about pregnancy and childbirth make a difference in care processes. Consider the different choices that might be made if pregnancy is seen as an essentially normal, healthy experience or if it is believed to be a dangerous time in need of management. Some believe that women's bodies are capable of giving birth; others think that intervention is needed in the preparation for labor and the "delivery" of the baby (Martin, 1992). Engaging in a process of data collection about oneself is essential to becoming a practitioner who provides competent, individualized, midwifery care.

THE TIME-LIMITED VISIT AND CULTURALLY COMPETENT CARE

One of the first areas of contact between a provider and a pregnant woman may be during the health history. It is understood that all participants in the health care system desire and deserve respect. Even without cultural or linguistic fluency, it is possible to obtain an adequate and respectful health history. If skilled interpreters are available, they may offer suggestions about the culturally appropriate way to approach sensitive subjects. A practitioner oriented to public health goals can collaborate with community representatives. In linking with communities, the practitioner emphasizes the value of the community as well as the importance of prenatal care (Boxes 15-1 and 15-2).

The following suggestions may be beneficial to clinicians who are stretched between ever-increasing demands to provide care that is relevant to the woman in her own context and ever-decreasing amounts of clinical encounter time in which to meet those demands are provided.

1. Assume permanency. Relationships with clients last a long time, and the entire family is affected by the health care that any one person receives. The clinician should not assume that an individual with a history of migration is a transient client.
2. Be geographically correct. Caribbean immigrants may speak Spanish, Dutch, French/French Creole, or English, so providers should not make the mistake of assuming that one particular language is spoken. Providers should know the difference between Iraq and Iran and where they are. Jordanians do not wish to be confused with Egyptians, although both are Arabs and speak the same language. Hispanic is a catchall term that does not indicate the vast differences between South Americans, Central Americans, Mexicans, Cubans, and others of Latin descent.
3. Promote education to students. Midwives should reach out not only to prospective clients but also to future midwives, nurses, and physicians.

Box 15-1 *Use of Interpreters*

1. Be patient. An interpreted visit may easily take twice as long as an ordinary visit because careful interpretation requires long explanations.
2. Before the session, meet with the interpreter to explain the purpose of the visit.
3. If possible, have the interpreter meet with the patient before the session to learn about educational level and attitudes toward health and health care and to determine the depth of information and explanation needed.
4. Speak in short units of speech. Do not use long, involved sentences or paragraphs or complex discussions of more than one topic in a single session. Plain but accurate speech is easier to interpret. In addition, monolingual women who are learning English will understand much more if you speak plainly.
5. Use simple language. Avoid technical terms, abbreviations, professional jargon, colloquialisms, abstractions, idiomatic expressions, slang, and metaphors.
6. Encourage translation of the patient's own words as much as possible rather than paraphrasing in professional jargon. The patient's own words provide a better sense of ideas and emotional state.
7. Encourage the interpreter to refrain from inserting his or her own ideas or interpretations or omitting information.
8. Check the patient's understanding and the accuracy of the translation by asking her to repeat the message or instructions in her own words, facilitated by the interpreter.
9. During the interaction, look and speak directly to the patient, not the interpreter.
10. Listen to the patient, watching such nonverbal communication as facial expressions, voice intonations, and body movements to learn about emotion associated with the topic.

Adapted from Lipson J, Dibble S, Minarik P: *Culture and nursing care,* San Francisco, 1996, UCSF Nursing Press.

Box 15-2 *When There Is No Trained Interpreter*

Interacting with women and their families without the use of an interpreter is unavoidable. It should be minimized, and when it is necessary, it is important to remember a few points.

1. Be sensitive to the fact that a family member or friend may be acting "out of role" as an interpreter. This may be acutely uncomfortable for children who are asked to interpret for their parents, men who interpret for women, or friends who are communicating information that is considered sensitive or embarrassing. When possible, it is important to select the friend or family member who will have the least role conflict in the situation.
2. Untrained interpreters are far more likely to base their messages in both directions on their own perceptions of what is best for the situation. Concern for role maintenance, attempts to avoid embarrassment, or social norms may lead the interpreter to omit information. Repetition of information, use of written information, and having the patient explain in her own words may help.

4. Modify data forms to include subpopulations and country of origin.
5. Conduct needs assessment surveys within your own clinic setting.
6. Identify barriers to care in the community. Before criticizing women for arriving late or missing appointments, the clinician should develop an understanding of the limitations of public transportation in the area. Clinics should also develop a mechanism for assessment of services from the client's viewpoint. Procedures or policies that clash with cultural expectations

necessitate system changes to meet client needs.

7. Establish appointment times that meet the needs of women in the community. Migrant clinics find that they need to have late hours so that women can be seen after working in the fields. Agricultural workers are not paid if they are not working, and a mother's participation in the family work force may be necessary to their economic survival. Evening and weekend appointments also are appreciated by women who have difficulty arranging child care during the day but who have a partner who is home in the evening.
8. Establish walk-in slots during each clinic session. Many factors may serve to make women "get there when they get there." The vagaries of public transportation, difficulty obtaining child care or transportation, and different cultural orientation to time may make rigid appointment slots a barrier.
9. Ensure the availability of translation services. Many clinics are creating incentives for staff to become bilingual to better meet the needs of the community.
10. Keep learning by consuming the literature. Research on minority health too often examines the cultural and genetic factors that affect health and ignores the socioeconomic, environmental, and political factors that may have significant influences. Look at research literature closely to determine whether findings can be generalized to your clinic population. Consider participating in research that explores the health care experiences of women during their childbearing years.

SUMMARY

The purpose of this chapter has been to disrupt the view of and from the "center." It is an invitation to each reader to consider how clinical practice might be conducted if there were no "central childbirth experience" against which to create a margin. Childbirth is made up of socially constructed attitudes, experiences, and beliefs that are embodied in daily practices around the world. There are consequences to those practices that affect the health and well-being of individuals, families, communities, and populations. As old barriers and boundaries are broken, it is necessary to continue to search for challenges to go beyond "individualizing" plans for care using the culturally embedded perspective of the white, Eurocentric, middle class, educated, married woman. There is a sense of urgency to prepare midwives to attend childbearing women in the "global villages" now being discussed. Childbearing is universal, although its expressions are situated in local customs and beliefs. The work of the midwife is to attend to women in all of their diversities and in childbirth in all of its forms.

References

New shot in welfare battle: take kids, *San Jose Mercury News,* January 11, 1997.

Adams D: *Health issues for women of color,* Thousand Oaks, Calif. 1995, Sage.

Chapin J, Pereles SA: Women's access to the health care system. In Horton JA, editor: *The women's health data book,* Washington, DC, 1995, Elsevier.

Green JW: *Cultural awareness in the human services,* Englewood Cliffs, NJ, 1982, Prentice Hall.

Hannaford I *Race: the history of an idea in the west,* Baltimore, 1996, The Johns Hopkins University Press.

Keeney RL, Von Winterfeldt D, Eppel T: Eliciting public values for complex policy decisions, *Manage Sci* 36(9):1011-1030, 1990.

Lipson J, Dibble S, Minarik P: *Culture and nursing care,* San Francisco, 1996, UCSF Nursing Press.

Martin E: *The women in the body: a cultural analysis of reproduction,* Boston, 1992, Beacon Press.

Meleis A et al: *Diversity, marginalization, and culturally competent health care: issues in knowledge development,* Washington, DC, 1995, American Academy of Nursing.

Morgan R: Dispatch from Beijing, *MS* 6(4):12-21, 1996.

Sheffield W, Sheffield L: Changing ways for determining values, *College Student J,* February-March, 1975, pp 49-54.

Simon SB, Howe LW, Kirschenbaum H: *Values clarification,* New York, 1978, A & W Publishers.

Spector R: *Cultural diversity in health and illness,* San Mateo, Calif, 1991, Appleton & Lange.

Stevens P, Hall JM: A critical historical analysis of the medical construction of lesbianism, *Int J Health Serv* 21(2):291-307,1991.

Unit III

Labor, Birth, and Postpartum Period

Chapter 16

Anatomic and Physiologic Aspects of Labor and Birth

> The last few hours of pregnancy are described by thunderous uterine contractions that effect dilation of the cervix and force the fetus through the birth canal. Much energy is expended during this time, and hence the use of the term labor to describe the process. (Cunningham et al., 1997, p. 261).

The process of labor involves anatomic and physiologic transitions that facilitate the woman's ability to actively and safely birth her baby. Many structural and biochemical adaptations prepare the maternal system for the birth process. Research findings continue to increase our knowledge of the maternal biochemical factors associated with the initiation and maintenance of labor, but the fetal factors remain poorly understood in humans. This chapter presents an overview of the adaptations that occur before the initiation of labor, the hormonal changes believed to initiate labor, and the physiology of the contractile activity associated with labor and birth.

UTERINE ADAPTATIONS FOR LABOR

From conception until labor the body of the uterus and the cervix provide very different functions. The uterine body must remain relatively passive while expanding during fetal growth, and the cervix must remain rigid to prevent premature dilation. With labor these functions reverse. The myometrium of the uterus must actively contract to cause cervical dilation and descent of the fetus, whereas the cervix must soften and open to facilitate birth. Throughout pregnancy uterine smooth muscle cells are bundled with few cell-to-cell contacts. Connective tissue holds the cells end-to-end or side-by-side, but actual contact zones called gap junctions do not appear until late in pregnancy (Figure 16-1). Gap junctions are low resistance bridges or intracellular connections where ions and molecules can be exchanged between cells. The increased ability to generate electrical stimulation is necessary for synchronization of contractions (Fuchs and Fuchs, 1996). Animal studies suggest that the formation of gap junctions is stimulated by estrogen and prostaglandins; conversely, progesterone and prostaglandin inhibitors are thought to inhibit gap junction formation.

The cervix, with its composition of smooth muscle cells, collagen, elastin fibers, and a ground substance containing dermatan, must resist increasing pressure from the enlarging uterus throughout pregnancy in order to remain closed. Dermatan binds with the collagen fibers to maintain a firm consistency. During the last few weeks of pregnancy collagen is broken down by proteolytic enzymes, and the glycosaminoglycans, including dermatan, are replaced by hyaluronic acid. The hydrophilic characteristics of hyaluronic acid result in increased water content of the ground substance, with resultant softening of the cervix. This process is known as ripening. The softening of the cervix may be associated

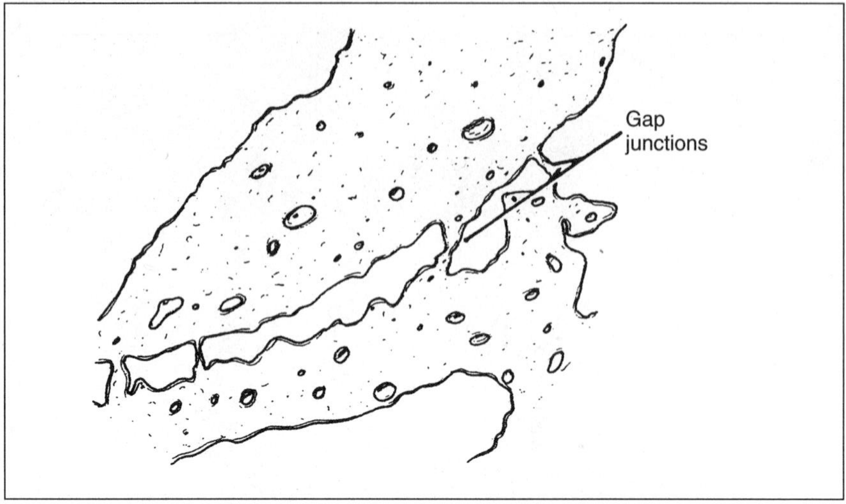

Figure 16-1 Gap junctions.

with dilation that releases the "mucous plug," the thick mucus that seals the cervix during pregnancy.

Progesterone is believed to be the primary hormone that inhibits ripening during pregnancy. Estrogen and relaxin are thought to promote ripening. The role of relaxin is poorly understood. Relaxin is produced by the corpus luteum, yet in women with ovarian failure and donated embryos, ripening can occur without exogenous relaxin. The exogenous hormone most commonly used for cervical ripening is a prostaglandin (PG) E_2, which is thought to act directly on the connective tissue. Ripening alone does not result in the thinning and dilation of the cervix in labor.

In primigravid women ripening and effacement usually occur simultaneously. These changes may be linked to the increase in gap junctions and the resulting myometrial activity. Contractions of the muscle fibers in the cervix and lower uterine segment draw the cervix upward, thus incorporating its components into the lower uterine segment (effacement). Therefore the internal os of the cervix functionally becomes part of the lower uterine segment. The extent of effacement is usually noted by the examiner by estimating the length of the cervix in centimeters or by estimating the percentage of thinning that has occurred, with the average 2-cm long cervix considered uneffaced and the paper-thin, fully effaced cervix considered 100% effaced. Pressure on the ripe, effacing cervix may lead to dilation before active labor. In multiparous women ripening occurs without concurrent effacement, yet the soft cervix may still dilate under the pressure from the gravid uterus and direct pressure of the presenting part before active labor.

Increased Braxton-Hicks contractions and the cervical softening lead to descent of the fetus into the pelvis. Primigravid women typically experience this descent (lightening) about 2 weeks before labor. Although lightening is usually a gradual process, the woman may suddenly have the feeling that she can breathe easier and that the fundus has "dropped." Lightening usually leads to increased perception of pelvic pressure, increased frequency of urination secondary to pressure on the bladder, and at times pressure or discomfort on the thighs. Multiparous women with decreased pelvic muscular support often carry their fetuses deeper in the pelvis and usually do not experience any significant lightening.

FETAL ADAPTATIONS IN PREPARATION FOR LABOR

During the first half of pregnancy maternal cortisol in the fetal circulation is thought to inhibit corticotropin-releasing hormone (CRH) from the fetal hypothalamus. This results in low production of pituitary adrenocorticotropic hormone (ACTH), which prevents activation of the cortisol-producing cells of the adrenal gland. During the latter half of pregnancy estrogen stimulates an increase of conversion of cortisol to cortisone in the placenta, leading to a decrease in maternal cortisol in fetal circulation. Since the inhibitory effects of circulating cortisol are diminished, fetal CRH rises. About 3 to 4 weeks before labor the fetal hypothalamus signals the pituitary to increase release of ACTH, thereby activating the synthesis of enzymes by the adrenal gland that is necessary in the conversion of pregnenolone to cortisol. Estrogen also influences the fetal tissues to convert cortisol to cortisone which, since it is biologically inactive, has no inhibitory effect on release of ACTH from the pituitary (Sweet, 1997).

As the fetal adrenal increases in its ability to synthesize cortisol, the liver, lungs, and adrenal medulla develop the capacity to convert cortisone to cortisol. Cortisol is instrumental in maturation of the hepatic systems that allow for synthesis of glycogen and production of enzymes necessary for metabolism of carbohydrates, proteins, and lipids. Hepatic glycogen increases dramatically from 36 weeks' gestation until birth, and during the first 12 to 24 hours of life the neonate depends on these glycogen stores to prevent hypoglycemia. In addition, cortisol plays a key role in stimulating surfactant biosynthesis, a process that is necessary for initiation and maintenance of respirations.

HORMONAL INFLUENCES ON LABOR

Uterine contractions are primarily the result of hormonal rather than neural factors. The fact that paraplegic women and women who have had bilateral lumbar sympathectomies experience normal, though painless, contractile patterns in labor supports this finding. Cervical ripening may be mediated by sympathomimetic innervation, but this has yet to be confirmed in humans. Manipulation of the cervix, including "stripping" the membranes, results in release of PGs, an action that may be the result of catecholamines releasing PGE_2 from nerve endings (Fuchs and Fuchs, 1996). The only other proposed neural factor in labor is the increased oxytocin release in response to pressure on nerve fibers in the vagina (Ferguson reflex). This reflex has been demonstrated in animal studies but has not been replicated in human studies.

Myometrial contractures occur throughout pregnancy, and labor occurs with a transition from a contracture to contraction pattern of activity. Contractures are characterized by long-lasting, low-amplitude myometrial activity and typically have a slower pattern of tightening and relaxation. The switch to synchronized high-amplitude contractions is closely associated to the woman's nightly increases in plasma estrogen and oxytocin levels. One theory regarding initiation of labor is that estrogen prepares the myometrium through its stimulation of oxytocin receptors and oxytocin actually causes the transition to contractions (Nathanielsz, 1994; Olson, Mijovic, and Sadowsky, 1995).

Steroids and oxytoxic hormones comprise the hormonal factors in labor. The steroids estrogen and progesterone stimulate the synthesis of cell-surface receptors, phospholipids, and other lipids that are the precursors for PG synthesis. Steroid production shows distinct diurnal variation. Animal studies have identified that estrogen has a morning peak stimulated by maternal androgen secretion and a nocturnal peak stimulated by fetal secretion of dehydroepiandrosterone. The morning peak may play a role in stimulation of the formation of gap junctions and oxytocin receptors in the myometrium. Gap junctions are nonexistent in nonpregnant women but increase to 1000 per cell in labor. Myometrial oxytocin receptors increase 80- to 100-fold in early labor. The nocturnal peak of estrogen parallels the nocturnal peak in oxytocin and is associated with increased myometrial activity. Endogenous oxytocic agents include oxytocin, PGE and PGF, and alpha-adrenergic agonists. The nocturnal peak in oxytocin, usually occurring at nightfall, coincides with women's reports of increased uterine activity in the evening.

Estrogen levels increase at 34 to 36 weeks' gestation. Estrogen has been shown to promote the formation of gap junctions; increase oxytocin and estrogen receptor sites in the myometrium; enhance lipase activity and release of arachidonic acid, which stimulates PG synthesis; increase the binding of intracellular calcium; and increase myosin phosphorylation. Myosin is one of three protein myofilaments that are responsible for the contractility of the myometrium. Phosphorylation is a process whereby the myosin filaments are bound to actin, a second protein monofilament, to produce a contraction that exerts a large force over a short distance at low velocity. This smooth muscle contractile pattern allows the myometrium to sustain strong contractions over many hours (Blackburn and Loper, 1992). Although estrogen is produced by the placenta, fetal adrenal precursors influence its synthesis. Concentrations of estradiol and estrone increase in amniotic fluid 15 to 20 days before both term and preterm labor. The chorion and decidua produce estrone, resulting in a shift in the progesterone-to-estrogen ration. Local effect of estrone may also promote the production of PGF_{2a} and the formation of the gap junctions. Nathanielsz (1994) has suggested that certain stressors may result in increased amounts of precursors for placental estrogen production, which may help explain the occurrence of preterm labor in association with social, nutritional, and physical stressors.

Progesterone inhibits uterine irritability throughout pregnancy. Studies in animals have suggested a decrease in progesterone as a triggering factor in labor, but this effect has not been demonstrated in humans. Progesterone levels remain fairly stable in humans, but there may be localized decrease in progesterone activity as a result of progesterone-binding protein that may be induced by the rising levels of estrogen at term. Other researchers have hypothesized that fetal cortisol competes with the action of progesterone in the regulation of CRH and thereby blocks action of progesterone (Karalis and Majzoub, 1995).

PGs are influential in initiation and maintenance of labor through their roles in forming gap junctions and increasing calcium levels in the cytoplasm of the myometrial cells. PG receptors function somewhat differently than oxytocin receptors in that stimulation by another hormone is not necessary for their proliferation and action. PG receptors are present and capable of stimulation for contractions at any time during pregnancy. Maternal and fetal tissues have varying forms of PGs. The amnion has high concentrations of PGE_2, but little of it crosses the chorion intact since enzymes in the chorion rapidly convert PGs to inactive metabolites. The placenta and umbilical cord produce PGE_2, PGD_2, PGI_2, and thromboxane A_2. PGI_2 is produced in the myometrium and vascular compartment. The decidua produces high concentrations of PGI_2 and lesser amounts of PGF_{2a} and PGE_2. Enzymes in the decidua convert PGE_2 to PGF_{2a}, an activity that is enhanced by oxytocin. Research suggests that the decidua is a major source of PGs during and after labor. Decidual cells obtained immediately after a spontaneous birth have PGF_{2a} concentrations approximately 30 times greater than those found after elective cesarean section. Actions of these PGs are summarized in Box 16-1.

The exact triggering factors for initiation of labor remain illusive. Most investigators agree that both maternal and fetal factors are necessary and that these factors are mediated by oxytocin. Research findings have included:

1. Initiation of labor can be delayed or stopped in early stages by agents that inhibit oxytocin release (ethanol) or agents that inhibit PG synthesis (acetylsalicylic acid, indomethacin). However, as evidenced in cases of preterm labor, the inhibition of labor appears to be a temporary effect.
2. The levels of PGE and PGF in amniotic fluid are not increased above normal pregnant levels at the beginning of labor but increase as labor progresses.
3. Plasma oxytocin levels are increased in early labor and precede the increase in plasma PG metabolytes, which increase as active labor progresses.
4. Uterine responsiveness to oxytocin increases significantly as pregnancy progresses and reaches its peak at term; uterine responsiveness to PGs remains fairly stable throughout pregnancy.
5. Induction of labor with oxytocin is accomplished with plasma doses in the physiologic range of endogenous oxytocin. Induction of labor with PGs requires plasma levels that greatly exceed physiologic levels, regardless of route of administration.
6. Chorion has an active PG dehydrogenase system that permits only a small proportion of amniotic PGs to pass through without alteration (Fuchs and Fuchs, 1996).

Previous investigators have argued that oxytocin has no role in initiation of labor and that PGs released from the amnion are the stimulus for myometrial contractions. This theory seems to be disputed by the findings documented in previous paragraphs. Fuchs and Fuchs (1996) argue that the maternal and fetal signals are integrated into the decidua, which uses PGs for transmission of those signals to the myometrium.

Box 16-1 *Prostaglandin Actions*

PGE_2
Necessary in formation of gap junctions; involved in cervical ripening by relaxing cervical smooth muscle; has little influence on myometrial activation caused by desensitization of the uterus to oxytoxic effects of PGE_2

PGF_{2a}
Stimulates myometrial contractions by increasing intracellular calcium both by opening calcium channels and releasing calcium from intracellular vesicles; increases excitability of myometrial cells at concentrations lower than those required for contraction leading to enhancement of other oxytoxics; no changes in cervical resistance; prime protanoid released during labor

PGI_2
Vasodilator; inhibits platelet aggregation; relaxes smooth muscle but has no uterine effect

TX_{A2}
Vasoconstrictor; platelet aggregation factor

Oxytocin is a highly potent hormone that is released in a pulsed pattern. Pulsed activity increases in late pregnancy, and research suggests that women with lower concentrations of oxytocin before labor are more likely to experience dysfunctional labors (Dawood et al., 1979). Fuchs, Behrens, and Liu (1992) found that the pulse frequency before labor averaged 1.3/min, with a threefold to fourfold increase in early labor and a further threefold increase in the second stage of labor. During the third stage of labor they found a 60% decrease in frequency, with frequency remaining well above the prelabor levels. Injections of 2 to 8 mU of oxytocin intravenously produced similar results. Research has demonstrated that pulsed administration of oxytocin is more effective in maintaining contractions than continuous infusion (Dawood, 1989; Randolph and Fuchs, 1989).

The fetus is also a source of oxytocin (Chard, 1989; Chard et al., 1971; Dawood et al., 1978). Oxytocin concentration in the umbilical artery is twice that of the umbilical vein, which has a concentration similar to the maternal concentration. It is estimated that the fetus contributes oxytocin equivalent to an infusion of 2 to 3 mU/min, which doubles the amount of oxytocin available to the uterus in a typical labor.

Low concentrations of oxytocin receptors in the endometrium and myometrium are found in the nonpregnant uterus. By 17 weeks' gestation, there is a sixfold increase in the number of receptors, and by term there is an 80- to 100-fold increase. In early labor the concentration of receptors increases two to three times that of the concentration immediately before labor. The concentration in the fundus, body, and upper part of the lower segment are similar. The concentration in the lower segment is dramatically less (about 28% the concentration of the body of the uterus). Cervical concentration is minimal. It appears that estrogen stimulates the formation of oxytocin receptors, but the contribution of progesterone is unclear.

With so much of labor under hormonal influence, it stands to reason that emotional, psychologic, and environmental factors can facilitate or inhibit labor progress. It has been well documented that mammals require a sense of safety to deliver their young. When mammals are disturbed in labor, uterine contractions are inhibited. This phenomenon is noted in women when they leave their homes to go to the hospital or other site of birth. Women often report experiencing regular contractions that increase in intensity and frequency; yet, when they enter the birth site, the contractions decrease. This most likely is a result of high levels of maternal serum catecholamines, which have a direct inhibitory effect on myometrial contractility.

Research continues to identify specific triggers for initiation of labor. Further understanding of the multiple factors that are involved in the process will not only guide clinicians in facilitating normal labor but will provide necessary knowledge to prevent or inhibit preterm labor as well as more effectively intervene in postdates gestations when medically indicated.

CHARACTERISTICS OF LABOR CONTRACTIONS

During labor the upper part of the uterus is the active segment, and the lower segment remains relatively passive. The point at which the fibers of the upper and lower segments meet is the physiologic retraction ring (Figure 16-2). The active segment becomes progressively thicker as regular contractions continue into the active phase of labor. Conversely, the lower segment becomes increasingly thinner to facilitate descent of the fetus. This differentiation enhances the forces necessary for dilation and expulsion.

Myometrial cells in the upper segment contract and retract in a way that maintains constant tension around the uterine contents. If this were not accomplished, the repeated relaxation of the muscle fibers would inhibit cervical change and descent of the fetus. Myometrial cells in the fundus contract and never return to their original length. This shortening leads to thickening of the myometrial wall, which reaches its maximum thickness immediately after the birth of the baby. This action of contraction and retraction depends on the simultaneous changes in the lower segment. The myometrial fibers of the lower segment stretch with each contraction and remain fixed at the longer length.

The differentiation between the myometrial cells in the upper and lower segments leads to the specific progression of the contractile wave. The following pattern must be present for effective contractile activity:

1. The contraction is propagated from the fundus downward to the lower segment.
2. The duration of the contraction is longest in the fundus and decreases progressively downward.
3. The intensity of the contraction is strongest in the fundus and diminishes progressively downward.

These characteristic contractile patterns are referred to as the triple descending gradient. If the uterus were a closed system without these differences in contrac-

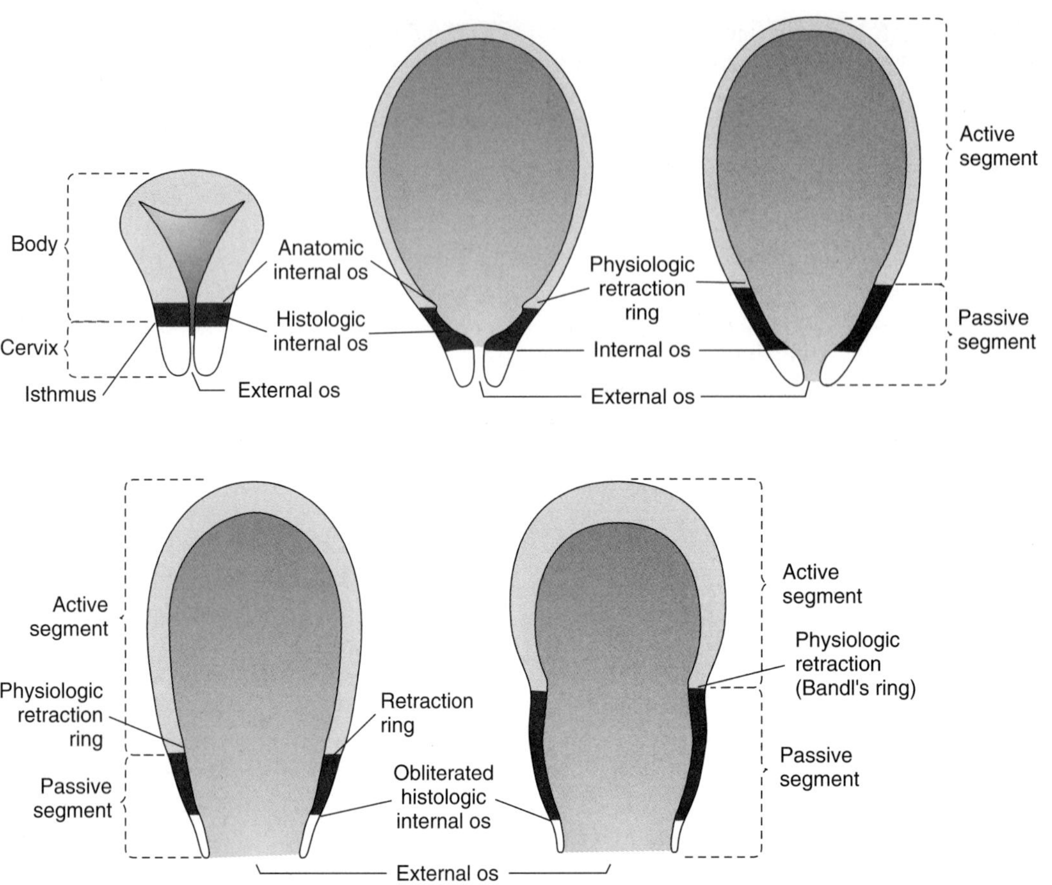

Figure 16-2 Development of the segments of the uterus during pregnancy.

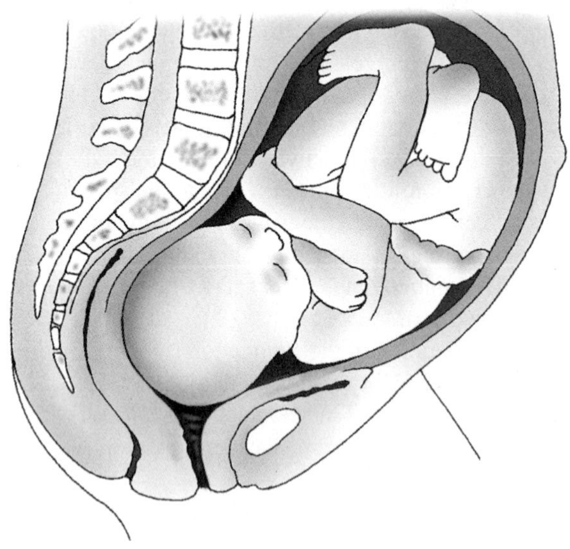

Figure 16-3 Uterus at complete dilation.

tile waves, there would be no dilation or descent of the fetus.

Not only must the coordinated contractile pattern from the fundus to the lower segment be present, but uterine contractions must exert sufficient pressure to dilate the cervix and expel the infant (Figure 16-3). Use of frequency, active pressure, and duration of the contractions has been proposed as a means to measure uterine activity since 1927. Development of technology that allows direct measurement of pressure through the use of intrauterine catheters has increased the ability to differentiate between normal and abnormal labor patterns. It is estimated that contractions must increase intrauterine pressure at least 30 mm Hg above the usual resting tone of 8 to 10 mm Hg to affect cervical change. Intrauterine pressure of greater than 50 mm Hg is usually seen in a normal active labor pattern.

Caldeyro-Barcia and Poseiro (1959) proposed using the frequency and amplitude of contractions to determine the montevideo unit (MVU). MVUs are calculated by determining the peak pressure above resting tone during each contraction. Pressures for all contractions in a 10-minute period of time are added to obtain the total MVUs. For example, if a woman experiences three contractions in 10 minutes, each with intensity of 60 mm Hg, the MVU would be 180. Labor usually begins when a woman's contraction pattern reaches 80 to 120 MVUs. Greater than 200 MVUs is considered verification of normal contractile pressures.

Even with quantification of uterine contractions, labor progress cannot always be predicted. Size and position of the fetus and characteristics of the pelvis may inhibit progress to spontaneous birth. The wise clinician will consider numerous factors when assessing whether a particular labor is progressing normally.

References

Blackburn ST, Loper DL: *Maternal, fetal and neonatal physiology,* Philadelphia, 1992, WB Saunders.

Caldeyro-Barcia R, Poseiro JJ: Oxytocin and contractility of the human pregnant uterus, *Ann NY Acad Sci* 75:813-830, 1959.

Chard T: Fetal and maternal oxytocin in human parturition, *Am J Perinatol* 6(2):145-152, 1989.

Chard T et al: Release of oxytocin and vasopressin by the human foetus during labor, *Nature* 234(5328):352-354, 1971.

Cunningham FG et al: *Williams obstetrics,* ed 20, Stamford, Conn, 1997, Appleton & Lange.

Dawood MY: Evolving concepts of oxytocin for induction of labor, *Am J Perinatol* 6(2):167-172, 1989.

Dawood MY et al: Fetal contribution to oxytocin in human labor, *Obstet Gynecol* 52(2):205-209, 1978.

Dawood MY et al: Oxytocin in maternal circulation and amniotic fluid in pregnancy, *J Clin Endocrinol Metabol* 49(3):429-434, 1979.

Fuchs AR, Behrens O, Liu HC: Correlation of nocturnal increase in plasma oxytocin with a decrease in plasma estradiol/progesterone ratio in late pregnancy, *Am J Obstet Gynecol* 167(6):1559-1563, 1992.

Fuchs, AR, Fuchs F: Physiology and endocrinology of parturition. In Gabbe SG, Niebyl JP, Simpson JL, editors: *Obstetrics: normal and problem pregnancies,* ed 3, New York, 1996, Churchill Livingstone.

Karalis K, Majzoub JA: Regulation of placental corticotropin-releasing hormone by steroids: possible implications in labor initiation, *Ann NY Acad Sci* 771:551-555, 1995.

Nathanielsz PW: A time to be born: implications of animal studies in maternal-fetal medicine, *Birth* 21(3):163-169, 1994.

Olson DM, Mijovic JE, Sadowsky DW: Control of human parturition, *Semin Perinatol* 19(1):52-63, 1995.

Randolph GW, Fuchs AR: Pulsatile administration enhances the effect and reduces the dose of oxytocin required for induction of labor, *Am J Perinatol* 6(2):159-166, 1989.

Sweet BR: *Maye's midwifery: a textbook for midwives,* ed 12, Philadelphia, 1997, WB Saunders.

Chapter 17

Mechanisms of Labor

Birth requires that the fetus successfully negotiate through the pelvis to the extrauterine environment. This navigation is influenced by the three "Ps": passenger, passage, and powers. Some authors also consider a fourth P—maternal psyche—since there are associations between psyche and progress of labor. This chapter explores factors related to the passage and the passenger that enhance or inhibit the birth process.

Mechanisms of labor, or cardinal movements, refer to the changes of position of the fetus that facilitate the movement through the birth canal. The funnel-shape of the bony pelvis, coupled with the shift in direction of the birth canal as the fetus passes through the outlet of the pelvis, requires specific fetal rotations to allow the diameters of the head, shoulders, and in some cases, hips, to effectively pass the planes of the pelvis. Rotation is enhanced by both the resistance inherent in the pelvic musculature and in the loss of resistance once the presenting part is birthed.

It is helpful for the beginning midwife to remember that birth is a process that follows principles of physics—mass and force. Late in pregnancy the fetus begin to settle into a position influenced by pelvic shape, uterine characteristics, and shape and size of the fetal head. Some women describe the sensations as feeling like the baby is trying to find the "best fit" into the pelvic inlet. If resistance is met, the fetus rolls into a different position. For example, if the anterior part of the pelvic inlet is compromised (small), the fetal head rotates posteriorly in an effort to find a better "fit." In addition, gravity plays a part in this preparation for labor. The fetal head, with its bony structure and increased size relative to adult proportions, is the heaviest part of the fetus and tends to present at the pelvic inlet because of the effects of gravity. Contractions provide force that pushes the fetus downward. Through the entire process, as resistance is met, fetal position often changes to a less resistant orientation.

FETAL POSITIONING

As the fetus nears term, it fills the uterus more, encouraging further flexion of the extremities. This posture, or relationship of extremities to the body and head, is referred to as the *fetal attitude*. The *lie* of the fetus refers to the relationship of the long axis of the fetus to the long axis of the mother. Over 99% of fetal lies at term are longitudinal, meaning that the long axis of the fetus is parallel with the long axis of the mother. Occasionally the lie can be transverse when the long axis of the fetus is perpendicular to the long axis of the mother. Oblique lies occur when the fetal and maternal axes cross at 45 degrees. These usually shift to longitudinal lies as labor progresses and the presenting part descends into the pelvis. Gravity, the ovoid shape of the uterus, and good abdominal muscle tone promote longitudinal lies.

The fetal part that enters the pelvis determines the *presentation.* In longitudinal lies the presenting part is either the fetal head (cephalic) or the fetal buttocks (breech). Cephalic presentations are further categorized by the attitude (i.e., the relationship of the fetal head to the fetal body). When the head is well flexed, the chin rests on the thorax, and the presentation is considered to be vertex or occipital. During a vaginal examination, if there is cervical dilation or if the lower uterine segment is extremely thinned out, the examiner can identify the posterior fontanelle and the occipital bone. Approximately 96% of presentations are vertex. When the head is hyperextended so that the occiput rests on the fetal back, the face is the presenting part. About 0.2% of presentations are face presentations. With deflexion that is not as pronounced as the face presentation, the anterior fontanelle (sincipital or military presentation) or the brow (brow presentation) may present.

In breech presentations the thighs and knees may both be flexed, leading to a complete breech presentation. When the thighs are flexed but the knees are not, the legs extend over the anterior part of the fetal body, and the fetus is in a frank breech presentation. An incomplete breech presentation (footling breech) is when one or both feet are presenting in the lower uterine segment (Figure 17-1). At term 3% to 3½% of presentations are breech.

When there is a transverse lie, the shoulder presents in the inlet. Vaginal birth is not possible with this presentation, and allowing labor to continue without attending to change the fetus to a longitudinal lie will only cause further impaction of the fetal shoulder and upper body in the pelvic inlet.

When the fetus assumes a breech, sincipital, brow, face, or shoulder presentation, it is said to be in a malpresentation. Each malpresentation is associated with distinct increased risks for the woman and her infant. Maternal factors associated with malpresentation include decreased uterine length/height secondary to anomalies, masses, or placental placement; lax abdominal tone; and compromised pelvic inlet diameters. Fetal conditions that are associated with malpresentation include prematurity, hydramnios, increased or decreased fetal mobility, and fetal anomalies, including hydrocephalus, anencephaly, and autosomal trisomies.

Position is determined using a distinct landmark (denominator) on the fetal presenting part and describing its orientation to the maternal pelvis. The landmark used in vertex presentations is the occiput, the bony prominence behind and inferior to the posterior fontanelle. The occiput may be on the maternal left or right and may be anterior, transverse, or posterior. The positions describing vertex presentations are illustrated in Figure 17-2. The denominator used in breech presentations is the fetal sacrum, and the denominator used for face presentations is the chin (mentum). Shoulder presentations use the scapular as the landmark. Figures 17-3 and 17-4 illustrate positions found in breech and face presentations.

Fetal positioning is first assessed during the abdominal examination. A skilled clinician should be able to

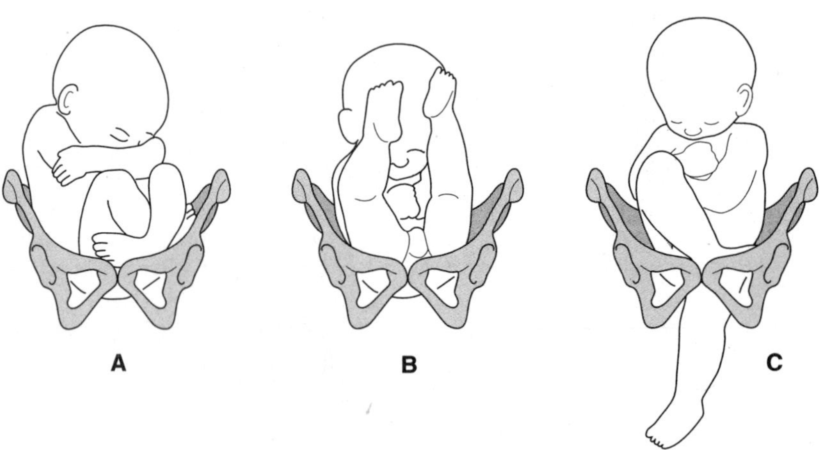

Figure 17-1 Presentations. **A,** Complete breech; **B,** frank breech; **C,** footling breech.

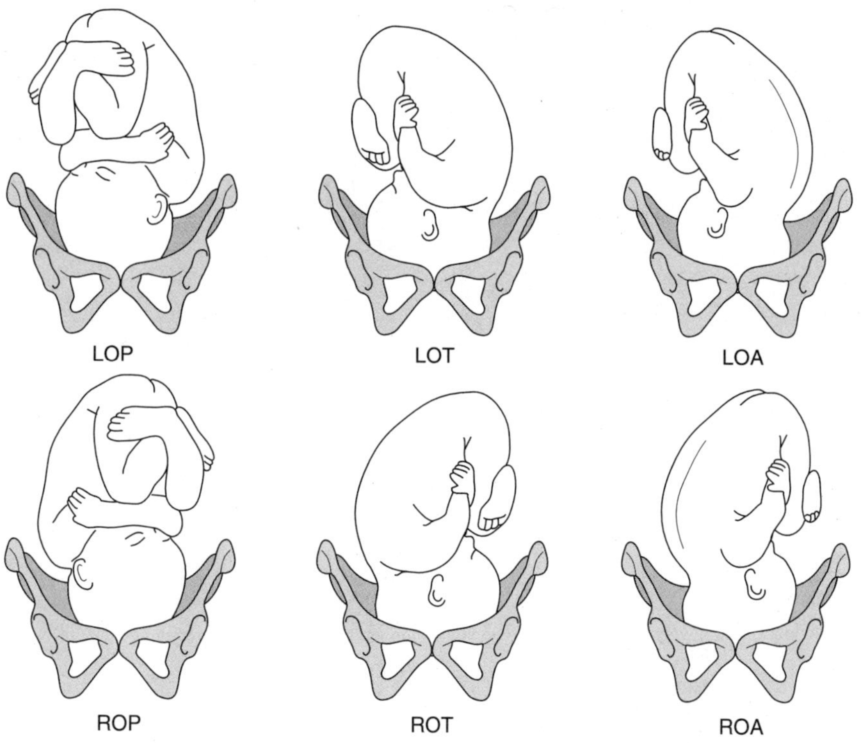

Figure 17-2 Fetal positions—vertex. *L,* Left; *O,* occiput; *P,* posterior; *T,* transverse; *A,* anterior; *R,* right.

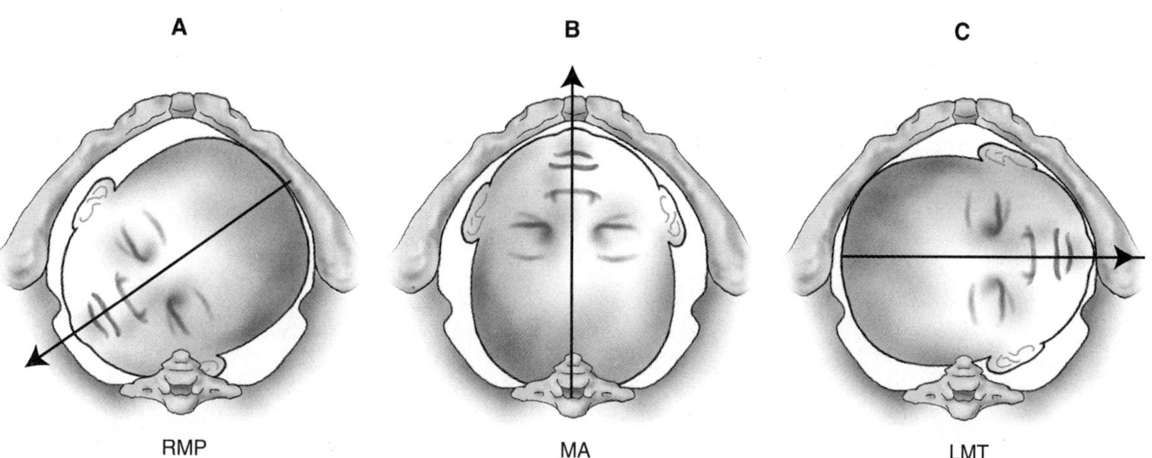

Figure 17-3 Fetal positions—face. **A,** Right mentoposterior *(RMP);* **B,** mentoanterior *(MA);* **C,** left mentotransverse *(LMT).*

Sacrum anterior
RSA
LSA
RST
LST
RSP
LSP
Sacrum posterior

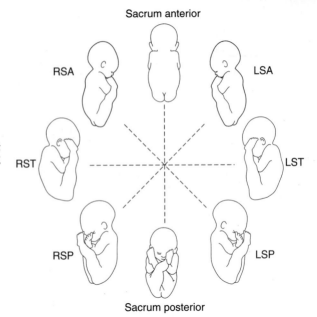

Figure 17-4 Positions—breech. *RSA,* Right sacrum anterior; *RST,* right sacrotransverse; *RSP,* right sacroposterior; *LSA,* left sacroanterior; *LST,* left sacrotransverse; *LSP,* left sacroposterior.

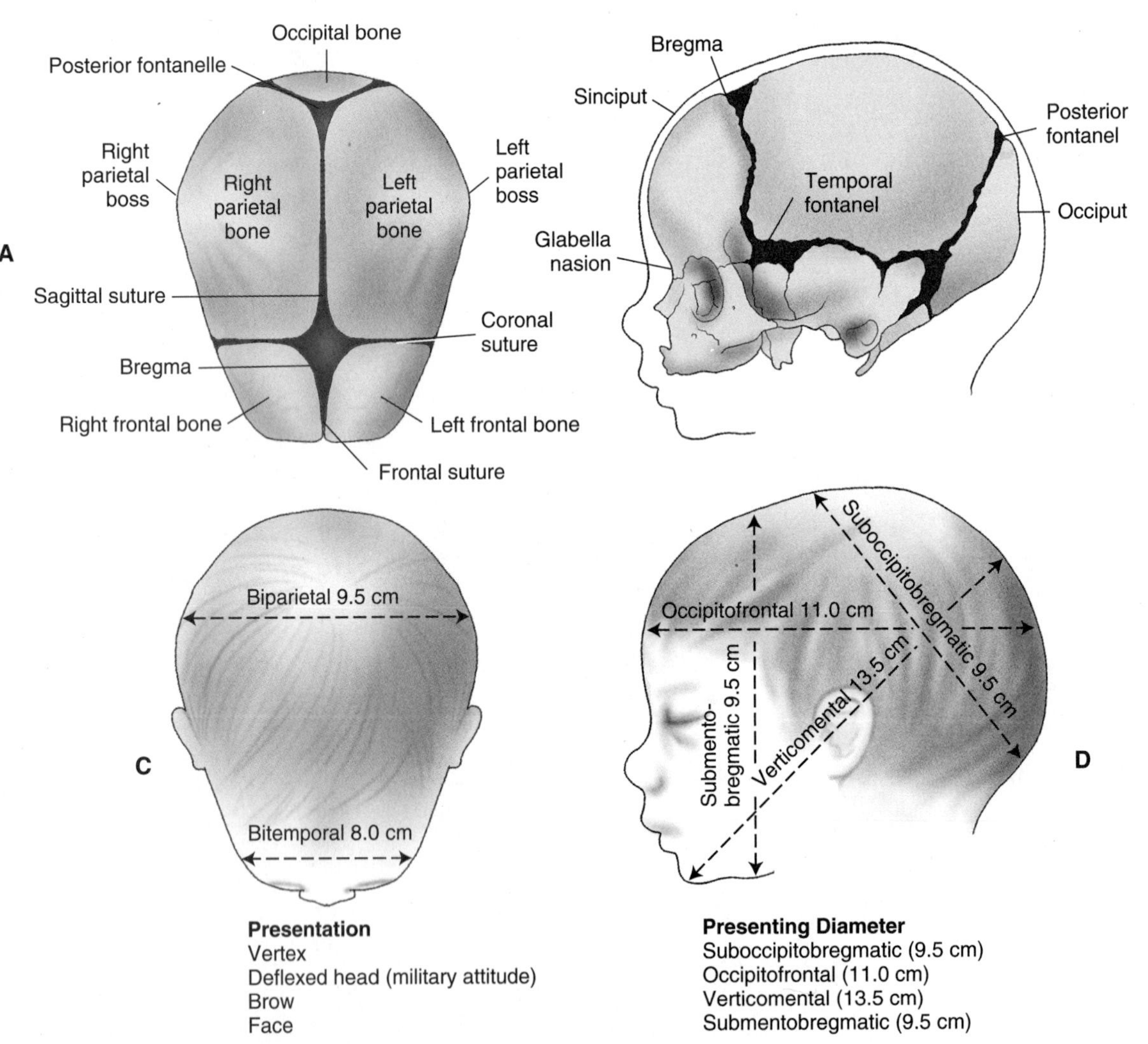

Figure 17-5 Fetal skull landmarks. **A,** Vaginal "touch" picture; **B,** side view; **C,** transverse, **D,** anteroposterior diameters.

Table 17-1 *Presenting Diameters for Cephalic Presentations at Term*

Presentation	Presenting diameter
Vertex	Suboccipitobregmatic (9.5 cm)
Sincipital	Occipitofrontal (11.0 cm)
Brow	Verticomental (13.5 cm)
Face	Submentobregmatic (9.5 cm)

identify the presentation and position abdominally unless the abdominal musculature is extremely strong, there is excess adipose tissue, or there is excess amniotic fluid. Vaginal examination serves to either confirm the abdominal examination or accurately identify position when it is difficult to palpate the fetus. During the vaginal examination for a cephalic presentation, the examiner seeks to identify the sutures and fontanelles on the fetal skull (Figure 17-5). Once the position is identified, the examiner can estimate the presenting diameters for the fetal head (Table 17-1). It is clear that, when the fetal head is not well flexed, the presenting anteroposterior diameters increase, which may inhibit descent in the pelvis. Most fetuses that present with brow or sincipital presentations experience further flexion into vertex presentation as labor progresses, unless there are other factors that interfere with flexion.

In vertex, sincipital, and brow presentations, it is also helpful to determine the presence of synclitism or asynclitism. If the fetal head is synclitic, the sagittal suture is midway between the maternal symphysis pubis and the sacral promontory. In anterior asynclitism the sagittal suture is closer to the maternal sacral promontory, and a larger proportion of the anterior parietal bone is palpable compared to the posterior parietal bone. Conversely, in posterior asynclitism the sagittal suture is oriented toward the maternal symphysis pubis, and a greater proportion of the posterior parietal bone can be palpated. When a woman has normal abdominal tone, the fetal head usually enters the pelvis with slight posterior asynclitism. This is actually a favorable position since the force of the contractions result in descent in the true direction of the pelvic angle. When abdominal tone is lax so that the fetus is not supported well, anterior asynclitism can alter the presenting diameters enough to inhibit descent (Figure 17-6).

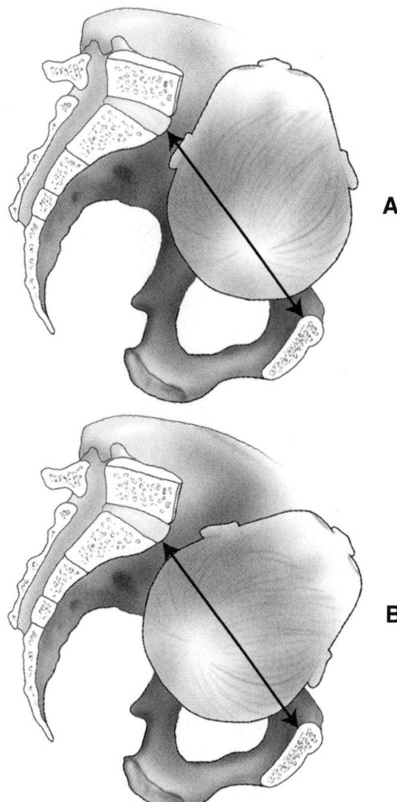

Figure 17-6 **A**, Posterior asynclitism; **B**, synclitism.

FETAL SKULL

The fetal skull is composed of the cranial vault, the face, and the base. At term the bones of the face are heavier that those of the vault and are fused. The bones of the vault remain unfused, allowing for changes in shape as the fetal head (molding) accommodates to the maternal pelvis. The vault consists of two frontal bones on the anterior aspect of the fetal head, two parietal bones on each side, and one occipital bone on the posterior aspect of the head. The base of the skull consists of two temporal bones.

The membranous spaces between the bones of the vault are the *sutures*. The sagittal suture lies between the parietal bones and provides the anteroposterior demarcation along the central aspect of the top of the skull. The frontal suture lies between the frontal bones, and it is usually not as prominent as the parietal suture. The coronal sutures lie between the parietal and frontal bones. The lambdoidal sutures lie between the occipital bone

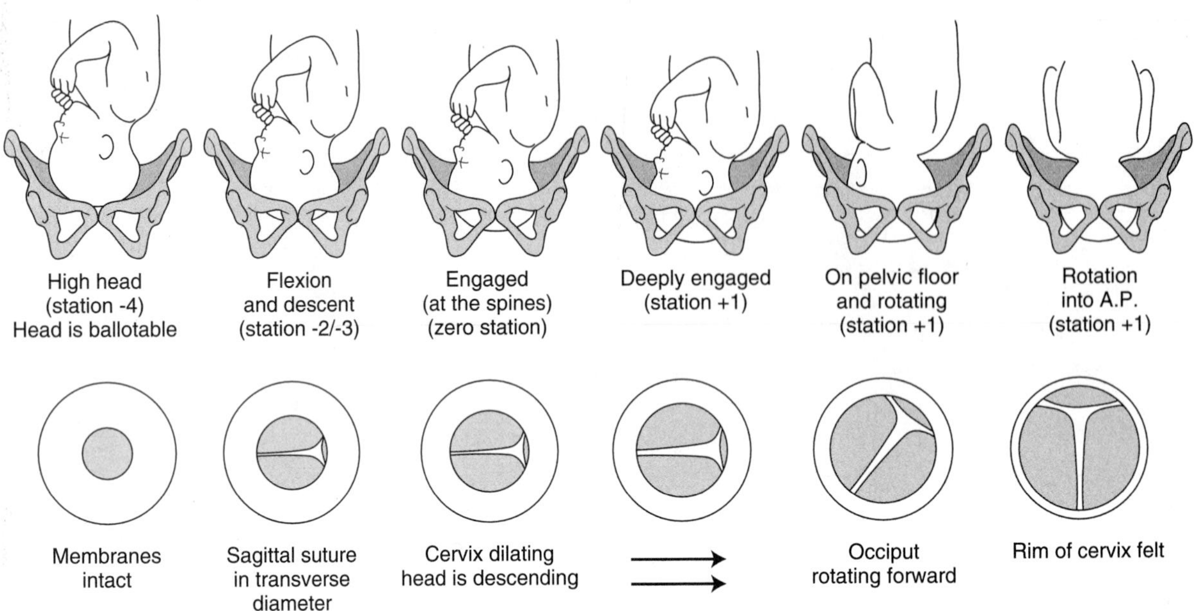

Figure 17-7 Positions of the sagittal suture.

and the parietal bones (see Figure 17-5). The *fontanelles* are the membranous spaces created where sutures intersect or converge. The anterior fontanelle (bregma) is bordered by the frontal and parietal bones and lies where the sagittal, coronal, and frontal sutures converge. The junction of the four bones and sutures creates a diamond shape. The average size of the anterior fontanelle at term is 2 × 3 cm, and closure usually occurs 12 to 18 months after birth. The posterior fontanelle (lambda) is located at the intersection of the lambdoidal and sagittal sutures and is bounded by the occipital and parietal bones. This triangular-shaped fontanelle averages 0.5 to 1 cm at its widest point. The posterior fontanelle usually closes by 6 to 10 weeks after birth. Open sutures are important during the rapid growth of infancy since they allow for growth of the cranium over the enlarging brain.

The fontanelles and the sagittal sutures are the most common landmarks used in determining fetal position during a vaginal examination when the fetus is in a vertex presentation. The sagittal suture can be identified as anteroposterior, transverse, or oblique. When it is palpated obliquely from the maternal left anterior aspect of the pelvis to the maternal right posterior aspect, it is said to be right oblique. When it is palpated from the maternal right anterior to the left posterior aspect of the pelvis, it is said to be left oblique (Figure 17-7).

Diameters of the fetal skull are determined using landmarks in the bony structure. There are two transverse diameters, the larger of which is the biparietal diameter. This is the measurement between the two parietal prominences, and it averages 9.5 cm at term. The bitemporal diameter is the measurement between the lateral aspects of the temporal bones, and it averages 8 cm at term.

The suboccipitobregmatic diameter is the shortest anteroposterior diameter of the flexed fetal head (9.5 cm at term), and it is measured from the point just under the prominence of the occipital bone to the center of the anterior fontanelle. When there is less flexion, the occipitofrontal diameter presents in the pelvis (11.5 cm at term). This is measured from the prominence of the occipital bone to the point where the frontal bones define the nasal cavity. With no flexion, the occipitomental diameter presents (12.5 cm at term), and it is measured from the prominence of the occipital bone to the chin. When the fetal head is hyperextended (face presentation), the presenting diameter is the submentobregmatic diameter from the junction of the neck and jaw to the bregma (9.5 cm at term).

MECHANISMS OF LABOR—VERTEX PRESENTATION (LEFT OCCIPITOANTERIOR)

When considering the movements of the fetal presenting part through the pelvis, it is important to keep in mind that they may not be distinct, separate movements. Some occur at the same time; others flow very smoothly, one to the other, without any interruption.

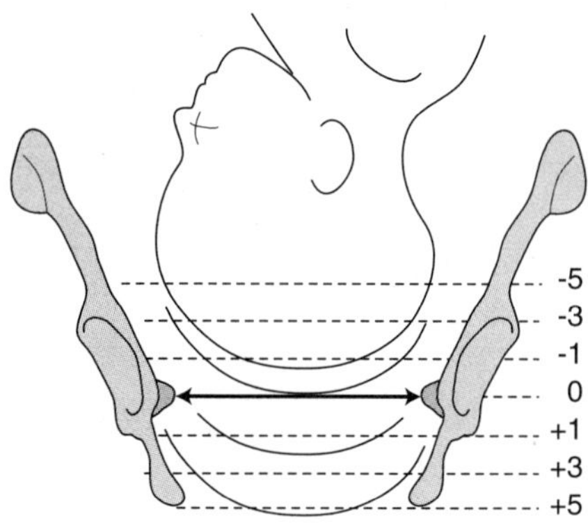

Figure 17-8 Stations of descent.

Descent

Descent has usually occurred to some degree before labor. Descent is described by estimating the *station* of the presenting part. Station is an estimation of the position of the presenting part in relation to the ischial spines in the midpelvis. When the lowest point of the presenting part is at the level of the spines, it is determined to be at zero station. In a term fetus, when the occiput is at the level of the ischial spines, the biparietal diameter has descended to a plane below the level of the pelvic inlet. This degree of descent is termed *engagement.* Engagement can be suggested by abdominal examination when the examiner notes that the fetal head has "dipped" deep into the pelvis and is no longer movable, but it can only be confirmed by vaginal examination. Engagement may occur up to 2 weeks before labor in nulliparous women and may not occur until active labor in multiparous women.

When the presenting part is at a level above the spines, measurement is indicated by a negative number; when below the spines, a positive number is used. There are several methods for estimating station. Some examiners estimate the number of centimeters the presenting part lies above or below the ischial spines. However, this cannot be an exact measurement because of the effect of the curving of the pelvic structure (Figure 17-8). Others recommend dividing the areas above and below the spines into fifths. Thus, if the fetal occiput is at the pelvic inlet, it would be considered to be at −5 station. If it were crowning, it would be +5. This method has become confusing since other examiners divide the space above and below the spines into thirds, so the crowning fetus would be +3. Because of this, some authorities recommend noting the station as a fraction so that others will know which fractional system is being used (e.g., $-\frac{2}{5}$ or $+\frac{1}{3}$) (Cunningham et al., 1997). It is important that examiners be clear about which system is being used and that the same system be used consistently.

Descent does not follow a steady, continuous pattern. Typically the greatest rate of descent occurs during the deceleration phase of first stage of labor and during the second stage of labor.

Flexion

Flexion also begins before labor. As the fetal head meets resistance of the bony structure of the pelvis and the pelvic musculature, it is forced into a more flexed attitude. Flexion of the head against the thorax is possible because the fetal chin and mandible are typically very small in relation to other aspects of the face and can easily be pushed back further and because relaxin may promote more flexion of the cervical vertebrae than will be possible following birth. Factors that inhibit flexion include multiple nuchal cords and masses such as fetal goiter or other fetal anomalies.

In the LOA position, descent and flexion bring the fetal head into the pelvis with the posterior fontanelle on the maternal left and the sagittal suture running obliquely from the left anterior quadrant to the right posterior quadrant of the pelvic plane (Figure 17-9, *A*).

Internal Rotation

When the fetal head has descended to the level at or below the ischial spines, it meets the resistance of the coccygeus and ileococcygeus muscles of the pelvic floor. This resistance causes passive rotation of the fetal head 45 degrees anterior so that the occiput rests directly under the symphysis pubis. This rotation brings the transverse diameter into the widest diameter of the midplane and outlet of the gynecoid pelvis. During this rotation the head rotates independently of the body, and the shoulders remain in the oblique diameter (Figure 17-9, *B*).

Extension

As the fetal head emerges through the introitus, several factors force it from flexion to extension. The forces of the contraction push the fetus downward while the resistance of the pelvic musculature forces it anterior, following the normal curve of the birth canal. With birth of the head, there is no further resistance, and the head easily pivots under the symphysis pubis into an extended position (Figure 17-9, *C*).

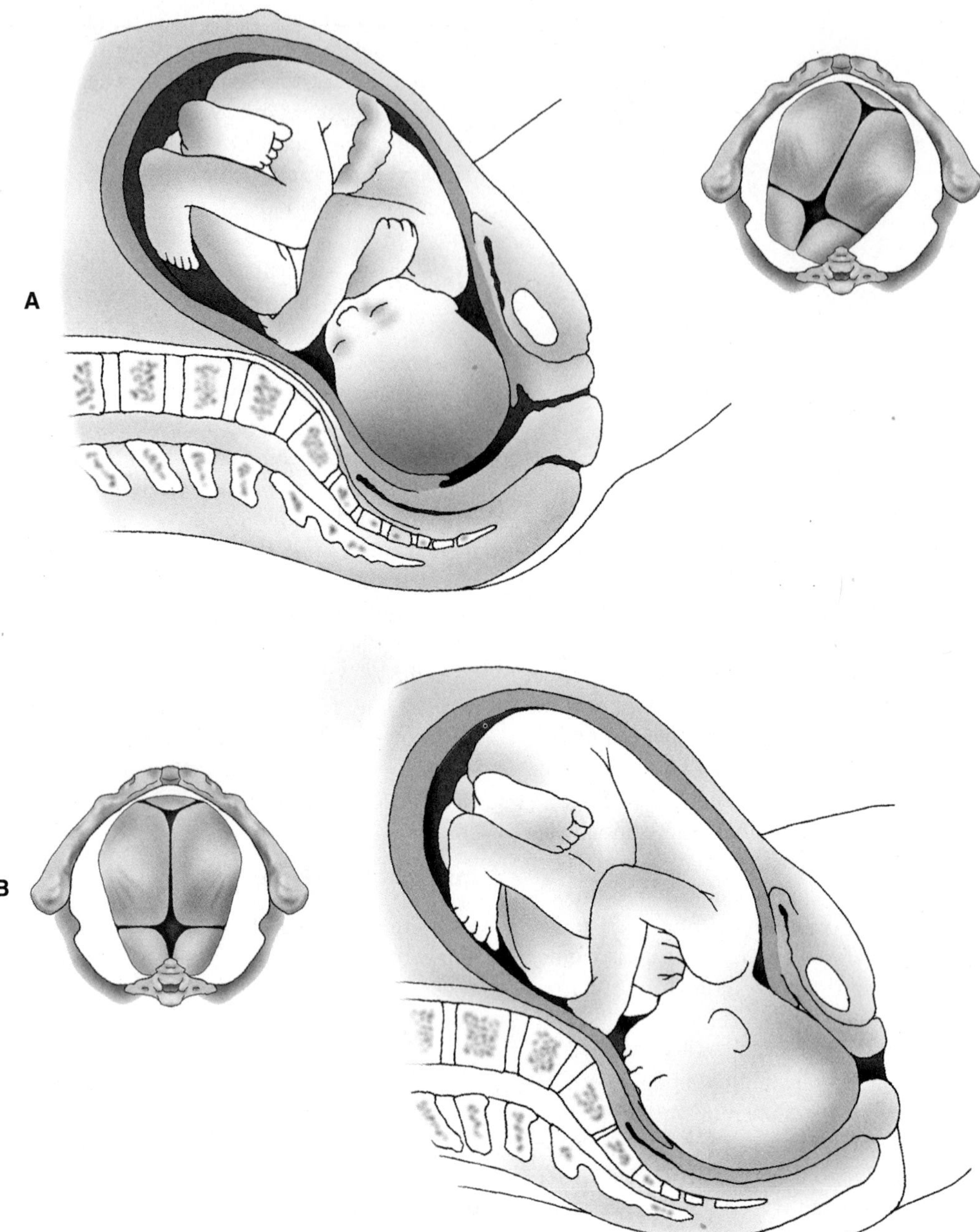

Figure 17-9 Mechanisms of labor—**A**, Left occipitoanterior; **B**, internal rotation to occipitoanterior.

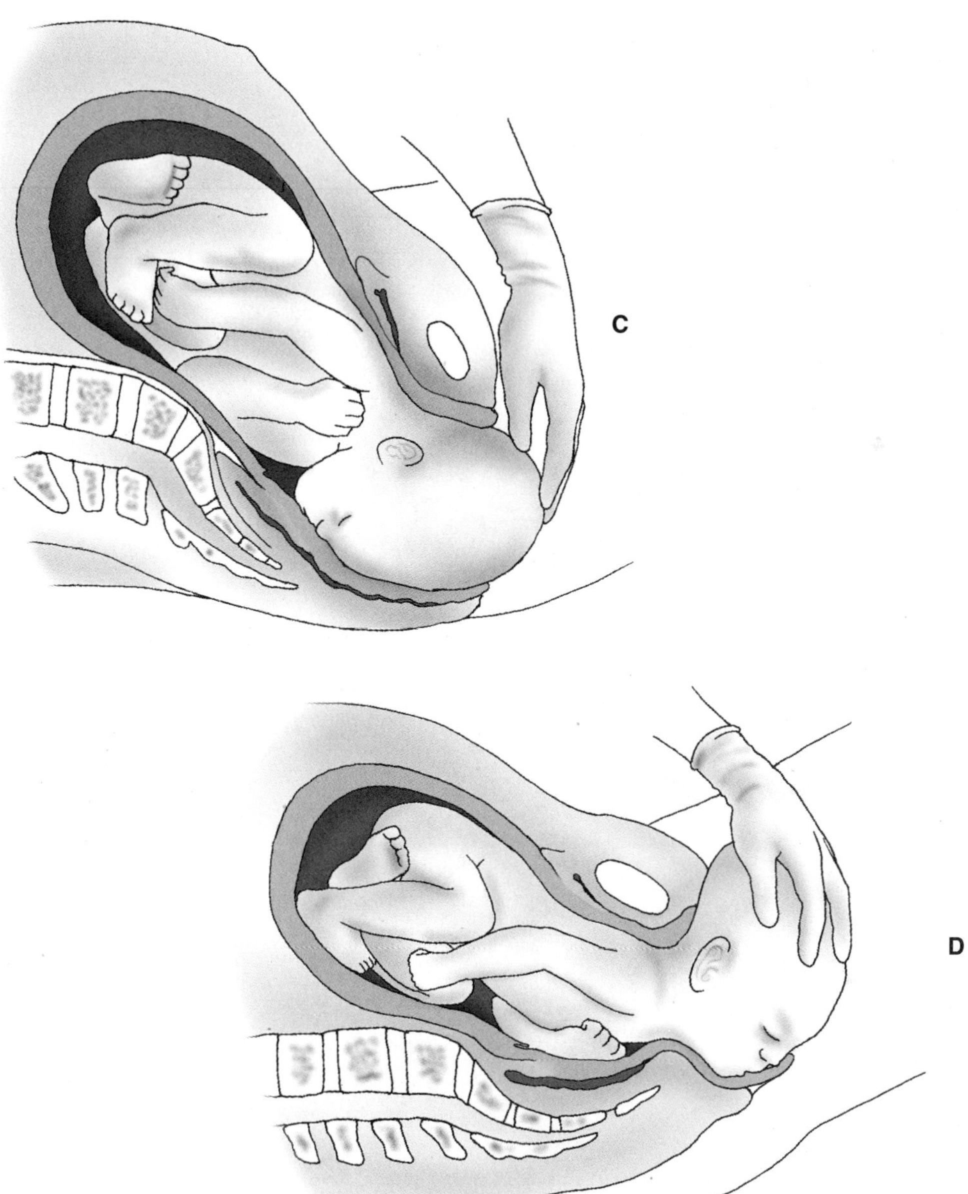

Figure 17-9, cont'd Mechanisms of labor—**C,** fetal neck impinging under maternal symphysis pubis with fetal head still in flexion; **D,** birth of head by extension.

Continued

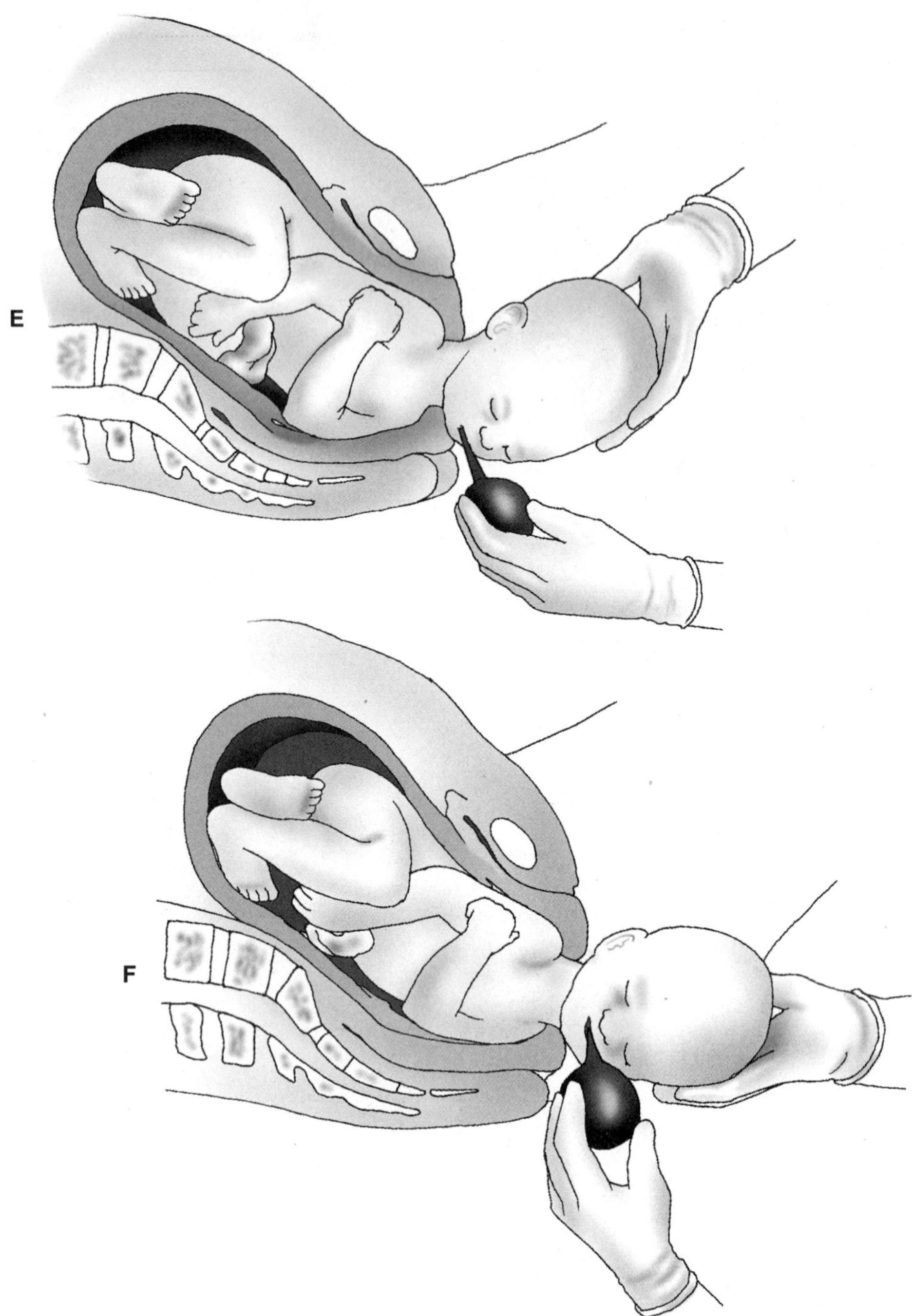

Figure 17-9, cont'd Mechanisms of labor—**E,** restitution; **F,** external rotation.

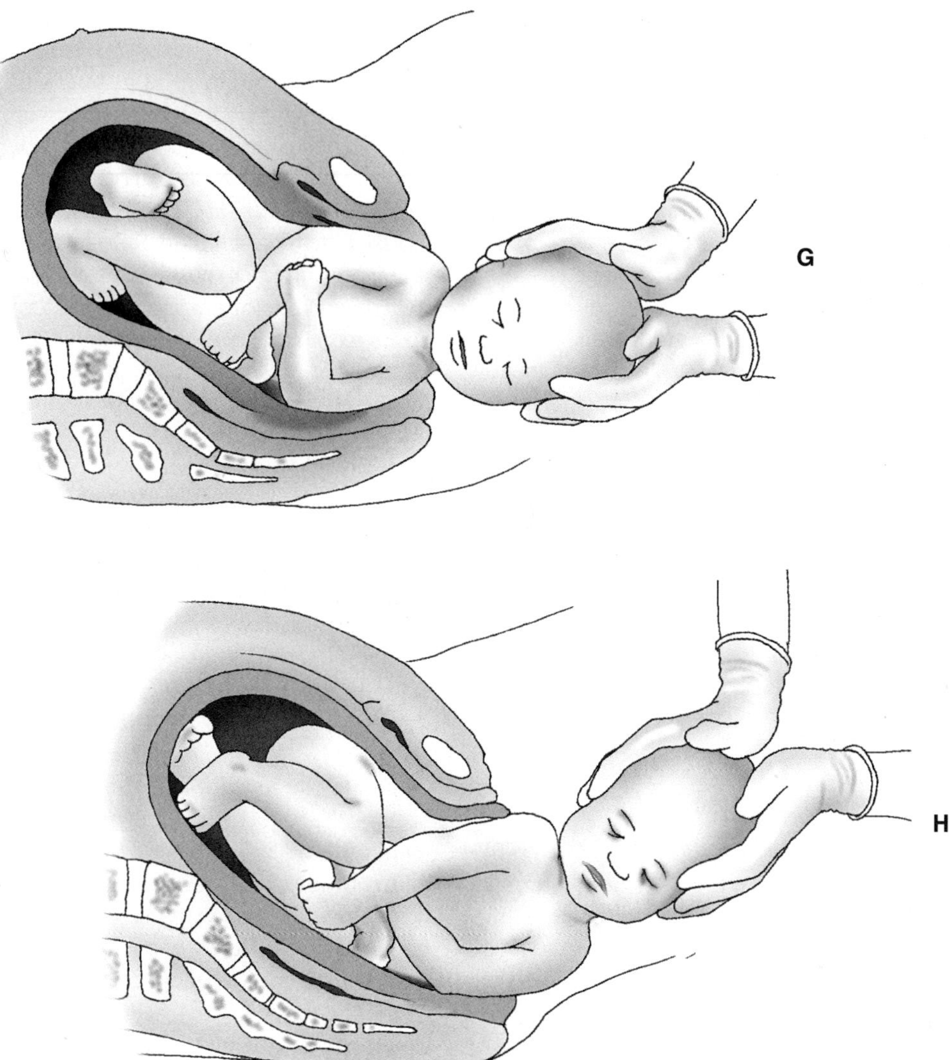

Figure 17-9, cont'd Mechanisms of labor—G, delivery of anterior shoulder; H, delivery of the posterior shoulder.

Restitution

When the head is birthed, the lack of resistance allows it to spontaneously rotate 45 degrees to the left, thereby putting it into alignment with the body (Figure 17-9, *E*).

External Rotation

For the transverse diameters of the shoulders to enter the widest diameter of the pelvic outlet, the anteroposterior diameter, the fetus's body needs to rotate 45 degrees further to the left. This brings the sagittal suture into the left transverse position and the anterior shoulder directly under the pubic arch. The anterior shoulder is usually delivered first, quickly followed by the posterior shoulder (Figure 17-9, *F-H*).

Expulsion

Once the shoulders are delivered, the rest of the body is birthed quickly. Birth of the trunk occurs by lateral flexion, following the normal curve of the birth canal.

MECHANISMS OF LABOR—VERTEX PRESENTATION (RIGHT OCCIPITOANTERIOR)

When the fetus is in the right occipitoanterior (ROA) position, it follows cardinal movements similar to those in the LOA position. The fetus enters the pelvis with the occiput in the maternal right anterior aspect of the pelvis and the sagittal suture in the left oblique position. With descent and flexion the fetus negotiates the inlet and midpelvis and then meets the resistance of the pelvic floor. Internal rotation involves rotation of the fetal head 45 degrees anterior so that the occiput is directly under the symphysis pubis. Birth of the head is by extension, and the fetal head then restitutes 45 degrees to the right, where it is realigned with the body. External rotation brings the sagittal suture into the transverse position with the shoulders in the anteroposterior position. Expulsion occurs with delivery of the shoulders and birth of the body by lateral flexion. Figure 17-9 illustrates the mechanisms of labor for the fetus in ROA position.

MECHANISMS OF LABOR—VERTEX PRESENTATION (LEFT OCCIPITOPOSTERIOR)

When there is a roomy posterior pelvis or there is compromise in the diameters of the anterior pelvis, the fetus assumes a posterior position. In the left occipitoposterior (LOP) position, descent and flexion bring the fetus into the pelvis, with the occiput in the maternal left posterior aspect of the pelvis and the sagittal suture in the left oblique position. The fetal head does not conform to the diameters of the maternal pelvis as well as when there is an anterior position, so the head may be somewhat deflexed. This increases the diameters of the presenting part and may inhibit descent. When the fetal head meets the resistance of the pelvic floor, it rotates either anteriorly or posteriorly, depending on the size and shape of the maternal bony pelvis and the size and shape of the fetal head.

Anterior Rotation (Long Arc Rotation)

With the resistance of the pelvic floor, the fetal head rotates 45 degrees anterior, bringing it into the left occipitotransverse position. Anterior rotation continues until the occiput lies directly under the symphysis pubis. The total rotation from LOP has been 135 degrees. From this position the mechanisms of labor are similar to the birth of fetuses in the anterior vertex positions. Birth of the head is by extension, and the head restitutes to align with the body. With long arc rotation the body may rotate somewhat, bringing the shoulders into the anteroposterior position. In this case further external rotation is unnecessary since the shoulders are already in the diameter with the largest dimensions for birth. If the fetal body has remained in the previous LOP position, external rotation from the oblique position of the shoulders to the anteroposterior position is necessary. Once delivery of the shoulders is accomplished, the remainder of the body is delivered by lateral extension. Figure 17-10 summarizes long arc rotation.

Posterior Rotation (Short Arc Rotation)

When the posterior portion of the pelvis is the roomiest part, the fetal head rotates posteriorly 45 degrees so that the occiput lies over the coccyx. Since the fetal head cannot rotate smoothly under the symphysis pubis as in anterior positioning, birth of the head occurs by flexion rather than extension. The clinician can assist the delivery of the head by maintaining counterpressure, ensuring complete flexion until the biparietal diameters pass through the introitus. Once the widest transverse diameter of the head has been born, the head passively extends and restitutes back to the LOP position. Further 45-degree rotation anteriorly then completes external rotation, and the shoulders rest in the anteroposterior position. The anterior shoulder pivots under the symphysis pubis, and the posterior shoulder is delivered. Expulsion of the body is by lateral flexion. Figure 17-11 summarizes short arc rotation.

MECHANISMS OF LABOR—VERTEX PRESENTATION (RIGHT OCCIPITOPOSTERIOR)

With descent and flexion the fetal head enters the pelvis with the occiput in the right posterior aspect of the maternal pelvis and the sagittal suture in the right oblique position. The fetal head rotates either anteriorly or posteriorly, similar to the mechanisms of the LOP position. If the fetal head rotates anteriorly, it then follows the anterior mechanisms of extension, restitution, external rotation, and expulsion. If the fetal head rotates posteriorly, it is delivered by flexion, the shoulders are delivered following restitution and external rotation, and the expulsion delivers the rest of the body.

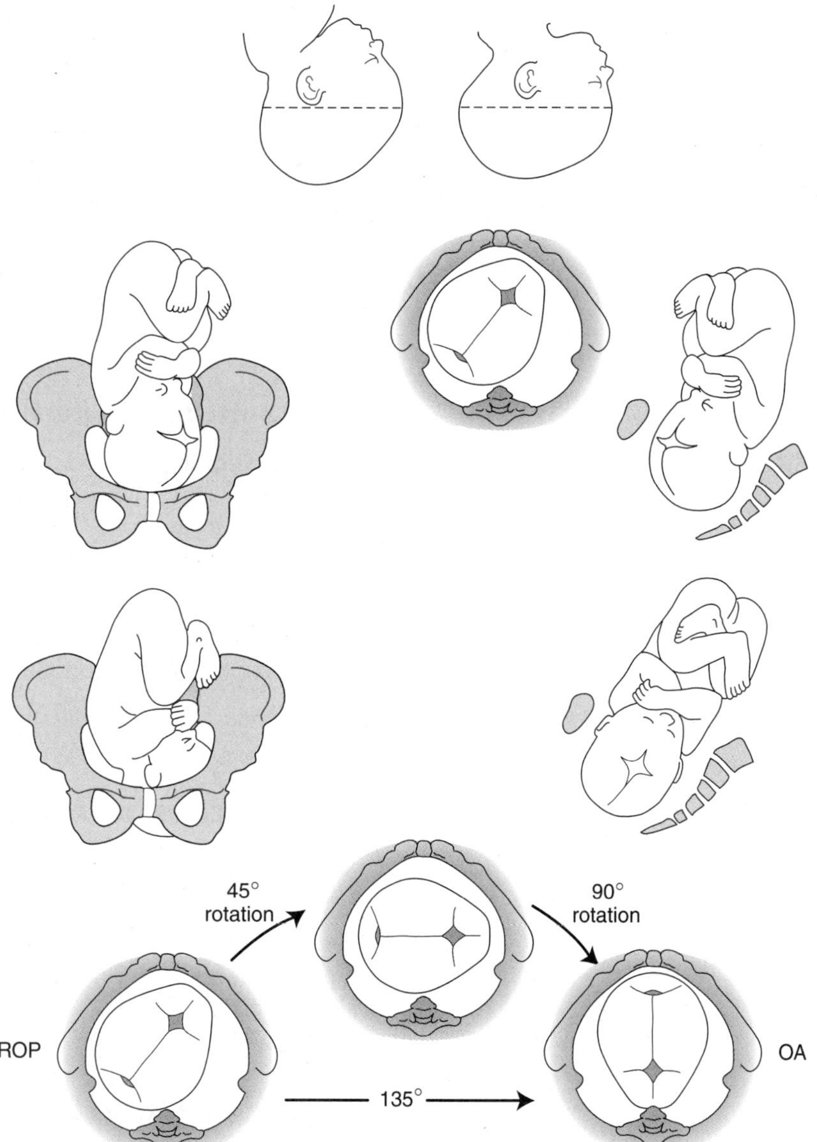

Figure 17-10 Long arc rotation.

MECHANISMS OF LABOR—BREECH PRESENTATION (RIGHT SACROANTERIOR)

When the fetus enters the pelvis in breech presentation, several factors affect the progress of labor. First, the buttocks in frank breech and the feet and buttocks in complete and footling breeches are not as effective dilators as the round, firm fetal head. Second, when the fetus is in frank breech presentation, the legs that are extended against the trunk act like a splint, decreasing the maneuverability of the fetus as it negotiates the curve of the birth canal. Finally, the after-coming head does not have the opportunity to mold, so that the head remains round with larger diameters than if it had molded. Birth of the fetus in breech presentation requires mechanisms of labor to deliver three diameters and planes: (1) the buttocks and lower limbs, (2) the shoulders, and (3) the head. Figure 17-12 illustrates the cardinal movements for breech birth.

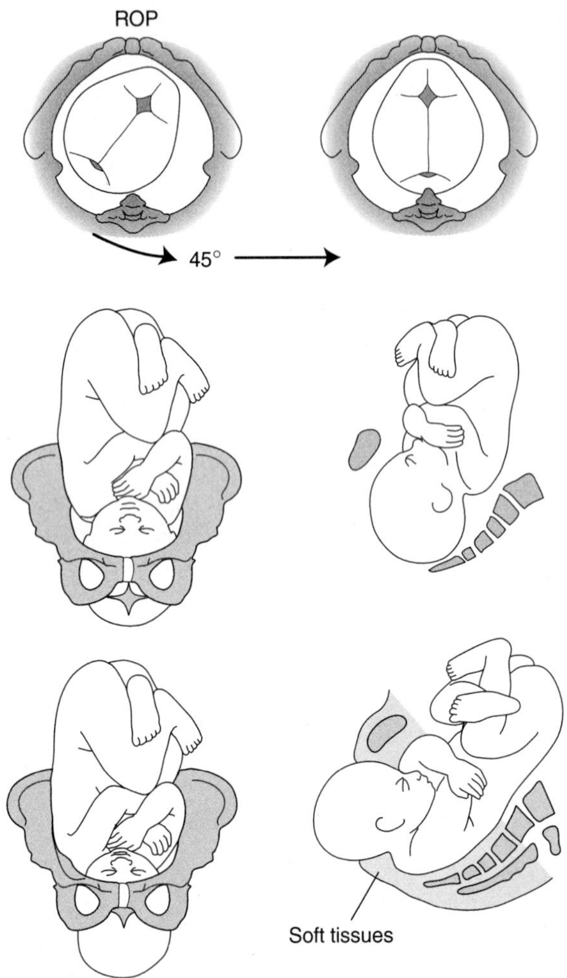

Figure 17-11 Short arc rotation.

Descent

Fetuses in breech presentation usually enter the pelvis with the bitrochanteric diameter in the oblique diameter of the inlet. In right sacroanterior (RSA) the sacrum is in the right anterior aspect of the maternal pelvis, and the bitrochanteric diameter is in the right oblique diameter. The presenting part becomes engaged when the bitrochanteric diameter passes the pelvic inlet. At this point vaginal examination may reveal that the station of the presenting part is −2 to −4 (in the system using fifths) since there is not much mass to the fetal buttocks. Descent may be very slow, and in some cases the buttocks may not descend to zero station until full dilation and rupture of the membranes.

Flexion

Lateral flexion as the fetus negotiates the midpelvis and pelvic outlet assists the descent.

Internal Rotation of the Breech

As the anterior hip meets resistance of the pelvic floor musculature, the hip rotates 45 degrees anterior. This brings the bitrochanteric diameter into the anteroposterior diameter and the sacrum into the right transverse position (right sacrotransverse [RST]).

Birth of Buttocks by Lateral Flexion

The anterior hip impinges against the symphysis pubis, and the posterior hip is pushed anteriorly. Once the posterior hip passes through the introitus and there is no further resistance, the hips shift toward the anus, and the right hip slides under the symphysis.

Engagement of the Shoulders

With further descent of the fetus, the shoulders enter the inlet in the right oblique diameter. This is considered engagement of the shoulders, and, when this occurs, the sacrum rotates from RST to RSA.

Internal Rotation of the Shoulders

As the anterior shoulder meets resistance at the symphysis pubis, it rotates 45 degrees anteriorly, bringing the bisacromial diameter into the anteroposterior position.

Birth of the Shoulders by Lateral Flexion

With the anterior shoulder impinged against the symphysis, the posterior shoulder delivers over the perineum. This movement flexes the body first anteriorly; then with posterior flexion the anterior shoulder slides under the symphysis and is delivered.

Descent and Engagement of the Fetal Head

As the shoulders are birthed, the fetal head enters the inlet of the pelvis. The occiput is in the right anterior aspect of the pelvis, and the sagittal suture is in the left oblique diameter.

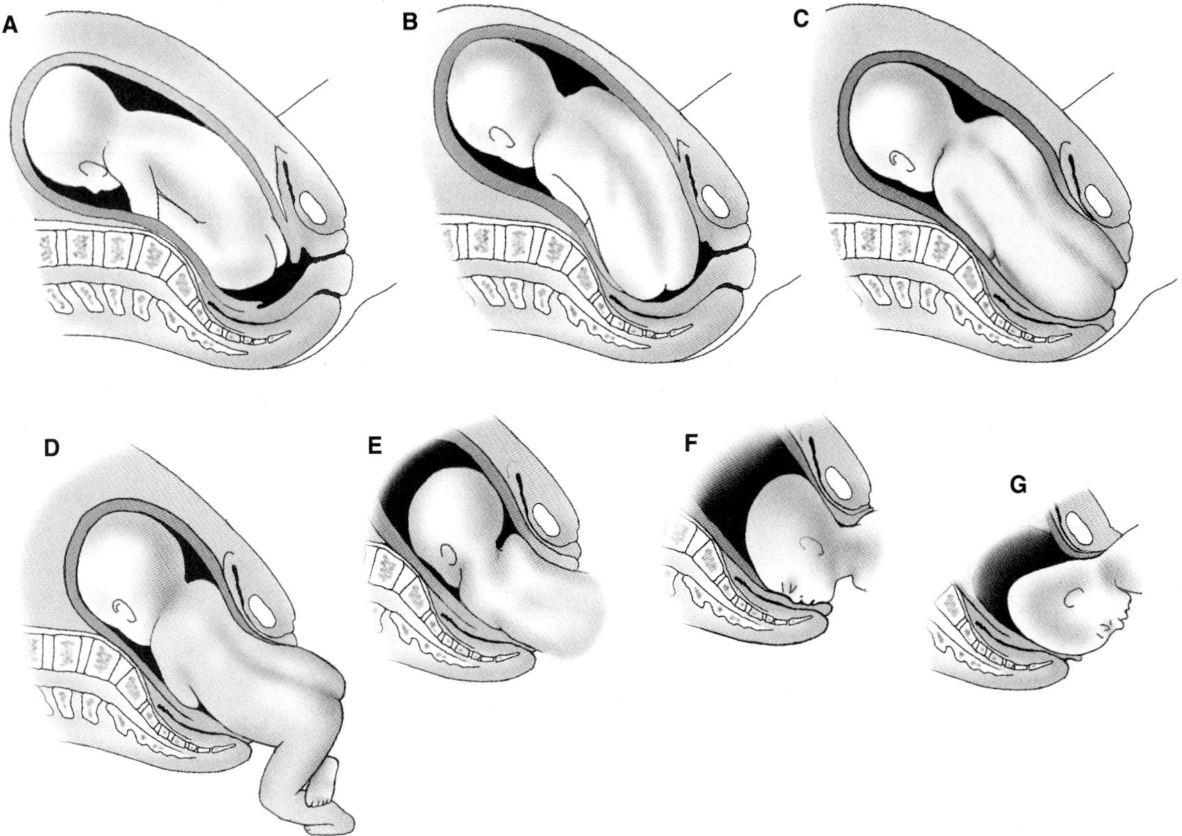

Figure 17-12 Mechanisms of labor—breech. **A,** Breech before onset of labor; **B,** engagement and internal rotation; **C,** lateral flexion; **D,** external rotation or restitution; **E,** internal rotation of shoulders and head; **F,** face rotates to sacrum when occiput is anterior; **G,** head is born by gradual flexion during elevation of fetal body.

Flexion

Flexion has been encouraged by the pressure of the uterine fundus before labor and the small chin with poor neck control in the fetus. Flexion must be present to decrease the diameters of the fetal head.

Internal Rotation of the Fetal Head

As the mass of the cranium meets resistance at the level of the pelvic floor, the occiput rotates anteriorly, bringing it under the symphysis pubis. The sagittal suture is then in the anteroposterior position, and the brow is in the posterior pelvis. The fetal back is anterior ("back up").

Birth of the Head by Flexion

The occiput pivots under the pubic arch, and the fetal face slips over the perineum, with the head remaining in a flexed position.

MECHANISMS OF LABOR—BREECH PRESENTATION (LEFT SACROANTERIOR)

The mechanisms of labor for the fetus in the left sacroanterior position are similar to those of the RSA, except that the hips, shoulders, and head rotate from the maternal left rather than the right.

MECHANISMS OF LABOR—BREECH PRESENTATION (SACROPOSTERIOR)

If the fetus rotates so that the head enters the pelvis in a posterior position, the fetal face impinges on the symphysis, and the occiput is in the hollow of the sacrum. In this position it is easy for the fetal head to extend, resulting in more pronounced impingement of the chin on the symphysis. In a term infant delivery in this position is almost impossible. For this reason, even if the fetus has entered the pelvis in the right or left sacroposterior position, once the hips are birthed, assisted rotation so that the back is anterior is necessary to facilitate the vaginal birth.

MECHANISMS OF LABOR—FACE PRESENTATION (LEFT MENTOANTERIOR)

Face presentation is associated with anomalies; thus, when it is suspected before labor, ultrasound anatomy scanning is recommended to identify structural anomalies that may influence management of labor (Figure 17-3). In about one third of face presentations anencephaly is present (Seeds and Walsh, 1996). Diagnosis of face presentation can be made by abdominal palpation when the cephalic prominence is noted on the same side as the fetal back, but only about 5% of infants in this position are identified this way (Seeds and Walsh, 1996). Vaginal examination identifies the soft face, which can be confused with a breech presentation. Eliciting a suck response when the examiner's finger is inserted into the mouth is diagnostic. Ultrasound imaging confirms the diagnosis.

In 60% to 70% of infants in face presentation, the mentum is anterior. Some of those with mentum transverse or mentum posterior will rotate during labor into the mentum anterior position. The chance of a successful vaginal delivery in a term pregnancy is nearly impossible when the mentum is posterior.

Descent

The fetus descends into the pelvis with the chin in the left anterior aspect of the maternal pelvis and the forehead in the right posterior aspect of the pelvis. When the chin is at the level of the ischial spines, the widest diameters of the fetal head have not yet entered the inlet.

Internal Rotation

When the chin meets resistance of the pelvic floor, it rotates 45 degrees anteriorly and rests under the symphysis pubis. This internal rotation may not occur until immediately before the birth.

Flexion

Similar to posterior vertex positions, the head is birthed by flexion. With the submental aspect of the fetal neck impinged behind the pubic arch, flexion allows the head to pivot around the symphysis. As the head flexes, the mouth, nose, forehead, vertex, and occiput slide over the perineum.

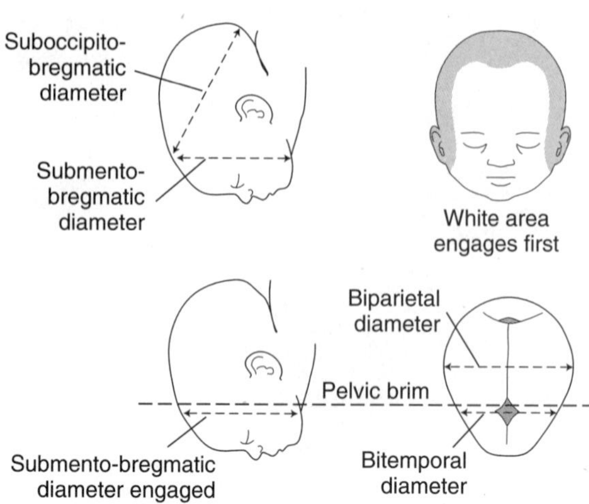

Figure 17-13 Fetal head diameters—face presentation.

Restitution

Once the resistance of the pelvic musculature is gone, the head rotates 45 degrees toward the left, aligning it with the fetal body.

External Rotation

As the anterior shoulder meets resistance at the pelvic floor, it rotates anteriorly, bringing the bisacromial diameter into the anteroposterior diameter of the pelvis. The chin rotates to the left mentotransverse position.

Expulsion by Lateral Flexion

Once the shoulders are in the anteroposterior diameter, they are delivered similarly to births with vertex presentation. The anterior shoulder passes under the pubic arch, and the posterior shoulder delivers over the perineum. The rest of the body is then birthed in lateral flexion, following the normal curve of the birth canal.

REFERENCES

Cunningham FG et al: *Williams obstetrics,* ed 20, Stamford, Conn, 1997, Appleton & Lange.

Seeds JW, Walsh M: Malpresentations. In Gabbe SG, Niebyl JR, Simpson JL, editors: *Obstetrics—normal and problem pregnancies,* New York, 1996, Churchill Livingstone.

Chapter 18

Maintenance of Comfort and Management of Pain

Barbara Petree, RN, MSN
and Linda V. Walsh, CNM, PhD

Although the biologic aspects of labor and delivery are universal, the perception of comfort and distress during the birthing process is mediated by culture. Jordan (1993) and Lozoff, Jordan, and Malone (1988) argue that a biosocial framework considers that the biologic function of birth and the sociocultural matrix of behaviors surrounding birth need to be analyzed together to understand a woman's birth experience. Pain is a "recognized and expected part of the birth process in almost all societies" (Jordan, 1993), but it is the personal perception of the pain, the external behaviors demonstrated in response to the pain, and the cultural understanding of the role of pain in the birthing process that vary among communities. The cultural role of the birth attendant and the acceptance of interventions that influence pain and response to pain reflect the beliefs held by members of a society.

Jordan's classic studies of birth in the Yucatan, the Netherlands, Sweden, and the United States (1993) provide dramatic illustrations of the differing expectations and approaches to discomfort during parturition. In the United States pain relief is available but controlled by the medical attendant. The woman needs to convince the birth attendant of her need for pain relief (i.e., the well-prepared woman who has attended childbirth classes chooses a physician who is known to recommend epidural analgesia as soon as the contractions become regular and strong, or the unprepared, fearful woman cries out as she finds she cannot cope). This is in contrast to care in Sweden, where medication is widely used, but the decision to use any intervention is totally in the hands of the laboring woman. The Dutch and Mayan women studied held vastly different views of the childbearing process. In these cultures birthing is seen as a natural function of the woman's body, and it is expected that women will be able to cope with the support of others in the birthing room. In these cultural contexts medication is used only in extremely unusual, medically complicated cases.

Because of the strong influence of culture on the woman's experience during birthing, it is important that the provider consider more than Western medicine's interpretation of the safety or effectiveness of a given intervention during labor. Comfort measures such as ambulation or use of pharmacologic agents may conflict with the woman's belief system, thereby causing internal conflict that may affect her perception of the experience and her transition to her maternal role.

This chapter reviews the biologic and cultural aspects of comfort and pain in labor and delivery, as well as present commonly used approaches for maintenance of comfort and relief of pain.

ETIOLOGY OF PAIN IN LABOR

Anatomic and Physiologic Components of Pain

Perception of pain depends on an intact neurologic network. The neurophysiology of pain follows a predictable process:

1. Noxious stimuli are introduced through receptors found in the skin, subcutaneous tissue, joints, muscles, periosteum, fascia, and viscera. Nociceptors (pain receptors) are terminals of small A delta fibers that are activated by mechanical or heat stimuli and C afferent fibers that are activated by mechanical, thermal or chemical stimuli (Bonica and McDonald, 1995). The nociceptive stimuli below the level of the head are transmitted across these afferent fibers to the dorsal horn of the spinal cord.
2. Stimuli are then transmitted through extremely complex structures containing a variety of neurons and synaptic arrangements that facilitate a high degree of processing of sensory input. Some of the impulses are then transmitted through internuncial neurons to the anterior and anterolateral horn cells, where they stimulate neurons that supply skeletal muscles and sympathetic neurons that supply blood vessels, viscera, and sweat glands. Other nociceptive impulses are transmitted to ascending systems that articulate with the brain stem.
3. Impulses ascending to the brain stem are then routed to the hypothalamus which regulates the autonomic system and neuroendocrine response to stress, and to the cerebral cortex which provides a cognitive function that is based on past experience, judgment and emotions (Bonica and McDonald, 1995).

During the first stage of labor, pain is primarily experienced because of stimulation of nociceptors in the adnexa, uterus, and pelvic ligaments. Most studies support the theory that first-stage labor pain is the result of dilation of the cervix and lower uterine segment, with resultant distention, stretching, and trauma to the muscle fibers and supporting ligaments in those structures (Bonica and McDonald, 1995) proposes that the following factors support this theory:

1. Stretching of smooth muscles has been shown to be a stimulus for visceral pain. The intensity of pain experienced with contractions is associated with the degree and rapidity of dilation of cervical and lower uterine segment.
2. The intensity and timing of pain is associated with the build-up of intrauterine pressure which contributes to the dilation of the structures. Early in labor, there is a slow build-up of pressure, and pain is perceived approximately 20 seconds after the initiation of the uterine contraction. Later in labor, there is a faster buildup of pressure with a resulting minimal lag time before perception of pain.
3. When the cervix is dilated quickly in nonlaboring women, they experience pain similar to that which is felt during uterine contractions.

Although mechanical stimulation of the nociceptors is most likely the primary source of the impulses, the presence of chemical nociceptive mediators, including bradykinins, prostaglandins, serotonin, and lactic acid, has also been suggested (Brownridge, 1995).

First-stage labor stimuli are transmitted from the afferent fibers through the inferior, middle, and superior hypogastric plexus, the lumbar and lower thoracic sympathetic chain, to the posterior nerve root ganglia at the level of T10 through L1. Pain may be referred from the pelvic area to the umbilicus, upper thighs, and midsacral area. With fetal descent, usually in the second stage, the stimuli are transmitted via the pudendal nerves through the sacral plexus to the posterior nerve root ganglia at levels S2 through S4.

During the early part of second stage of labor, when there is no further resistance from the cervix, pain is still experienced because of the continued distention of the lower uterine segment. However, as the fetus descends in the pelvis, pain caused by distention of the anterior third of the vagina and the perineum replaces the deep visceral pain. Pressure and trauma to the fascia, subcutaneous tissues, and skeletal muscles stimulate the nociceptors and shift the locus of pain externally. Pressure on the roots of the lumbosacral plexus leads to pain in the thighs, legs, vagina, perineum, and rectum (Brownridge, 1995) (Figure 18-1).

Other factors may influence the perception of pain during labor. Age, with its many confounding social variables, may increase incidence and severity of pain. Extremely young and older mothers report higher levels of labor pain. Parity may influence pain perception, with primiparae experiencing more pain in early labor and multiparae experiencing increased levels of pain later in the labor process with rapid descent in second-stage labor. It has been suggested that women with contracted pelves, higher weight for height, large babies, or babies in abnormal presentations report higher levels of pain. There is also evidence that women with a history

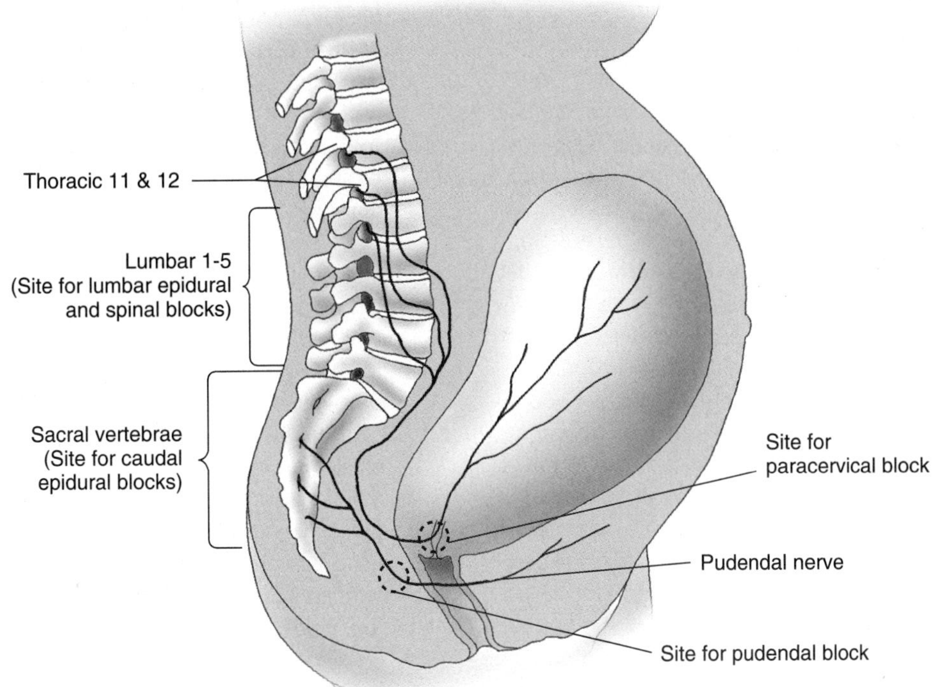

Figure 18-1 Pain pathways in labor.

of dysmenorrhea may experience increased perception of pain, possibly because of the production of excess prostaglandins. Time of day has also been found to be associated with severity of labor pain: significantly lower ratings of pain were noted in labors in which the second stage started at night (Harkness and Gijsbers, 1989).

Research suggests that anxiety is associated with increased pain in labor. The influence of preparation for birth, beliefs and values, and support will be addressed below in the cultural context of coping and pain. However, it should be remembered that excessive anxiety may produce increased nociceptive stimuli at the level of the cerebral cortex, as well as increased catecholamine secretion that will further increase nociceptive stimuli in the pelvis because of decreased blood flow and increased muscle tension (Lowe, 1996).

Physiologic responses to pain include hyperventilation, which may lead to maternal hypocarbia ($PaCO_2$ 15 to 20 mm Hg) and respiratory alkalosis (pH 7.55 to 7.60) (Brownridge, 1995). These changes can further lead to nausea, fatigue, mental confusion, tetany, pallor, and sweating. Pain-mediated stimulation of the autonomic nervous system may contribute to further delay in gastric emptying time and decreased intestinal peristalsis.

Several theories have been proposed to understand the nature of pain perception, coping, and control in labor. Perhaps best known is the gate control theory, which proposes that stimuli can be modified at the levels of the spinal cord, brain stem, and cortex to effectively block the processing of the impulse in the brain. It is thought that cells in the gray matter of the spinal cord, substantia gelatinosa, block transfer by limiting the action of the T cells that are responsible for transmitting the impulses. This mechanism can be initiated through separate stimulation of the skin (e.g., massage or acupressure) or stimulation of the brain stem, thalamus, and cerebral cortex (e.g., conscious relaxation, alterations in sensory stimulation).

Endogenous pain control theory proposes that chemicals released from the pituitary gland (enkephalins) bind to opiate receptors, where they inhibit neuron transmission of painful stimuli. Endorphin is the most well known of these chemicals. Endorphin levels are known to increase as labor progresses, and it has been proposed that many of the nonpharmacologic approaches to pain relief may further facilitate production. Conversely there is evidence that exogenous opiates may inhibit normal endorphin levels by binding with the available receptor sites.

Cultural Aspects of Coping and Pain Perception

How a community conceptualizes birth shapes the decisions made regarding the appropriate site, attendant, and process of care that a woman chooses for her birth experience. As noted above, birth is expected to be a stressful but normal part of family life in the Yucatan; a natural process in the Netherlands; and an intense, fulfilling achievement in Sweden (Jordan, 1993). In the United States the medicotechnical approach to birth has become the norm, and use of medically provided interventions to relieve pain (as well as control the process of labor) is expected (Davis-Floyd, 1993; Jordan, 1993). Even interventions such as prepared childbirth, which were developed in response to the perception of overuse of medical technology, have become a part of the medical approach to birth, as evidenced by the number of hospital-sponsored classes that inform the participants of the usual interventions to expect. It is important for providers to remember that our Western, American approach may clash with the beliefs held by women who bring other cultural values to their childbearing experiences.

Areas that may provoke cultural clashes include the following:

1. *Authority figure in the birthing process.* The American medical system places the obstetrician in the central role of decision-making during childbearing. Professional position papers, editorial opinions, and testimony regarding regulatory activities argue that, because of the years of specialist medical training, the obstetrician is the most appropriate expert—the "captain of the ship." This approach fails to recognize the importance of other specialist and nonspecialist attendants during birth, including the woman's family, neighbors, and friends. Many U.S. hospitals now allow laboring women to have a specified number of support people (rarely more than three), but restrictions on whom those individuals can be still exist. In many cultures the authority figure for the woman may be a respected elder or traditional healer. Or, as in Sweden, the woman may be respected as the expert regarding her needs in labor, and, although the professional is expected to give objective information about all options, the woman is the one who makes the decision if and when medication will be used.
2. *Site of birth.* Although there is a small but increasing proportion of births occurring in out-of-hospital settings in the United States, the norm for site of birth is still considered to be the hospital. This environment may be very different from that of the home or community clinic expected by some women. The hospital may represent illness or death, when the cultural belief is that birth is natural and best supported without medical intervention, unless there are complications.
3. *Activity during the birth process.* Although there appears to be an increase in acceptance for ambulation during labor in the United States, it is still the norm for hospitalized laboring women to be restricted to bed rest. Cultures that view birth as natural often expect that the woman will continue her usual activities until discomfort causes her to seek support from others. Often that support then will include massage and other physical approaches by nonprofessional individuals. Restriction in activity may increase the woman's discomfort, thereby lessening her coping abilities.
4. *Beliefs about parts of the body.* Non-Western cultures may hold beliefs that conflict with common interventions used in Western, American birth. For example, piercing or cutting the body may be considered improper because of fear of harming an area that holds the soul. Thus surgery or injections hold a very different meaning to women in this context.
5. *Pharmacologic intervention.* The perceived need for and use of medication for the pain of childbirth must be considered in the cultural context of the woman's belief system. Dutch women who retain their cultural beliefs regarding birth neither expect nor request analgesia. In contrast, in Sweden, pain relief and sedation are common, but the woman expects a variety of options rather than one particular approach. In the United States there is a high reliance on pharmacologic agents to relieve pain, and it has been argued that women have internalized the need for medicated births (Davis-Floyd, 1993). When women migrate to other cultures, the degree of acculturation needs to be considered when evaluating the desire and need for pharmacologic intervention.

Ideally the provider should have the opportunity to begin discussion about beliefs about childbirth during the prenatal period. It is important to establish the woman's expectations before she presents to the labor and delivery unit in pain. The woman's beliefs, desires, and concerns should be documented on the prenatal record so that intrapartal personnel will be made aware of any possible clashes.

NONPHARMACOLOGIC APPROACHES TO MAINTENANCE OF COMFORT AND PAIN MANAGEMENT

Prepared Childbirth

Although childbirth preparation in the medical model of care was introduced in the 1930s by Grantly Dick-Read, the educational process of preparation for childbirth came to the forefront in the late 1960s and early 1970s as consumers increasingly sought alternatives to heavily medicated, obstetrically managed birth. Most prenatal educational programs propose that, when a woman approaches labor and delivery with knowledge, confidence, a positive attitude, and practiced conditioned responses to discomfort, she will experience less obstetric intervention and will have greater satisfaction with her labor experience. Childbirth preparation programs usually incorporate a variety of nonpharmacologic approaches to pain relief.

Physical Presence

By their very presence, care providers usually provide reassurance to the laboring woman. The association between presence of another, even a stranger, has been shown to decrease length of labor and improve birth outcomes. Professional caregivers—clinicians, nurses, and doulas—are commonly seen as experts by the woman and her family, and thus their interventions, recommendations, and encouragement are usually sought during labor. A well-conducted meta-analysis that evaluated 14 randomized control trials found that "... the continuous presence of a support person reduced the likelihood of medication for pain relief, operative vaginal delivery, cesarean delivery, and a 5-minute APGAR score less than seven" (Hodnett, 2000).

The ability of professional caregivers to provide a consistent physical presence is strongly associated with the institutional staffing in the birth site. Midwives and birth assistants attending births in homes are most likely to provide ongoing one-to-one care. Out-of-hospital birth centers also are likely to provide consistent midwifery and nursing support. Midwives and nurses practicing in hospitals, especially busy perinatal units, are more likely to have assignments that include two or more women in labor. In addition, it has been found that, even when nurses are assigned in a one-to-one model of staffing, they spend little of their time providing supportive care practices (Hodnett, 1996; McNiven, Hodnett, and O'Brien-Pallas, 1992).

Relaxation and Distraction

Conscious relaxation has been found to be associated with decreased muscular tension, decreased heart rate, decreased respiratory rate, and decreased metabolism rate. Relaxation has been used in all areas of health care to decrease stress and anxiety. Conscious relaxation of muscles throughout the body during labor appears to increase the effectiveness of the uterine contractions. Preparation for conscious relaxation usually involves practice of cognitive exercises that lead to decreased tension in voluntary muscles. Relaxation can be further enhanced through control of the environment. A quiet room, soothing music, comfortable temperature, and comfortable maternal positioning all promote comfort.

The provider should be aware of the process the woman has used for her conscious relaxation to more effectively support her efforts. Even when a woman has not prepared before the birth, the provider can enhance relaxation through control of the environment and coaching through each cycle of contraction and rest. When combined with slow-paced breathing, relaxation can help the laboring woman cope more effectively with her contractions and rest more fully between contractions.

Imagery

Imagery or visualization is often taught in conjunction with conscious relaxation during childbirth preparation classes. When used effectively, imagery allows the laboring woman to substitute the immediate feelings of discomfort or pain with pleasant images that encourage relaxation. Similar to relaxation, imagery can lead to decreased muscular tension and heart and respiratory rates and a more general sense of well-being. It appears that it is more effective when practiced before labor. However, the provider or other support individual can coach the untrained woman by having her close her eyes and visualize a place where she has felt rested and safe. Concentration on the feelings she experienced when in that space will then facilitate her transferring those feelings of well-being to the present. The one study that explored the effect of teaching imagery-assisted relaxation (IAR) found no significant difference between groups when analyzing state anxiety after training, perception of intensity of pain, use of pain medication, timing of pain medication, and 1-minute APGAR scores. Physiologic measures of the woman suggested a greater degree of relaxation in the imagery assisted relaxation group, and 5-minute APGARs of infants in the IAR group were higher. However, the study was limited by small sample size and no power analysis (Lindberg and Lawlis, 1988).

Maternal Position and Position Changes

Cross-cultural study of women's choices of positions during labor suggest that women tend to select a variety of positions and frequent position changes during labor and delivery. The medical tradition of assuming bed rest during labor rests more in the perceived sick role of the laboring woman and the resulting difficulty in moving about when interventions such as intravenous hydration, continuous fetal monitoring, and sedation and anesthesia are the norm. When researchers have observed laboring women in an uncontrolled setting, they note the frequent position changes that tend to keep the woman's torso vertical. Position change, including ambulation, has been associated with less use of pain medication, more effective contractions, and greater maternal sense of control. Effects of position and position changes are summarized in Table 18-1.

Massage and Pressure

Massage is thought to assist in relaxation and decreased pain awareness by increasing blood flow to the affected areas, stimulating sensory receptors in the skin and underlying muscles, altering skin temperature, and providing a general sense of well-being associated with human closeness. Massage can vary from light stroking (effleurage) to deeper massage of skin and underlying structures. Hedstrom and Newton (1986), in their now classic study of the use of touch in labor, found that touch is universally used in labor for providing relief from pain. It is suggested that the stimulation of release of endorphins, the reduction of endogenous catecholamines, and the stimulation of afferent nerve fibers resulting in blocking of transmission of painful stimuli (gate control theory) may be instrumental in the effect of this intervention.

Acupressure

Acupressure is an ancient Eastern healing approach that uses massage of particular points in the body (meridians or energy flow lines) to decrease pain or alter organ function. Beliefs based in Eastern medicine support the explanation of its effect as facilitating the flow of energy or freeing a block in the flow through meridians. Others, more based in Western medicine, explain its success by suggesting that the pressure increases local endorphin levels. Practitioners who are more comfortable with Western medical approaches may use the term pressure point massage to describe this modality (Jungman, 1988). Research on the use of acupressure in labor is limited; however, its use for centuries in Asian countries and its inclusion in the original psychoprophylactic work done in Russia provide historical overviews of its effectiveness. One published study in an American medical journal has reported effectiveness in stimulating and inducing labor and inhibiting preterm labor (Tsueii, Lai, and Sharma, 1977)

The specific stimuli produced by acupressure are supplemented by the emotional and tactile presence of an individual support person. Additional support is generated by directed guidance that incorporates other modalities such as relaxation, visualization, and patterned breathing. The combined effect, then, is synergistic in nature.

Pressure should be applied with the fingertips or thumbs over the acupressure point, either as a nonmoving pressure or a force applied in small circular movements (Jungman, 1988). The laboring woman is expected to give feedback regarding whether the amount of pressure used is sufficient. The pressure is not directed onto a bone, but rather toward the bone, and, when applied properly, the woman may note tenderness or a tingling sensation. Pressure is usually exerted for up to 5 to 10 seconds.

During labor acupressure can be applied laterally down the length of the spine and along the arms and legs to enhance relaxation (Figure 18-2). This particular type of pressure point massage may have been taught during the couple's childbirth preparation class. The Chien-chin points, located on either side of the spine at the neck, are helpful for decreasing upper body tension. Pressure on the Shen-shu acupressure point, approximately 5 cm from the anterosuperior iliac spine on a line connecting it to the sacrum, relieves low back pain (Nichols and Zwelling, 1997). Several particular pressure points are helpful for relief of discomfort in labor. During late first-stage labor, pressure to the palm points and the Ho-Ku (Co4) points (Figure 18-3) may decrease pain. Ho-Ku points are located between the first and second metacarpals on the dorsal side of the hand. San-Yin-Chiao (Sp6) (Figure 18-4) is considered a point for difficult labors (Jungman, 1988). The point is three finger-

Table 18-1 *Physiologic Positions and Movements for Labor and Birth*

Position	Effect on labor efforts
Standing	Gravity contributes to descent of presenting part; fetal long axis is well aligned with pelvis; contractions are perceived as less painful and more productive; may increase urge to push because of better application of presenting part
Walking	Movement causes changes in pelvic joints, encouraging rotation and descent
Standing and leaning onto partner or firm surface	Relieves back pain; allows for access to back for massage and pressure; may allow for more rest in between contractions.
Leaning with swaying of body	Movement changes pelvic joints; embrace of loved one increases sense of well-being; back massage or pressure can be applied while moving
Lunge: one foot and knee flexed while the other is extended	May increase pelvic diameters
Sideway lunges done during contractions	May encourage rotation of occipitoposterior fetus
Sitting upright	Good resting position; provides some gravity effect; can be used with continuous fetal monitoring
Sitting on toilet	May help relaxation of perineum during pushing
Semisitting	Same as sitting upright
Sitting, leaning forward with support	Relieves backache
Hands and knees	Helps relieve backache; assists rotation of fetus from OP positions; facilitates pelvic rocking; takes pressure off hemorrhoids or vulvar varicosities
Kneeling with forward support	Provides less strain on hands and wrists than hands and knees
Side-lying	Provides very good resting position; convenient for necessary interventions; useful to slow a rapid second stage; easier to relax between contractions during late first and second stage of labor

Adapted from Simkin P: Reducing pain and enhancing progress in labor: a guide to nonpharmacologic methods for maternity caregivers, *Birth* 22: 161-171, 1995.

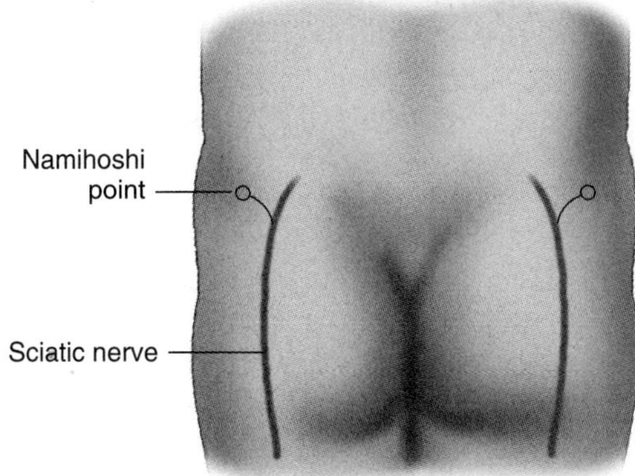

Figure 18-2 Acupressure points—spine. (From Nichols FH, Zwelling E: *Maternal-newborn nursing: theory and practice,* Philadelphia, 1997, WB Saunders, p. 839.)

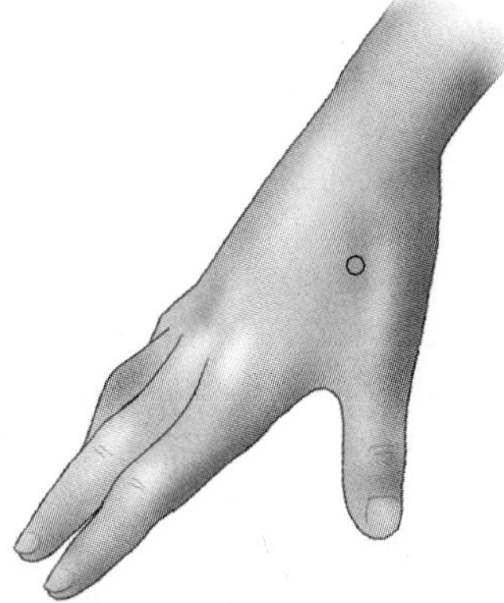

Figure 18-3 Acupressure palm points. Co4.points.

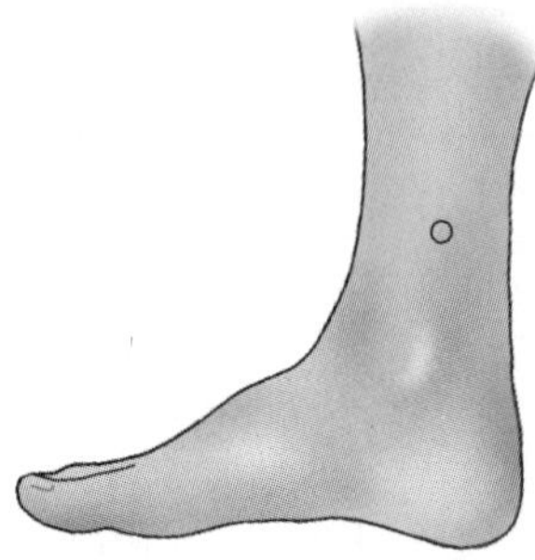

Figure 18-4 Acupressure SP6 point.

breadths superior to the inner ankle, posterior to the tibia. Pressure on both the San-Yin-Chiao and Ho-Ku points has been shown to be effective for induction of labor. For this reason, couples should be instructed not to apply pressure before 37 weeks.

Acupressure also should not be used over any tissue surface that is inflamed, irritated, or infected. Pressure and massage to the legs should be avoided in the presence of varicosities with the potential for thromboembolic activity.

Use of Local Heat and Cold Applications

Application of heat compresses to tense, painful areas is thought to relieve pain by reducing muscle spasms caused by ischemia, stimulating neurons that block further transmission of painful stimuli and causing vasodilation and increased blood flow to the area (Nichols and Zwelling, 1997; Simkin, 1995). Heat application is particularly helpful when the laboring woman is experiencing back pain caused by fetal occiput posterior position or generalized tension in the back muscles. Heat can be applied using warm moist compresses or a hot water bottle or heating pad.

Application of cold compresses decreases discomfort by reducing the sensitivity of the skin and superficial muscles by stimulation of sensory neurons (gate control theory) and by reducing inflammation or stiffness (Nichols and Zwelling, 1997). The use of cool washcloths is also soothing since the woman experiences increased heat production and resulting perspiration during active labor and pushing. Ice packs on local areas of pain or tension (e.g., with back pain) can also decrease discomfort.

Care must be taken to protect the skin and underlying tissues when using topical heat and cold. Pain thresholds can be altered during labor, and the laboring woman may not notice extreme temperatures that could produce burn or frost damage.

Hydrotherapy

It has long been recognized that immersion in water leads to muscle relaxation, increased vasodilation with resulting increased blood flow, and a general feeling of well-being. Warm baths, showers, and whirlpools most likely facilitate relaxation by stimulating cutaneous nerve endings, leading to reversal of sympathetic nervous system response (Simkin, 1995). Shower spray and whirlpooling additionally activate thermal and tactile receptors, thereby transmitting stimuli to the dorsal horn of the spinal cord and inhibiting transmission to the cerebral cortex. Historical study of childbearing support in the early twentieth century found examples of tub bathing both for relief of the discomfort of labor and stimulation of labor when the woman's stress was contributing to poor progress (Walsh, 1992). The use of water jet hydrotherapy may provide even greater relief than simple immersion since the flow of water can be directed at distinct areas of discomfort. Research exploring the safety and effectiveness of hydrotherapy has been limited by small sample sizes and numerous descriptive rather than experimental studies. One randomized control trial found that women who used the tub during labor were less likely to use narcotic or epidural analgesia, less likely to require instrumental assistance at delivery, and more likely to deliver over an intact perineum (Rush et al., 1996). A meta-analysis of three randomized control trials evaluating use of water immersion during labor found that immersion during first stage of labor was associated with a trend to decreased use of pain relief methods, and the authors concluded that, although no adverse effects were reported, further research is necessary to determine safety of immersion on the fetus and newborn (Nikodem, 2000).

Use of hydrotherapy may be limited by lack of access to tubs and institutional concerns regarding safety and liability. The CNM Data Group (1998) reported use of hydrotherapy in only 15% of labors in their nine institutions. Fear of an increase in infection, especially in cases with ruptured membranes, is often cited as a reason to prohibit bathing. One systematic review (Simkin, 1995) found no increase difference in chorioamnionitis, endometritis, or neonatal infections when comparing patients who used tubs in labor and those who did not. Obviously a rigorous cleaning procedure with evaluation by periodic cultures is necessary for infection control. Concerns are also raised regarding fetal assessment while the woman is laboring in water. Intermittent fetal monitoring can be continued using a doptone or fetoscope.

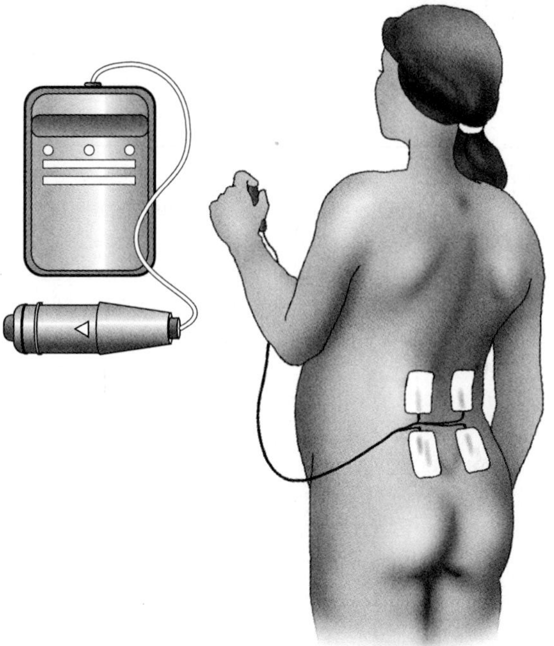

Figure 18-5 TENS unit.

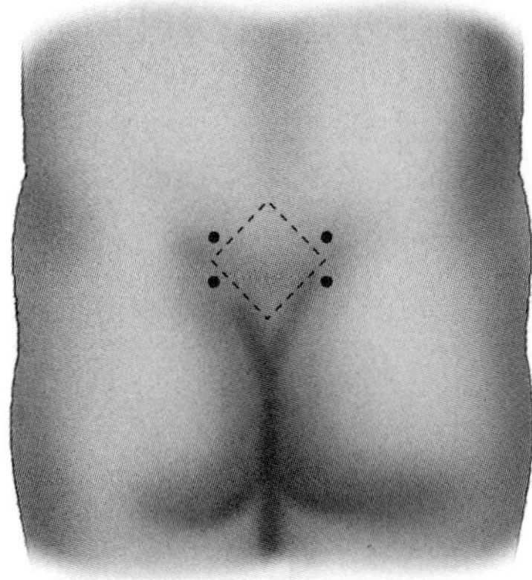

Figure 18-6 Sterile water papule injections.

Transcutaneous Electrical Nerve Stimulation (TENS)

Although transcutaneous electrical nerve stimulation (TENS) is primarily being used in physical therapy for chronic pain and postsurgical patients, it is sometimes used in labor. TENS units are handheld, battery-operated devices that are connected to the skin of the lower back at the level of T10 to L1 by two pairs of electronic pads (Figure 18-5).

When the electrodes are activated, the unit delivers pulsed alternating current to the muscles, and the woman senses a tingling feeling in the tissues being stimulated. It is theorized that analgesia is achieved either by blocking impulses to the pain through the increase in afferent neuron transmission (gate control theory) or by stimulating local release of endorphins (Harrison, et al., 1986). The results of randomized control trials suggest that women who use TENS have decreased use of epidural analgesia and are generally satisfied with its use (Simkin, 1995). An occasional side effect is skin irritation caused by the electrode leads. Furthermore, the trials found no untoward fetal or neonatal effects. TENS seems to be most helpful when women have been taught how to use and control the device during the prenatal period and when it is initiated early in labor. TENS units are available only through prescription and are usually distributed through the physical therapy departments of agencies/institutions.

Intradermal Injections of Sterile Water

Approximately one third of laboring women experience back pain with labor, and the intensity is often described as severe. Administration of narcotics is often ineffective in relieving this type of pain. TENS has been shown to be effective, but the procedure requires special apparatus and is most effective when women have practiced the technique before labor. Epidural and spinal analgesia and anesthesia may be effective but require specially prepared medical personnel and equipment. Several investigators in Europe have explored the use of intradermal injections of sterile water over the skin of the lower back, and findings suggested that the procedure significantly decreased pain scores—often dramatically (Ader, Hansson, and Wallin, 1990; Trolle et al., 1991). It is proposed that the mechanism of action is that the sterile water injection stimulates endogenous endorphins and/or provides stimulation to the rami of T10-L1, thereby preventing further transmission of the stimuli from the cervix and lower uterine segment.

Two injections are administered bilaterally over the posterior superior iliac spines; additional injections are administered bilaterally 2 cm inferior and 1 cm medial to the first (Figure 18-6). The sites correspond with those used for TENS and acupressure. Lytzen, Cederberg, and Moller-Nielsen (1989) note that "no great accuracy was required." Sterile water (0.1 ml) is injected intracutaneously using a Mantoux syringe; the injection produces a small white papule. Women experience a sharp burning pain with the injection, with relief in about 30 seconds. Relief of back pain usually occurs within several minutes and lasts for at least 2 hours.

PHARMACOLOGIC APPROACHES TO PAIN MANAGEMENT

Physiologic Considerations in the Use of Pharmacologic Agents

Physiologic and anatomic changes in pregnancy must be taken into account when one is considering use of pharmacologic agents in labor and delivery.

Pulmonary Changes. It is important that pulmonary changes be considered when considering general anesthesia or medical management of medical complications in pregnancy. Venous engorgement and mucosal edema increase the risk of airway obstruction or trauma during intubation. Changes in the diameters of the chest cavity—increased chest circumference, elevated diaphragm, increased abdominal pressure on the diaphragm—make ventilation via mask and intubation more difficult. Stress of labor with increased minute ventilation may increase the normal slight alkalotic shift to frank respiratory alkalosis. In this situation the resting time between contractions may result in hypoventilation secondary to decreased respiratory drive in response to CO_2 (Driver, 1997). When the maternal PaO_2 falls below 70 mm Hg, the fetus may experience decreased PaO_2 with resultant late decelerations. Partial relief of pain (e.g., with narcotics) decreases hyperventilation but may further depress respirations between contractions.

Cardiac changes. Much of the increased cardiac output is directed to the uterine-placental unit. Consequently, uterine hemorrhage can lead to rapid exsanguination (Driver, 1997). Cardiovascular instability can rapidly affect renal and liver blood flow and functioning, thereby affecting the metabolism and excretion of drugs. Uterine contractions increase cardiac load through the extrusion of 250 to 300 ml of uterine blood into the central system. In the absence of analgesia, this may cause an increase of 20 to 30 mm Hg in the systolic and diastolic blood pressures (Driver, 1997).

Neurologic changes. Pregnancy predisposes women to increased sensitivity to volatile anesthetic agents and local anesthetics. Sensitivity to narcotics, barbiturates, and benzodiazepines is not altered. The mechanism for the noted sensitivity is unclear but may include increased serum and central nervous system (CNS) progesterones, increased β-endorphins, and decreased serum bicarbonate (Driver, 1997).

Gastrointestinal changes. Pain increases the release of gastrin, which leads to an increase of gastric acid secretion. Anxiety and stress increase gastric emptying time, which is further inhibited by the recumbent position.

In addition to normal physiologic changes in pregnancy, one needs to consider factors influencing absorption, transport, and excretion of agents. Lipid solubility, degree of ionization, protein-binding properties, molecular weight, and pH may effect both maternal effect and fetal uptake of the drug.

The primary mechanism of transfer of pharmacologic agents across the placenta is simple diffusion, the movement of molecules from higher concentration to lower concentration. Simple diffusion is effective for the transfer of small molecules through the cell wall. Since placental cell walls have high lipid content, some lipid-soluble substances are transported directly through the lipid regions. Larger molecules that are not fat soluble, such as certain muscle relaxants used in anesthesia, cannot be transported effectively. Narcotics, barbiturates, and anesthetics all are transferred through simple diffusion. Epinephrine diffuses easily but may not reach significant levels in the fetus because of enzymatic deamination in the placenta.

The chemical characteristics of analgesics and anesthetics influence transfer across the placenta. Lipid-soluble, unionized, low-molecular-weight, and poor protein-binding drugs all have increased transfer properties. Drugs with large molecular weight, certain enzyme-bound properties, and red blood cell bound properties are inhibited from transfer. In addition, factors that influence uterine blood flow affect the transfer of substances through the placenta.

The decision regarding route of administration should include consideration of factors that influence absorption, transport, and fetal uptake of the agent. Oral administration is rarely used in labor, but, when it is desired, the clinician needs to consider the effect of the gastrointestinal changes during pregnancy and labor. Increased gastric acid levels and decreased stomach emptying time may affect absorption. In addition, the vomiting experienced in active phase may prevent absorption. Intramuscular administration may deliver varying amounts of the agent because of tissue changes, including edema and altered blood flow. When regional anesthesia is used, intramuscular drugs should be given in the arm rather than the leg or buttocks because of the vascular changes caused by autonomic neural blockage. Intravenous injection of drugs should be timed at the beginning of a contraction since decreased placental perfusion during the contraction allows time for the maternal blood levels to stabilize, thereby lowering the concentration gradient from mother to fetus.

Sedatives/Tranquilizers

Sedatives refer to drugs that lead to restfulness or sleep. Tranquilizers usually refer to drugs that have a calming effect, usually the psychotropics or benzodiazepines. The use of sedatives and tranquilizers has been proposed for labor and delivery because of the recognition that labor is often accompanied by fear and apprehension. Fear and apprehension are best approached with prenatal preparation for the birth and ongoing support through the childbearing experience. However, in cases of severe anxiety, use of these medications may be warranted.

Barbiturates. Short-acting sedatives (secobarbital and pentobarbital) can be useful in early labor to decrease anxiety or facilitate rest. When used at dosages of 50 to 200 mg, the effect is usually that of relaxation rather than analgesia. These medications are not effective once labor has progressed to active phase labor.

After oral administration, barbiturates peak within 1 to 1½ hours and last for 4 hours. Although the drugs can be administered intramuscularly or intravenously, they are rarely used by those routes in labor. The recommended doses have no physiologic effects on the maternal system. They may have a beneficial effect on labor by reducing anxiety and promoting rest.

The drugs appear in fetal circulation within minutes of maternal administration and may have a synergistic depressant effect on infants suffering asphyxia or other depressive conditions. For this reason, these drugs are not recommended for preterm birth. Newborns who are exposed to these medications in the face of other stressors may be depressed for 2 to 4 days after birth.

Benzodiazepines. Benzodiazepines produce sedation, decreased anxiety, and muscle relaxation. In addition, they may be used for their anticonvulsant properties. Because of their long half-life, they are not drugs of choice during childbearing. They are contraindicated in early pregnancy because of increased risk of malformations, including cleft lip and palate. Two neonatal effects are found with use of diazepam. First, neonates exposed to diazepam intrauterinely are less capable of controlling normal body temperature, and this effect may persist for up to 1 week. Second, diazepam binds to albumin, thereby competing with bilirubin and putting the neonate at increased risk for hyperbilirubinemia.

Phenothiazines. Promethazine and propiomazine are useful in labor because of their antianxiety properties. Their mechanism of action is believed to be the blocking of receptors to dopamine and norepinephrine in the brain. Intravenous doses of 25 to 50 mg produce an anxiolytic effect, but their use is limited to early labor because of their antianalgesic effects. They are preferable to other phenothiazines (chlorpromazine, promazine, prochlorperazine) since the latter drugs are more likely to cause hypotension.

Hydroxyzine. The mechanism of action of this drug is unclear, yet it is accepted that its administration at doses of 25 to 50 mg relieves anxiety, and doses of 75 to 100 mg produce hypnotic effects. Research suggests that hydroxyzine increases the analgesic effects of narcotics by at least 50% (Driver, 1997). It is also useful for its antiemetic effect. Use in early pregnancy is not recommended because of malformations noted at high dosages in animal studies.

Use of tranquilizers may cause a minor decrease in beat-to-beat variability in the fetus. When given close to delivery, they may be associated with CNS depression in the neonate.

Opioids

Opioids produce a physiologic effect on every organ in the human body. During labor and delivery the most important effect is that on the CNS. Effects on the CNS can include analgesia, euphoria, dysphoria, sedation, drowsiness, emesis, dizziness, hypoventilation, myosis, and pruritus. Different opioids produce differing effects, and individuals may experience differing effects over time. Opioids function as agonists that bind with receptors presynaptically and postsynaptically. Opioid receptors include a binding site that interacts with the opioid molecule and a triggering site that causes the chemical reactions that in turn cause the final analgesic effect (Driver, 1997). The basic effect of opioids is neuronal inhibition caused by changes in the Ca^{++} channels (Table 18-2).

Following intravenous injection or absorption into the vascular system after administration through other routes, the effect of opioids is modified by pH and the individual binding properties to plasma proteins. Lower protein-binding characteristics, lower ionization, and higher lipid solubility facilitate diffusion from plasma into tissues, including the CNS. Fentanyl enters the brain quickly because of its high diffusion potential; likewise it leaves the brain rapidly. Meperidine, be-

Table 18-2 *Opioid Equivalents*

Opioid duration	Equivalent parenteral dose (mg)	Equipotent oral dose (mg)	(hr)
Morphine	10	20-30	4-5
Meperidine	75	150	3-5
Hydromorphone	1.3	4	4-5
Buprenorphine	0.3	N/A	4-8
Codeine	130	100	4-6
Methadone	10	10-20	4-8
Nalbuphine	10	N/A	3-6
Propoxyphene	N/A	130	4-6
Oxycodone	N/A	15	4-5
Fentanyl	0.1	N/A	1-2

From McCormack J et al.: *Drug therapy—decision-making guide*, Philadelphia, 1996, WB Saunders.

cause of its lower diffusion potential, enters the brain more slowly and has a slower reverse process. Morphine has very low diffusion potential, but its transfer to the brain is facilitated by its low lipid solubility that results in less drug needed for the same effects (Benedetti, 1995). The effect of concentrations of opioids in plasma, cerebrospinal fluid, and CNS tissues varies among individuals. The minimum effective analgesic concentration (MEAC) is the minimum plasma level that will relieve severe pain in an individual (Benedetti, 1995). MEAC remains fairly constant in individuals but varies dramatically between patients. Studies have suggested that subjects report an eightfold difference in the MEAC for meperidine.

Opioids lose their activity in the body through enzymatic transformation in the liver and kidneys and elimination through the renal system. Drug metabolites formed in the liver may be excreted through the gastrointestinal tract.

Systemic use of opioids in labor decreases uterine activity. When given during latent phase, opioids will decrease or stop contractions for the duration of action. Used this way, they can provide therapeutic rest for the woman experiencing prolonged latent phase. Therapeutic doses given during active phase do not appear to have this effect on uterine activity.

All opioids have the potential to cause neonatal depression since they pass readily to the fetus and have a direct depressant effect on the respiratory center of the CNS. When given intramuscularly or subcutaneously, the peak effect in the neonate occurs 2 to 4 hours after administration. When administered intravenously, the effect occurs within minutes. It does not appear that the dosages used for epidural analgesia exert this depressant effect on the baby. Depressant effects in the neonate can continue for 2 to 4 days after birth and are more pronounced in cases complicated by prematurity, hypotension, prolonged labor, cesarean section, and trauma. Decreased beat-to-beat variability in fetal heart rate will also be noted after administration of opioids. This loss of variability is seen approximately 10 minutes after administration of meperidine in labor and lasts for around 30 minutes. Opioids can also stimulate a sinusoidal fetal heart rate pattern, though this drug-induced pattern has not been associated with any pathologic response in the fetus.

Morphine. Morphine can be administered via subcutaneous (SC), intramuscular (IM), intravenous (IV), epidural, or spinal routes. Dosages of 5 to 10 mg intramuscularly or subcutaneously provide therapeutic levels of analgesia. When given intramuscularly or intravenously, morphine may produce hypotension since it has a vasodilating effect.

Meperidine. Merperidine is perhaps the most commonly used opioid in labor and delivery. It can be administered orally, intramuscularly, or intravenously, although absorption from the oral route is 50% less effective than the parenteral route. Onset of action after IM administration occurs in 15 minutes, with peak action evident in 40 to 60 minutes. Duration is 2 to 4 hours, almost 50% shorter than that of morphine. A single dose of 50 mg intramuscularly provides satisfactory analgesia for more than 80% of women in early labor. The IV route is preferred in labor since IM absorption can be erratic and lower IV doses can be used for the analgesic effect. Usual IV dose is 25 mg slow IV push, and analgesia onset occurs in 3 to 5 minutes. Intravenous duration is 2 to 3 hours. Rapid intravenous administration will cause vasodilation, possibly through histamine release.

Neonatal depression occurs 2 to 4 hours after maternal dosing, and the degree of depression depends on gestational age and presence of asphyxia. Elimination half-life in the neonate is 18 hours, compared with 2.4 hours in the mother. Ninety-five percent of meperidine is eliminated from the neonate in 2 to 3 days (Benedetti, 1995).

Fentanyl. Fentanyl is approximately 80 to 100 times as potent as morphine. It can be administered intravenously and has been used in epidural analgesia since 1980. Usual dosage during labor is 50 to 100 μg intravenously. Sufentanil, which is 8 to 10 times more potent than fentanyl, is used in combination with bupivacaine for epidural analgesia.

Butorphanol. Butorphanol is an agonist-antagonist opioid that has greater analgesic effectiveness with fewer side effects than other agonist-antagonist preparations. Its potency is 5 times that of morphine and 40 times that of meperidine. It is less likely to cause nausea and vomiting than morphine. It can be administered intramuscularly or intravenously, with the usual dose being 1 to 2 mg intravenously. Onset of action occurs 2 to 3 minutes after IV administration and persists for 3 to 4 hours. Maternal half-life of elimination is 2.7 hours. Metabolization of butorphanol occurs in the liver, and excretion is primarily via the renal system. Although butorphanol rapidly crosses the placenta, no neonatal neurobehavioral effects have been reported.

Nalbuphine. Nalbuphine, also an agonist-antagonist preparation, can be administered intramuscularly, subcutaneously, or intravenously. The usual IV dose is 2 to 4 mg, with onset of action at 2 to 3 minutes after administration with a duration of 5 to 6 hours. It is metabolized in the liver and excreted through the kidneys. Analgesia is produced 45 to 60 minutes after IM administration and lasts 4 to 5 hours. Like butorphanol, nalbuphine produces sedation. Nalbuphine is less commonly used than butorphanol.

Opioid Antagonists

Opioid antagonists displace opioid agonists (e.g., morphine, meperidine, fentanyl) from the receptor sites, thereby reducing or eliminating their effect. Naloxone rapidly reverses respiratory depression caused by the opioids and is particularly effective in treating neonates who may be depressed from intrauterine exposure. Neonatal dosage is 0.01mg/kg intravenously. Maternal dosage is 0.4 mg intravenously. The drug should be given slow IV push (2 to 3 minutes) since rapid infusion causes nausea and vomiting. Other side effects include tachycardia, hypertension, pulmonary edema, and cardiac dysrhythmias, most likely the result of the stimulation to the sympathetic nervous system. Naloxone is short-acting (30 to 45 minutes), and repeated doses may be needed when counteracting longer-acting opioids. Naltrexone acts similarly to naloxone but has an effect up to 24 hours.

LOCAL AND REGIONAL ANESTHESIA AND ANALGESIA

Local Infiltration Block

Local infiltration of the perineum can be done before cutting an episiotomy or after the birth for the repair of the episiotomy or laceration(s). Infiltration of 5 to 10 ml of 1% lidocaine is usually sufficient to anesthetize the tissues that will be manipulated and sutured. Care should be taken to ensure that the solution is injected evenly in the tissue; otherwise effective approximation of tissues is more difficult.

Local infiltration block provides anesthesia in local tissues because the anesthetic agent has direct contact with nerves and prevents transmission of painful stimuli. The anesthetic agents used can be amide-linked agents (lidocaine and bupivacaine) or ester-linked agents (procaine, tetracaine, 2-chloroprocaine). Ester-linked agents are short-acting and do not pass readily into the fetal circulation. Amide-linked agents are longer-acting and pass more readily into the fetal circulation. Previous sensitivity to anesthetic agents must be determined before administration of any of these drugs (Figure 18-7).

Paracervical Block

Paracervical block is infiltration of an anesthetic agent lateral to the cervix and provides relief from pain through the direct effect on the inferior hypogastric plexus and ganglia as they cross the parametrium to transmit painful stimuli as the cervix dilates. When used in labor, it is most effective as the woman enters the acceleration phase of first stage. Maternal contraindications to the procedure include full dilation of the cervix, restlessness or uncontrolled movements that would interfere with safe infiltration of the anesthetic, conditions in which uterine perfusion may be compromised (e.g., hypertension, diabetes) and known sensitivity to amide or ester types of anesthetic agents. Fetal contraindications include presenting part at or below 2+ station, prematurity, and fetal intolerance of labor.

The provider first performs a vaginal examination to determine cervical dilation and station of the presenting part. Injection is accomplished through the introduction of an 22-gauge needle guarded by a sheath (Iowa trumpet) so that only 2 to 3 mm of the needle tip can extend into tissue. The examining fingers stabilize the guide at the 9 o'clock position in the lateral vaginal fornix, the needle is advanced into the vaginal mucosa no more than 2 to 4 mm, and aspiration is done to prevent intravascu-

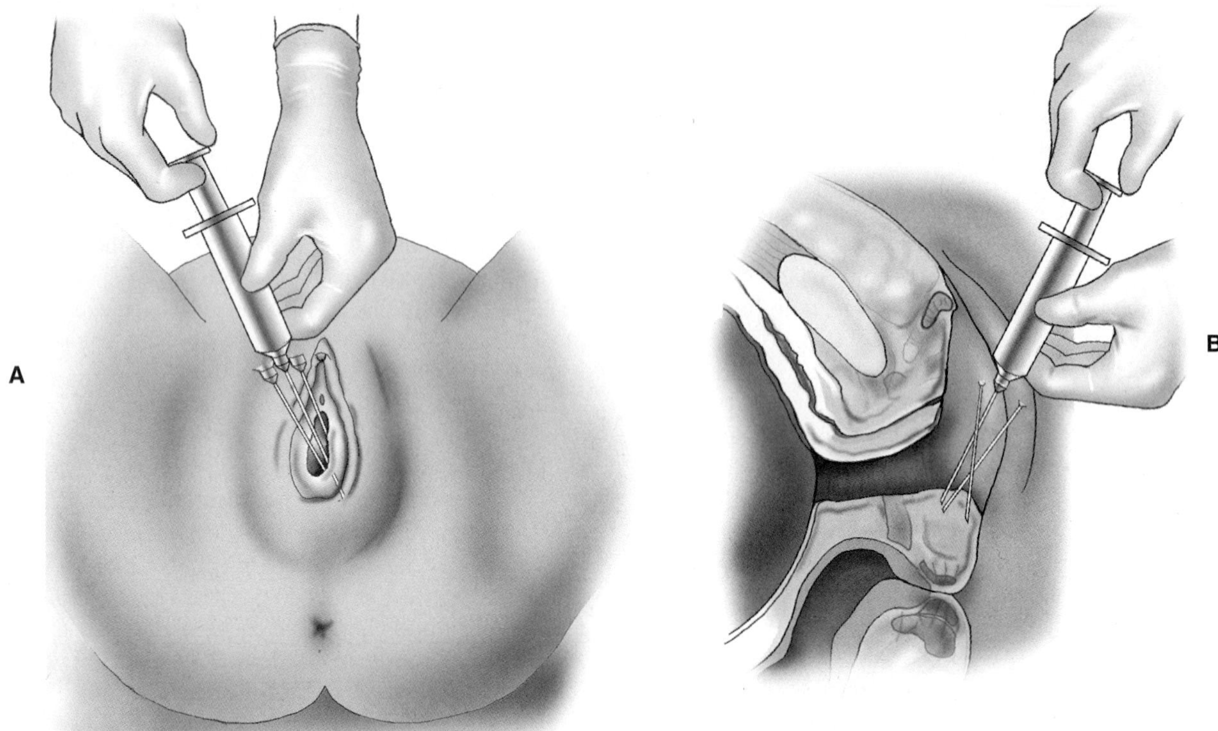

Figure 18-7 Local infiltration of the perineum. A, External view; B view of internal structures.

lar injection. Once placement is considered to be correct, 2.5 ml of chloroprocaine is injected slowly. (Amide-linked agents are more likely to be associated with fetal bradycardia; mepivacaine and lidocaine are vasoconstrictors that can affect uterine perfusion.) The needle is then withdrawn slightly, and the needle guard is readjusted to aim downward toward 8 o'clock. After aspiration another 2.5 ml is injected. The needle system is then withdrawn, and the fetal heart rate is observed through two contractions. If fetal distress occurs, no further block is introduced. If the fetus appears stable, injection is then carried out on the opposite side at 3 o'clock with redirection toward 4 o'clock.

Paracervical block is rarely used because of its association with fetal bradycardia and the availability of other modalities for pain relief. Fetal bradycardia results from inadvertent intravascular injection of anesthetic, simple diffusion through the uterine artery, and vasoconstriction caused by the anesthetic action or mechanical compression of the vessels (Figure 18-8).

Pudendal Block

Pudendal block can be a very effective anesthetic for second-stage labor, instrumental delivery, and perineal repairs following birth. The pudendal nerve is in close approximation to the ischial spines, and injection of 10 ml of 1% lidocaine or 0.25% bupivacaine at that point produces rapid block for the lower vagina and perineum. Side effects are few, but the following complications have been reported: systemic toxic reaction if injected vascularly, local nerve trauma, vaginal hematoma, infection through the greater sciatic foramen into the joint capsule of the ipsilateral femur, and abscess formation (Bonica and McDonald, 1995).

Since pudendal block is used just before delivery, there is no effect on labor. However, because it is administered late in labor, the technique may be difficult because of the descent of the fetal head. After inserting the second and third fingers of the opposite hand from the side of the block into the vagina, the birth attendant palpates the ischial spine. Using a needle guide, the attendant guides the needle to the vaginal mucosa immediately medial to the ischial spine. The needle is inserted approximately 1 cm. Resistance will be felt as the needle passes into the sacrospinous ligament. A 2-ml amount of anesthetic is injected into the ligament after determining through aspiration that there is no blood return. Infiltration of the sacrospinous ligament anesthetizes the inferior hemorrhoidal nerve, which is not a branch of the pu-

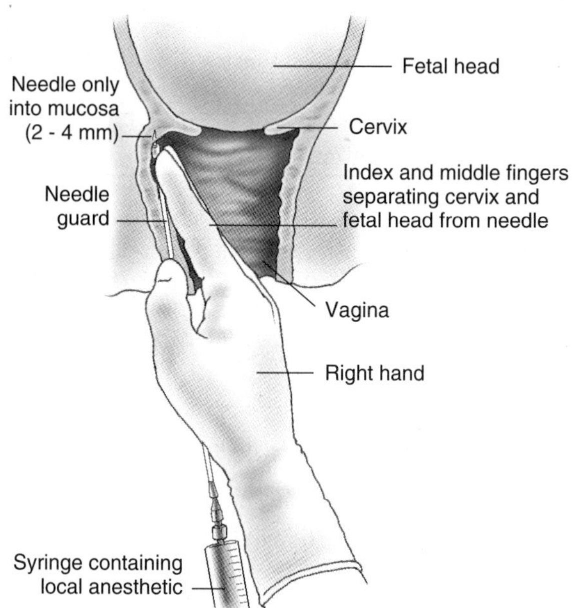

Figure 18-8 Paracervical injection site.

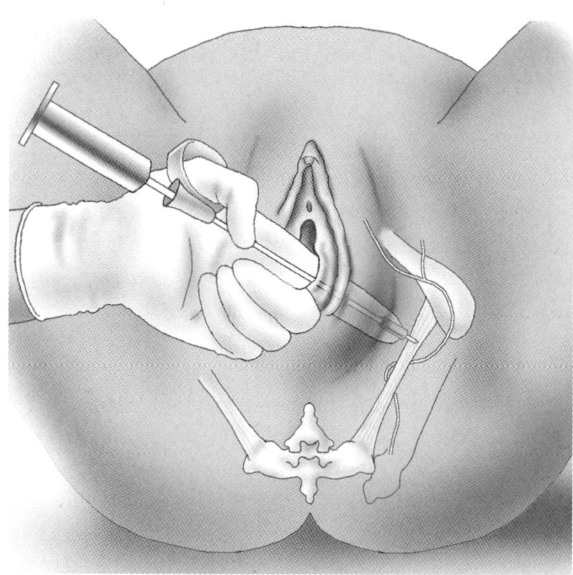

Figure 18-9 Administration of pudendal block.

dendal nerve and therefore is not included in the pudendal block. The practitioner then advances the needle and will feel a loss of resistance as the needle enters the plane behind the ligament (Alcock's canal). Following aspiration, 6 to 8 ml of anesthetic is slowly injected over 20 to 30 seconds into the canal. Inserting the needle more than 1 to 2 mm may result in passing through the canal and into the gluteus muscles. The woman and her fetus should be observed for several minutes to ensure that there are no untoward effects; if both are stable, injection of the opposite side can be accomplished. Approximately 3 to 4 minutes after infiltration, the successful block causes anesthesia in the lower vagina and posterior vulva (Figure 18-9).

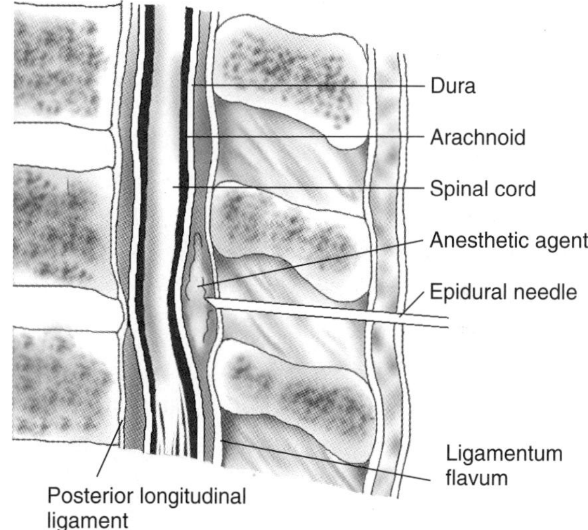

Figure 18-10 Membranes and spaces of the spinal column.

Epidural Analgesia

The epidural space is a potential space that contains areolar tissue, fat, lymphatics, and the internal venous plexus. The venous plexus becomes engorged in pregnancy, thereby reducing the volume of the space. The epidural space is bordered by the ligamentum flavum and the dura, and it extends longitudinally from the skull to the end of the sacrum. The level anesthesia necessary for labor and vaginal birth is from the tenth thoracic vertebra (T10) to the fifth sacral dermatome (S5). Abdominal delivery requires a higher block to the level of T8. For these levels the introduction of the needle and catheter apparatus is between L2 and L4. Care is necessary to ensure that the needle has not punctured the dura since injection of the anesthetic dose used for an epidural block can cause respiratory paralysis and cardiovascular collapse (Figure 18-10).

Dosage is determined by considering the level of anesthesia desired, the concentration and volume of the drug, and the position of the woman. Most often, a combination of local anesthetic (bupivacaine) and narcotic (fentanyl) is used to decrease the potential loss of motor function while retaining the analgesic properties. Epidural blocks can be administered by a single injection or through continuous infusion through an indwelling catheter.

Advantages of epidural block are effective pain relief while the woman remains alert and relaxed and the ability to control the administration so that the infusion can be increased or decreased as necessary. Disadvantages include the side effect of hypotension, the occurrence of fetal bradycardia following injection, increased risk for instrumental and surgical births, and increased maternal temperature that may lead to inappropriate septic work-up of the infant. Hypotension is primarily caused by vasodilation throughout the lower abdominal and pelvic region secondary to the blocking of sympathetic nervous system impulses. The risk of systemic hypotension can be reduced by providing at least 500 ml of IV fluid before injection. However, even with preload of fluid, significant hypotension in the uterine vessels can lead to fetal bradycardia. The bradycardia usually resolves spontaneously after several minutes but may result in the necessity of immediate cesarean section. One investigation (Stavrou, Hofmeyr, and Boezaart, 1990) found that the incidence of prolonged bradycardia was 11% in the sample; however, all infants with the prolonged bradycardia had 5-minute APGAR scores of 7 or above. Two studies exploring uteroplacental blood flow using Doppler after placement of epidural analgesia for elective cesarean section suggest that epidural infiltration is associated with decreased blood flow and increased fetal heart rate abnormalities (Baumann, Alon, and Atanassoff, 1990; Olah and Gee, 1991).

Epidural anesthesia should be administered by an anesthetist skilled in obstetric anesthesia. Full resources for resuscitation should be readily available. The procedure is usually done with the woman in a sitting position, although it can be done with her positioned on her side. After obtaining informed consent, the baseline blood pressure, pulse, and fetal heart rate are obtained. The skin at the site of administration is cleaned with an antiseptic solution, and sterile draping is secured. A small amount of local anesthetic is usually injected over the site of injection. The anesthetist then inserts a 16-gauge Tuohy needle, advancing slowly until resistance of the ligamentum flavum is felt. A syringe filled with saline or air is attached to the needle, and, as the needle passes into the epidural space, there is loss of resistance that can be noted with depression of the syringe plunger. If no blood or cerebrospinal fluid is aspirated, the epidural catheter is threaded into the epidural space. A test dose of anesthetic is given. If no adverse effects are noted, the catheter is secured in place, and the first dose or continuous infusion is administered.

Blood pressure should be monitored every 5 minutes for 20 to 30 minutes, then every 15 minutes. Fetal heart rate should be monitored continuously. Signs of hypotension with resulting decreased placental perfusion include a 20% decrease in systolic pressure or pressure under 100 mm Hg, fetal bradycardia, or decreased beat-to-beat variability of the fetal heart rate. If severe hypotension occurs, the woman should be positioned on her side, her legs can be elevated, and oxygen should be administered via mask. Since an urge to void may not be noted, catheterization may be necessary to prevent overdistention of the bladder.

The use of narcotics in combination with anesthetic allows for a decrease in the amount of anesthetic necessary for pain relief. The narcotic binds with receptors along the spinal cord, blocking transmission of painful stimuli while allowing continuation of motor control. Patients who are able to support weight on their legs and who do not have any obstetric contraindication to ambulation can be allowed to ambulate. However, the use of intravenous fluids and continuous fetal monitoring limits this option.

Most studies comparing use of epidural anesthesia with length of labor suggest that women who use epidural anesthesia experience longer first and second stages of labor (Thompson and Breedlove, 1996). Data also suggest that use of epidural anesthesia increases the risk of cesarean section for dystocia, especially when the epidural is placed cervical dilation at 3 cm or less. Failure to descend, particularly in the second stage, results from relaxation of the muscles of the pelvic floor. This decrease in the resistance that aids in rotation of the presenting part can particularly hinder the rotation necessary for fetal heads in the occipitoposterior position. Failure to rotate leads to prolonged second stage and an increased rate of instrumental and cesarean deliveries.

Additional side effects of epidural anesthesia include pruritus, nausea, vomiting, and backache. Pruritus can be managed with diphenhydramine, 25 to 50 mg intravenously. Metoclopramide (Reglan), 10 mg intravenously or orally, can be administered for nausea and vomiting. Effects of epidural anesthesia/analgesia on newborn behavior have been explored with conflicting findings. Use of epidural has been associated with lower neurobehavioral scores during the first days of life, but lack of randomization limits the findings.

Contraindications for epidural anesthesia/analgesia include maternal hypotension (e.g., in hemorrhage), severe hypertension, neurologic disease, bleeding disorders, allergy to anesthetic agents, and infectious lesions near the site of skin puncture.

Intrathecal Narcotic Injection

Intrathecal narcotics have been used in obstetrics since the early 1980s. Pain relief is satisfactory for the visceral pain of first stage but will not be effective for the somatic pain of second stage. Common dosages include 25 μg of fentanyl, 10 μg of sufentanil, and 0.2 to 0.25 mg of morphine. Fentanyl and sufentanil are lipid soluble and therefore absorbed more rapidly into the CNS, producing shorter-acting effects. The analgesia usually takes effect in 3 to 5 minutes and lasts for 1.5 to 3 hours. Combinations of morphine and fentanyl are sometimes used to take advantage of the longer effect of morphine. A combination of intrathecal injection and epidural anesthesia is being used in some centers.

Advantages of intrathecal narcotic injections include rapid and effective pain relief, maintenance of the sensation of "urge to push," and no loss of motor control of the lower body. Intrathecal narcotic injections may be particularly effective in facilities where resources for epidural anesthesia may not be readily available. Disadvantages include pruritus, nausea and vomiting, urinary retention, and postdural puncture headache. The pruritus associated with fentanyl can be easily controlled with 25 to 50 mg of IV diphenhydramine.

Spinal (Subarachnoid) Block

Infiltration of local anesthetic into the subarachnoid space has been used in obstetrics for decades. Its use is rare in spontaneous labors and vaginal births, but it is still used for cesarean births in many centers. Complications associated with spinal block include maternal hypotension, total spinal block, postdural puncture headache, and bladder dysfunction. Preload of intravenous fluid decreases the risk of severe hypotension. Maternal hypotension may lead to fetal compromise. Use of postpartum ergotamine drugs may increase hypotensive response. In total spinal block paralysis of the respiratory muscles occurs with resultant respiratory support necessary. Spinal headaches can be treated with analgesics and/or the use of a blood patch at the site of dural puncture.

General Anesthesia

General anesthesia is rarely necessary for vaginal and cesarean births. It may be necessary when there are contraindications to regional blocks (including patient refusal) and rapid delivery is necessary for fetal indications. It may also be needed when rapid relaxation is necessary for emergency procedures such as shoulder dystocia.

SUMMARY

Preparation for comfort measures and pain relief interventions ideally begins in the prenatal period. The clinician should be aware of the philosophies and class curricula offered in the community so that she or he is able to address questions, concerns, or areas that may not be covered in classes. Women should be encouraged to maintain an open mind about comfort measures since rigidity on either extreme—the desire for NO medication vs. the desire for an epidural immediately—fails to take into account the fact that the type of labor a woman will experience cannot be predicted. During the labor the birth attendant should offer an honest appraisal of the maternal and fetal benefits and risks of the options available. The laboring woman's personal beliefs, cultural expectations, and perception of discomfort/pain and her decision(s) regarding what is best for her and her baby should guide the use of interventions during the birthing process.

References

Ader L, Hansson B, Wallin G: Parturition pain treated by intracutaneous injections of sterile water, *Pain* 41:133-138, 1990.

Baumann H, Alon E, Atanassoff P: Effect of epidural anesthesia for caesarean delivery on maternal femoral arterial and venous, uteroplacental, and umbilical blood flow velocities and waveform, *Obstet Gynecol* 75:194-199, 1990.

Benedetti C: Opioids, sedatives, hypnotics, ataractics. In Bonica JJ, McDonald JS, editors: *Principles and practice of obstetrics analgesia and anesthesia,* ed 2, Baltimore, 1995, Williams & Wilkins.

Bonica JJ, McDonald JS: *Principles and practice of obstetric analgesia and anesthesia,* ed 2, Baltimore, 1995, Williams & Wilkins.

Brownridge P: The nature and consequences of childbirth pain, *Eur J Obstet Gynecol Reprod Biol* 59 (suppl):S9-15, 1995.

CNM Data Group: Midwifery management of pain in labor, *J Nurse Midwifery* 43(2):77-82, 1998.

Davis-Floyd RE: *Birth as an American rite of passage,* Berkeley, 1993, University of California Press.

Driver RPJ: Practical obstetric physiology. In Dewan DM, Hood DO, editors: *Practical obstetric anesthesia,* Philadelphia, 1997, WB Saunders.

Harkness J, Gijsbers K: Pain and stress during childbirth and time of day, *Ethol Sociobiol* 10(4):255-261, 1989.

Harrison RF et al: Pain relief in labour using transcutaneous electrical nerve stimulation (TENS): a TENS/TENS placebo controlled study, *Br J Obstet Gynaecol* 93:739-746, 1986.

Hedstrom LW, Newton N: Touch in labor: a comparison of cultures and eras, *Birth* 13(3):181-186, 1986.

Hodnett E: Nursing support of the laboring woman, *J Obstet Gynecol Neonatal Nurs* 25(3):257-264, 1996.

Hodnett ED: Caregiver support for women during childbirth. In Review C, editor: *The Cochrane Library,* vol I, Oxford, 2000, Update Software.

Jordan B: *Birth in four cultures: a crosscultural investigation of childbirth in Yucatan, Holland, Sweden, and the United States,* Prospect Heights, Ill, 1993, Waveland Press.

Jungman R: Acupressure. In Nichols F, Humenick S, editors: *Childbirth education: practice, research and theory,* Philadelphia, 1988, WB Saunders.

Lindberg C, Lawlis GF: The effectiveness of imagery as a childbirth preparatory technique, *J Mental Imag* 12(1):103-113, 1988.

Lowe NK: The pain and discomfort of labor and birth, *JOGNN* 25(1):82-92. 1996.

Lozoff B, Jordan B, Malone S: Childbirth in cross-cultural perspective, *Marriage Fam Rev* 12(3-4):35-60, 1988.

Lytzen T, Cederberg L, Moller-Nielsen J: Relief of low back pain in labor by using intracutaneous nerve stimulation (INS) with sterile water papules, *Acta Obstet Gynecol Scand* 68(4):341-343, 1989.

McNiven P, Hodnett E, O'Brien-Pallas LL: Supporting women in labor: a work sampling study of the activities of labor and delivery nurses, *Birth* 19(1):3-8; discussion 8-9, 1992.

Nichols FH, Zwelling E: *Maternal-newborn nursing: theory and practice,* Philadelphia, 1997, WB Saunders.

Nikodem VC: Immersion in water in pregnancy, labour and birth. In Review C, editor: *The Cochrane Library,* Oxford, 2000, Update Software.

Olah KSJ, Gee H: Epidural analgesia—a cause for transient impairment of the utero-placental circulation, *Br J Obstet Gynaecol* 98:1174-1184, 1991.

Rush J et al: The effects of whirlpools baths in labor: a randomized, controlled trial, *Birth* 23(3):136-143, 1996.

Simkin P: Reducing pain and enhancing progress in labor: a guide to nonpharmacologic methods for maternity caregivers, *Birth* 22:161-171, 1995.

Stavrou C, Hofmeyr GJ, Boezaart AP: Prolonged fetal bradycardia during epidural analgesia: incidence, timing, and significance, *S Afr Med J* 77:66-68, 1990.

Thompson JA, Breedlove G: Epidural analgesia in labor: an evaluation of risks and benefits, *Birth* 23(2):63-82, 1996.

Trolle B et al: The effect of sterile water blocks on low back labor pain, *Am J Obstet Gynecol* 164(5, part 1):1277-1281, 1991.

Tsueii J, Lai Y, Sharma S: The influence of acupuncture stimulation during pregnancy, *Obstet Gynecol* 50:479-481, 1977.

Walsh LV: *A special vocation—Philadelphia midwives, 1910-1940,* Unpublished Doctoral dissertation, Philadelphia, 1992, University of Pennsylvania.

Chapter 19

First-Stage Labor

Catherine A. Carr, CNM, Dr.P.H.
and Alexandra Schott, CNM, MSN

INTRODUCTION

MISFLAP (a mnemonic standing for *M*aternal status, *I*ntake, *S*upport, *F*etal status, *L*abor status, *A*ctivity status, *P*ain/*P*syche/*P*rovider) is an approach to caring for women in labor. This approach identifies the woman in labor as the central point of context, thus changing the paradigm from what is considered to be "normal" to what is normal for this particular woman at this time in her experience of pregnancy and birth. Using MISFLAP reminds the midwife to look at the entire picture of the woman, fetus, and labor to gather the data needed to appropriately attend birth. This chapter uses MISFLAP to organize data collection when caring for women in the first stage of labor and discusses how to apply the art of midwifery to the data. Data alone (i.e., subjective and objective information that also considers the social and cultural environment of the woman) are insufficient in and of themselves. The MISFLAP approach is a means of data collection that may be used to enhance the basis on which decisions about care processes are made.

MATERNAL STATUS

Chart Review

Unless there is an emergency requiring immediate action or delivery is imminent, data gathering should begin with a complete review of existing records. The chart review provides the midwife with a base of information about the woman and her pregnancy and offers clues about how to approach this particular birth. Chart review begins with a review of the history of the current pregnancy and how the woman has experienced it.

History of the present pregnancy. *What was the quality of prenatal care received?* Timeliness and consistency of prenatal care is determined by noting the weeks of gestation at the initial prenatal visit and the number of return prenatal visits. The pattern of visits should reflect the community norm—either the traditional monthly, bimonthly, and weekly pattern or the modified schedule recommended by the Expert Panel on the Content of Prenatal Care. If there was late or inadequate prenatal care, the clinician should review any documentation that provides information about the reason for inadequate care.

Is this a term pregnancy? The clinician next notes the estimated delivery date (EDD) to determine whether this pregnancy is term or not. The EDD is actually the midpoint of the time span between 38 to 42 weeks when the baby may be expected to be born. There are many dating parameters used to select the best EDD, and all have limitations (see Chapter 7). Using several dating measures improves precision in estimating gestational age.

The date and findings of ultrasound examinations should be compared to the last menstrual period (LMP) and EDD. Ultrasound is most accurate for dating during the first trimester and least accurate during the third. Because ultrasound, like all of the dating measures, gives a range of time, findings should be compared to the EDD determined by other available methods to find the best available EDD.

Physical examination and clinical parameters are valuable correlates of EDD determination. If the first examination is early in pregnancy, an experienced clinician should be able to make a fairly accurate estimate of gestational age. Fetal heart tones may be heard with the Doppler between 10 and 11 weeks in a slender woman and by 13 weeks in a larger woman. By the end of the first trimester, a retroverted uterus has risen into the abdomen and is easier to auscultate. Unamplified fetal heart tones are usually audible by 18 to 20 weeks, depending on the woman's body habitus and the examiner's skill. It is important to note that 22 weeks of unamplified fetal heart tones indicates a term pregnancy. Quickening, or the maternal perception of fetal movement, is most often felt by multiparous women between 16 and 18 weeks and by primiparous women between 18 and 22 weeks.

Although careful review of dating information should have been done during the antenatal period, the conscientious provider checks to ensure that this did indeed occur and reassesses if necessary. Although it is tempting to use a preferred method of calculating the EDD, the clinician should review all information that is available on the chart and determine the accuracy of the information. Intervention or failure to intervene because of a miscalculated due date is a danger to be avoided if at all possible.

Has the woman experienced a healthy pregnancy, or have there been problems or deviations from normal? Total estimated or documented weight gain should be determined. There is a very wide range of normal weight and weight gain in pregnancy. However, extremes of weight gain may indicate other problems. A very low weight gain may be due to an eating disorder, insufficient resources to obtain needed food, anxiety about pregnancy, or current or recent illness. A very large weight gain may also indicate an eating disorder, preeclampsia and subsequent retention of large amounts of fluid, or poor dietary habits, or it may be normal for that particular woman. The overriding question is how the weight affects labor and fetal outcome. In periods of starvation or famine, fetal weight may be 500 g lower than normal. Macrosomic infants may be at higher risk for shoulder dystocia, traumatic delivery, and brachial plexus injury.

Deviations from normal parameters in pregnancy need to be identified. Deviations should be considered warning signs until proven otherwise. Blood pressure deviations should be evaluated using the woman's baseline blood pressure and the normal trend over time in pregnancy. Deviations in urine screening should be noted. Increased urinary excretion of protein in pregnancy is normal, and proteinuria is not considered an abnormality until levels exceed 300 mg in 24 hours. Reagent testing (dip stick) can detect proteinuria, but a high rate of false positives at low levels (one plus and trace) make results less easily interpreted. Proteinuria is a nonspecific late sign of preeclampsia and is correlated with poorer fetal outcome. The level of proteinuria and blood pressure elevation are only weakly correlated. Positive ketones and glucose on urine dipstick are rarely useful in labor if other parameters and history are normal (e.g., the woman had normal glucose screening in pregnancy, she is appropriately nourished and hydrated, and she is not vomiting).

Does it appear that this fetus has experienced normal growth and development? The midwife must be mindful of the mother/fetus connection during the history of this pregnancy. The following areas should be reviewed:

1. *Fundal growth.* Growth should have followed a consistent pattern. If deviations were identified, appropriate evaluative measures should have been taken in an attempt to explain the deviation. A decreasing fundal height in the last weeks of the pregnancy may be explained by a corresponding notation regarding the presenting part being deep in the pelvis.
2. *Presentation.* A history of frequently changing presentation or recent malpresentation should alert the provider to be particularly careful in assessing the current presentation.
3. *Estimated fetal weight (EFW).* When noted, the fetal weight estimates should be appropriate for

gestational age. If there is a deviation from the expected fetal weight for gestation, additional studies should have been done to further understand the fetal growth trend.

4. *Laboratory findings.* Laboratory results that indicate possible fetal effect should be noted. These would include indications of an infectious process that may affect the neonate immediately after birth. Group B streptococcus, recently acquired varicella, or recent primary genital herpes all increase the risk of infection in the neonate. Other conditions confirmed by laboratory testing such as maternal drug use, maternal diabetes, exposure to teratogenic substances, positive antibody screens, or untreated sexually transmitted infections require pediatric consultation and possible attendance at delivery.
5. *Diagnostic procedures.* The results of fetal screening and diagnostic procedures such as triple screen, nonstress tests (NSTs), amniotic fluid indices (AFIs), ultrasonic fetal anatomy screening, and amniocentesis should be reviewed. Deviations may require the presence of the pediatrics team at delivery.
6. *Maternal perception of fetal movement.* Consistent fetal movement patterns noted by the woman provide evidence of a healthy fetus. Any report of decrease in fetal activity may indicate potential fetal problems and potential intolerance of labor.

Past medical and surgical history. It is important to know whether there are medical problems that need to be addressed in labor. These could include cardiac disease, diabetes, thyroid disease, or asthma. The midwife should assess the need for obstetric consultation, co-management, or referral and whether it is necessary to inform the pediatrics team to be present for the birth. Changes in medical condition during the pregnancy are important considerations during the labor assessment. Women with cardiac disease or asthma may require pharmacologic intervention in labor. It is important that the medical history review include both substance abuse treatment and medical treatment for mental health problems since women may be on medication for these conditions.

Identification of any previous surgeries is essential, particularly identification of uterine incisions. Although vaginal births after cesarean (VBACs) are quite common, there are other reasons that a woman might have had surgery involving the uterus. Prior surgeries involving the uterus should be documented in the records, and it is most helpful if copies of operative records are available. The clinician must identify any prior surgery that might affect function of the uterus or the position of the fetus. Previous experience with anesthesia should also be noted, including any untoward effects of anesthesia. Previous problems should be communicated to the anesthesia team.

Social history. It is essential to identify any history of socioenvironmental problems. The clinician should identify the need for postpartum intervention if the social or economic situation warrants it. Domestic violence and abuse are not always discovered during prenatal care, particularly if the provider is uncomfortable about asking questions that might be considered sensitive or embarrassing. Therefore chart review should include a search for warning signs such as unexplained emergency room visits, late entry into care, or missed prenatal appointments. Chart review should also include a search for factors that may predispose the woman to psychologic dystocia. A woman's concerns and worries may affect the progress of her labor. If she has other children but is worried about their comfort, she is less able to be emotionally present for the labor. If a woman has a history of sexual abuse, she may have great difficulty with the inherent loss of control that occurs in labor (Seng and Hassinger, 1998; Rhodes and Hutchinson, 1994; Simkin, 1992).

Past obstetric history. The chart review should identify the length of time since the woman's last labor and the outcome of all prior labors and pregnancies. Events that have an increased risk of occurring with this pregnancy, including postpartum hemorrhage, preeclampsia, or other hypertensive disorders; rapid active labor; rapid second stage; and a large baby should be identified. Women usually remember dramatic events such as hemorrhage, unusually rapid labors, or whether the delivery was complicated. A careful history can often unravel even an uninformed recounting. Women who have experienced a very rapid active or second stage or who have had serious problems in labor may be anxious about being left alone.

It is also important to consider things that are less likely to repeat—cesarean delivery, a lengthy first stage in a primipara, long prodromal labor, premature rupture of membranes (PROM), meconium, or fetal distress. Women who experienced long prodromal labors, slow-slope active phase, or labors that were perceived as unusually painful may enter labor requesting epidural anesthesia for fear that history may repeat itself.

Chart review should also identify whether anesthesia or analgesia was used with prior births, including any unforeseen reactions to these interventions. A woman who has experienced only medicated labors in the past will need focused support in labor if she desires to avoid medication with this labor. Notation of whether an episiotomy or laceration repair was done for prior births should be done. Protection of the scar(s) will be an important part of the management of second stage in this labor.

Laboratory and special testing. All laboratory tests or screens should be reviewed. The clinician should identify whether there was follow-up on abnormal results. For example, documentation of treatment and a test of cure should follow a positive urine culture. Untreated or insufficiently treated tuberculosis or sexually transmitted infections may increase the risk to the fetus. Laboratory tests that may need to be followed in labor or may change management in labor need to be identified. For example, evidence of antenatal urinary tract infection with group B streptococcus is an indication for antibiotic prophylaxis in labor to prevent neonatal infection. The clinician should specifically look for documentation of blood type and Rh status and third trimester hemoglobin and/or hematocrit.

General Appearance

Chief complaint or concern. The clinician should determine why the patient contacted the midwife or came into the hospital or birth center. Contractions, cramping, pelvic pressure, pain, and rupture of membranes are common concerns. Less often reported but also common are fear and anticipation or need for reassurance. The midwife should ascertain the woman's perception of her labor or her status and compare her general appearance with her perception of the situation. If she is contracting, the midwife assesses whether her coping appears congruent with the intensity of the contractions. In most cases the midwife assesses the following areas:

Labor Activity A description of the onset and trend over time of labor activity should be obtained. The historical trend of frequency, duration, and intensity of contractions should be noted. The midwife ascertains how the laboring woman's coping mechanisms correlate with the assessment of intensity of her contractions. The laboring woman's ability to relax may be affected by anxiety, discomfort, stress, or fear as well as the discomfort of the contractions.

Maternal Concerns Each woman will arrive in labor with her own anticipations and goals as well as fears and concerns. The midwife reviews any previous documentation such as requests or concerns noted on the chart and birth plan and begins the discussion about labor expectations. Given the unpredictable nature of labor, it is important for the midwife, the client, and her family to understand that it may not be possible to fulfill all of her wishes. However, they need to be articulated and acknowledged in order to validate them and to demonstrate the expectation of the active participation of the woman in clinical decisions about her labor.

Vital signs. Maternal temperature should be determined on admission and every 4 hours as long as the woman remains afebrile. When fever is identified, temperature should be taken every hour. Pulse and respirations should follow the frequency of temperature. Blood pressure should be taken every 4 hours in normotensive women. More frequent blood pressure determination is necessary in hypertension or when specific interventions (e.g., epidural anesthesia) warrant close monitoring.

Physical assessment. A brief physical assessment provides the midwife with the opportunity to closely evaluate the woman's physical status. This can be done concurrently with the history and/or assessment of labor status. Throughout the examination, the clinician has further opportunity to observe the woman's general level of relaxation, her muscle tone, and her skin appearance, being alert for bruising, varicosities, lesions, evidence of injection drug use, and previously unexplained scars.

The physical assessment should include the following:

1. *Heart/lungs.* Auscultate for evidence of murmurs, clicks or other deviations from normal. In women with histories of respiratory problems (asthma, chronic bronchitis, smoking), the lungs should be auscultated for diminished respiratory effort.
2. *Breasts.* Evaluate nipples to identify flat or inverted nipples that may hinder nursing efforts. A woman with a history of breast implants may have questions about her ability to breast-feed and may need reassurance and guidance. Any masses found should be noted for immediate postpartum follow-up.
3. *Abdomen.* The abdominal examination should include identification of the fetal lie, presentation, position, and EFW. If the woman already

has electronic fetal monitoring (EFM) straps on, they *must* be removed to complete an appropriate abdominal examination. A cursory examination between and around straps may cause the clinician to miss a breech or other malpresentation. If scars are noted, they should be matched against the previously obtained history of prior cesarean delivery, appendectomy, or other abdominal surgery. Abdominal examination also includes palpation of contractions. Frequency, duration, and intensity should be determined by the examiner. It is not appropriate to rely on an external electronic fetal monitor to determine characteristics of contractions. Although the fetal monitor may identify frequency, depending on maternal habitus and fetal position, it does not accurately reflect duration or intensity.

4. *Extremities.* The clinician should identify any edema, noting location and the degree of swelling. Generalized edema, coupled with increased blood pressure and/or proteinuria, may reflect a hypertensive disorder of pregnancy. Deep tendon reflexes should be evaluated to establish a baseline. Varicosities should be noted; signs of tenderness, warmth, and/or swelling over the varicosity indicate the need for immediate medical consultation.
5. *Pelvic examination.* The external examination should identify signs of gross rupture of membranes, lesions, or any infectious process. It is particularly important to closely evaluate a woman with a history of herpes to identify current lesions or establish whether she has any feeling of impending lesion. The midwife should note evidence of bloody show and, if there is leakage of fluid, look for evidence of meconium. When checking for meconium, it is necessary to look for the color of meconium against a white towel, sheet, or pad. Light meconium is easy to miss against the commonly found light blue pads in labor and delivery areas.
6. *Sterile speculum examination.* A sterile speculum examination should be done before any digital examinations if there is any history or suspicion of ruptured membranes. Cultures for group B streptococcus should be done at the same time (Box 19-1).
7. *Digital examination.* The digital examination should serve to confirm a careful abdominal examination. The midwife should note effacement, dilation, position of the cervix, fetal station, presenting part, position and status of membranes. Clinical pelvimetry should be done at this point, particularly if the woman has a large baby or a prior pelvimetry is not noted.

There may be times when it is necessary to obtain an ultrasound examination before the speculum or digital examination. With excess bloody show or any history that might indicate risk for previa or abruption, an ultrasound examination is indicated to determine location of placenta and/or signs of premature separation of the placenta. Deferral of the digital examination should be considered with PROM and no labor or early labor.

Deviations from normal. The midwife must evaluate the need for consultation, co-management, or referral. Depending on the site of the birth and the situation, the midwife will need to inform the obstetric consultant, appropriate nursing staff, and/or pediatrics personnel of the findings. Deviations from normal may be minimal and require fairly small interventions, such as inability to retain fluids, necessitating parenteral fluids. It is important to keep in mind that commonplace treatments (intravenous [IV] fluids, artificial rupture of membranes, fetal scalp electrode) are nonetheless interventions and should not be used indiscriminately but only when there is a deviation from the normal. Any deviation from the normal may also include a need to evaluate the site of birth.

INTAKE/OUTPUT: FEEDING THE MOTHER

Intake

Labor is an active physical event, and the laboring woman needs an energy source for optimal progress and outcome. Left to their own decision-making, women tend to eat and drink during labor, with the amounts diminishing as the labor progresses and nears second stage. The practice of withholding oral fluids and food during labor is fairly recent and is based on unsupported data and anecdotal information. Before the 1940s, women were encouraged to eat and drink during labor to have sufficient energy to withstand the physical exertion required. In the 1940s Mendelson (1946) ascribed the cause of intrapartum anesthesia deaths to the aspiration of regurgitated acidic stomach contents and recommended that women be denied oral feedings during labor to reduce the

Box 19-1 *Evaluation of Ruptured Membranes*

Ruptured membranes are evaluated with history, appearance of leaking in gross rupture, nitrazine litmus paper, and the slide ferning test.

History

The client may give a history of a large gush of warm fluid from her vagina or may simply feel more wetness or leaking. Variability in the history may be due to rupture of a forebag, a high leak that then seals off, heavy mucus discharge, urinary incontinence, or grossly ruptured membranes. Although a history of a large watery gush followed by leaking leaves little doubt of the diagnosis, it is still important to verify that the fluid was indeed amniotic fluid. If the woman calls from home, she should ascertain the character of the leaking, its color, odor, and amount. Color can be noted by pressing a clean white towel or washcloth against the perineum or by wearing a sanitary pad. Amniotic fluid has a particular musty smell and can be differentiated from the smell of urine. An obviously foul odor may be indicative of an infectious process.

Examination

Examination for ruptured membranes, whatever the setting, should be done carefully to avoid iatrogenic chorioamnionitis. The client should sit or lie on clean white material to evaluate the color of the fluid. The presence of meconium is difficult to evaluate if it is on the blue or blue-green waterproof pads commonly seen in hospitals. If there is obvious leaking from the woman's vagina or fluid is seen on her legs, a nitrazine paper may be directly touched to the fluid, and a cotton swab is used to plate a microscope slide.

Tests for Ruptured Membranes

If there is a suspicious history but no obvious rupture, a speculum examination is done using a sterile speculum and sterile gloves.

Pooling is the presence of amniotic fluid literally pooling in the vagina, usually seen in the posterior fornix or flowing from the cervix. If pooling is not observed, a Valsalva maneuver by the woman may cause the obvious discharge of fluid. Using a sterile cotton swab, a sample of the fluid is plated onto a microscope slide. A second swab is used to obtain a sample to roll across a small strip of nitrazine paper, or the paper may be touched to the fluid on the speculum after it is withdrawn. If there is no obvious pooling, the samples are taken from the vaginal discharge in the posterior fornix. *To avoid increasing the risk of infection, digital examinations are not done at this time.*

Nitrazine paper is a gold-colored litmus paper that turns dark blue on contact with amniotic fluid as a result of the alkaline pH of the fluid (7.0 to 7.5 as opposed to the normal vaginal pH of 4.5 to 5.5 in pregnancy). Nitrazine paper comes in a nonsterile roll and should not be inserted into the vagina. A false-positive result may be the result of cervical mucus, meconium, blood, semen, or vaginal infections that raise the pH of the vagina.

Ferning is the distinctive fernlike pattern seen on a microscope slide that has been plated with amniotic fluid. The ferning, or arborization, is a frondlike pattern caused by the presence of salts and protein in amniotic fluid. The slide should be completely dry before examination. Ferning is unaffected by blood, mucus, or meconium.

risk of aspiration of stomach contents. This became the standard of care, and is still seen in many maternity units.

Subsequent research has failed to find that aspiration of gastric contents is a contributor to maternal mortality and has noted that, even without oral intake, the stomach is never empty (Ludka and Roberts, 1993; O'Sullivan, 1994). The decline in anesthesia-related maternal deaths is most likely the result of improved anesthesia induction techniques, significantly increased use of regional anesthesia, and a decrease in the use of narcotics during active labor.

General considerations for oral intake during labor include:

1. *Gastric emptying time.* Gastric emptying time may be unpredictably increased during labor, with great individual variation. Fats, cold liquids, larger volumes of solids, and narcotic analgesia delay gastric emptying time (Ludka and Roberts, 1993; O'Sullivan, 1994).
2. *Need for nutrition.* The energy needs of women during labor have been compared to those of an athlete (Ludka and Roberts, 1993; O'Sullivan

1994). These comparisons, though interesting, are theoretic since there are no published studies of the energy requirements of laboring women (Enkin et al., 1996). O'Sullivan (1994) identifies comparable physiologic changes in performing athletes and laboring women, including increased cardiac output, minor delay in gastric emptying time, and increased oxygen consumption. Further using the athletic comparison, she notes that performance is enhanced with hydration and carbohydrate consumption during the performance. Advantages to oral intake during labor include physiologic factors (i.e., maintenance of blood glucose and decreased use of muscle glycogen) and psychologic factors since women often perceive enforced food and fluid restriction as very unpleasant.

3. *Ability to retain fluids and food.* As a general rule, women in labor should be encouraged to take a full range of fluids and eat lightly, particularly during early and early active labor. Choices should be mindful of causes of delayed gastric emptying—fat content, temperature, volume, and pH of the food or liquid consumed. Appropriate choices could include easily digested carbohydrates such as toast, crackers, cereal, fresh fruit, or low-fat yogurt and a full range of liquids. Women tend to self-select for eating and drinking in labor, with greater amounts early and decreasing as labor and cervical dilation progress. Contraindications for eating during labor would include women at increased risk for cesarean delivery and women receiving narcotic anesthesia or analgesia. Women unable to retain food may be able to drink fluids, particularly room temperature or warmed, and often find this comforting. Complete inability to retain fluids or food may indicate the need for intervention in the form of IV fluids, particularly if the labor is over 12 hours long.
4. *Fluid volume in labor.* Pregnancy is a hypervolemic state, with the healthy term woman superhydrated and thus well adapted for periods of minimal fluid intake (O'Sullivan, 1994). Excess fluids, however have been well documented to cause fluid overload and complications such as hyponatremia, maternal hyperglycemia, fetal hyperinsulinemia, and increased fetal blood pH (from glucose solutions). When IV hydration is necessary for the essentially normal laboring woman, normal saline or an electrolyte solution (e.g., Ringer's lactate) should be used. Because of the risk of fluid overload in laboring women, there should be clear need for IV therapy and careful attention to intake and output.

The use of IV fluids is indicated in certain situations in an otherwise essentially normal labor. Maternal conditions and events include imminent operative or assisted delivery, high risk of postpartum hemorrhage, inability of the woman to retain any oral fluids, need for oxytocin induction, severe anemia, use of epidural anesthesia in labor, and use of narcotic analgesia. Fetal indications include evidence of fetal distress, intrauterine growth retardation or any fetal condition that would significantly increase the risk of emergency or operative delivery. It is appropriate to use a saline "lock" for women who may need an IV access quickly but are otherwise normal, such as a with a VBAC.

Output

On admission urine should be evaluated to check for protein and ketones. Unless the client has hypertension or evidence of a urinary tract infection, a microscopic analysis is probably not necessary, although it may be required by hospital admission policies. Whether using a microscopic or reagent (dipstick) evaluation, it is important to look at the total picture with which the client presents. A microscopic evaluation is unlikely to offer immediate results, and most maternity settings and practices rely on the dipstick assessment of urine. The inherent inaccuracies of dipstick evaluation of protein and ketones must be remembered, particularly when the specimen is voided. The midwife should continue to focus on the total picture of the woman in labor rather than narrow information from a urine dipstick for management decisions.

Proteinuria of 2+ or over, particularly in an individual who has not previously had this finding, may be an indicator of preeclampsia and is an abnormal finding. Proteinuria is a late sign of hypertensive disorders or renal problems, however, and in the normotensive woman it is more likely to be the result of contamination of the urine by blood or mucus. Reagent or dipstick evaluation of lower levels of proteinuria is notoriously inaccurate, with a 25% false-positive rate with a trace reaction and a 6% false-positive rate with a 1+ reaction (Enkin et al., 1996). Catheterized specimens or carefully voided clean-catch specimens may be considered to be accurate at levels over 1+. It is sensible to attempt to obtain a clean-catch specimen on admission, but is probably unreasonable to ask a woman in labor to continue to provide clean voided urine during active labor. Catheterization is uncomfortable and increases the risk of urinary tract infections and should be reserved for women who have clear indications of a need for this type of urinalysis. It is unlikely that catheterization would be needed for urinalysis in a normal labor.

Ketonuria. It is unclear whether ketonuria during normal labor is a worrisome sign or a physiologic state that accompanies physical exertion. It is important to remember the difference between ketonuria, which is evidence of a shift to fat use, and ketoacidosis, which is a change in the pH of the blood and indicative of metabolic acidosis. Pregnant women are prone to ketosis due to the heightened demands of the fetoplacental unit and fat use. This tendency increases during labor with increased physical exertion. Ketonuria occurs in normal labors, and evidence is lacking that this is a harmful state, particularly in a patient who is otherwise healthy. Like proteinuria, ketones measured by urine dipstick tend to have a high false-positive rate, even when blood levels are normal. High levels of ketonuria, particularly if accompanied by inability to maintain oral fluid intake, may indicate a need for IV fluids. Correcting poor hydration and ketosis by IV administration in otherwise healthy women cannot be considered completely safe in light of the maternal and fetal side effects of IV fluid therapy. The midwife should attempt oral fluids and rehydration before routinely beginning IV infusion in the otherwise normal labor (Enkin et al., 1996; Ludka and Roberts, 1993; O'Sullivan, 1994).

Voiding in labor. The venerable Maggie Myles in early editions of a *Textbook for Midwives* (1975) always maintained that a good midwife *never, ever* let a woman get to second stage with a full bladder and to let this happen was tantamount to poor practice and generally sloppy care (Lee, 1978). The bladder at term has a smaller capacity and may be distended with relatively small amounts of urine. Distention is uncomfortable for the woman and may slow labor progress if the bladder impedes the ability of the presenting part to descend into the pelvis. In the event of a shoulder dystocia, a distended bladder could make delivery of the shoulders more difficult and increase the risk of trauma to the bladder itself. In the immediate postpartum period, a full bladder impedes the ability of the uterus to contract, making postpartum bleeding more likely.

Laboring women should be evaluated for bladder distention every 1 to 2 hours. The woman may be sufficiently focused on her labor that she does not feel the urge to void, or she may feel disinclined to move for fear of increased discomfort. Every abdominal examination should look for the revealing suprapubic bulge of a full bladder. In general, an appropriately hydrated woman should void over 100 ml every 1 to 2 hours.

Ambulating to the toilet is the most effective way for a laboring woman to void. She has more privacy, is able to void "normally," and is likely to be far more comfortable than she would be on a bedpan. In addition, the movement and gravity involved assist the progress of normal labor. Prohibiting ambulation to the toilet should only be in cases in which there is a risk of prolapsed cord (e.g., ruptured membranes with a high presenting part), placenta previa, preeclampsia, or other high-risk situations. Active labor itself is not a contraindication for ambulation to the bathroom. If a laboring woman is unable to ambulate because of risk factors, a bedside commode is the next most comfortable option. The use of the bedpan should be the last consideration.

Inability to void is not unusual in times of stress, discomfort, or anxiety—all distinct possibilities during labor. The sound of running water, warm water poured over the perineum, putting the woman's hands in warm water, or a few drops of oil of peppermint in the bedpan all may make it easier for her to void. Catheterization is invasive and uncomfortable and significantly increases the risk of urinary tract infection. Therefore it should be limited to occasions when the woman is unable to void, as with epidural anesthesia or preparation for operative delivery; or when the effort would be contraindicated, as with severe preeclampsia.

Emesis in labor. Emesis in labor is quite common and in the normal labor with an appropriately hydrated woman does not pose risk other than discomfort. It is most common during the late active phase. Preventive measures include encouraging the woman to eat low-fat meals in early labor and low-fat snacks thereafter. Cool washcloths, ice chips, and sips of carbonated beverages may help decrease nausea during labor. If the woman does vomit, helping her with the emesis basin, offering wet washcloths to clean up, and immediately changing a soiled gown and linens will increase her comfort. Reassurance that vomiting harms neither her labor nor her baby is important. Occasionally a laboring woman has unremitting vomiting in labor. If she is unable to retain fluids at all and delivery is not imminent, IV fluids will prevent dehydration and will probably make her feel better, despite the discomfort of having an IV started. Occasionally an antiemetic may be necessary to decrease unremitting vomiting.

SUPPORT STATUS: HELP FOR THE WOMAN

Direct support in the care of women in labor has always been the hallmark and pride of midwifery care. The very title is an old Anglo-Saxon word meaning "with woman." Support as described in this section is direct and at the woman's side and includes her family and companions.

Traditional societies provide support in out-of-hospital situations. In different cultures there may be various versions of who is the support (e.g., men may not be allowed; the presence of mother, sister, or mother-in-law may be required; and the presence of the midwife may be appropriate only at the time of the birth itself). Childbirth is a moment in time; the age of the mother leads to a different psychologic perspective, additionally filtered through her own beliefs, culture, experiences, fears, and hopes (Chalmers and Meyer, 1994). Every birth situation has a variation on the variables of the care provider, the mother and infant, and her partner/family situation/social support.

- The midwife brings her or his life experiences, birth experiences (both personal and professional), and social and professional values.
- The mother brings her life experiences, birth experiences, social values, experiences with her partner/support people, and feelings about her own and her infant's vulnerability.
- The partner and support people bring their own values, goals for the labor, fears for the woman and her infant, and often a sense of being the protector of the laboring mother.

Superimposed on these personal aspects are the practices and regulations of the institution, which may range from "baby friendly" to distinctly unwelcoming and counterproductive to the normal progress of labor and childbirth. It is the role of the midwife to identify the expectations, desires, and fears of the various participants; to facilitate their working together smoothly; and to negotiate the impasses that may arise when needs and desires conflict. At the same time, the midwife is expected to provide appropriate care for all laboring women under her charge at the time. This seemingly Herculean task is both learnable and doable.

Each midwife must learn to be both "with woman" and "with labor" as a support person. Participants in the birth process who are uncomfortable with their ability to provide support may withdraw from the woman and focus instead on tasks—charting, observing the monitor, or reading the chart. Support for the woman in labor can be organized into the provision of three components: physical care, supportive presence, and information. There are myriad ways that these may be provided, and the experienced midwife continues to accumulate tools for support.

Preparation for Labor and Birth

Midwives must always be aware that even multiparous women will have anxiety about birth. The capacity to be anxious is a biologic function necessary for survival. It can serve to mobilize energy and marshal forces to meet a challenge, but, if extreme, it can also be frightening or even debilitating. Normal fears of women in labor include death, pain, suffering, exposure, "breaking down," humiliation, loss of self, and fear for the unborn infant. Facing these fears and coping with the anxiety and sensations of childbirth can be a peak experience.

The midwife can help reduce the anxiety level by introducing a vocabulary of birth and providing reassurance and support for the woman's concerns. Women need to be taught how to be *with* birth, rather than how to *give* birth. The physiology of labor will take care of the birth, and reminding women that their bodies are programmed to do this task may relieve them of the feeling that they are responsible for correctly performing a complex function that they do not understand.

Important things to teach include permission to be active, to use a variety of comfort measures, and to make requests of the staff and institution. Although it is self-serving to "teach to the hospital" so that the mother arrives prepared to acquiesce to institutional procedures, it is unfair for her to enter the place of birth not knowing what to expect. The midwife is the liaison between mother and institution, and is in the position to interpret, facilitate, and soften the interface between them. Walking this fine line requires that the midwife maintain a sense of the needs of the woman and her family, the normalcy of the labor, and the needs of the staff. A healthy sense of humor, good negotiating skills, and flexibility are essential.

Midwifing the Labor

Discover the issues for this woman. If the midwife has provided prenatal care, she may already be aware of issues. If not, they may be in the prenatal records, as with a significant historical event or if she has expressed particular fears or concerns. More often, the midwife will need to discover through asking the laboring mother, in conversation with support people, and by observation.

Educate, reframe, and offer empowering options. Providing as much control as possible gives the woman in labor the ability to decide for herself what is most helpful. Assuring her that options are available and giving her the control of timing and selection help decrease the institutionalization and vulnerability that women often feel in a hospital. However, options must be realistic, so that she does not feel lied to or patronized. Laughter, praise, and encouraging a belief in birth all reframe the notion of birth as a fearsome and dangerous event.

Create the optimal environment to maximize the physiology of labor. An important role of the midwife is to protect the birth process from intrusion—providing quiet, dimmed lighting, privacy, and decreased stimuli. This helps decrease anxiety, which in turn reduces catecholamine production and allows the physiology of labor to progress unimpeded.

Provide coping measures for pain, from less to more, keeping in mind the normalcy of the labor and the desires of the mother. Present coping mechanisms as a range of options from relaxation and gentle touch to epidural anesthesia. Discuss with the woman and her family that the goal is a healthy birth. If the mother is concerned about the availability of pharmacologic relief, she should be reassured that medication is available, but the goal is to reduce the total dosage and postpone the epidural when possible for the health of both mother and infant. When both woman and midwife are able to be open and flexible about what comfort measures to use and when to initiate them, the experience is far more likely to be positive for all concerned.

Use the strength of a supportive presence. Several studies indicate that the simple presence of a supportive person provides the laboring mother with a sense of security (Hodnett, 1999). Labor support may include such things as massage, fanning, cool cloths, music, and acupressure; but the importance of the companion who simply sits with the mother and offers reassurance and praise cannot be overlooked (Research Box 19-1).

Be aware of your own background—the fears, biases, desires, conditioned reactions to events—as all of these affect the situation at hand. Each midwife needs to develop self-awareness of her or his own "hot buttons" or areas of particular concern or stress. Awareness helps the provider stay attuned to the needs and nuances of the current situation.

Supporting the support system. In the United States most women labor with at least one support person. The range of knowledge and ability varies considerably and may include friends or family members who have little understanding about how to attend birth. As with any situation, it is important to identify expectations of the mother for her supporters as well as the skills and interest of the supporters. Following that, the midwife can proceed to assist the labor companions in supporting the laboring woman.

Well-prepared companions who have good communication with the mother need little more than an orientation to the room and facilities so that they will be able to find such things as the bathroom, washcloths, ice, and drinks. For less well-prepared supporters, simple, specific, and straightforward instructions work well, particularly when accompanied by a brief explanation of why the comfort measure is helpful. Comfort measures that are quick and easy to explain include massage, cold cloths, fanning, and assistance with walking.

Encouraging family/support participation serves to empower the family, reframes the birth experience as a normal event, and helps to reduce anxiety for both the family members and the mother. Ongoing reassurance for the mother and her support is important. The midwife can remind the family that birth is an intense experience and may be uncomfortable and hurt. Pain may be unavoidable, but the midwife and the supporters are there to help the mother cope. Praise for the mother and for her supporters and frequent observations about how she is doing and how the baby is doing help reduce fears (Figure 19-1).

Supporting Survivors of Childhood Sexual Abuse

A commonly cited statistic indicates that approximately one in four women are sexually abused before the age of 18 years (Jamieson and Steege, 1997; Hinds and Baskin, 1999). Given such numbers, the midwife will find herself or himself attending these women in labor. Although many women have had sufficient time, distance, and therapy to cope with the abuse, many others exhibit posttraumatic stress disorder, which can be triggered in labor (Herman, 1992; Seng and Hassinger, 1998). Behaviors may include fighting labor, extreme stoicism, complete surrender to the authority of the provider, or withdrawal to a near catatonic state. If the woman has indicated prenatally that she is a childhood sexual abuse survivor, the midwife can ask her if she has particular needs or wants in labor. Common requests include self-insertion of speculum, very limited vaginal

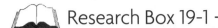

Research Box 19-1

Scott KD, Berkowitz G, Klaus M: A comparison of intermittent and continuous support during labor: a meta-analysis, *Am J Obstet Gynecol* 180(5):1054-1059, 1999.

Background

Randomized control studies have found that the presence of a female doula or labor attendant significantly reduces length of labor and need for oxytocin augmentation and decreases operative deliveries among healthy childbearing women. However, study findings have not fully explored the effect of the actual duration of support during labor.

Research Question

What are the effects of continuous and intermittent social support during labor on childbirth outcomes?

Methods

Eleven randomized control trials that explored the effect of female labor support on birth outcomes were identified using MEDLINE, the American Psychological Association data base, and Dissertation Abstracts International. Subjects in the studies were required to be at or near term. The independent variable was duration of social support in labor. Dependent variables were use of any analgesia, use of oxytocin augmentation, forceps delivery, cesarean delivery, and length of labor. Studies were allocated to the continuous or intermittent support group. Studies were weighted by sample size, and odds ratios were calculated for each of the dependent variables.

Sample

Five trials were determined to represent continuous support models and represented 1809 subjects. Six trials were determined to represent intermittent support and represented 2582 subjects. Of interest are the facts that the continuous support persons were consistently lay women and in all but one trial the intermittent support persons were midwives or student midwives.

Results

Findings suggest that the presence of a female labor support person on an intermittent basis is not significantly associated with decreased rates for any of the five dependent outcomes when compared to no support controls. The continuous presence of a doula significantly decreases all outcome variable rates when compared with no additional support. Continuous support reduces the odds of analgesia by 36%, oxytocin augmentation by 71%, forceps delivery by 57%, and cesarean delivery by 51%. Length of labor was significantly decreased (by 1.5 hours) in the continuous support group. Because of the difference in training of the support persons represented by the two groups, duration of labor may be a proxy indicator for style of support or role perception. The difference in site of studies and potential differences in obstetric styles of practice and cultural aspects of birthing may also explain the differences noted when the trials were allocated to continuous and intermittent groups.

Clinical Application

Because the presence of a continuous labor support person who is not also fulfilling the role of birth attendant appears to be associated with significant reductions in obstetrical interventions, findings suggest that a team approach between medical personnel and lay doulas may lead to benefits for mothers and infants. Further study is needed to understand the support styles of different doulas/attendants to design programs that are most effective in decreasing unnecessary intervention.

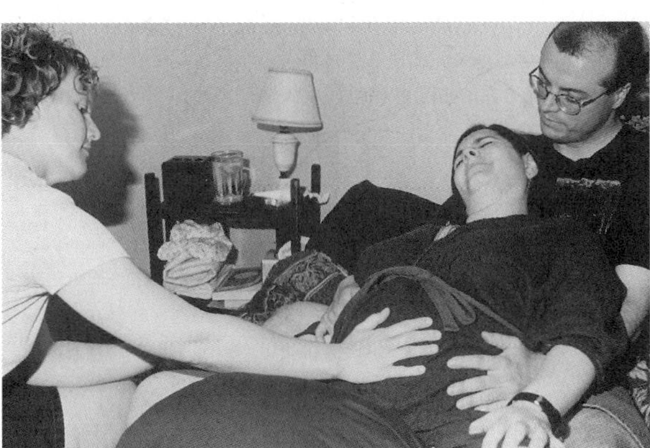

Figure 19-1 Support people helping woman cope with contractions. (Courtesy Caroline E. Brown.)

examinations, and extensive preparation for any invasive procedures.

The midwife may be unaware that the client is an abuse survivor until something triggers a reaction in labor. Women may be silent, unaware of or unable to confront traumatic experiences, and may attempt to avoid triggering memories. If unexpected memories or reactions occur, the midwife can try to ease the situation by addressing a few of the woman's most current needs. Labor is not the time to address sexual abuse, nor are midwives the appropriate people to initiate therapy. However, it is important to acknowledge the woman's history as she presents it and reassure her that she is safe and supported. She may have had the experience before and may know what helps reduce her anxiety. Privacy is very important as it gives the woman control and concentration. Involving her in management decisions also provides control. It is important to explain every step of every process since the hallmark of sexual abuse is a sense of having been invaded without permission. A matter-of-fact manner and calm attitude are reassuring. Abuse survivors do better with a consistent presence during the birth process (Simkin, 1992).

When Support Is Not Supportive

On occasion, the laboring woman's support system is not supportive. Companions may arrive under the influence of alcohol or drugs or may simply be unable or unwilling to provide the attention that the mother wants. When the midwife suspects a lack of support, it is necessary to ask the mother if she would like some intervention. This is done in private. Family and friends can be asked to step out of the room briefly while the midwife checks the woman or assists her to the bathroom. In the role of liaison, the midwife can offer to try to involve the unhelpful supporter or even "be the heavy" and limit the people in the room to those of the woman's choosing.

Turning off the television "so she can concentrate on her labor" gives supporters the message that the laboring mother is the central person and turns the focus to her. Often support companions want to help but are unsure what to do. The midwife can provide guidance, role modeling, and reassurance that a quiet presence is also helpful. This may be especially important when companions are overly energetic and seem bent on filming everything from the admission paperwork to every vaginal examination on the way to the birth. Again, the midwife asks the mother what she wants and tactfully conveys this information to would-be movie makers to negotiate a way to preserve memories of the birth as well as the mother's dignity and desire for privacy.

Working With Doulas

In today's environment of managed care, the midwife may find herself caring for several women in active labor at the same time in a busy labor and delivery unit. This reality must be addressed by midwives who work in high-volume practices. This sometimes necessitates a role shift from one-to-one supporter to something akin to stage manager. A trend in some areas is for families who want formal support in labor to contract with a doula. "Doula" is a Greek word that means a woman caregiver of another woman. In the United States doulas usually have taken a formal education program that includes both theoretic and clinical components. The doula's role is to be an advocate for the woman in labor, to provide physical and emotional support, and to be a resource for intrapartum and postpartum information (Zhang et al., 1996).

The use of doula support in labor may be difficult for the midwife who sees her highly valued role being taken over by another. Even when the workload makes it impossible for the midwife to offer a high level of individual support, it is often painful to surrender a large part of what makes midwifery a unique profession. Midwives who successfully work with doulas suggest that it is possible to have doula care and still be true to the "art and soul" of midwifery labor support.

The prenatal period is the optimal time to discuss the use of doula support with the client and her partner. If possible, the doula should attend a prenatal visit and meet at least one of the midwives in the practice. This offers an opportunity to orient the practice and the doula to each other and to discuss the expectations of the client, midwife, and doula. Avoiding territorial battles, preserving the calm of the labor environment, and making united efforts to support the mother and her family should be the goals of all providers working with pregnant women. The doula is a new and formalized version of the experienced labor companion. Ideally the doula and midwife support each other in their work to achieve a healthy birth outcome. Although the midwife may feel wistful at the loss of her role, in a busy managed-care practice she is unable to fulfill the role. When the midwife and doula work in an atmosphere of mutual respect and clear communication, the client benefits from the skills and support of both professionals.

FETAL STATUS

When evaluating the fetal status, it is important to maintain a continuing awareness of the fetus as part of a maternal-fetal unit. The health and well-being of the fetus are greatly affected by the health and well-being of the mother.

Maternal and fetal conditions before labor may or may not carry over into the labor, but should always be considered. Chronic diseases such as diabetes or hypertension are correlated with an increased incidence of intrauterine growth restriction, which in turn reduces the ability of the fetus to tolerate the stress of labor. Gestational age, whether early, within the range for term, or late, is a strong indicator of potential health or problems.

Chart Review

Fetal surveillance. Fetal surveillance refers to use of modalities to assess fetal well-being, from the more traditional methods such as fetal movement counts to the latest medical technologic imaging. Historically the primary objective of antepartum fetal surveillance was to identify fetuses at increased risk of fetal death. As methods to identify and treat fetal conditions during the antepartum and intrapartum periods have been introduced, surveillance procedures are increasingly used to identify fetuses at risk for a wide variety of adverse perinatal outcomes (Ananth, Smulian, and Vintzileos, 1997). However, there is no published evidence showing that antepartum fetal testing reduces neonatal complications related to intrauterine asphyxia. Cunningham and colleagues (1993) note that, despite the invention of increasingly complex testing methods, abnormal results are seldom reliable, prompting most clinicians to use antenatal testing to forecast fetal wellness rather than illness.

Chart review should include asking the question, "Why was the testing done?" to better ascertain the risk of an individual fetus for complications in labor. Common indications for antenatal testing include postdates gestation, fetal growth restriction, maternal hypertension, vascular disease, antiphospholipid antibody syndrome, insulin-dependent diabetes, PROM, vaginal bleeding, decreased fetal movement, Rh disease, nonimmune fetal hydrops, fetal arrhythmia and maternal hyperthyroidism, systemic lupus erythematosus, poor prior obstetric history, and twin gestation. Fetal testing includes the following interventions:

1. *Fetal activity counts.* Documentation of reported fetal movement during the last 6 weeks of pregnancy provides a baseline for determining fetal health. Studies report a strong correlation between good perinatal outcome and positive maternal perception of fetal movements (Moore and Piacquadio, 1989). The recent ACOG Practice Bulletin (1999a) recommends further fetal testing in the absence of a reassuring count. However, a formal program of fetal movement assessment is not recommended because of the lack of consistent evidence that it will result in a reduction in fetal deaths.
2. *Nonstress testing.* Nonstress testing is a surveillance technique that provides information related to the immediate condition of the fetus. Most testing schemes currently endorse twice-weekly evaluations in at-risk or high-risk pregnancies. In general, clients with a reactive antepartum NST have a tenfold lower risk for intervention for presumed distress during labor than fetuses that display a nonreactive "abnormal" pattern. However, the specificity of the nonreactive pattern is usually less than 50%. Given the poor specificity of a nonreactive NST, additional backup testing such as the biophysical profile (BPP), modified BPP, or contraction stress test is beneficial to provide a better understanding of the antepartum fetal status (Miller, Rabello, and Paul, 1996).
3. *Biophysical profile.* The BPP is based on the association between chronic fetal compromise and changes in fetal heart rate (FHR) patterns, decreased fetal body and breathing movements, and reduction in fetal blood flow and fetal oliguria, causing less amniotic fluid. The impact of the BPP on obstetric interventions, length of hospitalizations, serious neonatal morbidity, and parent's satisfaction is undocumented. A review of the small number of randomized control trials found in the literature concluded that there are insufficient data to reach any definite conclusion about the benefit or otherwise of the BPP as a test of fetal well-being (Alfirevic and Neilson, 1998).
4. *Amniotic fluid volume.* The AFI is an assessment of amniotic fluid volume using a four-quadrant summation of measurements of pockets of fluid. Antepartum testing for high-risk pregnancies includes not only an NST but also an AFI. This combination is called a modified BPP. Recent studies have suggested that the incidence of abnormal perinatal outcomes (fetal distress, cesarean section, meconium staining, low APGAR scores) was higher among clients with oligohydramnios even when the NST was reactive. This would indicate a greater predictive value for fetal tolerance of labor. Oligohydramnios with term and postterm pregnancies usually warrants intervention to expedite labor (Manning et al., 1990; Rutherford et al., 1987).

Fetal size. Fetal size depends on multiple variables, including genetics; ethnicity; chronic maternal conditions such as diabetes, hypertension, Crohn's disease, anemia, and malnutrition; pregnancy-related maternal conditions such as parity, gestational age, preeclampsia, gestational diabetes, excess weight gain, multiple gestation, and social circumstances such as substance exposure and poor environment. Infants at the extremes of birth weight (i.e., birth weight less than 2500 g or greater than 4000 g) face increased risks for perinatal problems. The variables that place a fetus at risk for low birth weight may be categorized as gestational, infectious, chromosomal, environmental, vascular, or nutritional. The primary contributor to low birth weight or very low birth weight is preterm birth. The incidences of low-birth-weight (<2500 g at birth) and very low–birth-weight (<1500 g at birth) deliveries have changed little since 1975, despite the availability of pharmacologic agents to inhibit preterm labor.

Approximately 75% of preterm births occur spontaneously after preterm labor or preterm PROM, and more than one-half of these births occur in women who have no apparent risk factors (Gabbe, Niebyl, and Simpson, 1996). A small-for-gestational-age infant (<tenth percentile for gestation on population curves) usually indicates a stressed uteroplacental environment during the pregnancy. This may be the result of an underlying vascular condition such as vasoconstriction associated with cigarette smoking, hypertension, preeclampsia, or multiple gestation. Chronic malnutrition associated with excessive alcohol intake, drug abuse, anorexia or bulimia, Crohn's disease, and inadequate financial resources impacts on birth weights. The Collaborative Perinatal Study documented that low birth weight occurred four times more frequently among women who gained less than 14 pounds than among women who gained from 30 to 35 pounds (Singer, Westphal, and Niswander, 1968).

On the other side of the fetal weight continuum is the large-for-gestational-age (LGA) fetus. Most sources define LGA as birth weight above the 90th percentile in population-based growth charts. Macrosomia is defined by some investigators as a birth weight in excess of 4000 to 4500 g (Delpapa and Mueller-Heubach, 1991). Excessive fetal growth resulting in macrosomia has long been recognized as a contributing factor to perinatal morbidity and mortality. At delivery the large fetus is at risk for shoulder dystocia, traumatic injury, and asphyxia. The most common identifiable conditions leading to excessive infant birth weight are maternal diabetes and maternal obesity (Gabbe, Niebyl, and Simpson, 1996). Accurate detection of the LGA fetus would allow for appropriate intervention for a timely vaginal birth or optimal selection of the route of delivery to reduce the likelihood of birth trauma. However, there is poor clinical identification of large fetal size, with only 35% of large infants being identified by fundal height measurements. In addition, ultrasonography has limited predictive value to identify the macrosomic fetus. The sensitivity and positive predictive values of ultrasonographic EFWs at term ranged between 50% and 60% (Chervenak et al., 1989; Pollack, Hauer-Pollack, and Divon, 1992; Johnstone, 1997).

Fetal Assessment in Labor

The mother's awareness of her fetus is a baseline for determining fetal well-being. A report of reduced activity or simply a generalized feeling of concern is a reason for greater need in determining current fetal health.

Fetal weight is one of the factors that determine the fit of the passenger (the fetus) with the passage (the pelvis). The average fetal weight of a term fetus (between 38 and 42 weeks) is between 3000 and 3800 g. The clinical estimation of fetal weight is based on Leopold's maneuvers. Even with easy sonographic availability, estimation of fetal weight by the clinician and even the mother is at least as good as sonographic estimation with a normal-term infant (Gabbe, Niebyl, and Simpson, 1996).

Regardless of fetal size, it is the relationship between that fetus and the maternal pelvis that strongly influences the fit. Fetal position is assessed abdominally using Leopold's maneuvers and confirmed with a cervical examination that identifies the presenting part and its landmarks. Determinations of fetal presentation, position, and estimated weight are essential in anticipating the course of labor and the possible interventions and/or consultations that will be necessary. Malpresentation requires obstetric consultation with either referral or comanagement determined by the professional relationship between clinicians, the institutional policies, and the experience of the providers. Malposition and extremes in estimated weight may require obstetric and/or pediatric consultation, depending on institutional policies and the provider's own practice guidelines.

Fetal Heart Monitoring

The FHR pattern in labor reflects the fetus's current status and tolerance of the forces of labor. The assessment should include a review of the baseline, the response to fetal movement and/or contractions, and heart rate changes over time. The heart rate may be monitored by auscultation with a fetoscope or Doppler, or by external or internal electronic monitoring that produces a tracing. The midwifery model of care provides a framework for appropriate use of technology in low risk and at risk pregnancies. The American College of Nurse-Midwives position statement on the appropriate use of technology in childbirth states, "In order to achieve the optimal outcome for the mother and/or infant at risk for conditions that deviate from normal, the ACNM supports the use of appropriate technologic interventions where the benefits of such technology outweigh the risks" (1997). In addition, the ACNM notes that, "when interventions are used, their benefits and risks should be thoroughly explained to the woman, and an attempt should be made to adapt such interventions to her social and cultural practice" (1997). It is incumbent on the midwife to base decisions on the mode of fetal assessment in labor on the effectiveness determined by science, not by ritual or routine of a given obstetric setting.

Routine continuous electronic FHR monitoring was introduced in the early 1970s. It was thought that this objective technique, when used in labor management of women at increased risk for poor perinatal outcome, would provide early evidence of fetal asphyxia. When fetal asphyxia was suspected, appropriate interventions could be initiated to protect the fetus and prevent intrapartum fetal death and morbidity. To "save the fetus from the hazards of labor," it was quickly accepted into obstetric practice before adequate research as to its validity or reliability. Continuous EFM is used in the management of labor and delivery in nearly three of four pregnancies in the United States (Albers and Krulewitch, 1993). Therefore, by its very use in both low- and high-risk pregnancies, its primary role has shifted from a diagnostic to a screening tool. This continues to be the case, despite recent agreement among policy makers and researchers that EFM is an ineffective screening tool. Effective screening tools are valid and reliable. Electronic fetal monitoring is neither. Validity refers to the accurate detection of the condition of interest: fetal asphyxia. However, there is little known about the actual relationship between EFM patterns and neurodevelopmental outcomes. Nor is the presence of abnormalities on the monitor strip indicative of a hypoxic event or, if there was such an event, the timing of that event. Epidemiologic findings show that asphyxia is far more likely to occur prenatally than intrapartally (Rosen and Dickinson, 1993). Reliability of a screening test refers to consensus among those who interpret the information. There is very little interobserver agreement in interpreting monitor strips. The two patterns where there is consensus, late decelerations and severe variable decelerations, are easily recognized with intermittent auscultation (Albers, 1994). Clinical utility of this screening tool is also called into question. What has occurred in the United States is excess use of operative intervention for suspect patterns without the use of additional procedures to diagnose fetal asphyxia. The blasé attitude about the use of fetal monitoring has minimized the needs of the laboring woman in favor of the presumed needs of the fetus.

A systematic review of randomized control trials of continuous EFM during labor found an increase associated with the use of EFM in the rate of cesarean delivery (relative risk 1.33), and an increase in total operative deliveries (relative risk 1.23) (Thacker and Stroup, 1998). Of particular significance is the finding that risk of cesarean delivery was greatest in low-risk pregnancies. Viewed with the knowledge that none of the nine published randomized control trials demonstrated a statistically significant difference between monitoring methods in the number of births with a 1-minute APGAR score below 7, the potential risk of an operative delivery in low-risk pregnancies because of an ineffective screening tool becomes apparent. The only complication with a decreased occurrence in the continuously monitored group was neonatal convulsions. No significant difference was observed in 1-minute APGAR scores below 7, rate of admissions to neonatal intensive care units (NICUs), and perinatal death. The review concludes that the benefits once claimed for EFM are clearly more modest than once believed and appear to be primarily in the prevention of neonatal seizures. However, abnormal neurologic consequences were not consistently higher among children monitored by auscultation relative to those monitored electronically.

A second meta-analysis that included essentially the same randomized control trials found that continuous electronic FHR monitoring was associated with higher rates of operative and instrumental delivery than intermittent auscultation alone (Neilson, 1994). This difference was true even when EFM was complemented by selective fetal blood sampling and pH estimation.

The American College of Obstetricians and Gynecologists recommends that clients at increased risk for perinatal complications have either continuous EFM or intermittent auscultation every 15 minutes in the first stage of labor. Women experiencing healthy pregnancies can be followed with intermittent auscultation every 30 minutes in the first stage of labor for low-risk clients (ACOG, 1995). The Bulletin further states that "there is no comparative data indicating the optimal frequency at which intermittent auscultation should be performed in the absence of risk factors" (p. 3). The Society of Obstetricians and Gynaecolgists in Canada (SOGC) issued a major policy statement in October 1995, stating that "the preferred method of fetal surveillance for low-risk women during labor is intermittent fetal heart auscultation with a handheld ultrasound Doppler" (SOGC, 1995). In this area of labor management, clinicians can be models for the appropriate use of low technology with policy support by ACOG and SOGC; and midwives can validate the normalcy of birth while caring for women in an increasingly technocratic field.

Not all fetuses provide a reassuring FHR. It is important for the clinician to identify situations when continuously monitoring the FHR is warranted and to determine the appropriateness of external vs. internal FHR monitoring.

Interpretation of Electronic Fetal Monitoring

Fetal heart rate baseline. Baseline FHR is defined as the approximate mean FHR rounded off to increments of 5 beats/min during a specified 10-minute period of time (NICHDR, 1997). Baseline rate excludes periodic or episodic changes and periods of marked FHR variability. The normal baseline is between 110 and 160 beats/min. Persistent intervals of tachycardia or bradycardia are more likely associated with hypoxia than a normal heart rate. Fetal tachycardia is a rate above 160 beats/min for at least 10 minutes. Fetal prematurity, maternal fever, fetal infection, atropine administration, fetal tachyarrhythmias, maternal anxiety, idiopathic asphyxia, and maternal thyrotoxicosis are some of the underlying causes of fetal tachycardia (Gabbe, Niebyl, and Simpson, 1996). Fetal bradycardia is a FHR below 110 beats/min for at least 10 minutes. Mild bradycardia of 90 to109 beats/min without accelerations or decelerations may be seen in the second stage of labor (Cunningham et al., 1993). Complete heart block must also be considered with a FHR range of 50 to 70 beats/min with absent variability and decelerations. The causes of complete heart block are congenital heart disease, particularly ventricular septal defect, maternal disease such as lupus erythematosus, which may cause inflammation and fibrosis in the conducting system and fetal heart failure or hydrops (Gabbe, Niebyl, and Simpson, 1996). It is important to evaluate prior baseline FHR and variability in conjunction with a bradycardic episode to determine how onerous the episode is.

Fetal heart rate variability. Baseline FHR variability is deemed as fluctuations in the baseline FHR of two cycles per minute or greater. Amplitude changes are quantified as follows:

- Amplitude range undetectable—absent FHR variability
- Amplitude range <5 beats/min—minimal FHR variability
- Amplitude range 6 to 25 beats/min—moderate FHR variability
- Amplitude range >25 beats/min—marked variability (NICHDR, 1997, p. 1386)

Variability reflects central nervous system status and is the most important characteristic of the FHR pattern. Alterations in the nervous system, including fetal sleep, medications, alcohol, or congenital anomalies may affect variability. Periodically, variability may be absent or reduced in normal situations such as fetal sleep, narcotic or epidural administration, and maternal position. Maternal dehydration may also be associated with decreased variability. Such situations must be closely watched, and the underlying cause rectified if appropriate. Absent or minimal variability may also indicate fetal compromise secondary to poor fetal oxygenation with resulting acidosis. Therefore it is important to further evaluate and appropriately manage this condition. Further evaluation includes evaluation of the baseline FHR, periodic FHR changes, and scalp stimulation to evaluate fetal acid-base status. Clinical management is guided by this evaluation and could range from continued observation with support measures (e.g., oxygen administration, maternal position change, and/or a bolus of IV fluid) to immediate delivery.

Periodic changes in fetal heart rate: accelerations. Fetal heart accelerations are an abrupt increase in FHR of at least 15 beats/min and at least 15 seconds' duration. Before 32 weeks' gestation, accelerations are defined as increases of >10 beats/min for >10 seconds. Accelerations may be caused by fetal movement, stimulation of contractions, umbilical cord occlusion, and fetal stimulation. Accelerations represent intact neurohormonal cardiovascular control mechanisms that are linked to fetal behavioral states. The presence of spontaneous or evoked FHR accelerations is a common indicator of fetal well-being. This assures the clinician that labor may proceed without immediate intervention (ACOG, 1995; Elimian, Figueroa, and Tejani, 1997).

Periodic changes in fetal heart rate: decelerations. Fetal heart decelerations occur in response to contractions or other factors that significantly decrease fetal perfusion. They are categorized as three types: early, variable, and late.

Early decelerations are gradual decreases in FHR that occur with the onset of a contraction and reach a nadir <30 seconds after the onset of the contraction. The nadir of the deceleration occurs at the same time as the peak of the contraction (NICHDR, 1997). They occur with head compression that causes increased intracranial pressure and the resulting vagal response of a deceleration. They usually occur in the active phase of labor and resolve spontaneously as labor progresses. Early decelerations may be used as an indicator of labor progress, thus minimizing the need for repeated cervical examinations. As long as there is adequate variability and additional periodic changes are not observed, early decelerations can be observed throughout labor without alterations in fetal condition, acid-base status, or neonatal or long-term outcome (Gabbe, Niebyl, and Simpson, 1996).

Variable decelerations occur within 30 seconds of the onset of the contraction and characteristically have an abrupt onset. The decrease in FHR is >15 beats/min, lasting at least 15 seconds, and there is a return to baseline <2 minutes after the onset of the contraction (NICHDR, 1997). The usual cause of variable decelerations is cord compression. The umbilical cord occlusion causes increased peripheral resistance and stimulation of the baroreceptors and chemoreceptors and produces a vagal response of a deceleration. Variable decelerations are self-limiting in that after the contraction the FHR returns to baseline. With a resilient fetus moderate-to-severe variables may be accompanied by an erratic rebound acceleration known as "shoulders" before returning to baseline. Mild variables are any depth not less than 80 beats/min and last less than 30 seconds. Moderate variables are less than 80 beats/min and of any duration. Severe variables are less than 70 beats/min and last longer than 60 seconds. In some instances there may be an acceleration immediately preceding or following the abrupt slowing or recovery of the heart rate. This "overshoot" phenomenon may indicate a more significant hypoxia in the fetus, as is a gradual rather than abrupt return to baseline (ACOG, 1995; Gabbe, Niebyl, and Simpson, 1996).

Prolonged decelerations last >2 minutes but <10 minutes. Any decrease in FHR >10 minutes is considered a change in baseline (NICHDR, 1997). These changes are always a concern and may be caused by any mechanism that can lead to fetal hypoxia. The degree to which such decelerations are non-reassuring depends on the depth and duration, the lack of variability, the response of the fetus during recovery, and the frequency and progression of recurrence. An immediate search for the cause of the nonreassuring FHR pattern is imperative. A cervical examination to evaluate for prolapsed cord is appropriate if the client has ruptured membranes and to identify if there is a dramatic change in labor progress. An attempt at resolution of the deceleration is mandatory. This can be done by maternal position change, oxygen administration, and an attempt to quiet an overstimulated uterus through tocolytic drugs or discontinuation of oxytocin if indicated.

Late decelerations occur after the peak of the contraction and have a gradual onset with the nadir >30 seconds after the onset of the contraction. They are usually the result of diminished uterine blood flow during contractions that leads to critical reduction of Po_2 following the peak of the contraction and subsequent reflex and hypoxic slowing of the FHR. Late decelerations can be associated with obstetric and/or anesthetic procedures such as epidural anesthesia, supine hypotension, or uterine hypertonicity. They can also be associated with placental insufficiency secondary to intrauterine growth restriction, hypertensive disorders of pregnancy, placental abruption, and other causes. The seriousness is determined by their repetitive nature, the variability of the baseline, and the length of time it takes to return to baseline. Intermittent late decelerations are not uncommon during labor. This is especially true with epidural anesthesia and/or oxytocin stimulation. Persistent late decelerations mean that they are present with most of the contractions and are considered nonreassuring (ACOG, 1995). As with other nonreassuring tracings, identification of the underlying cause, if possible, is indicated, and fetal resuscitation is warranted.

Decelerations that contribute to a nonreassuring tracing indicate a change in fetal status and require immediate evaluation, followed by intervention and/or consultation with an obstetrician. Fetal resuscitation is implemented by maternal position change, oxygen administration of 8 to 10 L/min, a bolus of electrolyte containing IV fluids, and discontinuation of oxytocin. Concurrently an assessment of labor progress by cervical examination should be performed to evaluate length of time until expected delivery. Fetal resuscitation measures are performed to increase oxygen transport to the fetus. Maternal position change removes the possibility of arterial compression by the enlarged uterus and may move the fetus away from a positional cord compression. Oxygen administration increases the oxygen supply to the vascular system, and some authorities believe that such administration may provide significant increase in fetal oxygen. However, these conclusions were drawn from animal studies (Meschia, 1989). Others argue that oxygen administration does not change fetal Po_2, so oxygen administration may be performed more for medicolegal reasons. IV hydration increases the oxygenated fluid volume to the fetus. Assessment of labor progress provides an estimate of the length of time the fetus will undergo stress from contractions (Figure 19-2).

Amnioinfusion

Amnioinfusion is the transcervical instillation of normal saline into the uterine cavity. It is used therapeu-

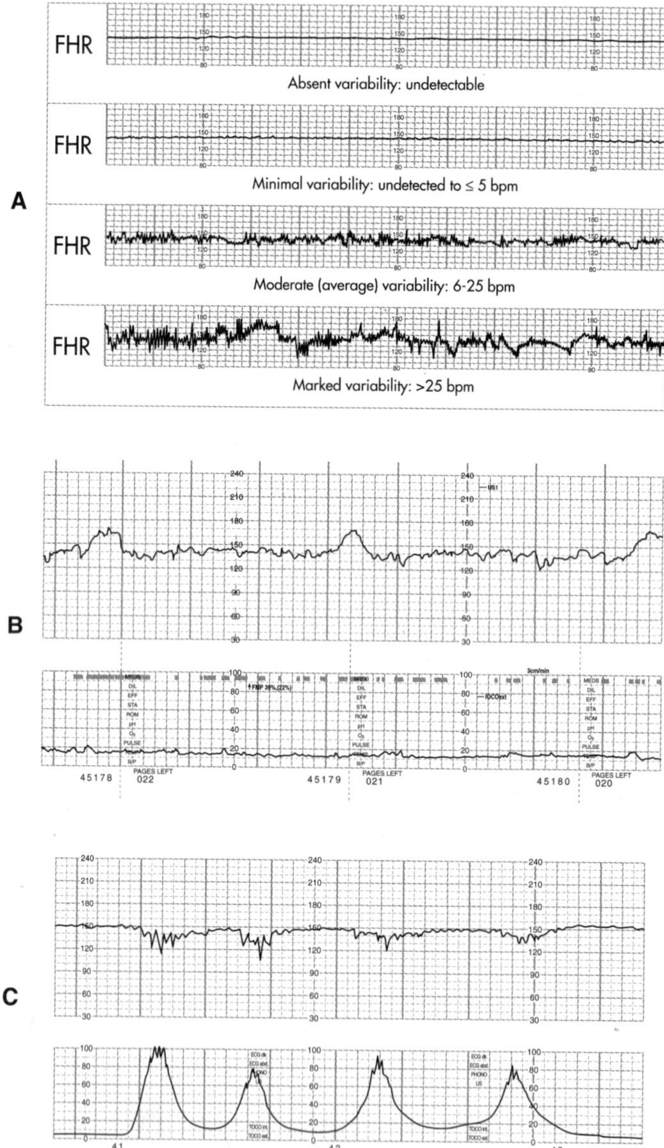

Figure 19-2 Fetal monitoring. **A,** Classification of variability; **B,** acceleration of fetal heart rate with fetal movement; **C,** early decelerations (actual tracings).

tically for repetitive moderate-to-severe variable FHR decelerations during labor and for the presence of moderate-to-thick meconium-stained fluid and oligohydramnios (Miyazaki and Nevarez, 1985; Spong, Ogundipe, and Ross, 1994). As previously noted, moderate-to-severe variable decelerations are often caused by umbilical cord compression, particularly when there is oligohydramnios. A review of randomized control trials assessing the effects of amnioinfusion on perinatal outcome concluded that amnioinfusion for potential or suspected umbilical cord compression reduces the occurrence of variable FHR decelerations (Hofmeyr, 1998). The most notable result is the significant reduction in cesarean births, accounted for by a reduction in surgery performed for "fetal distress" as diagnosed by FHR tracings. The findings also addressed the rare but serious maternal side effects of amnioinfusion. Several case reports have been published of amniotic fluid embolism following amnioinfusion, although a causal relationship has not been established.

Another review of the randomized control trials on the use of amnioinfusion for meconium-stained fluid in labor found a reduction in heavy meconium-stained fluid, variable FHR decelerations, cesarean section, 1 minute APGAR score <7, umbilical artery pH <7.20, meconium below vocal cords, meconium aspiration syndrome, neonatal ventilation, and NICU admission. An increase in oxytocin augmentation was noted as well as no measurable effect on narcotic or epidural analgesic use and labor duration (Hofmeyr, 1998). Many of the effects of amnioinfusion may be related to correction of oligohydramnios rather than dilution of meconium. Given this conclusion, it behooves midwives as clinicians to prevent iatrogenic oligohydramnios by advocating against routine amniotomies in labor.

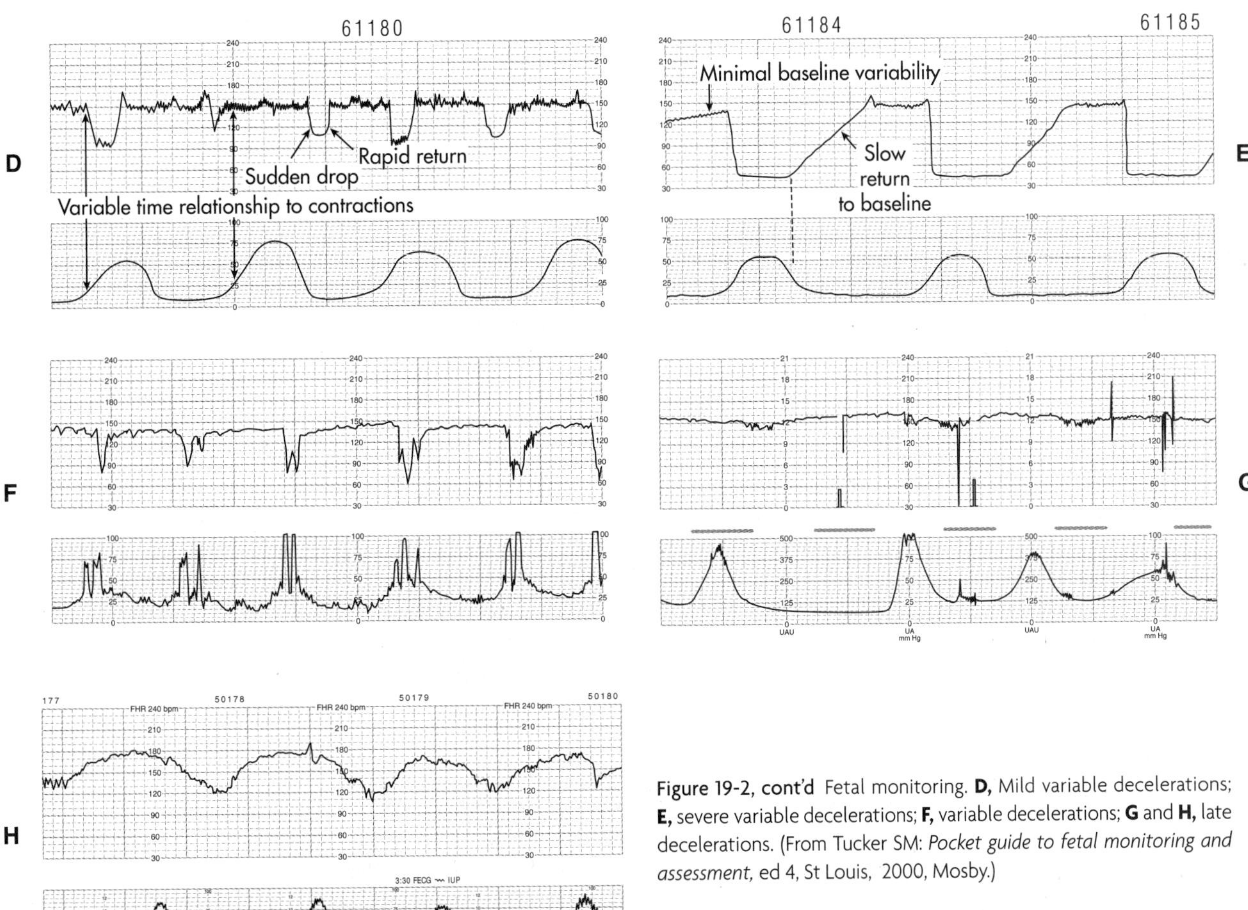

Figure 19-2, cont'd Fetal monitoring. **D,** Mild variable decelerations; **E,** severe variable decelerations; **F,** variable decelerations; **G** and **H,** late decelerations. (From Tucker SM: *Pocket guide to fetal monitoring and assessment,* ed 4, St Louis, 2000, Mosby.)

Amniotic Fluid Evaluation

The initial assessment of a client in labor includes an assessment of fetal membrane status. This is primarily done by interviewing the client about any leaking of fluid from the vagina, time when fluid was first noted, and color and volume of any fluid. If the client is unsure of the membrane status, a sterile speculum examination is performed for fluid evaluation by nitrazine paper and ferning and visual inspection of the posterior fornix for fluid pooling (see Box 19-1). The client readily notices membrane rupture with copious fluid, but sometimes there is a small leak that is hard to differentiate from urine or a copious vaginal discharge. In these cases it is best to see the client and obtain objective data to confirm membrane rupture.

Meconium-stained fluid may reflect multiple underlying conditions. For example, in many instances light meconium-stained fluid is an indicator of a healthy term fetus secondary to the higher chance for activation of the mature vagal system with excretion of meconium (Gabbe, Niebyl, and Simpson, 1996). Meconium-stained fluid may also indicate fetal compromise. A complete evaluation of the fetal status with appropriate fetal surveillance is imperative to rule out episodes of fetal hypoxia. When minimal fluid is encountered with membrane rupture, the risk of thick, tenacious meconium behind the presenting part is increased. Thick meconium-stained fluid may have significant neonatal consequences because it increases the risk of meconium aspiration syndrome. For this reason, amnioinfusion has been used to dilute the fluid. Clinical prudence in the use of this procedure is warranted, considering the rare possibility of amniotic fluid embolism.

LABOR STATUS

The dynamic process of labor includes four interwoven components that affect both the initiation and the progress of labor. These four components are the passenger (the fetus), the passage (the maternal pelvis), the powers (the uterine contractions), and the psyche (the emotional state of the mother).

What initiates labor remains unclear. However, the current theory hypothesizes a biochemical interaction between the fetus, the placenta, and the mother (Blackburn and Loper, 1992; Speroff, Glass and Kase, 1994). Once labor is initiated, the interaction between passenger, passage, powers, and psyche must be in synchrony for a spontaneous, vaginal birth to occur. In this section the passenger, the passage, and the powers are addressed.

The Passenger and Labor

The three cardinal aspects of passenger fit are fetal weight, fetal presentation, and the position of the presenting part in relation to the maternal pelvis. These three aspects must be looked at as a whole rather than as separate factors. For example, if all other variables are equal, an estimated 6-pound baby in an occipitoposterior position is a much more difficult fit than a 7-pound baby in an occipitoanterior position. The presentation of the fetus also has implications for labor progress. Any abnormal presentations must be identified as early as possible in labor if they have not been identified prenatally.

The Passage and Labor

No matter what the size and position of the passenger, it must fit the passage. The maternal pelvis is an important component of labor progress. Often the characteristics of the maternal pelvis will predicate fetal position and labor progress. The two types of pelves that offer a good prognosis for vaginal delivery are gynecoid and anthropoid. Android and platypelloid pelves have reduced diameters at the midplane and the inlet, respectively. Both types have compromised diameters that may prevent the fetus from entering the inlet, but with the platypelloid pelvis, if the fetus is small enough and in the correct position to navigate through the inlet and midplane, there is usually a rapid second stage. It is important to identify the woman's pelvic type/tendency using clinical pelvimetry in order to anticipate problems, provide appropriate client information, and appropriately introduce interventions that will facilitate descent of the presenting part. For example, a client with an anthropoid pelvis is more likely to have an occipitoposterior passenger because that is the best fit considering the long anteroposterior diameter. It would be expected that she may experience back labor; so early in labor this can be discussed, and appropriate modalities such as hot packs, Jacuzzi, and massage can be introduced.

Powers and Labor

The powers are the dynamic forces that move the passenger through the passage. These contractions that define labor are frequently monitored, biochemically manipulated, and made devoid of pain through analgesia and anesthesia. The two objective criteria used to evaluate the effectiveness of contractions are cervical dilation and descent of the fetal presenting part. Studies exploring the factors relevant to prediction of the length of the first stage of labor began in the 1930s with Calkins, Litzenberg, and Plass (1934). In 1941 his work culminated in an analysis that showed it was possible to predict the approximate length of the normal first stage on the basis of contraction intensity, cervical effacement, softening of the cervix, and engagement of the fetal presenting part (Calkins, 1941).

Emmanual Friedman continued to study the lengths of labor throughout the 1950s, and the Friedman curve continues to be used to evaluate normal progress of labor, despite the dramatic differences between current obstetric and social factors and those practiced in the 1950s (Albers, Schiff, and Gorwoda, 1996). As a tool, the Friedman curve does serve a function, despite the changes in practice and social attitudes. First, it provides a conceptual framework for an experience that is very personal. Each woman has her own labor experience, but the Friedman curve provides a common denominator from which all the players can speak. It divides labor into phases, which provides the client and the clinician with a time line that anticipates how labor should progress within certain statistical limits (Figure 19-3). This is important because labor is a stressful event both for the mother and the fetus. As with any stressful event, if it continues past maternal and/or fetal reserves, maternal and/or fetal compromise may occur. In addition, significant deviation on the Friedman curve serves as an indicator that the passenger, the passage, and/or the powers may be delaying or preventing a spontaneous vaginal delivery. This prompts the midwife to initiate further examination, assessment, and intervention as needed.

Phases of Labor

The first phase described by Friedman is the latent phase. This phase extends from the onset of labor, taken arbitrarily from the onset of regular uterine contractions, to the beginning of the active phase. The onset of this stage is a self-diagnosis, and women vary in their recognition and perception of painful contractions. The midwife should respect the woman's interpretation of the onset of her labor. Since latent phase is defined more by the woman's perception of contractions and their associated discomfort, she is the central figure in defining the onset of regular uterine activity (Figure 19-4).

The latent phase of labor is the preparatory phase. Its role is largely orientation and polarization of uterine contractions and preparation of the cervix for subsequent active dilation. On Friedman's graph it tends to be flat or nearly flat, and Friedman observed no statistical correlation between the length or slope of the latent phase and the remaining part of the labor (Friedman, 1967). However, the National Collaborative Perinatal Project data that used Friedman's 1958 to 1965 study population did show long-term abnormalities in newborns associated with prolonged latent phase, defined as >8 hours for nulliparous women and >5 hours for multiparous women (Chelmow, Kilpatrick, and Laros, 1993) (Table 19-1).

The contractions during the latent phase of labor are typically characterized as regular yet mild and of short duration. Women report being able to carry on with their

Table 19-1 *Comparisons of Active Phase of First-Stage Labor Identified by Different Investigators*

	Mean length (hrs)	Statistical Limit (hrs)
Nulliparas		
Friedman (1967)	5.8	12
Kilpatrick and Laros (1989):		
No conduction anesthesia	8.1	16.6
Conduction anesthesia	10.2	19
Albers, Schiff, and Gorwoda (1996)	7.7	19.4
Multiparas		
Friedman (1967)	2.3	6
Kilpatrick and Laros (1989):		
No conduction anesthesia	5.7	12.5
Conduction anesthesia	7.4	14.9
Albers, Schiff, and Gorwoda (1996)	5.7	13.7

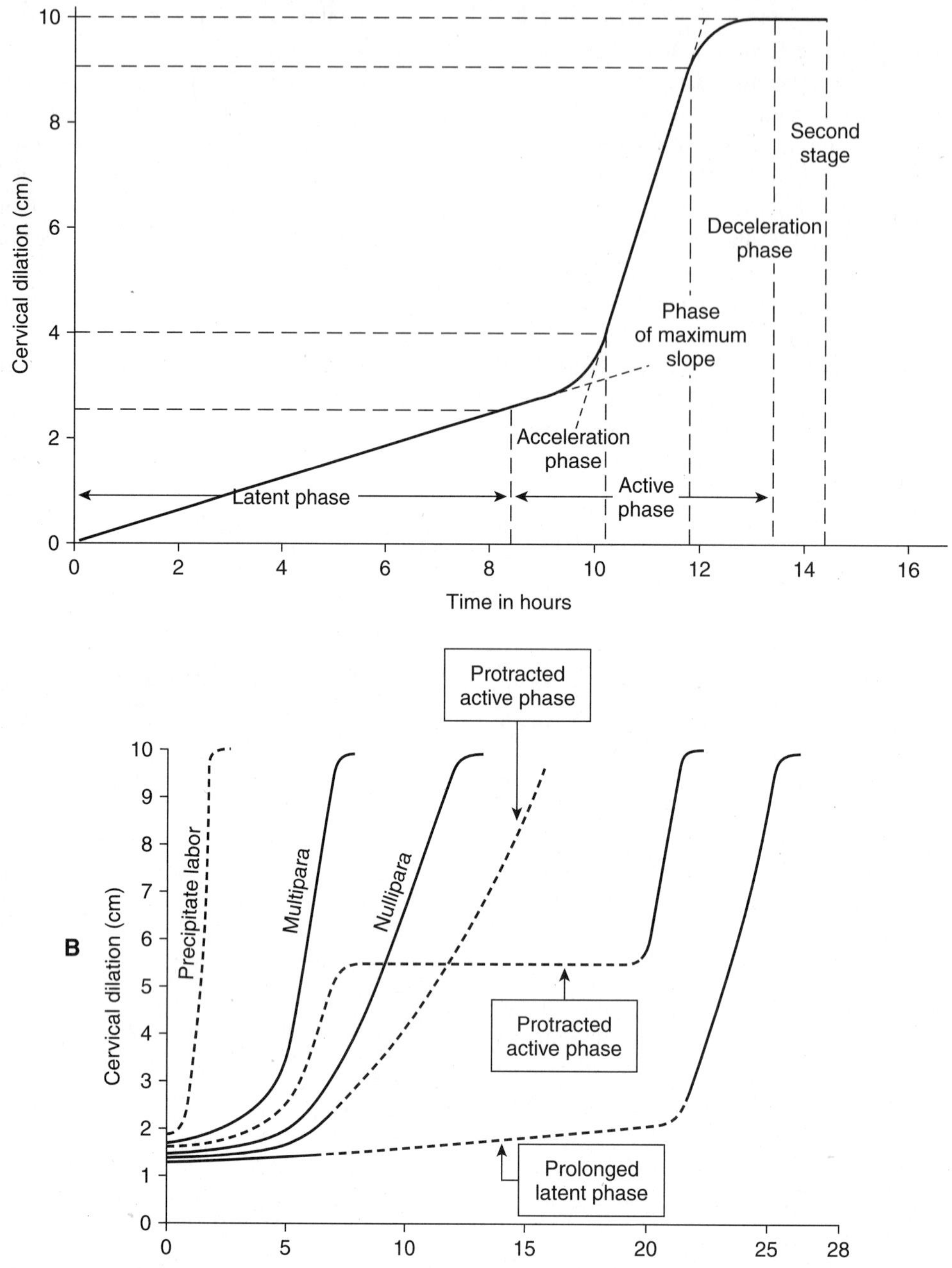

Figure 19-3 **A,** Phases of labor—nullipara; **B,** deviations from normal progress of labor.

daily tasks and are often able to sleep and/or rest between contractions. With a good support system and a sound knowledge base many women can stay home until the active phase of labor.

The duration of the latent phase is quite sensitive to outside interference and may be prolonged by heavy sedation or shortened with stimulation. This sensitivity to intervention affords clinicians opportunities to try to shorten a long latent phase. Provider philosophies and client desires are often the deciding factors in whether to intervene with sedation or stimulation. Currently both methods may be used to obviate a prolonged latent phase.

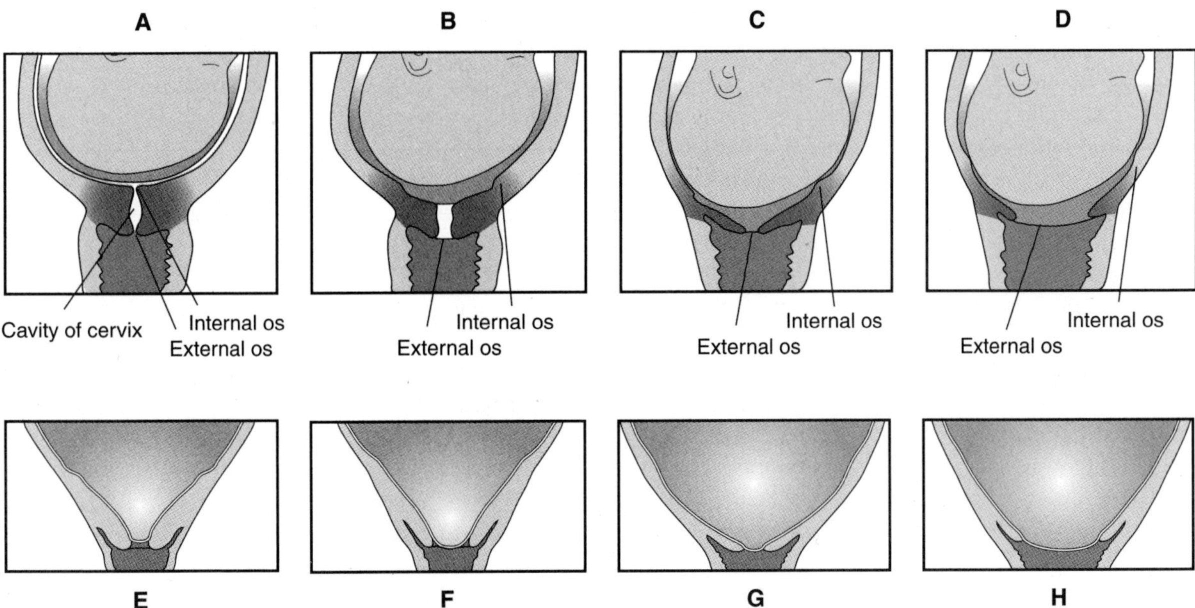

Figure 19-4, **A** to **H** Effacement of cervix.

Before categorizing a client as having a prolonged latent phase, the following questions are asked:

- *Was she ever in labor?* The contractions that the woman reports may be the asynchronous Braxton-Hicks contractions rather than the progressive contractions of labor.
- *Is she experiencing painful, regular contractions that have changed to a stronger, closer, and longer pattern?* These changes in contractile pattern suggest that she is progressing toward active phase of labor.
- *Is her contraction pattern the same regardless of activity?* Braxton-Hicks contractions tend to become more irregular and may cease with change of activity. True labor contractions tend to not be affected by changes in activity.
- *When was she unable to sleep through her contractions?* Inability to sleep through contractions suggests progression in labor. However, the clinician needs to evaluate the influence of anxiety and generalized discomfort secondary to fatigue on her inability to sleep.
- *Does she have a bloody show?* Bloody show may indicate progressive cervical dilation, particularly when there has not been a recent cervical examination.
- *Has there been a perceptible change in her cervix?* Ideally the same practitioner should do the cervical examinations to eliminate interexaminer variations in findings. Cervical changes during latent phase are often subtle. All changes—dilation, effacement, and station of presenting part—should be considered when assessing progress.

Many women experiencing a long latent phase have entered labor with an unprepared cervix. Thus the contractions of the latent phase soften and efface the cervix, changes that occur in the latter part of pregnancy for many women.

The management of choice for prolonged latent phase is therapeutic rest induced with morphine (15 to 20 mg). After several hours of rest, approximately 80% of treated women progress to active labor on their own, 10% require oxytocin augmentation, and 10% cease contractions (Cohen and Brennan, 1995). The rationale behind using augmentation is that the mother is in labor with an inefficient contraction pattern that requires additional oxytocin. If nonpharmacologic modalities are to be used to promote an effective contraction pattern, the clinician should consider using them early enough to evaluate their effectiveness. If ineffective, pharmacologic modalities may then be instituted in a timely fashion. Some nonpharmacologic interventions that may be considered to facilitate labor include hydration, caloric intake, hydrotherapy, ambulation, and relaxation techniques.

Active phase is the time in which most cervical dilation occurs and the fetal presenting part descends further into the pelvis. In Friedman's model of cervical dilation, the active phase of labor includes the acceleration phase, the phase of maximum slope, and the deceleration phase. The acceleration phase that begins the active phase of labor is commonly quantified at 4 cm if the laboring woman is having strong, regular, frequent contractions of 45 to 60 seconds' duration. Without an efficient contraction pattern, labor will not progress from the acceleration phase to the phase of maximum slope. The phase of maximum slope of active labor is a much finer measure of progress. It usually begins at 5 to 6 cm with rapid cervical progress. In Friedman's study population the average dilation for nulliparas was 3 cm/hr and 5.7 cm/hr for multiparas. The statistical limit (2 standard deviations) in terms of least dilation for continued "normal" progress in nulliparas was 1.2 cm/hr and for multiparas, 1.5 cm/hr. Descent of the fetal presenting part typically occurs during the deceleration phase. This phase begins at 8- to 9-cm dilation, with an average length of 54 minutes and 14 minutes, respectively, for nulliparas and multiparas (Friedman, 1967). As used in this system, deceleration refers to the deceleration of the rate of change of the cervix, not to a deceleration in the labor activity.

Recently Friedman's norms for the time interval for active phase of labor have come into question. Considering the difference in obstetric practice between the 1950s and the 1990s and the large number of high-risk clients he included in his original data, this challenge to his data is applauded. Albers, Schiff, and Gorwoda (1996) evaluated the length of active labor in normal healthy women and found the mean length for both nulliparas and multiparas to be much longer than that defined by Friedman. When Friedman reassessed his own data using only essentially normal primipara and multipara cases, the lengths of labor still showed a shorter time interval for the active phase of labor for primipara than the findings of more recent studies. His revisions using normal multipara cases showed no difference from his original study findings.

Expectant management using a valid curve for active labor should be considered as the primary management tool in caring for laboring women. Use of guides that underestimate the expected lengths of phases of labor increases the risks of misdiagnosis of dystocia and unnecessary interventions such as oxytocin augmentation, operative vaginal delivery, and cesarean delivery.

Traditionally it is expected that nulliparous women will dilate at least 1 cm/hr and multiparous women will dilate at least 1.5 cm/hr in the active phase of labor. A slow active phase occurs when these parameters are not met. Cephalopelvic disproportion contributes to 30% of the slow active phase group. The other 70% is associated with sedation, dehydration, exhaustion, pain intolerance, poor myometrial coordination, and the occipitoposterior position. The underlying cause of the slow active phase, whether it be inefficient uterine action, occipitoposterior position, or cephalopelvic disproportion, should be identified in order to intervene and consult appropriately.

Active management of labor (AMOL) is a multifaceted approach involving early amniotomy and early diagnosis of dysfunctional labor that indicates the need for augmentation with high doses of oxytocin. It was first implemented by O'Driscoll, Foley, and MacDonald at the National Maternity Hospital in Dublin, Ireland (1993) to help reduce the incidence of cesarean births and decrease the amount of time in dysfunctional labor. This protocol was coined "AMOL" over 20 years ago in the *British Medical Journal,* and the low rate of cesarean births (5% to 6%) at the National Maternity Hospital was attributed to the use of this protocol. An attempt to replicate these statistics using AMOL in the three randomized clinical trials in the United States has been unsuccessful. However, other results were noted. All the clinical trials showed a decrease in the length of labor and the incidence of prolonged labor with AMOL. Another consistent finding has been the decreased incidence of maternal febrile morbidity. None of the trials showed any increased incidence of complications associated with the use of AMOL.

Midwifery philosophy supports the belief in the normalcy of the labor process. This includes the belief that women have the intrinsic ability to labor normally and that the birth attendant's role is to facilitate their labors with activity, relaxation, support, and the judicious use of medical interventions. Using the medical intervention of AMOL only to shorten labor is not warranted in midwifery management. The AMOL removes the locus of control from the laboring woman and her family and gives it to hospital personnel whose primary interest may be "clearing the board." Staffing issues and patient census undermine the individual needs of women in labor. In this context AMOL benefits the institution far more than the client.

Common Intrapartum Interventions

Amniotomy. Most intrapartal interventions focus on two key components: establishing an efficient contraction pattern and providing adequate pain relief. Amniotomy is a common intervention implemented to increase frequency and/or strength of contractions. Rupture of membranes may facilitate transfer of amnion-derived PGE_2, resulting in a papcrine effect on the myometrium (McCoshen et al., 1990). This effect produces more frequent contractions, which in turn promote cervical dilation.

A meta-analysis of control trials examining the effects of amniotomy on rates of cesarean delivery and other indicators of maternal and neonatal morbidity show that a policy of early amniotomy appears to lead to an average reduction of labor duration from 60 to 120 minutes (Fraser et al., 1998). In addition, the report states that, although none of the trials assessed the effectiveness of amniotomy to treat established delays in labor progress, it is likely that amniotomy will be found to be beneficial in this context.

When considering this intervention, it is very important to appreciate all of its ramifications. This intervention *commits* the client to delivery in a "timely fashion." Because of this consequence, it is imperative that the client's progress in labor be accurately assessed in terms of all of the components: the powers, the passenger, and the passage. An amniotomy should not be performed under the following conditions: abnormal presenting part, an unengaged presenting part, in the latent phase of labor without other indications, and a progressing early active phase of labor with a reassuring FHR tracing. Early amniotomy is associated with an increase in the frequency of FHR abnormalities. In a secondary analysis of the results of a multicenter randomized trial of early vs. late amniotomy in labor, early amniotomy was associated with an increased hourly rate of severe variable and late decelerations (Goffinet et al., 1997). An amniotomy creates oligohydramnios, and the ramifications reviewed under the section concerning amnioinfusions is applicable in this context also. Indications for amniotomy include slow progress of active labor with a well-engaged presenting part; an imminent second stage with the clinician's desire to minimize body fluid exposure at the time of the birth; application of an internal scalp electrode to more closely evaluate fetal status; and introduction of an intrauterine pressure catheter to more accurately assess contractile forces.

Administration of oxytocin. Increasing oxytocin levels is another way to facilitate labor. Oxytocin levels may be increased with exogenous oxytocin via an IV infusion or through increasing endogenous levels via nipple stimulation. Currently nipple stimulation is used infrequently to augment labor, most likely because it requires more client education and more support staff to implement. Many physicians are uncomfortable with the fact that the effects of nipple stimulation cannot be controlled in the same way that administration of oxytocin can be controlled. One randomized prospective study comparing the effects of using nipple stimulation with the effect of using IV oxytocin augmentation found that the average and maximal uterine activity achieved was significantly higher in the oxytocin-stimulated group, without significant difference in the length of labor stages, cesarean birth rate, APGAR scores or umbilical artery pH (Stein et al., 1990).

Institutional customs and procedural fit have facilitated the widespread use of oxytocin infusion for augmentation of labor. Most women experiencing a hospital birth have an IV infusion of fluids in labor, regardless of the need for hydration or identified maternal and/or fetal complications. Therefore to begin an oxytocin infusion if the labor progress is less than expected becomes a simple addition. Fetal and maternal consequences are rarely considered. It is easy to forget that oxytocin is the most powerful uterine stimulant (i.e., 2500 times more potent than the prostaglandin PGF_2) (Fuchs et al., 1983). It contributes to tachysystole, FHR late deceleration patterns, and poor maternal pain tolerance. The incidence of these complications increases as high-dose infusions and rapid incremental increases become more popular. Uterine contractions closely resemble normal labor patterns when oxytocin is infused at a rate that establishes serum levels in the physiologic range ($<$16 mU/min) and when maximum steady-state contractile effects are reached between 30 and 60 minutes (Curtis and Safransky, 1988).

Most sources recommend starting oxytocin at 0.5 to 2 mU/min and increasing the rate by 1 to 2 mU/min every 15 to 30 minutes (ACOG, 1999b). An absolute maximum dosage has not been determined (ACOG, 1999b), but since oxytocin has antidiuretic action above 40 mU/min, most sources do not recommend dosages above 30 mU/min. The desired effect is to stimulate three strong, 45- to 60-second long contractions in 10 minutes and to maintain that pattern. With this type of pattern, cervical dilation should be expected to occur within the given norms. If this progress is not observed, the passenger and/or the passage need to be evaluated.

ACTIVITY STATUS

The activity status of a laboring woman may be as minimal as positional changes in bed or as much as hydrotherapy, ambulation, and moving with a birthing ball. The activity level women choose depends on a number of factors: culture, knowledge about labor, and perception of what may help the laboring process. The woman's choice also depends on maternal and fetal health. State of health is clearly measured by mobility and independence. Therefore, when a clinician encourages mobility, the cultural message that is heard goes beyond a walk in the halls. It states that one is healthy and one's baby is healthy. This message instills a level of maternal confidence that mere words cannot. The other unspoken message that is understood by the laboring family is that labor is normal. The psychologic benefit of normalizing labor is profound. The family becomes involved in the process, and contractions are viewed as a necessary activity for birth.

The clinician's role is to facilitate labor, guard maternal and fetal health, and validate the normalcy of labor and birth. One of the most effective ways of doing this is to encourage maternal activity. To remove the laboring woman from the sick room to engage with the outside world benefits the client, the family, and the support staff. It supports the appropriate use of intermittent monitoring, and it may prevent unnecessary interventions such as amniotomy and internal EFM. Furthermore, appropriate ambulation facilitates the judicious use of pain medication for labor.

Positioning

In the eighteenth century Mauriceau, the French obstetrician to the Queen of France, introduced the supine position for labor. This horizontal position was favored because it facilitated the management of labor by the accoucheur and *not* because it might be beneficial for the mother or the fetus. Throughout the late 1900s the dorsal recumbent position for labor has eclipsed the use of other positions for laboring women in the United States. This has become increasingly apparent as the use of routine electronic FHR monitoring becomes more standardized in obstetric practice. The increased use of technology and epidural anesthesia mandates a recumbent position since it is more difficult to maintain the smooth functioning of technology in alternate positions. This position in turn facilitates the increased use of technology and epidural anesthesia. Yet it is one that hinders rather than promotes the laboring process. It has been criticized for being unnatural, increasing fetal distress, slowing the progress of labor, and causing greater pain.

Through their impact on the hemodynamic status of the mother, maternal postural changes may enhance fetal well-being. Maternal cardiac output has been shown to decrease by 22% on average in the dorsal recumbent relative to the lateral-tilt position. In the supine position vena caval obstruction may impede venous return to the heart, causing a fall in maternal cardiac output and blood pressure and a decrease in uteroplacental perfusion (Kerr, Scott, and Samuel, 1964). This has the potential to result in FHR abnormalities. Albitol (1985) demonstrated reversal of late decelerations or late components on fetal monitoring in 24 of 126 participants when the lateral-tilt position was assumed. Most studies show no difference in incidence of decelerations between vertical and horizontal positions (Caldeyro-Barcia, 1979). Currently there is no evidence from clinical trials that upright posture in the first stage of labor results in differences in neonatal outcomes compared with recumbent postures (Figure 19-5).

Review of studies assessing the effects of maternal position in the first stage of labor show that, on average, the duration of labor was significantly shorter for those assigned the upright position vs. the dorsal-supine position by as much as 1.6 to 2.6 hours (Roberts, 1989). Trials that compared the upright to the lateral-tilt positions showed no significant differences between groups in first-stage duration (McManus and Calder, 1978; Calvert, Newcombe, and Hibbard, 1982), which may indicate that the lateral-tilt position is similar to the upright position as a means of promoting labor progress. Conversely, resting uterine pressure has been shown to be greater in the sitting rather than in the lying position. Both standing and lateral-recumbent positions are associated with stronger, albeit less frequent, uterine contraction than dorsal recumbent or sitting position (Diaz et al., 1980). However, a study on posture in labor performed at the Royal Maternity Hospital with 275 low- and high-risk participants concluded that the choice of ambulation may be caused by the ease of the labor rather that vice versa (Stewart and Calder, 1984). In terms of birth outcomes, a study examining the association of ambulation in labor with operative deliveries in a low risk sample of 1678 women found that women who ambulated for a significant amount of time during labor compared with those who did not ambulate had half the rate of operative delivery (Albers et al., 1997) (Research Box 19-2).

When promoting a labor position, the clinician must not forget the client's desires. Maternal preferences for positions during first-stage labor are reported in several studies. In one study in which women acted as their own controls to assess preference for position, up-

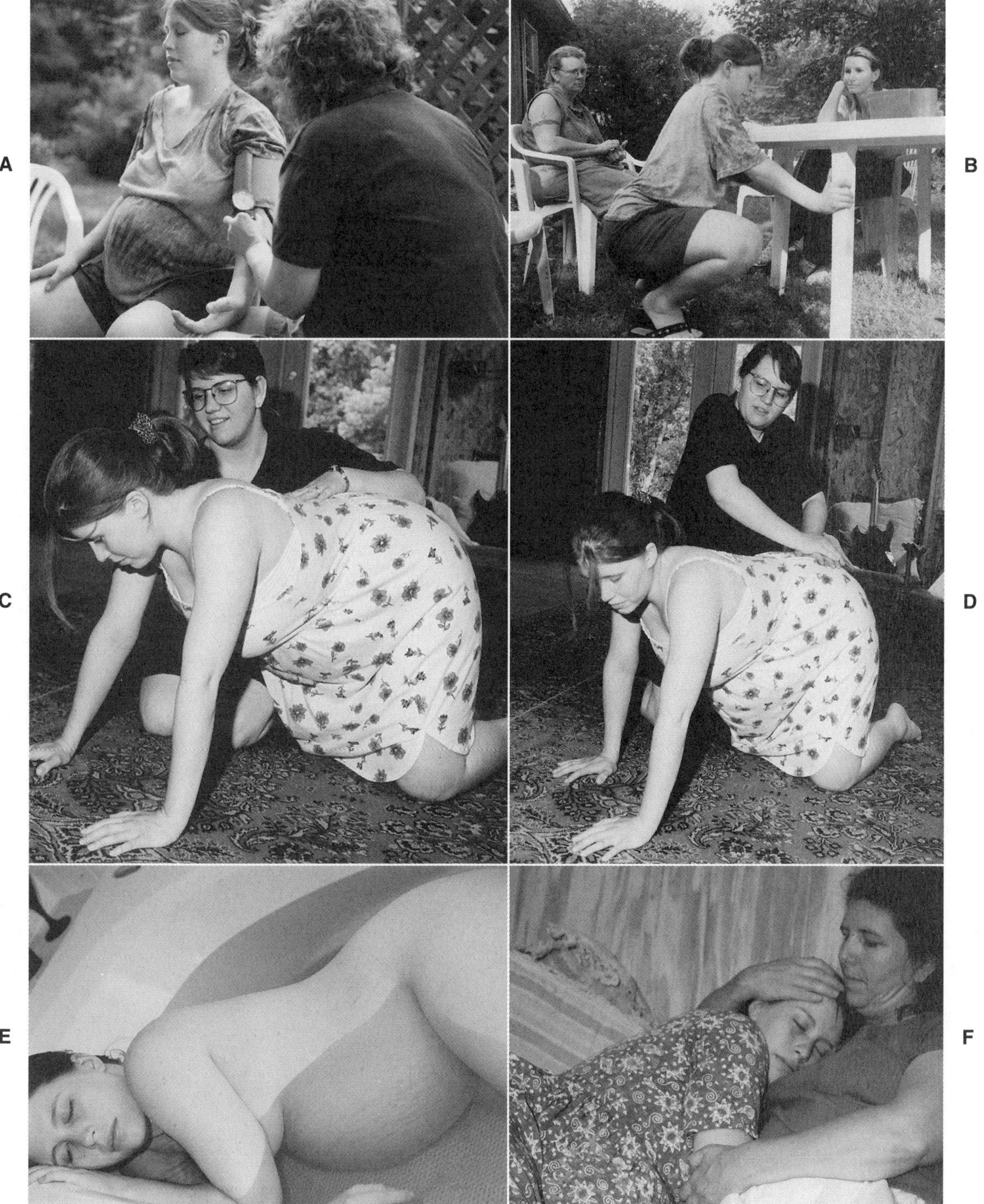

Figure 19-5 Woman in a variety of positions during labor. **A,** Sitting; **B,** squatting; **C,** on "all-fours"; **D,** on "all-fours" with counterpressure over sacrum; **E,** hydrotherapy; and **F,** lateral. (**A** to **F** courtesy Caroline E. Brown.)

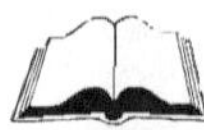

Research Box 19-2

Albers LL et al.: The relationship of ambulation in labor to operative delivery, *J Nurse Midwifery* 42(1):4-8, 1997.

Background

Physician-managed care during labor and birth is associated with restriction in maternal activity once the woman is admitted to the labor unit. Ambulation during labor has several potential benefits, including an increase in sense of control, distraction from pain, and support from another person. Studies that have assessed the influence of ambulation on labor and birth have been limited by small sample sizes, lack of randomization, and lack of control of confounding factors.

Research Question

What is the effect of ambulation in labor on the risk of operative delivery in healthy childbearing women?

Methods

Observational data were gathered on all intrapartum patients who began care with a certified nurse-midwife in three clinical sites and recorded on an abbreviated form of the Nurse-Midwifery Clinical Data Set. This study was a secondary analysis of data collected for a previous study. Ambulation in labor was recorded when "the patient was upright and mobile for a significant amount of time during labor, usually for at least half of the labor," and the decision to ambulate was ultimately the woman's, although the attending midwife may have suggested ambulation as an intervention. Operative delivery was defined as delivery by cesarean section, forceps, or vacuum extraction. Chi-square was used to determine statistical significance between groups. Confounding variables were analyzed using stratified analysis.

Sample

The sample consisted of 1678 healthy women at term (37 to 42 weeks' gestation) with a singleton pregnancy in vertex presentation and presenting in spontaneous labor. Women who had augmentation of labor by oxytocin and who chose epidural anesthesia were excluded from the sample. Forty-six percent of the women were ambulatory during labor.

Results

Ambulation was associated with decreased use of narcotic analgesia and less fetal distress. Women who were ambulatory in labor were more likely to have intermittent fetal monitoring, oral hydration, longer first stage of labor, and spontaneous vaginal deliveries. Ambulation was associated with a significant reduction in operative delivery (RR = 0.5, 95% CI = 0.3-0.9).

Clinical Application

Findings are limited by the fact that patients were not randomized into treatment and control groups, ambulation was not quantified, and self-selection for midwifery care may have produced a group that is inherently different from women who chose physician-managed care for childbearing. However, strengths of the study include the large sample of women at low-risk for operative delivery and the analysis of confounding variables. Operative delivery was relatively infrequent in the sample (4.2%), and ambulation was associated with further reduction of the operative delivery rate (2.7%). Findings suggest that ambulation in labor may have benefits that include decreased analgesia use, decreased fetal distress, and decreased operative deliveries.

right positions were preferred in early labor, and lateral-recumbent positions were chosen later in labor (Roberts, Mendez-Bauer and Wodell, 1983). Women who chose to ambulate usually returned to bed, on average, at about 5 to 6 cm of dilation. Maternal preference for ambulation may also be influenced by parity. Nulliparous clients are more likely to choose to stay in bed rather than ambulate, perhaps because of a lack of frame of reference regarding labor activity or perhaps because they are more likely to defer to institutional norms.

Clinicians are often faced with institutional norms that vary in supportive options for healthy laboring women. One study noted that women chose to stay in bed in the latter half of labor because the delivery room did not have comfortable chairs, and most of the women found ambulation inconvenient (Hemminki and Saarikoski, 1983). If the labor suite promotes ambulation with comfortable chairs and spacious areas for family support, women and their families are more likely to feel encouraged to move about. The clinician needs to consider the social environment surrounding the laboring woman and make suggestions about activity in a way that maximizes labor support while minimizing negative reaction by staff.

Hydrotherapy

There are reasons to believe that hydrotherapy has a beneficial effect during labor. The water transfers heat to the body, decreases the pressure on the abdominal muscles, and elicits pleasurable sensations. All these stimuli are able to close the gate for pain at the level of the dorsal horn, thereby decreasing the perception of pain. Moreover, hydrotherapy may diminish the emotional stress caused by labor and thereby decrease the release of catecholamine and cortisol, which adversely affect uterine activity and the progress of labor (Simkin, 1986).

There are few studies that explore the pain-relieving effect of a warm tub. One prospective study with a small study sample of 54 women found warm water to have beneficial effects during labor (Cammu et al., 1994). Bathing provided a temporal pain-stabilizing effect through relaxation, faster dilation, less labor augmentation, and higher consumer satisfaction. Interestingly, bathing did not provide objective pain relief as measured by a visual analog scale. Following that study, the investigators completed a larger, prospective study that found that whirlpool baths in labor decrease analgesia requirements and instrumental delivery rates, improve the condition of the perineum with fewer episiotomies and or lacerations, and give personal satisfaction (Rush et al., 1996). A small subset of participants who completed questionnaires about comfort measures had positive comments about the tub and about the fact that a companion or nurse remained with them during bathing. It is unclear whether the intervention of the tub or the added support was most beneficial. Benefit derived from support during labor has been substantiated in the literature; and the work of Rush and colleagues illustrates the difficulty of isolating the beneficial effects of the modalities used by clinicians in labor (Research Box 19-3).

Many components play into the dynamic process of labor. One that is rarely discussed is the placebo effect of the midwives' knowledge that a modality will work. Midwives, as labor experts, have a tremendous influence on how a client perceives the effectiveness of a recommended modality. It is easy to marvel at how quickly a laboring client progresses once she is placed sitting in the shower and counseled that the warm water will help her relax, thereby helping her dilate more effectively. It is not clear whether results occur because of the effect of the warm water, the reassuring word, and /or the trust in the expertise of the midwife.

In many institutions rupture of membranes is a contraindication for hydrotherapy because of the fear of intrapartal infection. Several investigations have not shown an increase in infection; however, they are limited by small sample sizes (Cammu et al., 1994; Church, 1989; Odent, 1983). It would seem reasonable that, with prolonged rupture of membranes of greater than 24 hours, a cautionary approach to bathing while in labor be adopted since the findings of some studies suggest a greater incidence of chorioamnionitis, FHR abnormalities such as tachycardia, and variable decelerations and desultory labor patterns with prolonged ruptured membranes.

Clinical trials show no difference between tub users and nontub users in 1- and 5-minute APGAR scores (Cammu et al., 1994). Many Doppler fetoscopes can now be immersed in water so that FHRs may be documented while the client is in the shower or bath.

Maternal contraindications to ambulation and hydrotherapy include any underlying pathology that warrants complete bed rest. These conditions are preeclampsia, HELLP syndrome, symptomatic cardiac disease, placenta previa, placental abruption, and/or poor placental perfusion, regardless of the underlying etiology. Fetal contraindications include any fetal condition with a high risk of prolapsed cord; thick meconium-stained fluid, which requires continuous monitoring with amnioinfusion; and FHR decelerations, which indicate poor oxygenation.

Ambulation with or without hydrotherapy is an effective midwifery tool to facilitate maternal well-being, fetal well-being, and labor progress. First, it reaffirms for the laboring client that she is not sick. Second, it facilitates the progression of labor by allowing for more efficient contractions and promoting appropriate alignment of the presenting part with the maternal pelvis. Third, with the use of hydrotherapy, relaxation occurs, and less analgesia is used. Fourth, fetuses are healthier because of less analgesic use, faster labors, and fewer operative applications.

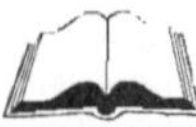

Research Box 19-3

Rush J et al: The effects of whirlpool baths in labor: a randomized controlled study, *Birth* 23(3):136-143, 1996.

Background

Showers, baths, and whirlpool baths are common interventions to alleviate pain and stress. Before this study there were only descriptive reports on the use of whirlpool baths in labor. Previous findings had suggested that hydrotherapy is associated with decreased use of analgesia and anesthesia and no increase in maternal or neonatal infection. The effect of hydrotherapy on length of labor has had conflicting results in previous studies.

Research Questions

(1) What is the pharmacologic pain relief experience among women who use the whirlpool tub during labor compared to those who experience conventional care (no bathing)? (2) Are there differences in length of labor, patient satisfaction, and other birth outcomes between the group that uses the whirlpool tub in labor and those who experience conventional care?

Methods

Participants were recruited in a large teaching hospital in Canada where there are approximately 3500 births annually with a cesarean delivery rate of 17%,and where approximately 85% of the births are attended by obstetricians. Women who consented to participation were randomly assigned to the experimental group (tub users) or the control group (conventional care). Eligible women were at term, afebrile, in active labor, and anticipating a vaginal birth. All women in the experimental group were offered the whirlpool tub; if the woman did not care to use the tub, the reasons were documented. Data collection included frequency and length of tub use, parity, gestational age, rupture of membranes, vaginal births after cesarean, presentation, labor length, birth position, birth outcome, status of the perineum, drug use, meconium, attendant, birth weight, APGAR scores, and signs of maternal or newborn sepsis. Data were collected by the attending nurse. A subset of participants were surveyed postpartum to determine use of and satisfaction with comfort measures during labor. Data were analyzed with appropriate statistical methods using an intent-to-treat approach.

Sample

Eight hundred women consented to participate in the study, and a total of 785 records was considered adequate for analysis. Characteristics of the study groups were similar, validating the random allocation. Forty-six percent of the women in the experimental group did not actually use the tub. The most common reasons for refusal of tub use were change of mind, pain or distress, early request for epidural anesthesia, and lack of availability of a tub. It was determined that a sample of 400 subjects per group would be necessary to detect a 15% reduction in rate of pharmacologic pain relief if 65% of the women used the tub, or a 20% reduction if 50% of the women used it.

Results

Women in the experimental group were significantly less likely to use narcotic analgesia or epidural anesthesia in labor. Birth outcomes were similar in both groups, and there were no differences in infections in mothers or neonates. Mothers expressed satisfaction with the tub, stating that the tub enhanced relaxation and pain relief.

Clinical Application

The relatively small proportion of women in the experimental group who used the tub limit the interpretation of findings. Although findings suggest that the tub may be an effective intervention to decrease analgesia and anesthesia in labor, further studies with larger sample sizes are necessary to fully evaluate the effect.

PAIN/PSYCH/PROVIDER

Pain Status

Most women experience pain in labor, and most women desire interventions—whether they be pharmacologic or nonpharmacologic—to assist them in coping with the experience. Although the experience of pain in labor is uniquely personal, cultural beliefs are instrumental in how pain is interpreted. The cultural component of childbirth is most dramatically seen in a woman's relationship with the pain of labor. As the culture becomes more comfortable with technology, the use of technology-intensive pain-relieving modalities becomes more of an expectation.

The midwifery challenge when evaluating the pain status of a laboring woman and suggesting interventions is to respect the client's wishes for pain relief and yet provide information as to what may be best for the labor, the fetus, and the client. This dialog requires critical and sensitive discussions and an assurance that the client is directing her labor experience. It is important when evaluating the pain status of a laboring client that the client's labor, expectations, and environment are appropriately assessed in order to obtain an accurate pain profile. The midwife's pain assessment should include: (1) duration, quality, and location of pain, (2) client attitude when not experiencing pain, (3) attitude of client's support concerning labor and pain relief modalities, (4) labor progress, (5) fetal status, (6) client-generated activities that lessen the pain, and (7) recognition of previous history of sexual abuse. This knowledge will direct the interventions according to the need to decrease fear and anxiety about labor, decrease the pain of the uterine contractions, and/or change fetal position. The goal in using any of these methods is to modify labor pain without causing ill effects to the mother and infant.

There have been many studies concerning expectations and experiences of pain in labor. The findings from one prospective study in England showed that, even in the 1990s, most women preferred to keep drug use to a minimum. This was true even though they expected labor to be "quite" or "very" painful. The study also found that anxiety about the pain of labor was a strong predictor of negative experiences during labor, lack of satisfaction with the birth, and poor emotional well-being postnatally (Green, 1993).

The importance of reducing anxiety through the presence of a doula, provision of information as to what to expect, and the use of therapeutic modalities for relaxation cannot be emphasized enough. As mentioned previously, one of the most successful measures for reducing labor pain and the length of labor is the continuous presence of a trained, experienced woman who focuses on the laboring woman throughout each contraction, softly speaking words of reassurance and encouragement, stroking her, holding her hand, walking with her, suggesting position changes, instructing her, and instructing and reassuring her partner. This birth attendant commits herself solely to the woman's emotional and physical comfort (Hodnett, 1999).

Nonpharmacologic methods of pain relief include patterned breathing, mental imaging, massage, therapeutic touch, activity and position change, baths or showers, music or audioanalgesia, and local applications of heat or cold. Many of these interventions, such as position change and hydrotherapy, have been addressed in previous sections.

The most commonly used pharmacologic agents for pain relief in labor are systemic narcotics and regional analgesics. Both modalities have certain benefits and risks. The systemic narcotics readily cross the placenta and can depress the infant. These side effects are dose and time related. Regional analgesia through an epidural or intrathecal administration of anesthetic agents or narcotics is the most effective means of pain relief. Approximately 85% to 90% of women who receive an epidural during labor report significant pain relief within 30 minutes (Howell and Chalmers, 1992). However, the complications that accompany this method are numerous. Although the randomized trials have mixed results as to the prolongation of the first stage of labor with epidural use, there is a clear relationship between epidural use and a prolonged second stage of labor. In addition, epidural analgesia is associated with a fourfold increase in the risk for an operative delivery, possibly because of the woman's inability to direct pushing efforts and possibly because of clinician impatience (King, 1997; Thorp and Breedlove, 1996).

The administration of pharmacologic methods for pain relief is never a singular intervention. Numerous procedures typically accompany the use of both systemic narcotics and regional analgesics. Given the sophistication of regional administration, this method by far supersedes systemic administration in terms of procedures, nursing support, and highly skilled provider time. However, both require bed confinement, IV fluids, continuous electronic monitoring, and often oxygen by mask. In addition, epidural analgesia usually requires restrictions on oral intake of food and fluids, oxytocin for labor stimulation, and an indwelling catheter. The research on epidural analgesia does not explicitly address this cluster of technical interventions, the combined use of which increases the cost of intrapartum care and the contributions to maternal morbidity of which are not fully appreciated (King, 1997).

Midwifery management of pain relief for women in labor tends to use both nonpharmacologic and pharmacologic modalities. These modalities are not mutually exclusive, and a combination may provide many women with adequate pain relief while minimizing worrisome side effects. The midwifery management of pain in labor was explored using a sample of 4171 patients experiencing hospital deliveries attended by certified nurse-midwives at nine hospitals in the United States in 1996. Approximately 90% of laboring women elected to use some type of pain management for labor. Many chose from an array of nonpharmacologic methods, with or without pharmacologic ones. As expected, the nonpharmacologic methods were preferred choices of multiparas, older women, and patients who were physically active during labor. Some preferences varied according to race and ethnicity. Hispanic and Asian women were more likely to use only nonpharmacologic methods, or no method at all, and black women were more likely to combine pharmacologic and nonpharmacologic choices. This finding reflects the cultural aspect of pain perception in labor. Epidurals were used in 18.7% of this low-risk patient population, with a modest but significant increase in operative delivery (CNM Data Group, 1998). The percentage of epidural use in this report, even though significant, is much less than reported nationally. Recent trends identify increasing use of epidural analgesia, with some hospitals reporting nearly 100% of patients using this approach for pain relief.

The timing of the administration of pharmacologic modalities is critical in terms of effectiveness and minimizing maternal and neonatal side effects. Most of the literature agrees that a laboring woman should be in active labor before systemic or regional analgesics are given. Meperidine (Demerol) and fentanyl are the most popular systemic analgesics for pain relief in labor. Meperidine has been recovered from the fetus within 2 minutes of administration to the mother. The degree of newborn depression is related to the quantity of the drug transferred to the fetus. Maximal depression of the infant occurs when delivery takes place 2 to 4 hours after maternal IV or intramuscular administration. Delivery of the infant within 1 hour of administration produces little evidence of newborn depression. Fentanyl is safer for the newborn since the terminal drug elimination half-life, after a single small dose, is 1 to 2 hours. Compared with neonates exposed to no narcotics or to other analgesics, no differences were found in the frequencies of low APGAR scores, depressed respirations, or abnormal neurologic and adaptive capabilities (Thorp et al., 1993). However, institutional guidelines rather than clinical judgment are primarily used when determining analgesic choice for pain relief in labor.

Provider Status

As Margaret Myles so eloquently stated in the *Textbook for Midwives* (1975):

> It has long been known that the personality and attitude of the midwife play an important part in influencing the behavior of the woman in labour. If the midwife is endowed with a calm, optimistic temperament, she is eminently suited from a psychological point of view for the work she is doing. (p. 227)

The cultural experience of labor is what the midwife is invited to share with her client and her elected family. This experience is filled with the laboring woman and her family's expectation, beliefs, and fears. How the midwife interacts within this cultural experience will impact the woman's labor and birth. This interaction comes from how the midwife views labor and birth. Health care professionals working with birthing women need to ponder the following questions to appreciate the personal values and beliefs that she or he brings to birth:

- Do you view labor from a point of sickness or wellness?
- Do you view the pain of labor as manageable or requiring anesthesia?
- Do you view labor from a point of work that must be done or work that must be managed?
- Do you view fetal health as frail and requiring constant vigilance or healthy and robust and requiring appropriate interval assessment?

The provider's attitude on entering the cultural domain of labor and birth are as critical to the promotion of maternal and fetal health and adequate labor progress as instituting oxytocin, ordering an epidural, or performing an episiotomy.

In comparing the first-stage labor duration of primiparas at three North American and three European hospitals for the past decade, median durations were found to be over an hour longer in the North American hospitals. This is despite more frequent labor stimulation with oxytocic drugs (Thomson, 1988). The one factor that is consistently found more frequently in European hospitals is the use of midwives for labor support.

Data continue to suggest that psychosocial support can affect labor duration. In one randomized trial involving 56 women in Hamilton, Canada, routine care was compared with a desired type of care (the Leboyer method) during labor and delivery. Median first-stage labor duration (from an unspecified onset point) was 7.6 hours in the desired-care group compared to 14 hours in the routine-care group (Nelson et al., 1980).

The routine care that is categorized in much of the scientific and obstetric literature is part of labor and delivery suite culture. Routine care is ritualized by hospital caregivers to maintain lines of authority and instill the notion that these practices provide a safe environment for labor and birth. It is the midwife's role to translate these practices in a meaningful way to the laboring woman so that decisions can be made regarding which practices are beneficial for her support and care. In collaboration with her client, the midwife should decide on the use of IV fluids, fetal monitoring, bed rest, oral intake, and the care of the newborn after delivery. For many midwives this requires a continuous dialog with support staff, consulting physicians, and colleagues. The institutional culture permeates all groups so that there may be many differences in practice styles among each midwife within a group practice.

Not only are individual practice styles different depending on where labor and birth fall on the continuum of wellness/sickness, but hospital practices also influence the labor experience. The AMOL has many supporters for a variety of reasons. A few authors have attributed short duration of labor at the Dublin hospital to the high frequent of stimulation with oxytocin (O'Driscoll, Foley, and MacDonald, 1993; Sheehan, 1987). However, the review of data concerning duration of labor in three North American and three European hospitals indicate the contrary. The rates of labor stimulation were relatively low at the Dublin hospital and also at the London hospital. In addition, black and Asian women had higher rates of stimulation and longer labors than white women at that hospital, although the timing and dosage of oxytocin stimulation should have been similar in all races (Thomson, 1988). This finding leads one to appreciate the difficulty in providing a cultural fit for a laboring woman from another culture confined to an institution. A common ground must be sought for incorporating individual and cultural practices that enhance each labor and birth. A common ground that supports the necessary institutional customs and yet is strong enough to embrace the uniqueness of each family is essential. This can be done with sensitivity is by asking the laboring woman, "What do you want for your birth?"

Our institutions, our society, our lives are dictated by *time.* Even labor is required to be timely. If not, there are interventions that will initiate or maintain cervical dilation. As a clinician, time becomes a delicate balance between expectant and active management. Once the client is admitted to the hospital, expectant management becomes harder to maintain the longer she is there. The clinician practicing with a midwifery philosophy must believe that allowing labor to progress naturally provides optimal maternal and fetal health. In this sense midwives are the facilitators of a natural and healthy process called *birth* for a healthy community of women.

References

Albers LL: Clinical issues in electronic fetal monitoring, *Birth* 21:108-110, 1994.

Albers LL, Krulewitch CJ: Electronic fetal monitoring in the United States in the 1980s, *Obstet Gynecol* 82:8-10, 1993.

Albers LL, Schiff M, Gorwoda JG: The length of active labor in normal pregnancies, *Obstet Gynecol* 87:355-359, 1996.

Albers LL et al: The relationship of ambulation in labor to operative delivery, *J Nurse Midwifery* 42:4-8, 1997.

Albitol MM: Supine position in labour and the associated FHR changes, *Obstet Gynecol* 65:1470-1475, 1985.

Alfirevic Z, Neilson JP: *Biophysical profile for fetal assessment in high risk pregnancies.* In Neilson JP et al, editors: Pregnancy and childbirth module of the Cochrane database of systematic reviews (updated December 2, 1997). Available in The Cochrane Library (database on disk and CD-ROM). The Cochrane Collaboration, Issue1, Oxford, 1998, Update Software. Updated quarterly.

ACNM Board of Directors: The appropriate use of technology in childbirth, Position Statement, Washington, DC, 1997, ACNM.

ACOG: Fetal heart rate patterns: monitoring, interpretation and management, *ACOG Tech Bull 207,* July 1995.

American College of Obstetricians and Gynecologists (ACOG): Antepartum fetal surveillance, *ACOG Pract Bull 9,* October, 1999a.

ACOG: Induction of labor, *ACOG Pract Bull 10,* November, 1999b.

Ananth CV, Smulian JC, Vintzileos AM: Epidemiology of antepartum fetal testing, *Curr Opin Obstet Gynecol* 9:101-106, 1997.

Blackburn ST, Loper DL: *Maternal, fetal, and neonatal physiology: a clinical perspective,* Philadelphia, 1992, WB Saunders.

Caldeyro-Barcia R: The influence of maternal position on time of spontaneous rupture of the membranes, progress of labor, and fetal head compression, *Birth Fam J* 6:7-15, 1979.

Calkins LA: On predicting the length of labor. I. First stage, *Am J Obstet Gynecol* 42:802, 1941.

Calkins LA, Litzenberg JC, Plass ED: The length of labor, *Am J Obstet Gynecol* 19:294, 1934.

Calvert JP, Newcombe RG, Hibbard BM: An assessment of radiotelemetry in the monitoring of labour, *Br J Obstet Gynaecol* 89:285-291, 1982.

Cammu H et al: "To bathe or not to bathe" during the first stage of labor, *Acta Obstet Gynecol Scand* 73:468-472, 1994.

Chalmers B, Meyer D: What women say about their birth experiences: a cross-cultural study, *J Psychosom Obstet Gynaecol* 15(4):211-218, 1994.

Chelmow D, Kilpatrick SJ, Laros RK: Maternal and neonatal outcomes after prolonged latent phase, *Obstet Gynecol* 81:486-491, 1993.

Chervenak JL et al: Macrosomia in the postdate pregnancy: is routine ultrasonographic screening indicated? *Am J Obstet Gynecol* 161:753-756, 1989.

Church LK: Water birth: one birthing center's observations, *J Nurse Midwifery* 34:165-170, 1989.

CNM Data Group: Midwifery management of pain in labor, *J Nurse-Midwifery* 43:77-82, 1998.

Cohen WR, Brennan J: Using and archiving the labor curves, *Clin Perinatol* 22:855-874, 1995.

Cunningham FG et al, editors: *Williams obstetrics,* ed 19, Norwalk, 1993, Appleton & Lange.

Curtis P, Safransky N: Rethinking oxytocin protocols in the augmentation of labor, *Birth* 15(4):199-204, 1988.

Delpapa EH, Mueller-Heubach E: Pregnancy outcome following ultrasound diagnosis of macrosomia, *Obstet Gynecol* 78:340-344, 1991.

Diaz AG et al: Vertical position during the first stage of the course of labor, and neonatal outcome, *Eur J Obstet Gynecol* 11:1-7, 1980.

Elimian A, Figueroa R, Tejani N: Intrapartum assessment of fetal well-being: a comparison of scalp stimulation with scalp blood pH sampling, *Obstet Gynecol* 89:373-376, 1997.

Enkin M et al: *A guide to effective care in pregnancy and childbirth,* ed 2, Oxford, 1996, Oxford University Press.

Fraser WD: Methodologic issues in assessing the active management of labor, *Birth* 20:155-156, 1993.

Fraser WD et al: *Amniotomy to shorten spontaneous labour.* In Neilson JP et al, editors: Pregnancy and childbirth module of the Cochrane database of systematic reviews (updated December 2, 1997). Available in The Cochrane Library (database on disk and CD-ROM). The Cochrane Collaboration, Issue 3, Oxford, 1998, Update Software. Updated quarterly.

Friedman EA: *Labor: clinical evaluation and management,* New York, 1967, Meredith Publishing.

Fuchs AR et al: Oxytocin and the initiation of human parturition. III. Plasma concentrations of oxytocin and 13,14-dihydro-15, keto-prostaglandin F_{2a} in spontaneous and oxytocin-induced labor at term, *Am J Obstet Gynecol* 147:497-502, 1983.

Gabbe SG, Niebyl JR, Simpson JL, editors: *Obstetrics: normal and problem pregnancies,* ed 3, New York, 1996, Churchill Livingstone.

Goffinet et al: Early amniotomy increases the frequency of FHR abnormalities, *Br J Obstet Gynaecol* 104:548-553, 1997.

Green JM: Expectations and experiences of pain in labor: findings from a large prospective study, *Birth* 20:65-72, 1993.

Hemminki E, Saarikoski S: Ambulation and delayed amniotomy in the first stage of labor, *Eur J Obstet Gynaecol Reprod Biol* 15:129-139, 1983.

Herman JL: *Trauma and recovery,* New York, 1992, Basic Books.

Hinds A, Baskin LS: Child sexual abuse: what the urologist needs to know, *J Urol* 162(2):516-523, 1999.

Hodnett ED: *Caregiver support for women during childbirth.* In Neilson JP et al, editors: Pregnancy and childbirth module of the Cochrane database of systematic reviews (updated December 2, 1997). Available in The Cochrane Library (database on disk and CDROM). The Cochrane Collaboration, Issue 4, Oxford, 1999, Update Software. Updated quarterly.

Hofmeyr GJ: *Amnioinfusion for intrapartum umbilical cord compression, 1996.* In Neilson JP et al, editors: Pregnancy and childbirth module of the Cochrane database of systematic reviews (updated December 2, 1997). Available in The Cochrane Library (database on disk and CD-ROM). The Cochrane Collaboration, Issue 4, Oxford, 1998, Update Software. Updated quarterly.

Hofmeyr GJ: *Amnioinfusion for meconium-stained liquor in labour, 1995.* In Neilson JP et al, editors: Pregnancy and childbirth module of the Cochrane database of systematic reviews (updated December 2, 1997). Available in The Cochrane Library (database on disk and CD-ROM). The Cochrane Collaboration, Issue 4, Oxford, 1998, Update Software. Updated quarterly.

Howell CJ, Chalmers I: A review of prospectively controlled comparisons of epidural with non-epidural forms of pain relief during labour, *Int J Obstet Anaesth* 1:93-110, 1992.

Jamieson DJ, Steege JF: The association of sexual abuse with pelvic pain complaints in a primary care population, *Am J Obstet Gynecol* 177(6):1408-1412, 1997.

Johnstone FD: Prediction of macrosomia in diabetic pregnancy, *Contemp Rev Obstet Gynecol* 2:113-120, 1997.

Kerr MG, Scott DB, Samuel E: Studies of the inferior vena cava in late pregnancy, *Br J Med* 1:532-533, 1964.

Kilpatrick SJ, Laros RK Jr: Characteristics of normal labor, *Obstet Gynecol* 74(1):85-87, 1989.

King T: Epidural anesthesia in labor: benefits versus risks, *J Nurse Midwifery* 42:377-388, 1997.

Lee L: Personal communication, 1978.

Ludka LM, Roberts CC: Eating and drinking in labor: a literature review, *J Nurse Midwifery* 38(4):99-207, 1993.

Manning FA et al: Fetal assessment based on fetal biophysical profile scoring. IV. An analysis of perinatal morbidity and mortality, *Am J Obstet Gynecol* 150:703-709, 1990.

McCoshen JA et al: The role of fetal membranes in regulating production, transport and metabolism of prostaglandin E_2 during labor, *Am J Obstet Gynecol* 163(5 pt 1):1632-1640, 1990.

McManus TJ, Calder AA: Upright posture and the efficiency of labour, *Lancet* 1:72-74, 1978.

Mendelson CL: The aspiration of stomach content into the lungs during obstetric anesthesia, *Am J Obstet Gynecol* 52:191-206, 1946.

Meschia G: Placental respiratory gas exchange and fetal oxygenation. In Creasy RK, Resnick R, editors: *Maternal fetal medicine: principles and practice,* Philadelphia, 1989, WB Saunders.

Miller DA, Rabello YA, Paul RH: The modified biophysical profile: antepartum testing in the 1990s, *Am J Obstet Gynecol* 174:812-817, 1996.

Miyazaki FS, Nevarez F: Saline amnioinfusion for relief of repetitive variable decelerations: a prospective randomized study, *Am J Obstet Gynecol* 153:301-306, 1985.

Moore T, Piacquadio K: A prospective evaluation of fetal movement screening to reduce the incidence of antepartum fetal death, *Am J Obstet Gynecol* 160:1075-1080, 1989.

Myles M: *Textbook for midwives,* ed 8, London, 1975, Churchill Livingstone.

National Institute of Child Health and Human Development Research Planning Workshop: Electronic fetal heart rate monitoring: research guidelines for interpretation, *Am J Obstet Gynecol* 177:1385-1390, 1997.

Nelson NM et al: A randomized clinical trial of the Leboyer approach to childbirth, *N Engl J Med* 302:655-660, 1980.

Neilson JP: Electronic fetal heart rate monitoring during labor: information from randomized trials, *Birth* 21:101-104, 1994.

O'Driscoll K, Foley M, MacDonald D: Active management of labor as an alternative to cesarean section for dystocia, *Obstet Gynecol* 63:485-490, 1993.

Odent M: Birth under water, *Lancet* 31:1476-1477, 1983.

O'Sullivan G: The stomach-fact and fantasy: eating and drinking during labor, *Int Anesthesiol Clin* 32(2):31-44, 1994.

Pollack RN, Hauer-Pollack G, Divon MY: Macrosomia in postdates pregnancies: the accuracy of routine ultrasonographic screening, *Am J Obstet Gynecol* 167:7-11, 1992.

Rhodes N, Hutchinson S: Labor experiences of childhood sexual abuse survivors, *Birth* 21:213-220, 1994.

Roberts J: Maternal position in the first stage of labour. In Chalmers I, Enkin M, Keirse MJ, editors: *Effective care in pregnancy and childbirth,* vol 2, Oxford, 1989, Oxford University Press.

Roberts JE, Mendez-Bauer C, Wodell DA: The effects of maternal position on uterine contractility and efficiency, *Birth Fam J* 4:243-247, 1983.

Rosen MG, Dickinson JC: The paradox of electronic fetal monitoring: more data may not enable us to predict or prevent infant neurologic morbidity, *Am J Obstet Gynecol* 168:745-751, 1993.

Rush J et al: The effects of whirlpool baths in labor: a randomized, controlled trial, *Birth* 23:136-143, 1996.

Rutherford S et al: The four quadrant assessment of amniotic fluid volume: an adjunct to antepartum fetal heart rate testing, *Obstet Gynecol* 7:146-149, 1987.

Satin AJ et al: Factors affecting the dose response to oxytocin for labor stimulation, *Am J Obstet Gynecol* 196:1260-1261, 1992.

Schott A: Measuring fetal movement. Maternal and Child Health Resources, Education Programs Associates, vol 10, issue 2, 1995.

Seng JS, Hassinger JA: Relationship strategies and interdisciplinary collaboration: improving maternity care with survivors of childhood sexual abuse, *J Nurse Midwifery* 43(4):287-295, 1998.

Sheehan KH: Caesarean section for dystocia: a comparison of practices in two countries, *Lancet* 1:548-551, 1987.

Simkin P: Stress, pain, and catecholamines in labor. Part 1: A review, *Birth* 13:227-233, 1986.

Simkin PT: Overcoming the legacy of childhood sexual abuse: the role of caregivers and childbirth educators, *Birth* 19:224-225, 1992.

Singer JE, Westphal M, Niswander K: Relationship of weight gain during pregnancy to birthweight and infant growth and development in the first year of life: a report from the collaborative study of cerebral palsy, *Obstet Gynecol* 31:417-423, 1968.

SOGC: Fetal health surveillance in labour, Policy Statement 41, October 1995.

Speroff L, Glass RH, Kase NG: *Clinical gynecologic endocrinology and infertility,* ed 5, Baltimore, 1994, Williams & Wilkins.

Spong CY, Ogundipe OA, Ross MG: Prophylactic amnioinfusion for meconium stained amniotic fluid, *Am J Obstet Gynecol* 171:931-935, 1994.

Stein JL et al: Nipple stimulation for labor augmentation, *J Reprod Med* 35(7):710-714, 1990.

Stewart P, Calder AA: Posture in labour: patient's choice and its effect on performance, *Br J Obstet Gynaecol* 91:1091-1095, 1984.

Thacker SB, Stroup DF: *Continuous electronic fetal heart monitoring during labor, 1998.* In Neilson JP et al, editors: Pregnancy and childbirth module of the Cochrane database of systematic reviews (updated December 2, 1997). Available in The Cochrane Library (database on disk and CD-ROM). The Cochrane Collaboration, Issue 1, Oxford, 1998, Update Software. Updated quarterly.

The Society of Obstetricians and Gynaecologists of Canada: Fetal health surveillance in labour, *J Soc Obstet Gynaecol Can* 17:865, 1995.

Thomson M: Different rates of prolonged first-stage labor in primiparas at two hospitals, *Birth* 15:209-212, 1988.

Thorp JA, Breedlove G: Epidural analgesia in labor: an evaluation of risks and benefits, *Birth* 23:63-83, 1996.

Thorp JA et al: The effect of intrapartum epidural analgesia on nulliparous labor: a randomized, controlled, prospective trial, *Am J Obstet Gynecol* 169:851-858, 1993.

Wheeler L: *Nurse-midwifery handbook: a practical guide to prenatal and postpartum care,* Philadelphia, 1997, JB Lippincott.

Zhang J et al: Continuous labor support from labor attendant for primiparous women: a meta-analysis, *Obstet Gynecol* 88(4, part 2):739-744, 1996.

Bibliography

Davis E: *Heart and hands: a midwife's guide to pregnancy and birth,* ed 3, Berkeley, Calif, 1997, Celestial Arts.

Klaus M, Kennell J, Klaus P: *Mothering the mother: how a doula can help you have a shorter, easier, and healthier birth,* New York, 1993, Addison Wesley.

Chapter 20

Second-Stage Labor

INTRODUCTION

The second stage, or "pushing stage," of labor is defined as the time from full dilation of the cervix until birth of the baby. Women often feel a surge of energy or an increased sense of control as they move into active pushing. The midwife's role includes continuing assessment for maternal or fetal risk factors; offering verbal and physical support of the woman's bearing-down efforts; and creating a safe, calm environment into which the infant will be born.

MATERNAL STATUS

General Appearance

Women without regional anesthesia note an increase in rectal pressure or an involuntary "urge to push" at the time of full dilation. A watchful birth attendant notes the beginning of involuntary bearing-down efforts at the peak of contractions as the cervix becomes fully dilated and the presenting part descends deeper in the pelvis. Perspiration may appear on the woman's upper lip, her facial expression may change, and she may express the feeling that "the baby's coming."

Some women may experience a decrease in frequency and intensity of contractions at full dilation, allowing them time to rest before the active pushing that will occur to birth the baby. This "peaceful interlude" has been called the latent phase of second stage (Nichols and Zwelling, 1997). Onnie Lee Logan, a granny midwife who practiced in Alabama for 53 years, notes in her oral history, *Motherwit* (1991):

> The contractions can leave awhile completely. . . . Give the mother time to rest between the contractions. This is a beautiful point about it. They gets so sleepy just befo' that baby is really fixin to crown on us yet, the mother gets so sleepy. . . You cain't stay awake to save yo' life. . . Befo' they get the urge to push that's when they get sleepy for a rest. (pp. 148-149)

During this interlude the fetus continues to descend in the pelvis, and the strong urge to push will occur when the fetal head applies pressure on the stretch receptors in the perineum, causing an increase in release of oxytocin.

Vital Signs

It is important for the midwife to remember that the second stage may last hours; thus continuation of pattern of vital signs based on maternal status is essential. It is not uncommon for the birth attendant and the nursing staff to get so involved in assisting the laboring woman with pushing efforts that several hours pass without monitoring of the blood pressure or temperature. Hourly temperatures are recommended for women who have prolonged ruptured membranes, borderline temperatures, or fetal or maternal tachycardia. Blood pressures are required hourly or more frequently when hypertension has been identified. In a healthy woman temperature, pulse, and blood pressure can continue to be taken every 4 hours.

Physical Assessment

The woman usually appears to be truly working during this part of labor. The midwife should note her bearing-down efforts and her coping mechanisms as she deals with the increased pelvic pressure. In multiparas rapid descent of the presenting part may cause bulging of the perineum, gaping of the anus, and opening of the vaginal introitus soon after full dilation has been reached.

Pelvic examination can be used to confirm that labor has progressed to the second stage. Initiation of the second stage is confirmed when no cervix is noted around the fetal presenting part. Station should be noted so the progress can be assessed over time. If the membranes have ruptured, continued assessment of the color of the amniotic fluid is essential. A change from clear to meconium-stained fluid during labor may indicate fetal stress, and further evaluation of fetal status is warranted.

The midwife should keep in mind that the verification of second stage by pelvic examination almost always occurs after the fact. It is extremely rare for the clinician to truly feel the last lip of cervix drawn up into the lower segment since there isn't continuous monitoring of the cervix. Pelvic examination can be used as a means to verify labor progress when the woman's verbal and nonverbal communication suggests that she has entered the expulsive stage of labor. However, since pelvic examination to determine cervical status can be uncomfortable and presents the risk of introducing pathogens into the genital tract, experienced midwives commonly support pushing efforts without pelvic examination, relying on the other maternal signs of second-stage labor.

INTAKE/OUTPUT: FEEDING THE MOTHER

The midwife should continue to monitor for signs of dehydration through second stage labor. Review of fluid intake and output is essential to ensure adequate hydration. Particularly in long labors, women may think they have been taking in sufficient fluids orally when in fact they may have had minimal intake. Poor urinary output (e.g., less than 100 ml every 1 to 2 hours) and concentrated urine give the clinician an indication of inadequate fluid intake.

Little research has assessed the actual fluid and nutritional needs of women in labor, and no studies specifically looking at those needs in second-stage labor were found. It stands to reason then that sufficient fluids should be given orally to prevent the development of increased urine specific gravity (greater than 1.020) as determined by urinary reagent strips. If the woman is unable to maintain hydration orally, use of intravenous hydration should be considered.

Monitoring of urinary output must be continued through second-stage labor. The birth attendant should be vigilant for signs of a distended bladder, since trauma to the bladder and urethra may occur during the birth process. In addition, an overdistended bladder may inhibit descent of the presenting part.

Many women expel stool with their pushing efforts. For this reason, some women may prefer to push while sitting on a toilet. The midwife should be quick to clean up any stool, for both aseptic and aesthetic reasons.

SUPPORT STATUS

Supporting the Woman

The beginning of the second stage may be exciting, but it may also be frightening to the woman. The overwhelming pressure experienced by some women or the feeling of being out-of-control may be very unsettling. The midwife can enhance a sense of security through calm, reassuring conversation and provide supportive physical care through the use of touch, massage, and warm or cool compresses.

Supporting the Support System

The beginning of the second stage often creates an air of excitement among the support people present. There is a sense that the birth will be soon, and supporters may begin to get ready for welcoming the baby. Cameras are made ready, audio tape recorders may be set, and, more recently, video cameras may be set up.

The midwife needs to counsel the family members and friends regarding the expected length of the second stage. With a first birth they need to understand that the second stage may last several hours and that ongoing support of the mother is still necessary. Supportive individuals can continue to help the woman assume positions of comfort that will enhance fetal descent and pushing efforts and provide massage and counterpressure to relieve musculoskeletal aches and pains. In multiparous women labor may progress very rapidly, and support individuals need to know that this is probably not the best time to go out for a meal or leave for other reasons.

As with the first stage of labor, cultural beliefs in the family system may influence the type of support given. In some cultures the male partner may be out of his cultural role in physically supporting the woman during this time. A female relative, often the woman's mother or mother-in-law, may be the expected supporter. Religious beliefs may proscribe the male from touching his wife or newborn baby because of the presence of blood products. It is important for the midwife to understand the expectations surrounding the birth process to appropriately coach the coaches.

FETAL STATUS

Fetal descent is often appreciated during the abdominal examination. Location of fetal heart tones may be noted lower on the abdomen, and palpation of the fetus may indicate descent of the presenting part deeper into the pelvis.

Fetal Monitoring

Intermittent auscultation of the fetal heart rate (FHR) using a fetoscope, doptone, or the external fetal monitor should be done every 15 minutes during the second stage in women at low risk for perinatal problems (ACOG, 1995). Auscultation should be done during the entire contraction and for a minimum of 30 seconds following the contraction. As the fetal head descends, head compression may lead to mild-to-moderate decelerations that return promptly to baseline at the end of the contraction. Prolonged and/or severe decelerations or slow return to baseline necessitates the use of continuous electronic monitoring to better evaluate fetal status.

Deviations from normal requiring medical consultation include the following:

1. *Baseline rate.* Baseline of fetal tachycardia (FHR >160 beats/min for greater than 10 minutes) or bradycardia (FHR <110 beats/min for greater than 10 minutes) suggest possible fetal compromise. Medical consultation is indicated, and consideration of consultation for pediatric attendance at delivery should be considered.
2. *Baseline variability.* If continuous electronic fetal monitoring is used, the midwife should assess the variability of the baseline. Absent or minimal FHR variability in a woman who has not been medicated with drugs that affect the FHR (e.g., narcotics) is an indication for medical consultation and consideration of pediatric attendance at delivery.
3. *Decelerations.* Recurrent late decelerations may be an indication of uteroplacental insufficiency and are an indication for medical consultation. Severe variable decelerations not alleviated with position change, particularly when associated with absent or minimal variability, warrant medical consultation for possible assisted delivery.

Amniotic Fluid Evaluation

If the membranes have not ruptured spontaneously during the first stage of labor, they will most likely rupture with the active pushing efforts of second stage. An advantage of intact membranes is that the fetal head is cushioned during descent and there is less likelihood of cord compression. A disadvantage of intact membranes is that it is difficult to determine the color of the amniotic fluid until the membranes bulge out of the introitus.

Although there are distinct fetal benefits for maintaining the fetal membranes, there are indications for amniotomy. Experienced clinicians have noted that, when the intact bag of waters bulges into the vagina in a way that does not facilitate stretching of the vaginal walls and descent of the fetal head, artificial rupture of membranes (AROM) may assist pushing efforts. Release of the bulging bag may serve to allow the fetal head to apply more direct pressure to the soft tissue structures and nerve plexus. AROM may also be done to assess amniotic fluid, especially if one plans to have a pediatric provider attend the birth if there is meconium-stained fluid. Assessment of the color of fluid is recommended if the FHR suggests fetal compromise.

Site of birth may also influence the decision to artificially rupture the membranes. In sites in which meconium-stained fluid is an indication to transfer the woman out of a birthing room to a delivery room or from an out-of-hospital site to an in-hospital site, the timing of AROM must allow for time for transfer if necessary. Therefore, with a woman experiencing a first labor with the fetal head at 0 station, it may be appropriate to perform the amniotomy at the beginning of the second stage. However, in a multiparous woman amniotomy may be done when she is 6 to 7 cm.

LABOR STATUS

Physical Assessment

Contractions tend to remain about 3 minutes apart and 60 to 90 seconds' duration during the second stage of labor. Some women experience a decrease in frequency at the time of full dilation, as noted previously. Intervention is rarely necessary when this occurs, since the frequency usually returns to the woman's norm within an hour. Monitoring the frequency, intensity, and duration of contractions can be continued using palpation. Although determination of intensity and duration may be seen as subjective, an experienced clinician can become quite adept at this technique. External monitoring using tocodynamometry measures the frequency of contractions by sensing the change in the shape and tone of the abdominal wall. Measurement of the intensity and duration of the contractions is influenced by maternal habitus and fetal position. Precise measurement of contraction patterns can be obtained through the use of an intrauterine pressure catheter, but this intervention should be limited to cases in which it is necessary to verify lack of progress in labor with documented adequacy of contractions.

Hospital-based nurses providing maternity care in the twentieth century have traditionally directed pushing during the second stage rather than encouraging spontaneous maternal bearing-down efforts. A maternity nursing text used at the time when birth was increasingly assisted in the hospital instructed the nurse, "At the beginning of a pain the patient should take a deep breath, close her lips, brace her feet and strain with all her strength" (Van Blarcom, 1937, p. 287). Practices such as encouraging long breath-holding and closed-glottis pushing, discouraging involuntary pushing, and the common cheerleading approach of telling the woman to "hold your breath, push, push, push," have persisted even in light of research findings that raise questions about the effectiveness and safety of these approaches (Petersen and Besuner, 1997). Many physicians and nurses argue that the directed, prolonged pushing efforts are necessary to hasten fetal descent and decrease the length of second-stage labor. However, the belief that there is an association between a prolonged second stage and poorer maternal and neonatal outcomes has been challenged by more recent research. Cohen (1977), in an early study to evaluate the relationship of length of second stage labor to maternal and neonatal outcomes, found no relationship between prolonged second stage and perinatal mortality when the FHR was monitored. Furthermore, the findings suggest that increased lower 1-minute APGAR scores and increased incidence of postpartum infection in women with second-stage labors greater than 2 hours is related to the interventions and management used by the birth attendant and not directly to the length of labor.

Some women without sensory blocks from anesthesia may feel the urge to push before complete dilation; others may not feel the urge until well after complete dilation, whereas still others may never feel a strong urge to push (Bergstrom et al., 1997; McKay, Barrows, and Roberts, 1990). The sensation of urge to push is closely associated with the station of the presenting part. Once the presenting part puts pressure on the pelvic floor, stimulation of stretch receptors located in the posterior vaginal wall cause the release of endogenous oxytocin, which increases the spontaneous pushing efforts. It appears clear that, when the presenting part is at or below the ischial spines (0 to +1 station), the laboring woman usually feels an urge to push, regardless of dilation. Thompson (1993) compared maternal and neonatal outcomes in a control group that experienced traditional directed pushing during second stage and an experimental group that received support for spontaneous pushing efforts. Results included the finding of a negative correlation between length of labor and venous cord pH in the control group but not the experimental group, suggesting that there was a disadvantage with longer second-stage labors only with directed closed-glottis pushing. Thompson found that women using spontaneous pushing had a significantly longer second stages of labor, but others have not found that to be the case. Parnell and colleagues (1993) found no difference in duration of second stage, umbilical artery pH, or perineal lacerations when comparing directed vs. spontaneous pushers. In a follow-up study Thompson (1995) sought to describe the characteristics of pushing efforts when the laboring woman was encouraged to "do what her body told her" (Thompson, 1995, p. 1030). Findings included the facts that none of the women so directed took a deep breath at the beginning of a contraction and that women used a combination of open- and closed-glottis pushing, often during the same contraction.

Bergstrom and colleagues (1997) have proposed a typology of second-stage labor that recognizes the woman's perception of the expulsive phase as part of the determination of phase of labor. A type I pushing situation occurs when the woman feels an urge to push but the cervix is not fully dilated. Traditionally professional staff have encouraged women experiencing type I pushing to pant or blow in order to not push with the sensation. A type II pushing situation is defined as the traditional second stage—the cervix is found to be fully dilated, and the woman experiences an urge to push. A type III situation is defined as the traditional first stage of labor—the cervix is not fully dilated, and there is no urge to push. A type IV situation occurs when the cervix is fully dilated and the woman feels no urge to push. Full dilation without an urge to push has also been described as latent phase of second-stage labor (Bergstrom et al., 1997). This classification validates the woman's perception of her experience of labor and provides a model more consistent with a midwifery paradigm than with the medical paradigm of birth.

One reason that spontaneous pushing support has not been adopted in many sites is that women who push instinctively often grunt or groan as they push. Particularly since the increase in use of regional anesthesia for labor, nurses and birth attendants have come to expect women to labor silently. One respondent to a survey exploring beliefs about second-stage labor support reported that she " 'was given a hard time' by coworkers if her 'patients got too noisy'" (Petersen and Besuner, 1997, p. 724). Other nurses express the concern that other patients or family members may be frightened by the sounds made by spontaneously laboring women. In light of the positive effects of spontaneous pushing techniques identified in the literature, it seems more appropriate to educate women and families about the normal sounds of birth than to try to maintain silence.

Pushing efforts are influenced by the position and size of the fetus. Occipitoanterior positions facilitate descent through the pelvis. Occipitoposterior positions may result in poor "fit" and may contribute to longer second-stage labor. The relationship between the presenting diameters of the fetal head and the maternal pelvis will also influence length of the second stage. Molding of the fetal skull facilitates passage of even relatively large infants through a pelvis that may have compromised anterior, posterior, or transverse diameters. A skilled midwife or physician learns the art of judging clinically when the molding becomes significant enough to warn that vaginal birth is not probable.

The assessment of whether the second stage is progressing normally must take into consideration the woman's parity, history of previous labors, coping abilities, and the response of the fetus to the expulsive efforts. Early research associated second-stage labors of longer than 2 hours with increased perinatal mortality and increased infection rates. However, close monitoring of the FHR to verify fetal tolerance of labor and monitoring of the mother to verify progress in descent and absence of signs of infection prevent unnecessary operative intervention (Research Box 20-1).

Protracted second-stage labor has been defined as descent less than 1 cm/hr in nulliparas and less than 2 cm/hr for multiparas (Friedman and Sachtleben, 1970). This definition correlates with the ACOG definition of protracted second-stage labor—longer than 2 hours in nulliparas without regional anesthesia, longer than 3 hours when regional anesthesia is used, and longer than 1 hour in multiparas. The diagnosis of protracted second stage or arrest of descent can be difficult, however, since estimation of station is less accurate than estimation of dilation. In addition, the length of the birth canal varies from 11 to 15 cm so that conversion of progressive change in station to descent in centimeters per hour is difficult (Gabbe, Niebyl, and Simpson, 1996). Progress in descent of the fetal presenting part is best determined by the same examiner over several hours. In addition to ascertaining the level of the presenting part in the pelvis, the examiner also must determine position and presence of molding or caput. The time needed for rotation of the fetal head from a posterior position to an anterior position can explain a prolonged second stage, thereby justifying deferring instrumental intervention as long as the woman and her fetus are tolerating the labor well.

As the second stage progresses, the midwife watches for visual cues that the birth is imminent. Bulging of the perineum confirms that the presenting part has descended to the level of the pelvic floor. The perineum progressively thins out and becomes increasingly distended. The anus pouches out, and rectal mucosa can be readily seen. The presenting part can then be seen at the introitus. The midwife must keep in mind that, particularly in multiparous women, these visible changes may occur rapidly, even during one contraction.

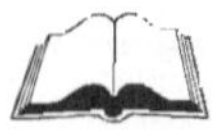

Research Box 20-1

Bergstrom L et al: You'll feel me touching you, sweetie': vaginal examinations during the second stage of labor, *Birth* 19(1):10-18, 1992.

Background

The role of birth attendants in the United States and other developed countries is a part of the social context of the birth experience. Increasingly the birth attendant is accepted as the "manager" of the labor and birth, with the resulting use of interventions that may or may not be of value during the birthing process. Sterile vaginal examinations are common procedures used to assess the progress of labor, but the use of these examinations in second-stage labor has not been rigorously explored. The wide variation in use of vaginal examinations in labor suggests that the culture of the birth attendant and birth setting rather than the actual process of labor and birth may determine the use of the procedure.

Research Question

What are the patterns of behavior and unwritten rules that defined the performance of sterile vaginal examination during the second stage of labor and guided caregivers' action and talk?

Methods

Women planning births in four settings—in-hospital and out-of-hospital—were recruited to participate in this ethnographic study of use of sterile vaginal examinations in second-stage labor. Videotaping of the second stage of labor began when the woman was found to be in second-stage labor by the provider or when the woman felt a spontaneous urge to push and continued through the birth of the baby. A trained transcriptionist completed transcripts of the interactions between the caregivers and the laboring women. Conversational analysis was used to analyze the content of the encounters.

Sample

Twenty-three women recruited during first-stage labor and consented to be videotaped during second-stage labor. Their ages ranged from 18 to 36 years, 36% were primigravidas, and all were accompanied by one or more nonprofessional support people. Women with medical complications were excluded from participation. Nine of the 23 had instrument-assisted deliveries. Care providers also gave consent to the videotaping and included registered nurses, student nurse-midwives, certified nurse-midwives, medical students, resident physicians, and attending physicians.

Results

Before the procedure the caregiver verbally or nonverbally informed the woman about the intended examination with the most common nonverbal sign being the donning of the sterile glove in the woman's line of vision. No women asked for clarification regarding the purpose or the necessity of the examination. The laboring woman's role was usually passive and permissive. During the examinations the caregivers often gave instructions to improve pushing techniques and rarely shared summary comments with the woman. When examinations were uncomfortable or painful for women, expressions of discomfort were either ignored or superficially acknowledged. Women were never warned about the possibility of pain when more complex examinations were anticipated. The investigators interpreted the interactions as recognition of the procedure as a type of ritual accompanied by personal disembodiment of the caregiver and a communication of the power relationship held between the care provider and the laboring woman. Frequent vaginal examinations in second-stage labor also communicate the message that the woman's body cannot be trusted to deliver the baby correctly or efficiently.

Clinical Application

By recognizing the social messages that use of the sterile vaginal examinations during labor convey, caregivers can mediate the negative aspects of the examination. Unless use of examinations is shown to have positive effects on the second stage of labor, such examinations should be kept to a minimum. Caregivers should clearly explain to the woman the rationale for the examination and allow for meaningful negotiation before performing it. Finally, caregivers should explain that the examination may be painful, acknowledge pain when it is experienced, and discuss findings with the woman. Findings from this exploratory study can be used to design research that can further assess the use of sterile vaginal examinations in second-stage labor and assess approaches that result in the woman being an active rather than passive participant.

ACTIVITY STATUS

Maintaining the laboring woman in a recumbent position during the second stage is a result of medical tradition and use of interventions that inhibit movement (e.g., electronic fetal monitoring). Historically women across cultures were encouraged to remain upright and actively move about through the first and second stages of labor. Early manuscripts and prints document the use of standing or squatting positions for birth and the use of birth stools or chairs. The use of the recumbent position for birth was proposed by physicians merely for their own comfort and for the ease of using instruments for assisted birth. European birth attendants increasingly used the left-lateral position for second stage labor; American physicians increasingly used the lithotomy position. Women attended by nurse-midwives in the United States most frequently push and give birth in either a sitting or side-lying position (Hanson, 1998). These are the positions that women most often chose when given the option of choosing their birth positions (Carlson et al., 1986; Rossi and Lindell, 1986).

The effect of maternal position during second stage on both maternal and fetal well-being has been well documented in the literature. When the woman is upright, the longitudinal axis of the birth canal straightens because the fundus shifts anterior. This shift in uterine alignment facilitates the passage of the fetal head into the inlet and midpelvis. With the upright position, the pelvis lies at a 90- to 120-degree angle to the spinal axis, further placing the fetal head in a better position for descent. This is in contrast to the 30-degree angle found when the woman is in the supine position (Holland and Smith, 1989) (Research Box 20-2).

The upright position results in increased inlet and outlet diameters. Progesterone-induced softening of the fixed joints of the pelvis and the effect of weight-bearing on the posterior sacroiliac joints leads to widening of the joints and shifting of the lower sacrum. This results in an increased intertuberous diameter. Other benefits of the upright position in second-stage labor include decreased pain with contractions, even with increased force during bearing-down efforts, and decreased use of analgesia and anesthesia.

It has been estimated that the squatting position may enlarge the outlet diameters by approximately 25% to 28% (Shermer and Raines, 1997; Sweet, 1997). Squatting forces the thighs against the abdominal wall, which may increase bearing-down efforts and facilitate fetal descent (Shermer and Raines, 1997). Squatting also causes stretching or separation of the symphysis pubis, increasing anterior pelvic outlet dimensions. However, American women rarely use squatting in their daily activities, so may not have the strength and flexibility in the legs and lower back to sustain squatting throughout second stage. Kneeling offers many of the benefits of squatting when squatting is not tolerated. Use of the birthing stool allows greater support and relaxation between contractions and maintains position similar to a true squat. Studies of the use of birthing stools and birthing chairs have reported conflicting findings in incidence or degree of perineal edema, perineal trauma, and maternal blood loss. Methodologic problems, including grouping the chair and stool together, small sample sizes, and lack of quantification of time using the support make interpretation of findings difficult. Shermer and Raines (1997) suggest that continuous pressure on the lower buttocks for extended periods of time may result in venous congestion and dependent edema. This can be prevented by suggesting frequent position changes when the laboring woman is using a birthing stool, birthing chair, or toilet during second stage (Research Box 20-2).

The upright position also has benefits to the fetus. Increased fetal oxygen saturation during labor, increased fetal/neonatal pH and Po_2 levels, and decreased fetal/neonatal CO_2 levels have been associated with neonates whose mothers labored in the upright position (Gupta, Brayshaw, and Lilford, 1989). Data suggest that there is no increase in molding of the fetal head or early variable decelerations when the upright position is used.

PAIN/PSYCHE/PROVIDER STATUS

The midwife continues to assess the woman's coping abilities throughout second-stage labor. Some women claim that being able to push "feels good," but others may be overwhelmed by the intensity of the sensations. Supportive physical and emotional care is essential to the continued well-being of the woman and her fetus.

Expulsive efforts are hard work. The woman will most likely perspire and may be comforted by a cool sponging of her face and neck. Frequent change of position will help to prevent muscle cramping or other positional discomforts. Some women experience leg cramps that can be relieved by extending the leg and providing counterpressure and dorsiflexion of the foot. Nonpharmacologic approaches that use stimulation to the skin and muscles are helpful in decreasing perception of pain, most likely because of the "gate control" theory of pain relief.

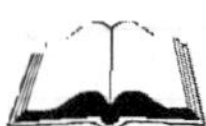

Research Box 20-2

Golay J, Vedam S, Sorger L: The squatting position for the second stage of labor: effects on labor and on maternal and fetal well-being, *Birth* 20(2):73-78, 1993.

Background

Women giving birth in the United States generally assume the recumbent and lateral positions for second-stage labor, whereas women in other countries often assume squatting or other vertical positions. The few studies that have explored use of upright position in labor have found decreases in pain, length of labor, and maternal and fetal morbidity. Squatting increases the diameter of the pelvic outlet, increases the urge to push, and enhances the alignment of the fetus in the birth canal. Even with these benefits, squatting is seldom chosen as a position for birthing by American women and their caregivers.

Research Question

Is there a difference between the effects of maternal squatting and semirecumbent positions during the second stage of labor on the evolution and progress of labor and the physiologic well-being of the woman and her baby?

Methods

This nonconcurrent cohort study compared the labor experiences of a group of women who assumed the squatting position for second stage of labor with a group who were primarily in the semirecumbent position. The practices/sites were chosen because of similar philosophies of practice, patient populations, and birthing facilities. However, the experimental group (squatting) received encouragement to practice squatting during the pregnancy and were more likely to use squatting during the birth. Data were collected using retrospective chart review. Charts were rejected if they did not contain a labor and delivery summary or if there was a cesarean delivery before second-stage labor. Every fifth obstetrics chart from the experimental practice was chosen for a total of 200 women, and every third chart was selected from the practice using primarily semirecumbent position for a total of 100 women. Demographic, obstetric, medical-surgical, antepartal, and intrapartum data were recorded on a preprinted instrument.

Sample

No statistical differences were noted between groups in gravidity, parity, and numbers of women with previous vaginal deliveries. The last factor was used for analysis rather than parity since the experimental group had a higher proportion of women who had a previous cesarean delivery. Other variables that differed between groups included maternal age (experimental group was younger) and attendance at childbirth preparation classes (experimental group was more likely to attend classes). The control group was more likely to have intravenous therapy in labor, artificial rupture of membranes, and continuous and intermittent external fetal monitoring.

Results

The experimental group had significantly shorter second stages of labor. First- and third-stage labors were similar in the two groups. There was no difference in rate of operative delivery between the groups. Of the women in the experimental group, 45% delivered over intact perineums compared to 18% in the semirecumbent group. Eight percent of the women in the experimental group had episiotomies, compared to 51% in the control group. There were no statistical differences in maternal or fetal/neonatal morbidity between the groups.

Clinical Application

Findings must be interpreted with recognition of the limitations of the nonconcurrent cohort design. Lack of randomization to groups and retrospective collection of chart data limit the comparisons of the participants. It is feasible that there are confounding variables that may have influenced the results. Further study using greater control to ensure similar group characteristics is necessary to determine whether the squatting position is an independent variable associated with shorter second stage, perineal integrity, and improved maternal and neonatal outcomes.

Professional support people can further enhance the woman's feeling of well-being by maintaining a calm, quiet environment for her. Between contractions the midwife, nurse, or doula should encourage the laboring woman in a calm and positive way. Efforts should be made to maintain privacy and modesty. Simple acts such as keeping the labor room door closed, limiting intrusion by other staff, and maintaining effective covering of the vaginal area conveys the sense of respect for the woman.

The birth attendant should continue to assess the woman's support system and intervene when appropriate. If the labor has been long, the primary support person may need relief to get something to eat or drink or to prepare emotionally for the birth. Professional staff can guide support individuals in ways to facilitate normal second stage. Suggestions for position changes, massage or counterpressure, and comfort measures such as compresses and oral fluids can facilitate the partner's or friend's effectiveness as a supportive other. Occasionally family and friends get so excited about the impending birth that their voices and activities become distracting to the woman. Professional staff should guide them in maintaining a calm, supportive environment in which the woman is the central figure.

PREPARING FOR THE BIRTH

An effective birth attendant begins to prepare for the birth in early labor. Consideration of the woman's obstetric history and the progress of this labor guides the midwife's assessment of expected time of birth. In a primigravida, materials needed for the birth can usually be prepared during second-stage as it becomes clear that the fetus has descended to the pelvic floor. In a multipara the midwife may recognize that materials need to be set up during late first stage if a rapid second stage is anticipated.

One of the professional staff should be responsible for checking emergency equipment, including oxygen delivery devices and suction apparatus. Medications for maternal or fetal emergencies must be readily available, including intravenous delivery systems when an intravenous infusion has not been used during the labor. Institutions vary in the equipment that is provided for the birth, but all sites should provide the following minimal supplies:

- Protective gown, mask, eye shields, and gloves for standardized precautions (Birth is an activity with high risk for exposure to body fluids, and protection against exposure for professional staff is essential.)
- Sterile drapes onto which the infant can be placed or on which instruments can be set (Birth itself is not a sterile procedure. However, internal examination of the laboring woman and surgical repair of lacerations or episiotomy must be done under sterile conditions to decrease risk of infection.)
- Two clamps for clamping the umbilical cord
- Two pair of scissors
- Needle holder
- One pair of pick-ups
- Two sponge sticks
- Placenta basin
- 4 × 4 gauze
- Clamp for the umbilical cord
- Suction catheter and/or bulb syringe

Determining Maternal Position for Birth

Most American-prepared birth attendants have been taught to use the semi-Fowler's or lithotomy position for birth. Although these positions may be most advantageous for the birth attendant, they may not be best for the woman or her infant. Both positions result in pressure on the inferior vena cava, thereby causing supine hypotension, decreased placental perfusion, and fetal hypoxia. These effects can be ameliorated with the use of a support wedge under one hip, with resulting displacement of the gravid uterus.

Midwives and laboring women have long recognized the usefulness of alternative positions for birth (Sweet, 1997) (Figure 20-1). Positions that may facilitate delivery of the baby through the effect of gravity include standing, squatting, kneeling, and sitting upright on a birthing chair or bed. Positions that enhance stretching of the perineum and decrease perineal trauma include left lateral and "all-fours" position. Left lateral and all-fours positions also provide for greater manipulation of shoulders when anticipating a large baby or tight fit.

Supporting the Delivery of the Infant

When it appears that the birth is imminent, the professional staff prepare to assist with the delivery of the infant. After donning protective goggles, the midwife or physician scrubs the hands and forearms, puts on the protective gown and sterile gloves, and sets up the equipment needed for the delivery. A small table or cart can be used for equipment, or a sterile drape or towel on which equipment can be placed can be put on the bed. A birth assistant should wash the perineal area to remove bloody show and other fluids.

The techniques used to assist the birth of the baby can only be learned by mentoring from an experienced clinician and experience. Hand placement and timing may vary among midwives and physicians, but several principles guide the process of a safe and satisfying birth experience (Figure 20-2).

Perhaps the most important principle is good control of the fetal head. Premature extension of the fetal head is associated with lacerations of the perineum and the ante-

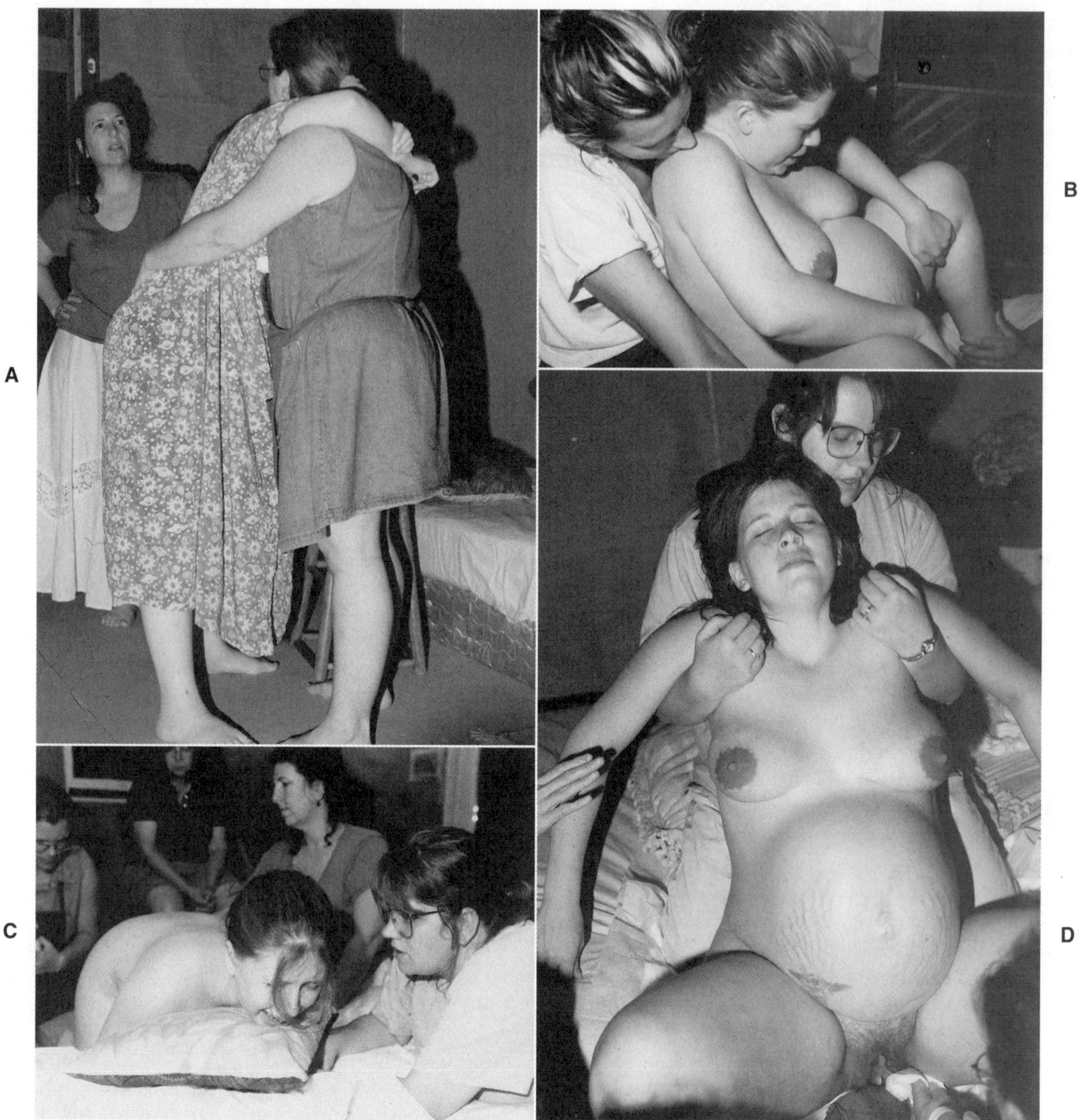

Figure 20-1 Pushing in a variety of positions. **A,** Supported standing; **B,** supported squat-sit; **C,** hands and knees; and **D,** supported squat. (Courtesy Caroline E. Brown.)

rior structures of the vulva. The clinician should coach the woman to slowly deliver the baby's head so that the perineum can stretch as necessary. Counterpressure against the fetal head, using the nondominant hand, may prevent premature extension. Factors associated with protection of the perineum include maternal positioning other than lithotomy or semi-Fowler's, verbal coaching of the woman, counterpressure on the fetal head to maintain flexion, use of warm compresses, and the clinician's unfavorable view of episiotomy (Albers et al., 1997; deJong et al., 1997; Flynn et al., 1997; Klein et al., 1995). Studies suggest that the use of perineal massage during the third trimester may decrease the need for episiotomy and occurrence of lacerations, particularly in women ages 30

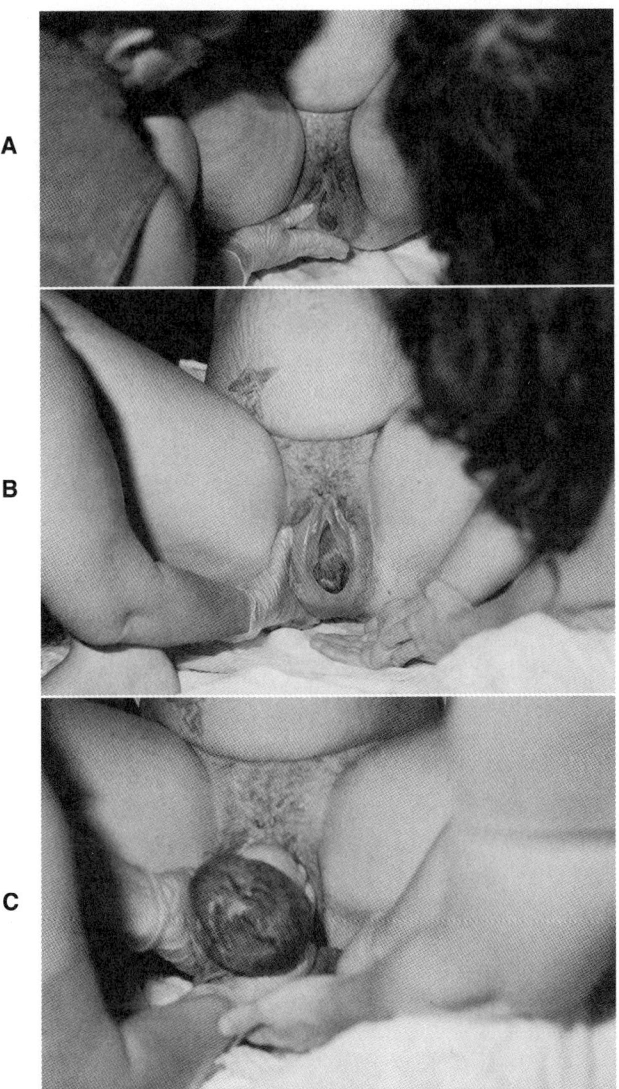

Figure 20-2, **A** to **C** Midwife's hand positions during birth of head. (Courtesy Caroline E. Brown.)

and older (Shipman et al., 1997). As the fetal head crowns, the woman usually experiences a burning sensation, and many women cry out with the final pushes. An effective birth attendant coaches the woman to maintain control of the final expulsive efforts but does not convey any sense that she is behaving poorly or inappropriately. During the last contractions the clinician determines whether an episiotomy is necessary (Research Box 20-3).

Episiotomy, the surgical incision of the perineum to enlarge the outlet, was introduced as an obstetric intervention on the late 1800s and made popular by DeLee's theory that its use would protect the perineum from severe lacerations. Obstetricians have also proposed that the use of episiotomy improves future sexual function and reduces urine and fecal incontinence. Research suggests otherwise. Episiotomy is associated with an increase in third- and fourth-degree lacerations (Henriksen et al., 1992; Klein et al., 1997) and increased postpartum pain when compared to spontaneous lacerations (Klein et al., 1997) (Research Box 20-3). Klein and colleagues, using data collected in a large randomized clinical trial, found that sexual functioning 3 months after delivery was more positive in women with intact perineums or spontaneous lacerations. They also found that pelvic urinary and bowel problems were similar in all groups, suggesting no protective value of episiotomy. Lede, Belizan, and Carroli (1996), in their review of the literature, conclude that there "is no reliable evidence that routine use of episiotomy has any beneficial effect; on the contrary, there is clear evidence that it may cause harm such as greater need for surgical repair and a poorer future sexual capability" (p. 1399). The Cochrane Pregnancy and Childbirth Group concluded that restrictive episiotomy policy rather than routine use of episiotomy is associated with less posterior perineal trauma and fewer complications, but carries an increased risk of anterior perineal trauma (Carroli and Belizan, 2000).

Although there is no maternal indication for episiotomy, there is fetal indication for the procedure. Because episiotomy does shorten the second stage of labor, it may be indicated in cases of fetal compromise. Use of episiotomy may shorten the second stage by several contractions, which may be a significant time period for an infant who will need resuscitation. If an episiotomy is necessary, a local anesthetic should be infiltrated at the site of the incision (Figure 20-3).

Using a sterile towel to protect against contamination from the anus, the clinician may use the dominant hand to protect the perineum (Figure 20-4). Slight counterpressure over the perineum gives the clinician a sense of the intensity of the expulsive efforts and the speed of descent and birth. The dominant hand can also be used to help slip the distended perineum over the baby's face or occiput.

Once the head is delivered, the clinician slips her or his fingers along side the fetal neck to determine whether there is a nuchal cord. Loose nuchal cords can easily be either slipped over the baby's head or enlarged so that the body can be delivered through the loop. Tight nuchal cords may necessitate clamping and cutting before delivery of the shoulders. The baby's face can be wiped with gauze to remove excess mucus. Suctioning of a healthy term infant is not necessary unless there is meconium-stained fluid. Suctioning of the oropharynx and nasopharynx in the presence of meconium-stained fluid be-

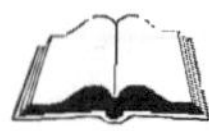

Research Box 20-3

Albers L et al.: Distribution of genital tract trauma in childbirth and related postnatal pain, *Birth* 26(1):11-15, 1999.

Background

Most vaginal births are associated with genital trauma from spontaneous lacerations, episiotomy, or both. The full extent of genital trauma is not known since clinicians may not completely assess the genital tract following birth, there is underreporting of some types of trauma, and there are significant practice variations in suturing vs. not suturing lacerations. Genital trauma experienced with vaginal delivery is associated with short- and long-term morbidity, including pain and its related impact on bowel, urinary, and sexual function.

Research Question

What are the range and extent of childbirth trauma and related postnatal pain at 2 days, 10 days, and 3 months in a low-risk population.

Methods

Data were collected during a randomized clinical trial to evaluate the outcomes of two distinct methods of perineal management—"hands on" or "hands poised." Data were recorded immediately after the birth by the attending midwife, at 2 and 10 days after delivery by midwives and mothers, and at 3 months after delivery by mothers. Sites of trauma and description of tissue layers involved were recorded by the attending midwife. The postpartum data included answers to the questions, "Have you had any pain in or around the perineum in the previous 24 hours?" at 2 days and 10 days postpartum, and "Have you had any pain in or around the perineum during the past week?" at 3 months after delivery.

Sample

The sample of 5404 women at term (37 to 42 weeks' gestation) experiencing spontaneous vaginal deliveries was recruited from two hospitals in southern England. Eighty-eight percent of the women were between 20 and 35 years of age, 94% were married, and 37% were experiencing a first birth. Ninety-nine percent were attended by midwives or student midwives.

Results

Approximately 15% of women experienced no genital trauma related to the birth. Women experiencing first births had a higher rate of trauma (77%) than those experiencing subsequent births (48%). The most common combination of trauma was first- or second-degree perineal plus outer vaginal lacerations (26%). Approximately two thirds of the sites of genital trauma were sutured. Reported pain levels were highest for trauma that included mid/upper vaginal lacerations and third- to fourth-degree perineal lacerations. Women without trauma also reported pain at each point in time but with less frequency than those who experienced trauma.

Clinical Application

The results of this study are influenced by the fact that almost all of the birth attendants were midwives and almost all women delivered their babies while assuming nonlithotomy positions. Therefore the findings may underestimate the frequency of genital trauma when physicians manage deliveries in hospital settings. The study provides baseline data that can be used when evaluating interventions that are anticipated to reduce trauma (e.g., different styles of pushing, different hand techniques during birth). The reports of pain provide valuable information for clinicians as they counsel women about pain and healing in the postpartum period. Of particular importance is the recognition that even women without genital trauma may experience postpartum discomfort secondary to the birth.

fore the delivery of the shoulders has been shown to decrease the incidence of inhalation of the meconium-stained fluid below the vocal cords.

Once restitution and external rotation have occurred, the birth attendant coaches the woman to deliver the baby's shoulders and trunk. Gentle posterior pressure on the baby's head guides the anterior shoulder under the pubis. Once the anterior axillar folds are seen, pressure is shifted anteriorly for delivery of the posterior shoulder. Many women instinctively reach toward their infants, and the birth attendant can help the mother grasp and receive her baby as long as the baby appears to be transitioning to extrauterine life well. Healthy babies may not cry immediately but may quietly rest on the mother's chest while initiating respirations and "pinking up" (Figure 20-5).

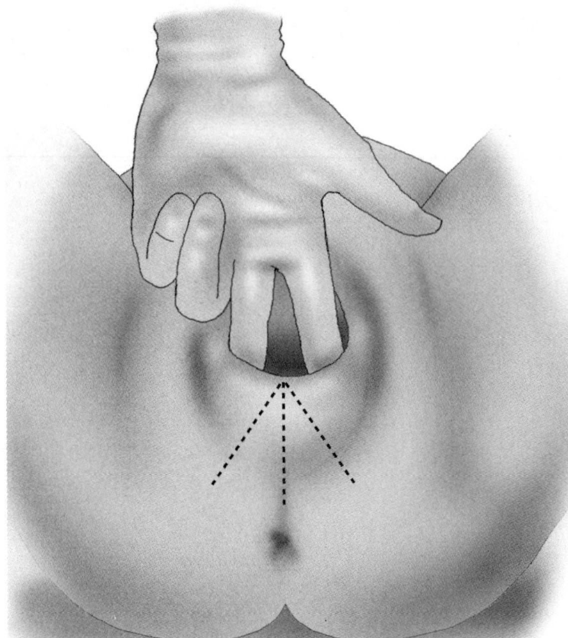

Figure 20-3 Episiotomy.

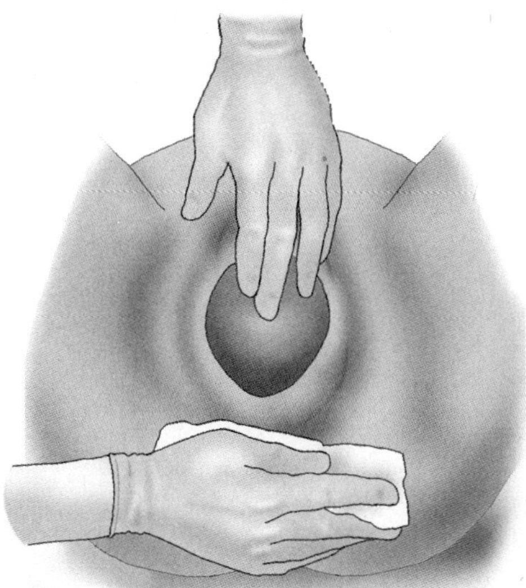

Figure 20-4 Maintaining flexion of the fetal head.

When the mother and infant are healthy without any problems requiring intervention, it is appropriate to allow the parents time to marvel at the miracle of the birth. Birth is usually a joyful event, and the parents and family members welcome the new infant in ways that are culturally appropriate for them. Similar to other times in the childbearing process, the midwife or physician should be aware of cultural expectations in order to support the parents' beliefs and wishes. For example, Muslim parents may want the first words the baby hears to be the prayers offered by the father. The birth attendant's role, then, is to maintain quiet until the prayers are complete.

Participation in the birth of a baby is an honor. A caring, respectful midwife or physician will guide the parents through this very intimate time in a way that facilitates their sense of control, safety, and readiness for their parenting role (Figure 20-6).

A

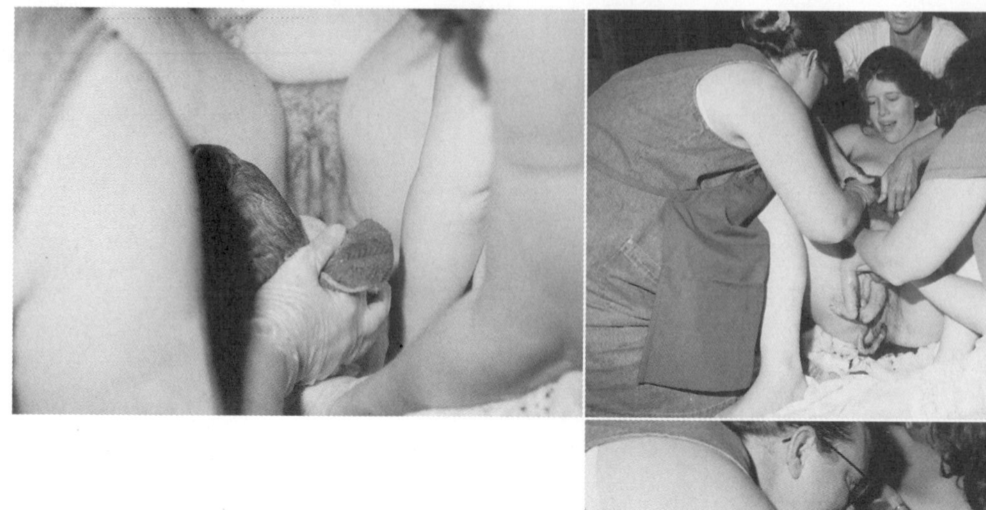

B

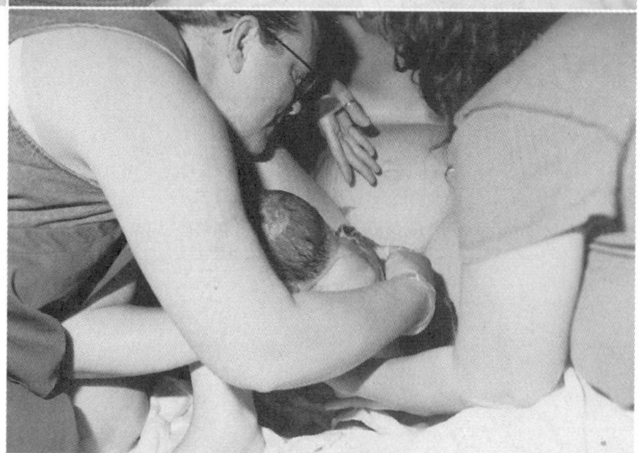

C

Figure 20-5, **A** to **C** Mother reaches down to receive her infant as she delivers the shoulders and trunk of the baby's body. (Courtesy Caroline E. Brown.)

A

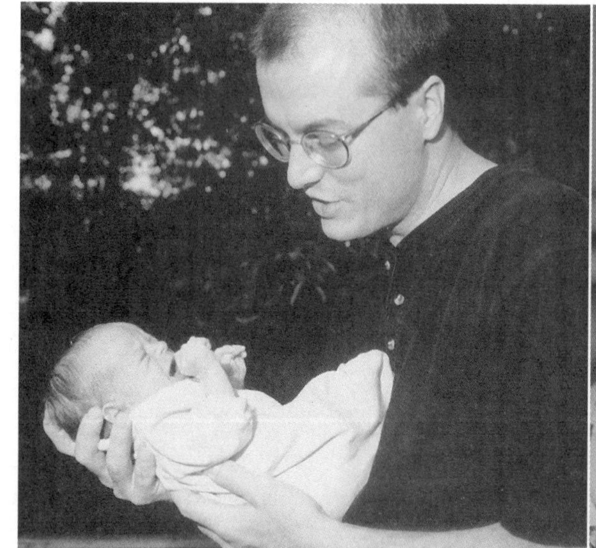

B

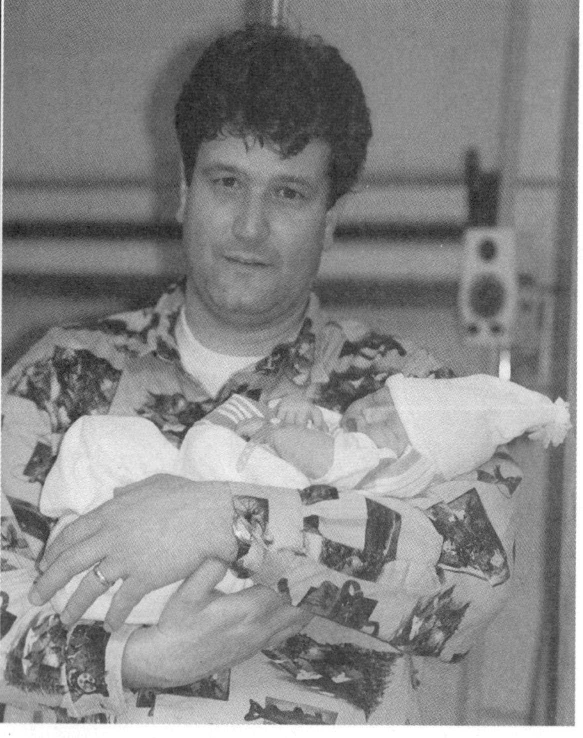

Figure 20-6, **A** and **B**, Father holding his new baby. (Courtesy Caroline E. Brown.)

References

ACOG: Fetal heart rate patterns: monitoring, interpretation, and management, *ACOG Tech Bull No. 207,* July 1995.

Albers LL et al: The relationship of ambulation in labor to operative delivery, *J Nurse Midwifery* 42(1):4-8, 1997.

Bergstrom L et al: "I gotta push. Please let me push!" Social interactions during the change from first to second stage labor, *Birth* 24(3):173-180, 1997.

Carlson JM et al: Maternal positions during parturition in normal labor, *Obstet Gynecol* 68:443-447, 1986.

Carroli G, Belizan J: *Episiotomy for vaginal birth (Cochrane Review).* In Neilson JP et al, editors: *Pregnancy and childbirth module of the Cochrane database of systematic reviews (updated December 2, 1997).* Available in The Cochrane Library (database on disk and CD-ROM). The Cochrane Collaboration, Issue 1, Oxford, 1998, Update Software. Updated quarterly.

Cohen WR: Influence of the duration of second stage labor on perinatal outcome and puerperal morbidity, *Obstet Gynecol* 49(3):266-269, 1977.

deJong PR et al: Randomised trial comparing the upright and supine position for the second stage of labor, *Br J Obstet Gynaecol* 104(5):291-292, 1997.

Flynn P et al: How can second stage management prevent perineal trauma? Critical review, *Can Fam Physician* 43(1):73-84, 1997.

Friedman EA, Sachtleben MR: Station of the fetal presenting part. V. Protracted descent patterns, *Obstet Gynecol* 36(4):558-567, 1970.

Gabbe SG, Niebyl JR, Simpson JL: *Obstetrics: normal and problem pregnancies,* ed 3, New York, 1996, Churchill Livingstone.

Gupta JK, Brayshaw EM, Lilford RJ: An experiment of squatting birth, *Eur J Obstet Gynecol Reprod Biol* 30(3):217-220, 1989.

Hanson L: Second stage positioning in nurse-midwifery practices. Part 1. Position use and preference, *J Nurse-Midwifery* 43(5):320-325, 1998.

Henriksen TB et al: Episiotomy and perineal lesions in spontaneous vaginal delivery, *Br J Obstet Gynaecol* 99(12):950-954, 1992.

Holland RL, Smith DA: Management of the second stage of labor: a review. Part II. Maternal positioning as it relates to the management of the second stage of labor is reviewed, *S D J Med* 42(6):5-8, 1989.

Klein MC et al: Determinants of vaginal-perineal integrity and pelvic floor functioning in childbirth, *Am J Obstet Gynecol* 176(2):403-410, 1997.

Klein MC et al: Physicians' beliefs and behaviour during a randomized controlled trial of episiotomy: consequences for women in their care, *Can Med Assoc J* 153(6):769-779, 1995.

Lede RL, Belizan JM, Carroli G: Is routine use of episiotomy justified? [see comments], *Am J Obstet Gynecol* 174(5):1399-1402, 1996.

Logan OL: *Motherwit, an Alabama midwife's story,* New York, 1991, EP Dutton.

McKay S, Barrows T, Roberts J: Women's views of second-stage labor as assessed by interviews and videotapes, *Birth* 17(4):192-198, 1990.

Nichols FH, Zwelling E: *Maternal-newborn nursing—theory and practice,* Philadelphia, 1997, WB Saunders.

Parnell C et al: Pushing method in the expulsive phase of labor: a randomized trial, *Acta Obstet Gynecol Scand* 72(1):31-35, 1993.

Petersen L, Besuner P: Pushing techniques during labor: issues and controversies, *JOGNN* 26(6):719-726, 1997.

Rossi MA, Lindell SG: Maternal positions and pushing techniques in a nonprescriptive environment, *JOGNN* 15:203-208, 1986.

Shermer RA, Raines DA: Positioning during second stage of labor: moving back to basics, *JOGNN* (6):727-734, 1997.

Shipman MK et al: Antenatal perineal massage and subsequent perineal outcomes: a randomised controlled trial, *Br J Obstet Gynaecol* 104(7):787-791, 1997.

Sweet BR: *Maye's midwifery,* Philadelphia, 1997, WB Saunders.

Thompson AM: Pushing techniques in the second stage of labour, *J Adv Nurs* 18:171-177, 1993.

Thompson AM: Maternal behaviour during spontaneous and directed pushing in the second stage of labor, *J Adv Nurs* 22:1027-1034, 1995.

Van Blarcom CC: *Obstetrical nursing—a textbook on the nursing care of the expectant mother, the woman in labor, the young mother and her baby,* ed 3, New York, 1937, Macmillan.

Chapter 21

Third-Stage Labor

Management of the third stage of labor from delivery of the infant until the delivery of the placenta requires understanding of the normal process of separation of the placenta from the uterine wall and the normal mechanisms to control bleeding. Mismanagement of third stage is the most common reason for atony and resulting postpartum hemorrhage. Patience and watchful waiting, coupled with appropriate anticipation of necessary interventions, are essential in assisting the woman through this stage of the birthing process.

MECHANISM OF SEPARATION OF THE PLACENTA

Birth of the baby, along with the loss of a significant amount of amniotic fluid, leads to contraction and retraction of uterine muscle around the remaining structures. This contracting leads to a decrease in the size of the placental site, forcing a buckling of the placenta once the site of implantation is diminished by half (Sweet, 1997). As part of the placenta separates, retroplacental bleeding occurs, leading to formation of retroplacental clot(s). It is thought that the contracting uterus forces some fetal blood back to the baby while maternal blood in the intervillous spaces is forced into the veins in the decidua basalis. Increased intravenous pressure ruptures the vessels, causing this retroplacental bleed. The amount of bleeding is controlled by the action of the uterine muscular fibers ("figure-of-eight ligatures") that contract around the vessels. Clotting at the sites of the torn vessels further protects against excess blood loss. The next coordinated uterine contraction forces further buckling, ultimately separating the entire placental structure (Figure 21-1). Early radiologic studies identified that placental separation usually occurs within 3 minutes of the birth of the baby. A more recent study (Combs and Laros, 1991) found that the mean length of the third stage was 6.8 minutes, with an intraquartile range of 4 to 10 minutes. Prolonged third stage, defined as longer than 30 minutes, was found in 3.3% of the deliveries and was associated with postpartum hemorrhage, blood transfusion, and dilation and curettage.

When placental separation occurs, the placenta is forced into the lower uterine segment and vagina. In about 80% of cases, the placenta separates centrally, and the fetal surface appears at the introitus (Schultz mechanism). If separation begins at the lower margin of the placenta, the maternal surface of the placenta presents at the introitus (Duncan mechanism). Signs of separation include (1) change in the shape of the uterus from a disk-shaped mass to a firm, ballottable globe, (2) a trickle or gush of blood, (3) a rise of the uterine fundus as the placenta moves into the lower uterine segment and vagina, and (4) lengthening of the cord at the introitus.

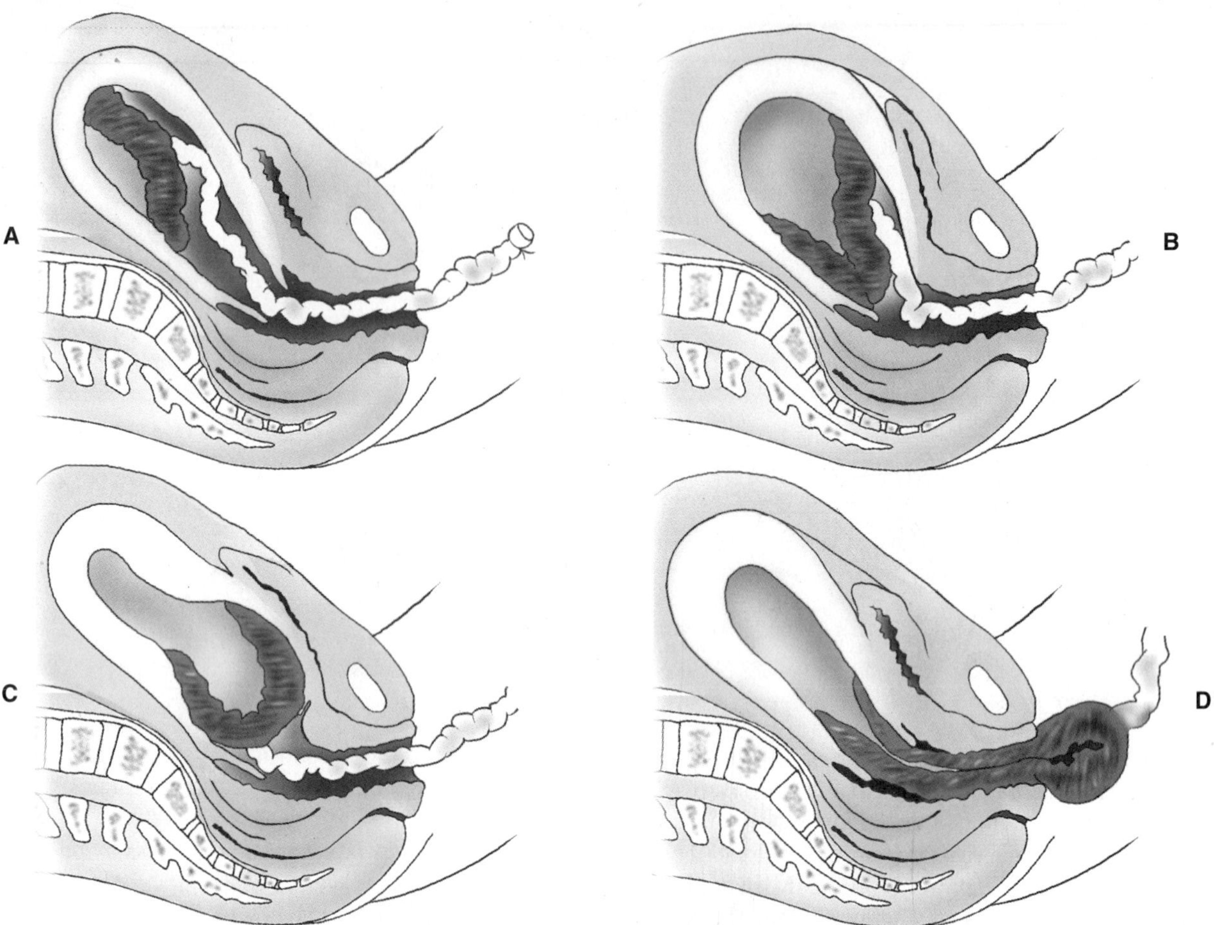

Figure 21-1 Delivery of the placenta. **A,** "Buckling of the placenta and formation of the retroplacental clot. **B,** Separation of the placenta. **C,** Descent of the placenta into the lower uterine segment. **D,** Delivery of the placenta (Schlutz mechanism).

DELIVERY OF THE PLACENTA

Management of the third stage of labor can be by the physiologic or expectant approach or by an "active" approach. The approach adopted by the clinician is determined by the woman's informed preference, the clinician's beliefs about management of labor, the clinician's skill and comfort with each method, and the absence or presence of factors associated with increased risk for postpartum hemorrhage.

Expectant (Physiologic) Management of Third Stage

There is relatively little research exploring the effect of the timing of clamping and cutting the cord. Delaying the cutting of the cord increases placental-fetal transfusion by 20% to 50%, depending on the positioning of the infant in relation to the level of the placenta (Linderkamp et al., 1992). The increased blood volume may increase risk for physiologic jaundice in the newborn, although studies have not shown a significant difference in rates of jaundice when comparing late vs. early clamping (Oxford Midwives Research Group, 1991). Clinicians who value the noninterventionist approach usually delay cutting the cord at least until cord pulsating has stopped. Because of the increased pressure in the vessels, delayed cord clamping is associated with increased risk of fetomaternal transfusion; thus it should not be used when the woman is Rh negative. Draining the cord does not appear to offer any benefit to decreasing fetomaternal transfusion (Thomas et al., 1990)

Following the birth of the baby, the clinician rests the less dominant hand gently on the fundus to palpate uter-

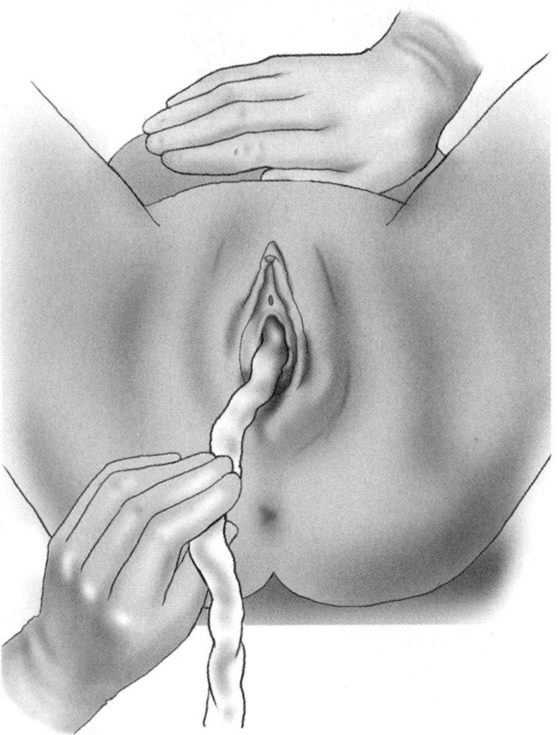

Figure 21-2 Hand placement during third stage.

ine contractions and note any increase in uterine size that would indicate bleeding and clot formation. IT IS ESSENTIAL THAT THE CLINICIAN NOT MASSAGE THE UTERUS OR TRY TO MANUALLY EXPRESS THE PLACENTA BEFORE THE NORMAL PROCESS OF SEPARATION. Monitoring the size and consistency of the uterus can also detect the presence of an undiagnosed twin. Premature traction on the cord can lead to partial separation of the placenta with resultant bleeding, cord detachment, and in extreme cases inversion of the uterus.

When signs of separation are noted, the clinician places the less dominant hand superior to the pubis and applies downward pressure to "guard" the uterus (Figure 21-2). The dominant hand applies firm traction to the cord, following the anatomic curve of the vagina and pelvis (curve of Carus). The woman can be coached to assist expulsion of the placenta by gently bearing down with the contraction. Some women actually feel an "urge to push" as the placenta descends into the vagina, and the clinician then coaches active pushing without any clinician intervention. As the placenta reaches the introitus, both hands can gently ease the placenta out of the vagina, taking care to deliver the membranes smoothly. Membranes can be assisted out by several techniques, the most common being the following:

1. Twisting the placenta and membranes as the placenta is lifted away from the introitus
2. Gently "teasing" the membranes using an up-and-down motion or twisting with a sponge forceps

Both of these techniques are helpful when the membranes start to tear before complete delivery or when part of the membranes still adhere to the uterine wall

Active Management of Third Stage of Labor

Active management of the third stage of labor has been proposed as a means of decreasing postpartum hemorrhage in women with factors that increase their risk of increased blood loss and has been supported by the World Health Organization (1994) as a means of decreasing postpartum hemorrhage when access to blood products and other resources are limited. Active management involves the use of oxytocin or ergotamine either with the birth of the anterior shoulder of the infant or immediately after the birth of the baby, early clamping of the cord, and controlled traction of the umbilical cord to facilitate delivery of the placenta.

Clinicians using active management in the United States usually give oxytocin, 10 U intramuscularly, and then gently rest the nondominant hand on the uterine fundus as noted in preceding paragraphs to determine the beginning of a uterine contraction. Once a contraction is palpated and there are signs of placental separation, the nondominant hand moves from the fundus to the symphysis pubis, where it exerts counterpressure upward on the uterus. The palm of the hand is toward the umbilicus. Controlled traction is applied to the cord until the placenta is at the vaginal introitus. If there is no descent of the placenta with a contraction, the clinician then waits for the next contraction, returning the resting hand to the fundus for light palpation.

Although some studies have suggested that active management of the third stage of labor decreases the incidence of postpartum hemorrhage and total blood loss (Khan et al., 1997; Prendiville, Elbourne, and Chalmers, 1988; Rogers et al., 1998), others have suggested either no difference in postpartum hemoglobins (Thilaganathan et al., 1993) or increase in other complications such as pain, hypertension, and secondary postpartum hemorrhage (Begley, 1990). When factors are present that increase risk of postpartum hemorrhage or when sufficient resources are not available to adequately manage a severe postpartum hemorrhage (such as in remote sites or

Table 21-1 *Examination of the Placenta, Membranes and Cord*

Structure	Findings
Placenta	
Size	Normal: usually about 1/6 the weight of the infant (400-500 g); diameter averages 18-20 cm; thickness averages 2-2.5 cm
	Small for infant size is associated with prematurity; intrauterine growth retardation; trisomy 17-18; rubella and other viral diseases
	Large for infant size is associated with Rh isoimmunization, congenital syphilis; toxoplasmosis; cytomegalic inclusion disease; polyhydramnios; congenital tuberculosis
Color	Deep "liver" red
Maternal surface	Normal has no/few infarcts and calcifications
	Missing cotyledons indicate incomplete expulsion
	Calcifications may indicate postdates; smoking.
Fetal surface	Normal is shiny, smooth, with normal pattern of vessels
	Dullness suggests amnionitis
	Ruptured vessels near insertion suggest fetal hemorrhage
Cord	
Length	Average length is 55 cm
Unusual findings	False knot; dilation of umbilical vessels causing unusual folds or loops
	True knot; more common with long cords
	Excessive twisting or lack of twisting; normal vessels twist in a counterclockwise direction with a ratio of 7:1
Insertion	Most commonly inserted centrally
	Velamentous insertion is insertion into the membranes with vessels dividing before the placental disk
	Interposition insertion is when the cord runs in the membranes parallel to the surface of the placenta before insertion into the placental disk
Membranes	
Size and site of rupture	Site of rupture distant from the placental edge indicates probable fundal placement of the placenta; rupture near the placental edge indicates probable low lying attachment
	Reconstruction of membranes should identify any obvious areas of tears or missing pieces
Color	Normal term membranes are translucent without pigment
	Green-staining of the amnion with no staining of the chorion indicates meconium passage 1-3 hours before the birth
	Green staining of the amnion in addition to the chorion indicates passage of meconium greater than 3 hours before the birth
	Brownish-yellow staining is consistent with pigments due to old blood, indicating possible abruption, circumvallation or decidual bleeding
	Opacity is consistent with chorioamnionitis
Unusual patterns	Amnion nodosa are nodules on the fetal side of the placenta and are caused by particulate matter (fetal epithelial cells, fibrin and lanugo) attaching to denuded areas; these are associated with oligohydramnios
	Amniotic bands indicate probable rupture of the amnion before 12 weeks' gestation.

underdeveloped countries), the benefits of active management appear to outweigh the risks.

Cord blood is often obtained while waiting for delivery of the placenta. This can be accomplished by placing the end of the cord in a sterile tube and releasing the cord clamp. A syringe and needle can also be used to obtain blood from one of the vessels with replacement of the cord clamp above the site of needle insertion. Although laboratory tests performed on cord blood may vary, depending on setting, it is usual for blood to be sent for type, Rh, and Coombs' (antibody screen) when the mother is Rh negative or when there is a history of ABO incompatibility in a previous pregnancy. If the placenta is delivered before collection of the blood specimen, cord blood can be aspirated from placental vessels.

Immediately after delivery of the placenta, the clinician palpates the uterus to ensure that adequate muscular contractions are present to control bleeding. If the uterus is "boggy," uterine massage usually stimulates adequate contractions. If the woman is planning to breast-feed, the initiation of breast-feeding stimulates release of oxytocin, facilitating the normal contracting mechanism of the uterus. If the infant does not show interest in nursing or if the woman is too uncomfortable to initiate breastfeeding, nipple stimulation can substitute for suckling. When the woman is not planning to breast-feed or when there is increased risk for uterine atony, the clinician may administer an oxytocic agent in an intravenous solution or intramuscularly.

Synthetic oxytocin (Pitocin) may be administered intravenously or intramuscularly. If an intravenous infusion is in place, 20 U of oxytocin can be added to 1 L of solution and administered at a rate of 10 ml/min until the uterus remains firmly contracted. If less than a full liter of intravenous fluid is already being administered, the dose of oxytocin should be altered accordingly. Sources vary in the recommended ratios, but there appears to be general agreement that if less than 500 ml is in the intravenous delivery system, only 10 U of oxytocin should be added. The rate of infusion can then be decreased to 1 to 2 ml/min until it is determined that the risk of excessive bleeding is minimal, at which time the intravenous infusion can be discontinued. Oxytocin should not be given as a bolus intravenously because of the risk of hypotension.

Ergonovine (Ergotrate) and methylergonovine (Methergine) are alkaloids available in solution for intramuscular use or in tablets for oral use. These drugs stimulate a tetanic contraction that occurs almost immediately with intravenous administration and within minutes after intramuscular or oral administration. Ergonovine and methylergonovine may stimulate a temporary but severe hypertension in women at risk for hypertension or in some women receiving conduction anesthesia. For this reason, these drugs should not be given when the woman exhibits hypertension.

Once it is clear that bleeding is controlled and mother and infant are stable, the placenta, cord, and membranes are inspected to determine completeness and identify any deviations from normal. Most clinicians find it most effective to spread the placenta out on a flat surface to completely examine both surfaces. Expected findings and common deviations are noted in Table 21-1.

Examination of the Perineum and Vagina

Once it is determined that the uterus is well contracted and bleeding controlled, the clinician should assess the woman's general status. Management of the fourth stage of labor, including repair of lacerations in the genital tract, is addressed in Chapter 22 and Appendix A.

References

Begley CM A comparison of 'active' and 'physiological' management of the third stage of labour, *Midwifery* 6(1):3-17, 1990.

Combs CA, Laros RK: Prolonged third stage of labor: morbidity and risk factors, *Obstet Gynecol* 77(6):863-867, 1991.

Khan GQ et al: Controlled cord traction versus minimal intervention techniques in delivery of the placenta: a randomized controlled trial, *Am J Obstet Gynecol* 177(4):770-774, 1997.

Linderkamp O et al: The effect of early and late cord-clamping on blood viscosity and other hemorrheological parameters in full-term neonates, *Acta Paediatr* 81(10):745-750, 1992.

Oxford Midwives Research Group: A study of the relationship between the delivery to cord clamping interval and the time of cord separation, *Midwifery* 7(4):167-176, 1991.

Prendiville W, Elbourne D, Chalmers I: The effects of routine oxytocic administration in the management of the third stage of labour: an overview of the evidence from controlled trials, *Br J Obstet Gynecol* 95(1):3-16, 1988.

Rogers J et al: Active versus expectant management of third stage of labour: the Hinchingbrooke randomised controlled trial, *Lancet* 351(9104):693-699, 1998.

Sweet BR: *Maye's midwifery: a textbook for midwives,* ed 12, Philadelphia, 1997, WB Saunders.

Thilaganathan B et al: Management of the third stage of labour in women at low risk of postpartum haemorrhage, *Eu J Obstet Gynecol Reprod Biol* 48(1):19-22, 1993.

Thomas IL et al: Does cord drainage of placental blood facilitate delivery of the placenta? *Aust NZ J Obstet Gynaecol* 30(4):314-318. 1990.

Chapter 22

Immediate Postpartum Period

Following birth, the woman experiences dramatic anatomic and physiologic changes as her body transitions to the normal nonpregnant state. Psychosocially she continues her process of maternal role attainment and infant attachment. Maternal behaviors are strongly influenced by personal beliefs and cultural expectations. Health care professionals best support the woman through this stage of childbearing by reinforcing the woman's ability to care for her child, validating cultural influences that are important to the woman and her family, providing appropriate guidance and counseling, and assessing the woman's physical and psychosocial state. When women have given birth in the hospital, much of this care occurs at the site of birth. When early discharge is experienced or when the birth has occurred in a birth center or at home, care is accomplished through home or ambulatory site visits. This chapter explores the adaptations that occur during the first 72 hours after delivery and the related care practices that enhance physical and psychosocial health status.

PHYSICAL CHANGES IN THE IMMEDIATE POSTPARTUM PERIOD

Reproductive System

The uterine, cervical, and vaginal transition from the pregnant to nonpregnant state is referred to as involution. The weight of the uterus at term is estimated to be 1000 g. By 1 week after delivery, the weight has decreased to 500 g, and by 2 weeks the weight is 350 g. By 6 weeks after delivery, the uterus has involuted to nonpregnant size by palpation, and the weight is approximately 50 to 60 g, the usual nonpregnant weight. The process of uterine involution includes three activities: (1) contraction of the uterus, (2) autolysis of myometrium cells, and (3) regeneration of epithelium (Blackburn and Loper, 1992).

Immediately after the birth, contractions decrease the size of the uterus to approximately 16 weeks' gestation, with the fundus approximately midway between the symphysis and the umbilicus. During the next 12 hours the fundus stabilizes at the level of the umbilicus, then decreases about 1 cm or 1 fingerbreadth per day, although there is considerable variability with the pattern of involution (Cluett, Alexander, and Pickering, 1997). The uterus usually becomes a pelvic organ at approximately 10 days after delivery. Uterine involution is slower with increasing multiparity and with conditions in which there has been overdistention of the uterus. Willms and colleagues (1995), using magnetic resonance imaging (MRI), found the mean length of the uterine corpus to be 13.8 cm (range 11.8 to 15 cm) less than 30 hours after delivery and the mean transverse dimension to be 12.8 cm (range 9.5 to 14 cm). The decrease in size of the uterus is accomplished through autolysis of excess intracellular proteins and cytoplasm within the myometrium. This results in a decrease in size without significant decrease in total number of cells. The waste products produced by this process are transferred into the maternal vascular system and eliminated through the kidneys.

Contractions decrease the size of the endometrial surface, and the placental site decreases from the placental diameter of 18 cm to approximately 9 cm. As the uterus continues to contract and decrease in size, the placental site becomes a raised rough area that is 4 to 5 cm in diameter. During the first few days after the birth, the endometrium and myometrium at the placental site are infiltrated with granulocytes and mononuclear cells. The basal layer of the endometrium remains intact, and by the seventh day after delivery there is evidence of regeneration of endometrial stroma and endometrial glands (Bowes, 1996). The placental site heals by exfoliation. The fundi of the endometrial glands grow upward, with simultaneous growth of endometrial tissue from the margins of the placental site, allowing healing to occur without scarring. Complete transition to normal endometrium at the placental site does not occur for at least 6 weeks. Development of normal endometrium in areas other than the placental site occurs within 2 to 3 weeks of the birth.

During the first day following delivery, necrosis of the decidua begins. It has been theorized that remaining healthy decidua contributes to the regeneration of the endometrium. Necrotic decidual cells are sloughed off in the lochia, and by 6 weeks after delivery no decidual cells remain. By invading the remaining decidua, polymorphonuclear leukocytes and lymphocytes create an antibacterial barrier during the first week after delivery (Bowes, 1996).

Hemostasis at the placental site is accomplished primarily by constriction of the vessels by the contracting uterus. Thrombosis of veins and hyalinization of the arteries provide further protection against blood loss. Thrombosed veins may be sloughed off along with the decidua, but arterial matter may remain at the site for weeks. Uterine discharge following the birth is termed lochia. Lochia during the first 2 to 4 days after delivery is lochia rubra, a red to reddish-brown discharge similar to a heavy menses and consisting of blood, decidua, and pieces of amnion and chorion. Similar to menses, lochia decreases in amount and changes in color over several days. By postpartum day 3, most women experience lochia serosa, a darker brownish-red color. Lochia serosa consists of old blood, serum, leukocytes, and tissue debris. The median duration of lochia serosa is 22 days (Bowes, 1996). Approximately 15% of women will still have lochia serosa at the time of the 6-week postpartum examination. The final transitional discharge is lochia alba, a whitish-yellow discharge that is composed of white blood cells (WBCs), decidua, epithelial cells, mucus, serum, and bacteria. The total amount of lochia produced ranges from 150 to 400 ml, with an average of 225 ml being reported (Blackburn and Loper, 1992).

During the first 2 to 3 days after delivery, a gush of blood from the vagina may be noted when the woman stands up or changes position. This is caused by pooling in the vagina and is usually not a cause of concern. Clots may also be expressed, with small clots being a normal finding. Once the lochia has changed to serosa, increased activity may be associated with a return of bright red bleeding. This is usually self-limiting, and women should be reassured that rest and breast-feeding should decrease the bleeding within 1 to 2 hours.

Immediately after the birth, laceration, ulceration, and ecchymosis of the cervix may be noted. Over the first 12 to 18 hours the cervix shortens and remains dilated 3 to 4 cm. Willms and colleagues (1995) found that the mean length of the cervix was 5.6 cm (range 3.8 to 7 cm) less than 30 hours after delivery. The greatest percentage change in cervical length occurs between 30 hours and 1 week after delivery. By 1 week after delivery the internal os is closed, and by 4 weeks after delivery the external os has closed with the shape of a slit. The cervical epithelium that had increased in thickness during pregnancy begins regressing within the first 4 days after delivery. The vascular hyperplasia and hypertrophy present in pregnancy recede after the first postpartum week.

Following vaginal delivery the vagina musculature is relaxed and edematous with minimal tone for several weeks. Rugae appear 3 to 4 weeks after delivery, and vaginal epithelium is restored by 6 to 10 weeks after delivery. Initial healing of episiotomy or laceration sites begins immediately after the birth and continues for 2 to 3 weeks. However, complete healing of an episiotomy may take 4 to 6 months in some women (Blackburn and Loper, 1992).

Immediately following the birth there is a decrease in estrogen, progesterone, human placental lactogen (hPL), and human chorionic gonadotropin (hCG), with resulting reversal of most pregnancy-related system changes. Hormones are first cleared from the maternal vascular system. Secondary clearance occurs as the hormones are mobilized from extravascular spaces. The speed of mobilization from extravascular sources determines the length of time that a substance will remain in the maternal plasma. hPL remains in the maternal plasma for only 1 to 2 days after delivery, whereas hCG can remain in the maternal system for up to 2 weeks. Plasma estradiol decreases to levels that are less than 2% of pregnancy levels by 24 hours after delivery. Estradiol levels similar to those found in the follicular phase of the menstrual cycle are reached by 1 to 2 days after delivery. Progesterone levels similar to those found in the luteal phase of the menstrual cycle are reached by 24 to 48 hours after delivery. Ovarian production of estrogen and progesterone remain low for the first 2 weeks after delivery. Prolactin secretion increases immediately after the birth and is maintained at increased levels with breast-feeding. In nonlactating women prolactin levels decrease and reach the nonpregnant range by 1 to 2 weeks after delivery. Ovarian changes occur later in the postpartum period and are discussed in Chapter 24.

Breasts

Nonlactating women experience involution of the breast tissue during the first week after delivery. By postpartum days 2 to 4, primary engorgement may be experienced as a result of the distention and stasis of the vascular and lymphatic systems. As milk distends the lobules and alveoli, secondary engorgement may be experienced. Lack of nipple stimulation leads to decreased prolactin levels, and milk production ceases.

Establishment of lactation. Physical and physiologic preparation for breast-feeding begins early in pregnancy. Shortly after conception the breasts increase in size, and the areolar pigmentation darkens. Sebaceous glands on the areolar surface (Montgomery tubercles) become more prominent, producing protective secretions that lubricate the nipple and areolar. Blood flow to the breasts increases, and the vessels become more visible. These pregnancy-induced changes result in an average increase in weight of 12 ounces for each breast. Increased estrogen levels stimulate the proliferation of the ductile system. Increased progesterone levels stimulate the increase in size of breast lobules. Prolactin, hPL, and hCG stimulate the growth of the glandular tissue in the alveoli. Growth hormone and adrenocorticotropic hormone further stimulate growth of the breasts. Proliferation of new alveoli, ducts, and lobule tissue continues through the second and third trimesters. Secretion of material that is similar to colostrum may begin in the second trimester (Figure 22-1).

Epithelial cells in the alveoli go through transition to secretory cells in the third trimester. These cells continue to proliferate after the birth under the influence of prolactin and the physical stimulation of suckling. Initiation of lactogenesis occurs through a complex neuroendocrine process (Blackburn and Loper, 1992). Prolactin is the primary hormone responsible for lactation. Growth hormone, insulin, cortisol, and thyrotropin-releasing hormone further contribute to the process. A high density of

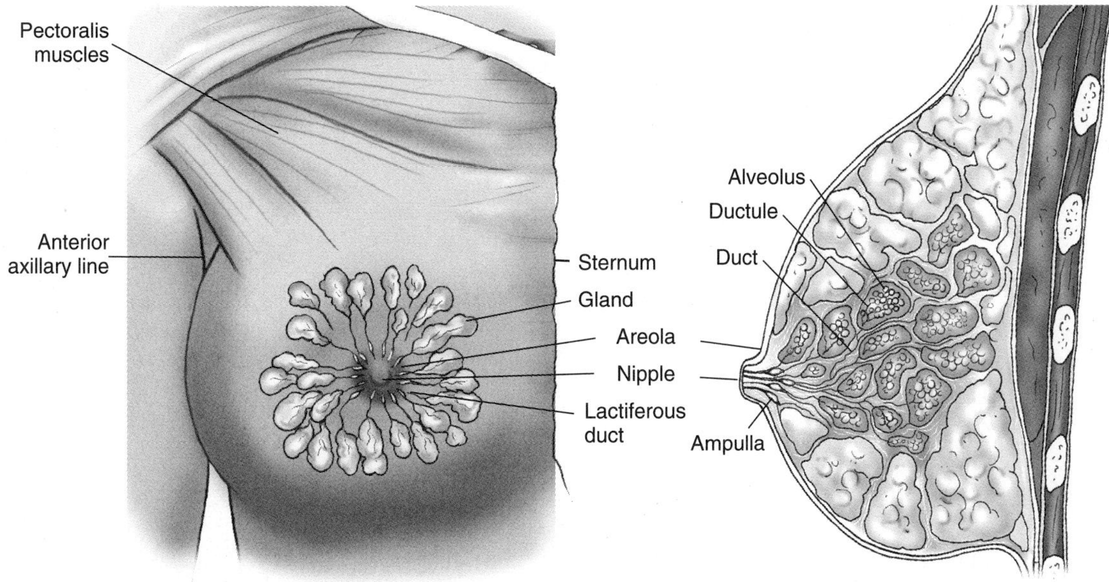

Figure 22-1 Anatomy of the breast.

sensory nerves beneath the nipple and areola provide the initial neural stimulation for lactation. Infant suckling stimulates the release of adenohypophyseal prolactin and neurohypophyseal oxytocin (Lawrence, 1994), at the same time sending neural stimulation through the spinal cord to the hypothalamus to suppress the release of prolactin-inhibiting factor (PIF).

Although prolactin levels increase during pregnancy, increased circulating levels of estrogen and progesterone inhibit lactation. Following the birth, estrogen and progesterone levels decrease dramatically, allowing prolactin to stimulate milk synthesis. In addition, decreased catecholamine levels suppresses the secretion of PIF from the hypothalamus. Prolactin levels increase dramatically with the birth, then stabilize at the baseline necessary for lactation by about 3 hours after delivery. Once the milk supply has been established, the base prolactin levels remain two to three times higher than pregnancy levels, and the level increases 10 to 20 times with suckling.

The prolactin level rises immediately with the initiation of suckling, and the amount of prolactin released and the volume of milk produced are directly associated with the amount of suckling (Chan, 1997). Prolactin secretion is influenced by circadian rhythm, with the highest levels occurring between 1 AM and 5 AM (Chan, 1997). Prolactin production is stimulated by sleep and sexual intercourse and is inhibited by severe maternal malnutrition and stress. Drugs and agents that stimulate prolactin production include neuroleptic drugs, thyrotrophin-releasing hormone, estrogens, phenothiazines, norepinephrine, histamine, and acetylcholine (Chan, 1997). Drugs and agents that inhibit prolactin production include L-dopa, ergots, clomiphene, monoamine oxidase inhibitors, and prostaglandins E and F (Chan, 1997). After 3 months postpartum, prolactin levels return to nonpregnant levels, and suckling produces minimal increase.

The milk ejection reflex ("let-down reflex") results in milk being ejected into the duct system and the sinuses. Sucking provides neural stimulation beneath the nipple that is then transmitted via the afferent neurons in the spinal cord to the hypothalamus, resulting in release of oxytocin from the posterior pituitary gland. Oxytocin stimulates the myoepithelial cells in the alveoli, resulting in contraction of the cells that squeezes the milk through the ductile system. The oxytocin release also stimulates uterine contractions, resulting in decreased postpartum blood loss. Mothers experiencing a first birth usually do not notice the contractions, but mothers experiencing second or subsequent births may experience mild-to-severe cramping with nursing. The reflex initially is unconditioned and requires the physical stimulation (Henschel and Inch, 1996). With continued nursing the reflex becomes conditioned, and it can be triggered by hearing a baby cry or thinking about the baby. Sexual arousal and orgasm also stimulate the hypothalamus, causing release of oxytocin and the resulting milk ejection reflex. Fear, anxiety, pain, and fatigue can inhibit the reflex.

Analgesia and anesthesia use during labor has been shown to have an effect on early breast-feeding efforts. Studies have found distinct relationships between analgesia and anesthesia and problems with nursing (Thorp and Breedlove, 1996). In addition, analgesia and anesthesia use increases the risk of other events that may negatively affect nursing efforts. These events include elevated maternal and infant temperatures, abnormal fetal heart patterns, maternal hypotension, increased use of oxytocin augmentation, prolonged second stage, increased use of instrumental delivery, and increased cesarean section rates (Walker, 1997). When mothers receive narcotic analgesia greater than 1 hour before the birth, infants experience depressed rooting and sucking instincts, resulting in increased time until effective suckling is established (Crowell, Hill, and Humenick, 1994; Nissen et al., 1995; Righard and Alade, 1990). Epidural anesthesia using bupivacaine alone has been associated with depression in motor abilities of neonates when those infants are compared to unmedicated controls (Murray et al., 1981; Sepkoski et al., 1992). Studies exploring epidural analgesia/anesthesia using bupivacaine and sufentanil or fentanyl lacked the rigor of inclusion of unmedicated control groups, but findings suggest subtle neurologic depression that has the potential for negatively affecting suckling (Copagna, Celleno, and Tomassetti, 1989; Loftus, Hill, and Cohen, 1995). Loftus, Hill, and Cohen (1995) found that the Neurologic and Adaptive Capacity Scores (NACS) of neonates exposed to epidurals containing bupivacaine and 80 to 265 μg of fentanyl were lower at 24 hours when compared to the NACS scores obtained at 2 hours after delivery. These findings were thought to reflect the slow clearance of fentanyl from the neonatal liver (Walker, 1997). These research findings suggest that when a woman has received analgesia or anesthesia during labor, the midwife, physician, or nurse may need to spend additional time with her and her infant to guide the initial nursing experience. It would seem even more important that, assuming the neonates are essentially healthy, these infants not be separated from their mothers and that they receive extensive skin-to-skin contact to foster the physiologic instincts for suckling.

Colostrum is the first substance produced by the secretory cells in the alveoli. This fluid can often be expressed in the latter half of pregnancy, and it is present until transitional milk is produced a few days following the birth. Colostrum is a clear, yellowish fluid that is higher in protein than true milk but lower in carbohydrate, fat, and calories (67 kcal/dl). The yellow coloring is the result of increased levels of carotene. Colostrum also contains immunoglobulins G and A, which offer protection to the newborn in the early weeks of life. Transition milk appears after 2 to 3 days; and it is higher in fat, lactose, and calories than colostrum. Mature milk is usually present by postpartum day 9 to 10, but in some cases it may not develop until as late as 28 days after delivery. Mature milk contains 75 kcal/100 ml, and it is composed of water (87.5%), carbohydrates (4.8%), fats (3.8%), and proteins (3.2%). Maternal nutrition affects the vitamin and fat content of mature milk.

Cardiovascular System

The decrease in blood volume is closely associated with blood loss experienced at delivery. Plasma volume initially decreases by 1000 ml because of blood loss and diuresis. After the third postpartum day, volume increases by 900 to 1200 ml as a result of a shift of extracellular fluid into the intravascular space. This results in a hemodilution that decreases hematocrit, hemoglobin, and plasma proteins. Total blood volume decreases 16% from the predelivery volume during the first 3 days after delivery. The estimated blood loss can be compared to the decrease in hemoglobin after delivery. A 500-ml blood loss will result in a reduction of 1 g of hemoglobin or 3 percentage points of hematocrit. The increased WBC level seen in labor decreases immediately after the birth to 6,000 to 10,000/mm^3, then stabilizes to normal range by 4 to 7 days after delivery. Platelets typically decrease with delivery, then return to normal nonpregnant levels at 3 to 4 days after delivery.

Pulse rate, stroke volume, and cardiac output remain elevated during the first 1 to 2 hours after birth. Immediately after the birth, cardiac output increases to a level 60% to 80% higher than prelabor levels, then begins to decline after 10 minutes (Blackburn and Loper, 1992). Cardiac output reaches the prelabor level about 1 hour after the birth and remains elevated above prepregnancy level for about 48 hours, when it begins to decrease. An increase in both diastolic and systolic blood pressure of approximately 5% is common during the first 4 postpartum days.

Blood pressure decreases during the first 2 days after delivery to the woman's late pregnancy norm. Continued low vascular resistance in the pelvis predisposes the woman to orthostatic hypotension with sudden position change from recumbent to sitting or standing.

Fibrolytic activity increases to its peak during the first 3 hours after delivery. Increases in fibrinogen, factor V, and factor VII occur, with return to normal by postpartum days 3 to 5. Other clotting factors decrease for 1 week following the birth when they reach normal prepregnant levels. Changes in the coagulation factors, along with decreased mobility, increase the risk of thromboembolic events in the immediate postpartum period.

Renal System

The shifting of extravascular fluid to the intravascular space within the first few days after delivery results in the maintenance of elevated renal blood flow during that time period. This elevated renal blood flow is associated with diuresis and natriuresis that eliminates the fluid and sodium retained during the third trimester. The sudden decrease in oxytocin contributes to this diuresis since oxytocin promotes resorption of free water (Blackburn and Loper, 1992). It is not uncommon to document urinary output of 3000 ml per 24 hours during postpartum days 2 through 5.

Mild proteinuria may be present for the first few days after delivery. The common glycosuria seen in pregnancy does not continue after delivery.

Resultant loss of sensation of the urge to void may lead to overdistention of the bladder, incomplete emptying, or inability to void. Bladder distention is associated with uterine atony with increase in lochia, displacement of the uterus to the right, and decreased urinary output. Trauma to the bladder during labor and birth may result in edema and submucosal hemorrhages.

It has been estimated that 30% to 60% of women develop urinary stress incontinence during pregnancy, and many of those women continue with the problem during the postpartum period. Relaxation of the urethral sphincter and decreased pelvic muscle strength contribute to the development of urinary stress incontinence. Some women develop urinary stress incontinence in the postpartum period without any previous history of the problem (Meyer et al., 1998).

Gastrointestinal System

Gastrointestinal tone and motility are decreased during the immediate postpartum period. Lax abdominal tone coupled with decreased motility may lead to gaseous distention 2 to 3 days after delivery (Blackburn and Loper, 1992). Decreased bowel activity, particularly following restriction in dietary intake during the previous 24 to 36 hours, may inhibit bowel movements for the first 1 or 2 days following the birth. Fear of pain at the site of lacerations, episiotomy, or hemorrhoids may further contribute to constipation in the first week after delivery. The woman's normal bowel pattern should resume during the first week.

MANAGEMENT OF THE IMMEDIATE POSTPARTUM PERIOD

Postpartum management should reflect sound understanding of the normal processes of stabilization in the healthy woman as her body goes through the transition to the nonpregnant state. Management should also reflect an understanding of the woman's and her family's beliefs and values. The health care professional can be perceived as a guide who recognizes and validates the individual's strengths and competencies as family members adjust to their new roles, while anticipating areas in which education and counseling are warranted.

During the first hour after delivery, pulse and blood pressure should be taken every 15 minutes, then every 4 to 8 hours if stable. Temperature should be taken at least every 4 hours (American Academy of Pediatrics and American College of Obstetricians and Gynecologists, 1997). The fundus, perineum, and lochia should be assessed at the same time as the vital signs. These assessments should be done more frequently when deviations from normal are identified or when increased risks for hemorrhage, infection, hypertension, or other problems have been identified. Activities should be done as nonintrusively as possible in order to not interfere with the woman's interaction with her infant and family. Once the vital signs have stabilized, they can be done every 4 to 8 hours until discharge from the hospital or birth center or for the first 2 days following a home birth.

If regional anesthesia has been used for labor and delivery, gross motor function of the legs should be assessed along with the vital signs. These frequent assessments should be done until the woman can raise her legs, flex her knees, and lift her buttocks off the bed without assistance. When general anesthesia has been used, mental orientation, respirations, and oxygen saturation levels should be assessed along with the vital signs. Any abnormal findings following regional or general anesthesia should be referred to the anesthesiologist.

When postpartum care is being given in a hospital, the fundus, lochia, and perineum should be evaluated at least once every 8 hours by a nursing staff member or the clinician. The fundus should remain firm. If atony is identified, massage should stimulate contractions and return the uterus to firm consistency. All women should be instructed in self-massage of the fundus to decrease the risk of continued atony, increase understanding of her body changes, and increase sense of control. In out-of-hospital sites, it is usual to instruct the woman to check her fundus and her lochia every 4 to 8 hours and to notify the provider if there is atony or increased vaginal bleeding. Further assessment may be done by the provider or other staff during home visits.

When there is increased risk for atony and/or the assessment identifies atony, endogenous and exogenous oxytocins should be considered. Increased infant suckling increases production of endogenous oxytocin and should be encouraged with all women who choose to breast-feed. Oxytocin USP (10 U) administered intravenously or intramuscularly stimulates phasic contractions of the uterus within 1 to 5 minutes (dependent on route). Care should be taken to reassess the fundus when the intravenous infusion has been discontinued or 30 to 60 minutes after intramuscular administration to ensure that atony has not resumed. Methylergonovine (0.2 mg), administered intramuscularly or orally, produces sustained tetanic uterine contractions. Prostaglandin 15 methyl F_2 (250 μg) administered intramuscularly also produces sustained contractions.

Vaginal bleeding is evaluated by observing the discharge during fundal massage and by assessing the amount of blood on the perineal pad. Saturating a pad within 15 minutes immediately after delivery is considered excessive blood loss. The commonly used hospital perineal pads become completed soaked with blood loss of 68 to 80 ml (Wong and Perry, 1998).

If there has been perineal trauma or development of edema, ice packs for the first 24 hours decrease discomfort. Droegemuller (1980) provides rationale for using cold or "iced" sitz baths rather than the traditional warm water sitz baths for relief of pain during the first 24 hours after delivery. Cold stimulation results in decreased excitability of free nerve endings and decreased nerve conduction, leading to an almost immediate relief of pain. Vasoconstriction caused by cold temperature also reduces edema and decreases muscle spasms. After 24 hours, warmth in the form of warm compresses or flow of water, sitz baths, a heat lamp, or a hair dryer increases healing through vasodilation of perineal vessels. Analgesia for perineal pain rarely needs to be stronger than nonsteroidal antiinflammatory drugs. Ibuprofen (600 mg) has been shown to be superior to acetaminophen for relief of incision/laceration pain and postpartum uterine cramping ("afterpains") (Windle, Booker, and Rayburn, 1989). Ibuprofen is safe during nursing since it has a low milk-to-plasma concentration ratio and a short half-life.

The healing placental site and sites of trauma in the vagina and perineum are potential sites of infection. For this reason, internal examinations should be kept to a minimum, and the perineal area should be kept clean and dry. Women can be instructed to rinse the perineal area with warm water after voiding and then patting the area dry with soft tissue from front to back. A clean perineal pad should be applied after voiding or defecating. Research has not identified any advantage to specific antiseptic solutions for rinsing.

If the woman experiences increasing pain or pain that seems out of proportion to the perineal trauma, the clinician needs to examine her to rule out hematoma. In addition, if bleeding seems to be brisk or a constant oozing, especially with a firm uterus, examination to rule out cervical or deep vaginal lacerations is necessary.

The woman should be encouraged to void within the first 4 hours after delivery. If she is unable to void or if a distended bladder is noted, catheterization should be considered. A distended bladder inhibits uterine contractibility and may be a cause of increased vaginal bleeding. When possible, the woman should be helped to the toilet for urination. Running water into the sink and directing flow of water from a squeeze bottle over the perineum may help her void. If she is unable to get out of bed, placing her on the bedpan with several drops of oil of peppermint in the pan may relax the urinary meatus and facilitate spontaneous voiding (Wong and Perry, 1998).

Bowel function usually resumes 2 to 3 days after the birth. Encouraging fluids and foods containing fiber facilitates bowel functioning. Women who experienced episiotomy or lacerations may benefit from stool softeners, especially if they have a history of problems with constipation or if they have hemorrhoids.

Immediately after birth, women often feel extremely hungry. If liquids are tolerated, progression to a full diet immediately after delivery is appropriate (American Academy of Pediatrics and American College of Obstetricians and Gynecologists, 1997). The clinician should be aware of cultural beliefs about nourishment after birth. Traditional Korean women may eat only seaweed soup and rice, believing that these foods regenerate the blood and encourage the flow of milk (Sich, 1981). Interestingly, seaweed is high in vitamin K and is a commonly prescribed by Korean physicians for cases of anemia and bleeding. Traditional Hmong women eat only warm chicken and rice with no fluids to prevent diarrhea and stomach cramps (Jambunathan, 1995). Chicken is prepared by boiling for the first 2weeks after delivery and is roasted thereafter. The boiling is thought to provide all of the liquid the mother needs for recovery. Asian and Latina women may hold beliefs regarding "hot" and "cold" foods and may consume only "hot" foods during the postpartum period because of the belief that the stress of labor and blood loss leads to a "cold" state.

Early ambulation decreases the risk of thrombophlebitis, so the woman should be encouraged to ambulate as soon as she feels that she is able. Because of the risk of orthostatic hypotension, another individual should be with the woman the first few times she gets out of bed.

Women who are Rh negative (D negative) and who deliver an Rh-positive infant should be offered 300 μg immunoglobulin D, even if they have had immunoglobulin D prenatally. It is recommended that the immunoglobulin D be administered within 72 hours of the birth. Women who are not immune to rubella should be offered rubella vaccine. Rubella vaccine is considered safe with breast-feeding but should not be administered when there are householders who are immune compromised since the virus is shed in urine and other body fluids.

Care of Women Following Cesarean Section

Women who have experienced cesarean section usually require medical management until discharge to their homes. In some settings midwives may co-manage the postpartum care of women who have had surgical deliveries. In other sites surgical delivery necessitates complete medical management. Regardless of the institutional policies covering management roles, there is still the need for midwifery counseling and guidance during the immediate postpartum period. Continuity of care with the midwife provides an opportunity for the woman to verbalize her feelings about the necessity of the surgical delivery, particularly when the cesarean section was not expected or planned. Midwives also provide necessary guidance for the normal transition to the mothering role, including support through initial maternal-infant encounters and assistance with breast-feeding. For this reason, when institutional policy requires post-cesarean medical management, many midwives continue to provide "midwifery rounds" to meet the many psychosocial and parenting needs of the women and her family.

Initiating Breast-Feeding

The benefits of breast-feeding for the woman and her infant have been well established. Maternal benefits include:

1. Decreased blood loss following delivery
2. Decreased levels of anxiety, stress, depression, fatigue, and guilt
3. Delay in resumption of ovulation with increased child spacing caused by lactational amenorrhea
4. Protection of iron stores caused by lactational amenorrhea
5. Decreased risk for osteoporosis
6. Decreased risk for breast cancer in women, particularly with breast-feeding greater than 3 months
7. Decreased risk for ovarian cancer
8. Financial savings for the family

Benefits for the infants who are breast-fed include:

1. Protection from infection, including gastrointestinal disease, respiratory illness, otitis media, necrotizing enterocolitis, and appendicitis
2. Decreased risk of sudden infant death syndrome
3. Increased concentration of docosahexanoic acid in the cerebral cortex phospholipids which is associated with greater capacity for neurotransmission in the cerebral cortex (This is thought to be associated with improved cognitive development.)
4. Decreased allergies related to cow's milk ingestion
5. Decreased childhood insulin-dependent diabetes
6. Decreased atopic dermatitis

Numerous expert panels and professional organizations have called for increased efforts to promote breast-feeding because of the many health benefits for children. Yet, it is estimated that only 59% of mothers breast-feed in the hospital after birth and only 21% of all mothers breast-feed for at least 6 months. Health care professionals are in the position to provide counseling regarding the benefits of breast-feeding. Unfortunately, many women do not receive counseling during the prenatal period. Izatt (1997) found that, in her sample of middle-class white women, only 23% reported receiving information about breast-feeding from their obstetricians. Midwives, physicians, and nurses caring for women during the perinatal period are in a position to offer advice about this beneficial practice to women who otherwise may not have considered it.

Health care professionals have the responsibility to provide an environment that supports the initial and ongoing breast-feeding efforts of the woman. In the past, hospital practices separated mothers and their infants and imposed rigid feeding schedules. When the woman and her infant are healthy, they should have continued contact that supports true "on demand" feeding. Family support and support from other women in the community should be identified, and any counseling should build on the mother's previous experiences with and beliefs about breast-feeding. Identification of cultural beliefs about breast-feeding should also be explored, and counseling tailored to meet those beliefs. For example, some traditional Asian groups believe that the infant should not be given colostrum. If the mother feels

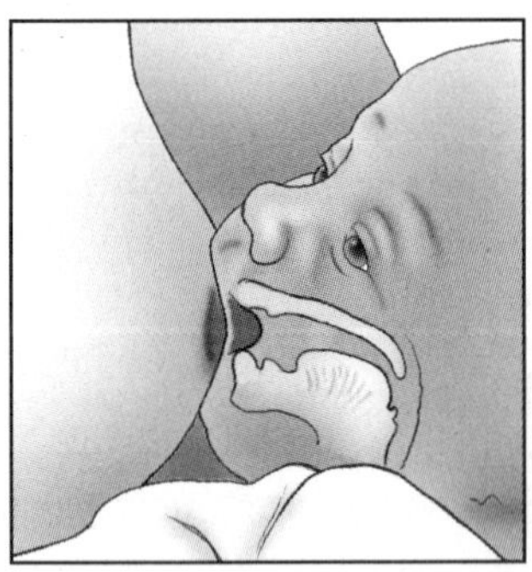

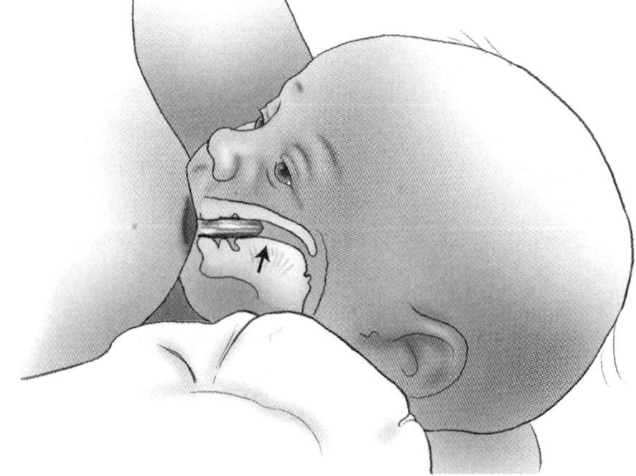

Figure 22-2 Proper latch-on of nursing infant.

strongly about following the instructions of her mother or mother-in-law, the option of pumping her breasts to stimulate milk production can be offered in lieu of putting the infant directly on breast.

Women breast-feeding for the first time will usually need assistance in using different infant positions for nursing. Henschel and Inch (1996) note, "Positioning a baby at the breast is . . . a skill to be learned, just as, for example, one needs to learn the individual movements of a dance or how to use the hands to shape the clay on a potters wheel." The health care professional practicing with a midwifery philosophy assists the woman in learning the skills of breast-feeding in several ways:

- Providing hands-on assistance when necessary
- Talking the woman through the practice of putting the baby on breast in such a way that the woman herself performs the task
- Leaving the woman to practice on her own or with other support individuals, if that is her preference (Henschel and Inch, 1996)

Breast-feeding should be thought of as a relaxing, mutually satisfying activity between the mother and her infant. The midwife assists the mother by helping her find a comfortable position to initiate nursing. Comfort in positioning is influenced by the type of delivery (vaginal vs. cesarean delivery), fatigue or muscle soreness from the birth, the woman's body shape, and the size and shape of the breasts and nipples. Positions may include sitting in bed propped by numerous pillows; sitting tailor fashion; sitting in a wide, comfortable chair; or lying on one's side. Stroking the infant's cheek should stimulate the rooting reflex, and, as her or his lips touch the nipple, it is sometimes helpful to move the head slightly away from the breast, which stimulates the infant to open his or her mouth even wider. As the mouth opens wide, the head can be brought back to the nipple, allowing the infant to take in as much of the nipple and areola as possible. The mother can determine whether her infant is correctly positioned if the following are observed:

- There is a strong and painless "drawing" of the nipple into the baby's mouth.
- If any of the areola is visible, there will be more above the baby's top lip than below the bottom lip.
- The baby's nose barely touches the breast.
- The chin is in contact with the breast.
- The angle of the corner of the baby's lips is more than 100 degrees.
- The whole lower jaw moves as the baby sucks (Henschel and Inch, 1996) (Figures 22-2 and 22-3).

If the infant is not well positioned, he or she will make little sucks rather than using the entire lower jaw to work the areola, he or she will purse the lips rather than having the lower jaw extended, the sucking will cause pain to the nipple, and the infant may appear frustrated at not being satisfied.

While gently guiding the woman in her efforts, the health professional can also use the time to point out the normal neonatal behavior during suckling and the unique aspects of the woman's infant. Individuals who are guiding the mother in the initial breast-feeding experiences should always reinforce the belief that the woman will be successful in breast-feeding. Subtle negative messages such as, "Your nipples may be too flat," or "With such a big baby, you'll probably want to supplement your feedings with formula," give the message that it is expected that she will not be successful in her nursing efforts.

Even with the known benefits to breast-feeding, there are some cases in which breast-feeding is contraindi-

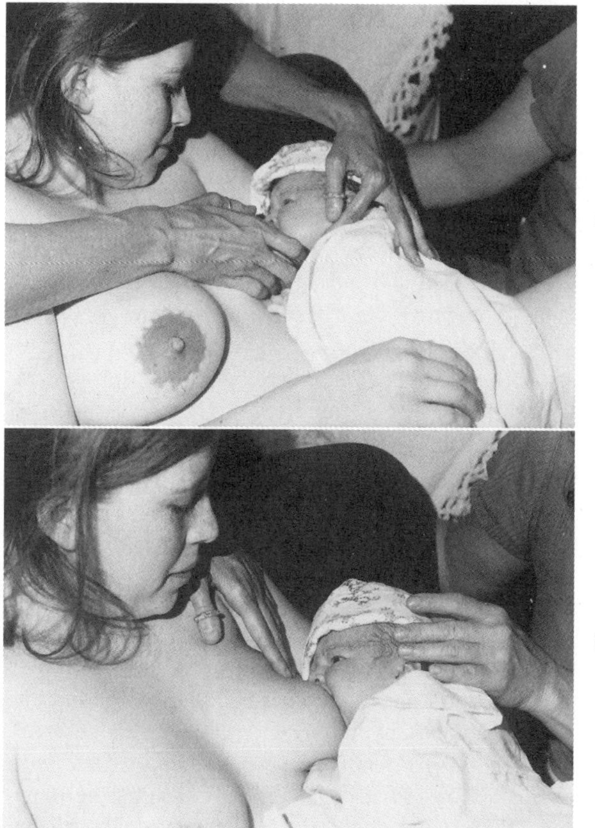

Figure 22-3 A and B, Initial breast-feeding. (Courtesy Caroline E. Brown.)

Box 22-1 *Common Drugs/Substances That Are Contraindicated in Breast-Feeding*

Alcohol (large doses)	Heroin
Amphetamines	Isotretinoin
Bromocriptine	Lithium
Cannabis	Methadone
Chloramphenicol	Methotrexate
Cocaine	Morphine
Cyclophosphamide	Phencyclidine
Cyclosporine	Phenindione
Doxorubicin	Radioactive iodine/ radiolabeled products
Ergotamine	
Gold salts	

Adapted from American Academy of Pediatrics and American College of Obstetricians and Gynecologists: *Guidelines for perinatal care,* ed 4, Elk Grove Village, Ill, 1997, American Academy of Pediatrics and Kacew S: Adverse effects of drugs and chemicals in breast milk on the nursing infant, *J Clin Pharmacol* 33:213-221, 1993.

cated. Women who use illegal drugs or abuse certain prescription drugs, women with untreated active tuberculosis, women in the acute phase of a primary outbreak of cytomegalovirus, and women infected with the human immunodeficiency virus (HIV) should be counseled that breast-feeding is not in the best interest of their infants. Women who test positive for hepatitis B surface antigen may breast-feed as long as their infants have received hepatitis B virus immunoglobulin and vaccine. In addition, women who are at high risk for undocumented infection with HIV (e.g., sex workers, partners of known HIV-positive individuals, intravenous drug users or partners of intravenous drug users) should be counseled regarding the risk of breast-feeding to their infants (American Academy of Pediatrics and American College of Obstetricians and Gynecologists, 1997). Box 22-1 identifies drugs that are contraindicated or not recommended during breast-feeding.

The World Health Organization (1989) and the United Nations Children's Fund (UNICEF) have developed the Baby-Friendly Hospital Initiative. This international effort provides guidelines for institutions to ensure that breast-feeding is considered the norm. Hospitals and other agencies are encouraged to become "baby-friendly," and to that end, *Ten Steps to Successful Breast-Feeding* have been proposed. These steps are summarized in Box 22-2.

Box 22-2 *Ten Steps to Successful Breast-Feeding in Hospitals and Birth Centers*

1. Have a written breast-feeding policy that is routinely communicated to all health care staff.
2. Train all health care staff in skills necessary to implement this policy.
3. Inform all pregnant women about the benefits and management of breast-feeding.
4. Help mothers initiate breast-feeding within a half-hour of birth.
5. Show mothers how to breast-feed and how to maintain lactation, even if they should be separated from their infants.
6. Give newborn infants no food or drink other than breast milk unless medically indicated.
7. Practice rooming-in—allow mothers and infants to remain together—24 hours a day.
8. Encourage breast-feeding on demand.
9. Give no artificial teats or pacifiers to breast-feeding infants.
10. Foster the establishment of breast-feeding support groups and refer mothers to them on discharge from the hospital or clinic.

From Saadeh R, Akre J: Ten steps to successful breastfeeding: a summary of the rationale and scientific evidence, *Birth* 23(3):154-160, 1996.

EMOTIONAL AND PSYCHOSOCIAL ASPECTS OF THE IMMEDIATE POSTPARTUM PERIOD

The literature exploring parent-infant attachment behaviors presents inconsistent terminology and definitions. In this chapter, the terms *attachment* and *bonding* will both be used to discuss the relationship that develops between parent and infant. Kennell and Klaus (1998) note that a "bond can be defined as the unique relationship between two people that is specific and endures through time" (p. 4). In addition, "parental bonds to their child can persist during long separations of time and distance, even though visible signs of their existence may not be apparent" (Kennell and Klaus, 1998, p. 4). Parental attachment begins during the prenatal period and increases in intensity shortly after the birth (Kennell and Klaus, 1998). Midwives, physicians, and nurses can facilitate the initial postdelivery attachment behaviors by providing an environment that fosters continued maternal and paternal contact and interaction with the newborn.

Attachment behaviors may be altered by a long and difficult labor, use of analgesia or anesthesia, and immediate postpartum status of the mother and baby. Attachment behaviors are also mediated by cultural beliefs. For example, southeast Asian women may not visually be demonstrative to their infants for fear that the "evil eye" will harm a wanted and loved infant. In addition to attachment behaviors, parental role attainment involves integrating parenting behaviors into one's identity of self, acquiring skills necessary for caring for the child, and finding pleasure and gratification in the role of parent (Mercer, 1985).

Healthy mothers and babies who have experienced no complications during the birth process should not be separated. Attachment requires proximity and interaction—factors that are not present when an infant is whisked away to the nursery for observation. The infant's initial alert state during the first 30 minutes of life is a perfect time to foster interaction. The lights in the room should be dimmed, and prophylactic antibiotic treatment of the neonate's eyes should be deferred so that eye-to-eye contact can be made between mother and infant. Studies have identified universal behaviors as mothers begin to explore their infants (Klaus et al., 1970). Women usually reach for their babies immediately, then proceed with exploring the baby's extremities with their fingertips. This is followed by full use of the palmar surface of the hand to explore the infant's trunk, then holding the infant close to the body. A similar pattern of touch has been identified in fathers (Eidelman, Hovars, and Kaitz, 1994; Rodholm and Larsson, 1979).

Recent research has provided an increased understanding of the newborn's contribution to the bonding process. The infant is not a passive recipient of attention. He or she actively participates in eye contact, listening for parents' voices, and responding to tactile stimulation. When the babies of unmedicated mothers are dried and put skin to skin on the mother's abdomen, they first rest and appear to be orienting themselves to their new surroundings. Crying is unusual during this time. At about 30 to 45 minutes of age, the newborn's mouth begins to make searching movements and he or she may begin to drool. The newborn then begins crawling movements that bring him or her toward the maternal nipple. Once in proximity of the nipple, the newborn opens the mouth and moves the face back and forth until the nipple is pulled into the mouth (Kennell and Klaus, 1998). This dramatic newborn behavior is rarely appreciated in hospital birth settings because the routines and rituals surrounding the birth and postpartum period interfere with this normal instinctive behavior.

It has been suggested that the release of oxytocin during breast-feeding provides a physiologic contribution to the development of attachment behaviors (Kennell and Klaus, 1998). Mothers who have skin-to-skin contact and nurse during the newborn's initial alert state are more likely to demonstrate positive behaviors toward their infants at 1 month of age. There are social triggers as well. Frodi and Lamb (1978) found that both mothers and fathers demonstrated physiologic changes, including increased pulse rate, increased respiratory rate, and heightened alertness when exposed to videotapes of distressed, crying babies. Once the videotaped babies were held and consoled, both mothers and fathers returned to a relaxed state.

During the first 1 to 3 days most mothers are in a dependent phase in which they may rely on others to respond to their needs for comfort, rest, and nourishment. This period of time was labeled the "taking-in phase" by Rubin (1963) in her classic research exploring maternal behaviors in the postpartum period. The woman may be very talkative at this time—reliving the birth experience, marveling at the infant, and seeking support from family and friends. She continues watching, touching, and smelling her infant. Providers can facilitate this process by pointing out normal newborn responses such as focusing on the maternal face or turning toward the mother's or father's voice. As she becomes more acquainted with her child, the woman then moves into developing skills needed in caring for the infant. Throughout this process the woman and her infant begin to learn to read each other's cues. This "cueing behavior" is necessary to meet the needs of both the mother and the infant. Sometimes mothers may feel negatively about certain cues and then feel guilty about not being good enough mothers. A woman who is not familiar with normal infant development may feel that her baby doesn't like her if he or she cries or that the infant is too demanding if he or she wants to breast-feed frequently. The health professional can gently explain neonatal behaviors and help the woman develop an appropriate understanding of those behaviors.

HEALTH EDUCATION NEEDS IN THE IMMEDIATE POSTPARTUM PERIOD

During the first 72 hours after the birth, the health care professional is responsible for assessing the woman's knowledge base regarding care of herself and her infant and providing education and anticipatory guidance as appropriate. The following areas of health care and promotion are usually covered in teaching efforts before discharge from the facility in which the woman has given birth or during a home visit on postpartum day 2 or 3.

Nutrition

A well-balanced diet is expected as the woman recovers from the physical exertion of birthing. If she is breast-feeding, a diet similar to that which she followed in pregnancy (at least 1800 kcal/day) is recommended (Food and Nutrition Board, 1992). Fluids should be encouraged to facilitate the cardiovascular and hemodynamic transitions occurring during the immediate postpartum period. Most clinicians recommend at least 8 to 10 eight-ounce glasses of water or nutritious fluids per day. Attention to protein helps with tissue repair; and fruits, vegetables, and other fiber sources assist the return to normal bowel function. If the woman has been anemic during pregnancy, if there was blood loss greater than 500 ml, or if she is at increased risk for anemia, a multivitamin supplement containing folic acid and supplemental iron should be considered, along with increased dietary intake of iron- and folic-acid containing foods.

Activity

Midwives have traditionally encouraged women to rest as much as possible following the birth. The term "lying-in period" refers to the historic tradition of keeping the woman resting for 4 weeks after the birth. During that time the midwife would visit and assist the mother and infant, and women in the community would take responsibility for meal preparation and care of other children. Most cultures provide relief from usual household or community responsibilities during the lying-in period. Traditional Mexican women may move into their mothers' homes for care, Filipino women are expected to care only for themselves and their babies while family members and relatives take care of the home, and southeast Asian women may be kept in bed in warm rooms to prevent long-term problems from cool winds. Although absolute bed rest is not wise because of the increased risk of thromboembolytic problems, the woman should be advised to rest whenever the baby rests. The midwife's instructions regarding "no cleaning, no cooking, no laundry, and no shopping" are almost always supported by other female relatives and community members.

Care of the Perineum

The woman should be instructed to rinse the area with warm water and apply a clean pad from front to back following urination or defecation. Sitz baths with plain warm water may be used for comfort during the healing process. Occasionally topical anesthetic creams or sprays may be warranted. Women should be advised to call the provider if there is increased pain in the area of any incision or lacerations, if it appears that the incision or laceration repair has broken down, or if there is any discharge from the incision or laceration.

Care of the Breasts

Breast-feeding women can be instructed to wash the nipples only with warm water and to wash their hands in preparation for breast-feeding. A well-fitting nursing bra provides support and increases comfort. A well-fitting bra provides support to the breasts without any areas of pressure or constriction. Underwired bras often apply pressure in a way that impedes milk flow through the ducts. Women who choose to bottle-feed only should be advised to wear a supportive bra and to not stimulate the nipples in any way. Medications to "dry up" milk are not warranted. Anticipatory guidance regarding engorgement and measures to decrease discomfort should be offered. These measures include applying ice packs to the breasts, using over-the-counter analgesics such as acetaminophen or ibuprofen, and using the shower to apply warm water to the breast. Stimulation of the nipple and pumping the breast to relieve discomfort should be discouraged. Reassurance can be given that the condition is self-limiting.

Sexuality

Women should be advised that resumption of sexual activity is a highly individual decision with a wide range of normal expression. In general, sexual intercourse can be safely resumed when there is no further red vaginal bleeding, when sutures feel healed, and when the woman emotionally feels like it. Breast-feeding women should be advised that vaginal lubrication may be decreased because of hormonal changes. An artificial water-based lubricant may decrease discomfort that is caused by vaginal dryness. Both breast-feeding and bottle-feeding women should be counseled to consider contraception as a means of protecting against closely spaced pregnancies (see Chapter 24). Women should be advised that, if they resume sexual activity before the traditional 6-week postpartum check-up, they should alert the provider to any area that is still tender or uncomfortable. Ideally counseling regarding sexuality can be done with the partner present. It should be stressed that types of expression other than intercourse can be considered throughout the perinatal period to maintain intimacy in the relationship.

Emotional Mood Changes

Providers should discuss the normal onset of "blues" and the more serious development of depression with all women (see Chapter 28). Women can be reassured of the normalcy of the "blues" and can be reassured that they are self-limiting. Depression and psychosis should be explained as serious conditions requiring professional intervention.

Postpartum Danger Signs

All women should be instructed to call their providers for the following deviations from normal:

- Fever of 101.4° F (38° C)
- Increase in vaginal bleeding that is not relieved with rest and nursing; saturating more than one pad per hour; change in character of lochia, including foul-smelling discharge or frothy discharge
- Localized pain in one or both breasts
- Pain over the uterus
- Pain with urination
- Pain, tenderness, or redness over veins
- Inability to care for self or baby; depression that interferes with activities of daily living

Follow-Up Care

A plan should be made for a follow-up assessment with the provider. Many midwives see their clients 2 weeks after delivery to assess transition to parenting and breastfeeding and to evaluate physical status. Other providers see clients for routine postpartum follow-up from 4 to 6 weeks after delivery.

DISCHARGE FROM THE FACILITY OF BIRTH

During the 1990s there has been much discussion about the concept of "early postpartum discharge." Hospital stay during the postpartum period decreased from 3 to 5 days in the 1960s to less than 48 hours in the early 1990s. In 1994 87.9% of postpartum stays in the western United States were 1 day or less (Declercq and Simmes, 1997). The move to discharge before 48 hours' postpartum was largely stimulated by third-party payers seeking to decrease health expenditures. Because of concerns raised by the increase in mothers being discharged at 24 hours' postpartum (often without their infants), consumers sought regulations to prevent premature discharge. Between 1995 and 1996 29 states passed laws that protected a stay of at least 48 hours in the hospital, and Public Law 104-204 requiring that insurance companies pay for hospital stays of 48 hours after a vaginal birth and 96 hours after a cesarean birth was adopted in September, 1996.

Although the debate over length of postpartum stay assumed that longer hospital stays (>48 hours) were preferable, there are little empiric data to support this position. Furthermore, this argument assumes that all women have similar needs in the postpartum period and that there is an ideal amount of institutional time that ensures that those needs are met. In reality, women's needs for support by health care professionals and institutional systems are quite varied. Studies exploring the experiences and perinatal outcomes of women birthing in out-of-hospital birth centers and at home have indicated that women who are healthy and who have adequate social support at home can safely receive care at home with only periodic assessments by professionals. Questions regarding appropriate length of stay and extent of provision of care by health care professionals seek answers rooted in system-centered rather than woman- and family-centered needs for care. In a midwifery model of care, the woman's needs and those of her infant become central, and length and scope of care are determined through a collaborative assessment of the family's needs and resources. In this model the woman is an active participant in the decision making and is central to the decision-making process. This approach differs from the ongoing policy debates that center on whether physicians or insurers should determine length of stay.

When length of stay less than 48 hours following delivery became more common, the lack of a sound system of home care and follow-up became apparent. Other developed countries support systems in which mothers and infants receive home visits by midwives or nurses, and during these visits assessments and education can be accomplished. For example, the United Kingdom provides up to 10 days of home visits by a midwife (Declercq and Simmes, 1997). During the reform of maternity care in Great Britain recently, the following standard was established:

> As far as practicable, the length of time spent in a postnatal ward should be discussed and agreed between the

Box 22-3 *Criteria for Early Maternal Discharge*

- Afebrile with pulse and respirations of normal rate and quality
- Blood pressure within normal range
- Amount and color of lochia appropriate for duration of recovery
- Fundus firm
- Urinary output adequate
- Surgical repair or wounds has minimal edema and no evidence of infection
- Ambulation with ease
- No abnormal physical or emotional findings
- Eating and drinking without problems
- Postpartum follow-up plan developed
- Education regarding self-care and deviations from normal completed
- Demonstration of readiness to care for self and infant
- Pertinent laboratory results available and within normal limits
- Immunoglobulin D administered if appropriate
- Support persons available for first few days after delivery

Adapted from American Academy of Pediatrics and American College of Obstetricians and Gynecologists: *Guidelines for perinatal care,* ed 4, Elk Grove Village, Ill, 1997, American Academy of Pediatrics.

Box 22-4 *Criteria for Early Neonatal Discharge*

- Antepartum, intrapartum, and postpartum courses for mother and baby uncomplicated
- Vaginal delivery
- Singleton birth at 38-42 weeks' gestation
- Vital signs within normal limits
- Urinating and passing meconium
- Completion of two feedings without problems
- Normal physical examination
- No excessive bleeding at circumcision site
- No evidence of jaundice in first 24 hours
- Mother able to care for infant
- Support individuals available to help mother in infant care
- Laboratory results within normal limits
- Screening tests done in accordance with state regulations
- Initial hepatitis B vaccine administered or appointment made for its administration
- Physician-directed source of continuing medical care for both mother and baby identified
- No family, environmental, and social risk factors identified

Adapted from American Academy of Pediatrics and American College of Obstetricians and Gynecologists: *Guidelines for perinatal care,* ed 4, Elk Grove Village, Ill, 1997, American Academy of Pediatrics.

> woman, the midwife and other professionals as necessary. The midwife can help the woman to assess her readiness to return home and to prepare her for doing so. For some women, after the first few days at home, it will be enough to know that they can contact their midwife for advice or a visit if they are concerned about themselves or their babies. For others, the visits of a familiar midwife, and their GP, in the period up to 28 days after birth of their babies will be essential to build confidence in their own abilities (Department of Health, 1993, quoted in Declercq and Simmes, 1997, p. 178).

ACOG and AAP note that "a shortened hospital stay (<48 hours after delivery) for healthy term infants can be accomplished but is not appropriate for every mother and neonate. Each mother-baby dyad should be evaluated individually to determine the optimal time of discharge" (American Academy of Pediatrics and American College of Obstetricians and Gynecologists, 1997, p. 165). Their guidelines make it very clear that their belief is that the physician is the most qualified individual to determine appropriate length of stay. Box 22-3 lists the criteria that should be met should the "physician and the woman want a shortened [maternal] hospital stay"; Box 22-4 summarizes the criteria for shortened neonatal hospital stay (American Academy of Pediatrics and American College of Obstetricians and Gynecologists, 1997).

As the health delivery system for childbearing women continues to evolve, it is important that traditional assumptions using a biomedical model of care

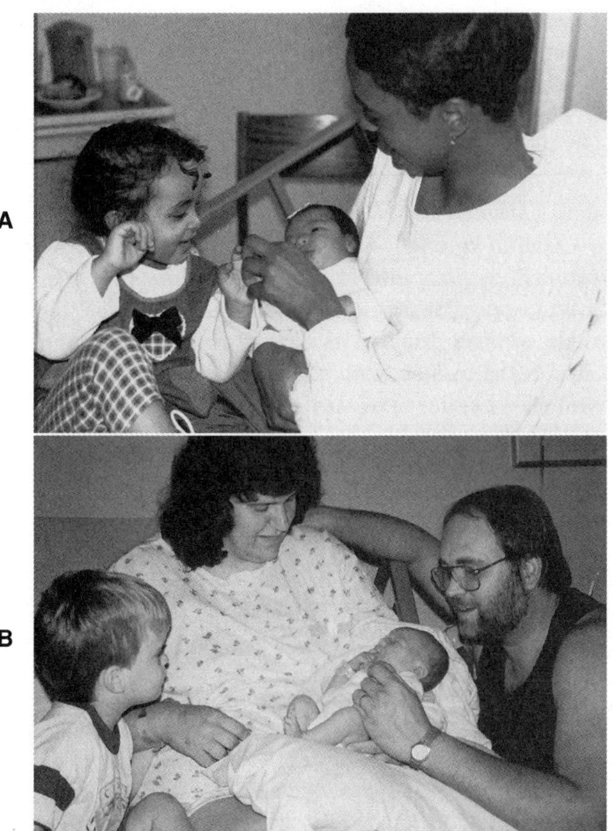

Figure 22-4, A and B, Support of family members/siblings is necessary during the postpartum period. (Courtesy Caroline E. Brown.)

suitable for illness rather than health be challenged. Research is needed to determine whether there is a significant period of time in which professional caregiving is beneficial. Continued exploration of the benefits and costs of models of care that use a variety of providers and sites of care will guide policy makers as the health care systems evolves. Possible advantages of early postpartum discharge include:

- Support of the belief that childbearing is a healthy state for most women and their infants
- Decreased chance of separation of parents and infant
- Decreased separation of the mother from other children and family members
- Promotion of involvement of family members/significant other in the care and support necessary during the postpartum period (Figure 22-4, *A* and *B*)
- Decreased exposure to pathogens in the institutional environment
- Decreased cost
- More appropriate use of acute care facilities (e.g., use of hospital beds for women with complications of the perinatal period)

Possible disadvantages of early postpartum discharge include:

- Discharge into an environment that is unsafe or not supportive
- Lack of support for household responsibilities when the mother may be fatigued or in pain
- Decreased opportunity for health education regarding care of self and infant, especially when the woman has experienced a first birth
- Maternal or neonatal complications that may not be identified in a timely manner
- Lack of continuity of care for mother and infant

The first 72 hours are a period of dramatic transition for the new mother. The health care provider practicing within a midwifery model of care is in a position to provide support in a way that increases maternal self-confidence and self-esteem. In the current health care environment in which hospital stays are shorter and in a social climate in which extended family support may not be available, the midwife continues in the historic role of health care provider and maternal counselor. Strong clinical skills, coupled with wisdom and respect for cultural beliefs surrounding birth and family, are essential to foster maternal, infant, family, and community health.

References

American Academy of Pediatrics and American College of Obstetricians and Gynecologists: *Guidelines for perinatal care,* ed 4, Elk Grove Village, Ill, 1997, American Academy of Pediatrics.

Blackburn ST, Loper DL: *Maternal, fetal, and neonatal physiology: a clinical perspective,* Philadelphia, 1992, WB Saunders.

Bowes WA: Postpartum care. In Gabbe SG, Niebyl JR, Simpson JL, editors: *Obstetrics—normal and problem pregnancies,* ed 3, New York, 1996, Churchill Livingstone.

Chan GM: *Lactation—the breast-feeding manual for health professionals,* Chicago, 1997, Precept Press.

Cluett ER, Alexander J, Pickering RM: What is the normal pattern of uterine involution? An investigation of postpartum uterine involution measured by the distance between the symphysis pubis and the uterine fundus using a paper tape measure, *Midwifery* 13(1):9-16, 1997.

Copagna G, Celleno D, Tomassetti M: Maternal analgesia and neonatal effects of epidural sufentanil for cesarean section, *Reg Anesth* 14: 282-287, 1989.

Crowell MK, Hill PD, Humenick SS: Relationship between obstetric analgesia and time of effective breastfeeding, *J Nurse Midwifery* 39:150-155, 1994.

Declercq E, Simmes D: The politics of "Drive-Through Deliveries": putting early postpartum discharge on the legislative agenda, *Millbank Q* 75(2):175-202, 1997.

Droegemuller W: Cold sitz baths for relief of postpartum perineal pain, *Clin Obstet Gynecol* 23(4):1039-1043, 1980.

Eidelman AI, Hovars R, Kaitz M: Comparative tactile behavior of mothers and fathers with their newborn infants, *Israel J Med Sci* 30(1):79-82, 1994.

Food and Nutrition Board, Institute of Medicine: *Nutrition during pregnancy and lactation: an implementation guide,* Washington, DC, 1992, National Academy Press.

Frodi AM, Lamb ME: Sex differences in responsiveness to infants: a developmental study of psychophysiological and behavioral responses, *Child Dev* 49(4):1182-1188, 1978.

Henschel D, Inch S: *Breastfeeding—a guide for midwives,* Cheshire, England, 1996, Books for Midwives Press.

Izatt S: Breastfeeding counseling by health care providers, *J Hum Lactation* (2):109-113, 1997.

Jambunathan J: Hmong cultural practices and beliefs: the postpartum period, *Clin Nurs Res* 4(3):335-345, 1995.

Kennell JH, Klaus MH: Bonding: recent observations that alter perinatal care, *Pediatr Rev* 19(1):4-12, 1998.

Klaus MH et al: Human maternal behavior at the first contact with her young, *Pediatrics* 46(2):187-192, 1970.

Lawrence RA: *Breastfeeding—a guide for the medical profession,* ed 4, St Louis, 1994, Mosby.

Loftus JR, Hill H, Cohen SE: Placental transfer and neonatal effects of epidural sufentanil and fentanyl administered with bupivacaine during labor, *Anesthesiology* 83:300-308, 1995.

Mercer RT: The process of maternal role attainment over the first year, *Nurs Res* 34:198-204, 1985.

Meyer S et al: The effects of birth on urinary continence mechanisms and other pelvic-floor characteristics, *Obstet Gynecol* 92(4):613-618, 1998.

Murray AD et al: Effects of epidural anesthesia on newborns and their mothers, *Child Dev* 82:71-82, 1981.

Nissen E et al: Effects of maternal pethidine on infants' developing breast feeding behavior, *Acta Paediatr* 84:140-145, 1995.

Righard L, Alade MO: Effect of delivery room routines on success of first breast-feed, *Lancet* 336:1105-1107, 1990.

Rodholm M, Larsson K: Father-infant interaction at the first encounter after delivery, *Early Hum Dev* 3(1):21-27, 1979.

Rubin R: Maternal touch, *Nurs Outlook* 11:828-831, 1963.

Sepkoski CM et al: The effects of maternal epidural anesthesia on neonatal behavior during the first month, *Dev Med Child Neurol* 34:1072-1080, 1992.

Sich D: Traditional concepts and customs on pregnancy, birth and postpartum period in rural Korea, *Soc Sci Med* 15B(1):65-69, 1981.

Thorp JA, Breedlove G: Epidural analgesia in labor: an evaluation of risks and benefits, *Birth* 23(2):63-81, 1996.

Walker M: Do labor medications affect breastfeeding? *J Hum Lactation* 13(2):131-137, 1997.

Willms AB et al: Anatomic changes in the pelvis after uncomplicated vaginal delivery: evaluation with serial MR imaging, *Radiology* 195(1):91-94, 1995.

Windle ML, Booker LA, and Rayburn WF: Postpartum pain after vaginal delivery: a review of comparative analgesic trials, *J Reprod Med* 34(11):891-895, 1989.

Wong DL, Perry SE: *Maternal child nursing care,* St Louis, 1998, Mosby.

World Health Organization: *Protecting, promoting and supporting breast-feeding: the special role of maternity services,* Geneva, 1989, World Health Organization, UNICEF.

Chapter

23

Healthy Newborn

Maureen Wolfe CNM, MSN

Historically the person attending childbirth cared not only for the woman giving birth, but for the newborn and other family members as well. Since the turn of the century, however, changes in our health care system have favored specialization. One obstetric provider cares for the woman and fetus during pregnancy and parturition, and a second pediatric provider takes over care of the newborn shortly after delivery. This is the model for the vast majority of births in the United States that take place in the hospital setting. Women who give birth out of hospital are more likely to have a single provider for both mother and infant throughout the processes of involution and adaptation to extrauterine life. Managed care calls for the return of a generalist to provide a broad base of care for the essentially normal woman and infant. A pediatric specialist is reserved for more complex care needs of the ill infant. The focus of this chapter is on the care of the healthy newborn from birth to 8 weeks.

EXTRAUTERINE ADAPTATION

A thorough understanding of the physiologic changes the neonate experiences at the time of birth is the basis for providing care to the newborn.

Cardiopulmonary Adaptations

At birth, changes in the respiratory and cardiovascular systems happen simultaneously to make the lungs rather than the placenta the main site of oxygen and carbon dioxide transfer. Circulation through the placenta is terminated, and the high-pressure pulmonary vasculature in the fetal system changes to a low-pressure system in the newborn. Functional changes occur in the first minutes of life, whereas anatomic changes may take up to 6 weeks.

In utero the fetal lungs are filled with fluid. During vaginal birth pressures applied to the thorax cause as much as 28 ml, or approximately one third of the fluid, to escape the upper respiratory tree. The rest is absorbed into the lymphatics of the lung. At the time of expulsion, chest recoil draws air (one fourth to one third of the residual capacity) into the airways, but does not fully expand the alveoli. The vigor of the first breaths determines how quickly air will replace fluid. High pressures of 30 to 40 cm H_2O are required for the first breath, whereas subsequent breaths require only approximately 15 to 20 cm H_2O. Tidal volume and minute ventilation increase most during the first 24 hours of life, but residual volume and lung compliance continue to increase over the first days of life.

Theories explaining the stimulus for the first breath remain elusive. Gasping may be a response to a drop in arterial Po_2 and rise in PCO_2 that happens when less blood flows through the umbilical cord. It is possible that neurosensory (touch, light, noise, cold) and proprioceptive (gravity) stimuli initiate respirations. Chemoreceptors in the aortic and carotid bodies and mechanical receptors of the lung regulate subsequent breaths. As air fills the lungs, alveolar fluid is resorbed into the capillaries and lymph ducts. Rales may be heard in the normal newborn for the first 20 minutes of life. The infant born by cesarean section may have rales for up to 1 hour.

Changes in the cardiovascular system occur simultaneously with the respiratory changes in the newborn. Three vascular shunts are operative in the fetal circulation—the foramen ovale, the ductus arteriosus, and the ductus venosus (Figure 23-1). The foramen ovale is an opening between the right and left atria of the heart. The ductus arteriosus connects the pulmonary artery with the descending aorta, bypassing the lungs. The ductus venosus connects the umbilical vein with the inferior vena cava. Oxygenated fetal blood flows from the placenta into the umbilical vein. Approximately 60% of this blood is shunted through the ductus venosus directly into the inferior vena cava and then to the heart. The remainder supplies the liver before it enters the inferior vena cava and heart. Once in the right atrium, 50% to 60% of the blood from the inferior vena cava flows through the foramen ovale and into the left atrium, bypassing the lungs before entering the left ventricle and aorta. The remainder of the blood from the right atrium flows into the right ventricle and then the pulmonary artery. From here, only 5% to 10% of the blood flows into the pulmonary bed because of the increased pulmonary vascular resistance. Instead, blood flows through the ductus arteriosus and into the descending aorta. From the aorta, blood supplies the brain and heart first and then other organs. Deoxygenated blood is returned to the placenta via the umbilical arteries.

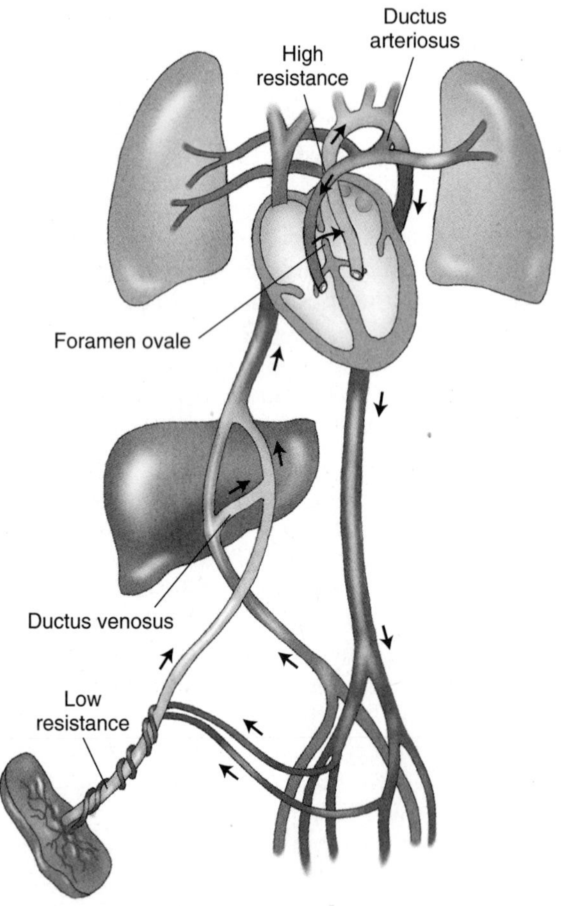

Figure 23-1 Fetal circulation.

Soon after birth, blood flow through the cord ceases, removing the low-pressure placental circulation and increasing the systemic vascular resistance (Figure 23-2). The ductus venosus may be anatomically patent for days but is not functional once the umbilical vein is occluded. With the first breaths, increased oxygen concentration in the alveoli causes vasodilation and a decrease in the pulmonary vascular resistance. Because of the decreased pulmonary resistance and the increased peripheral resistance, blood flows into the pulmonary artery and to the lungs rather than through the foramen ovale. The increased concentration of oxygen in the blood flowing through the ductus arteriosus causes constriction of the smooth muscle and functional closure of this shunt within the first 12 hours of life. Anatomic closure usually occurs within 1 month.

Thermoregulation

The newborn is particularly vulnerable to heat loss and limited in her or his capabilities to respond to cold stress. The four mechanisms of heat loss are conduction, radiation, convection, and evaporation. Conduction is loss of heat from a warm object in direct contact with a colder object. Radiation is the loss of heat from a warm object in close proximity (but not direct contact) with a colder object. Convection heat loss occurs as air currents sweep away the layer of warmed air that surrounds a warm body. Finally, heat is lost as fluids evaporate from skin.

The infant is born wet and is vulnerable to evaporative loss. The newborn also has a relatively large surface area in relation to body mass, providing more interface with the cooler environment. The neurologic immaturity of the infant makes shivering and purposeful increased muscle movements ineffective methods of heat production.

The newborn is equipped with brown fat, which provides an adaptive advantage. Brown fat makes up 2% to 6% of the infant's body weight. It is concentrated around the nape of the neck, upper spinal cord, and axillae and between the scapulae and around the great vessels and kidneys. Brown fat has more vascularity and sympathetic enervation than white fat and is a more efficient generator of energy. However, brown fat is a nonrenewable source of energy. Cold stimulation of skin receptors results in catecholamine release and oxidation of brown fat into fatty acids. Oxygen and glucose are required, but much heat is generated. When the infant experiences hypoglycemia, metabolism of brown fat is not efficient. Metabolism is regulated by the sympathetic nervous system and triiodothyronine (T_3). There is normally a marked increase in thyroid-stimulating hormone, thyroxine, and T_3 in the first 24 hours after delivery. Thyroid activity is not as great in infants born by cesarean section, so they are further compromised in their ability to regulate body temperature.

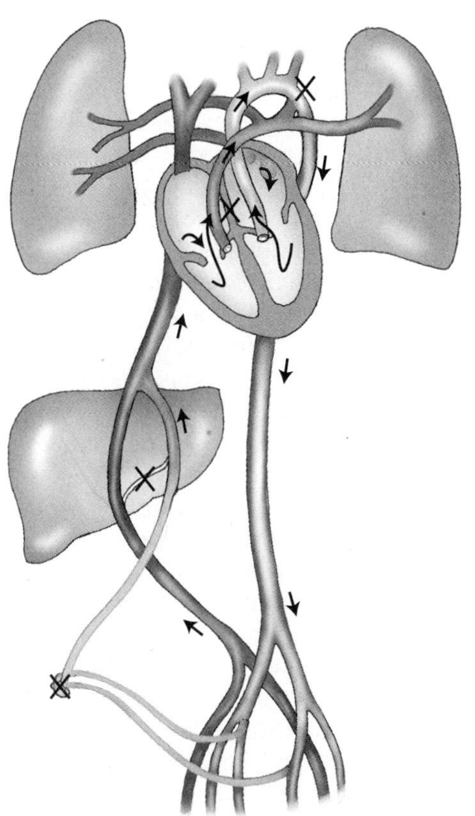

Figure 23-2 Neonatal circulation.

Normal axillary temperature is 36.5° to 37.5° C (97.7° to 99.5° F). Abdominal skin temperature is 36° to 36.5° C (96.8° to 97.7° F). Cold stress increases the respiratory rate and causes a threefold to fourfold increase in metabolic rate. The infant depletes energy stores in an attempt to maintain body temperature. Significant heat loss can lead to hypoglycemia, hypoxia, and acidosis. Thus it is critical that a neutral thermal environment be maintained for the infant. If the infant's temperature drops below normal, gradual rewarming is required. Rewarming too rapidly can cause apnea and further deplete energy stores.

The infant also has limited ability to tolerate overheating. Sweating is not an effective mechanism to dissipate excessive heat in the newborn. Tachycardia and/or disruption of metabolic processes results. Thus care must be taken not to overheat the infant. Normally by 2 days after birth the healthy newborn is able to stabilize body temperature adequately.

Fluid, Glucose, and Electrolyte Regulation

The neonate's need for water is great. At term, 78% of total body weight is water. A large part of this is interstitial fluid, which is high in sodium and chloride but low in potassium and magnesium. After birth much of this interstitial and intravascular water is mobilized and removed via the kidney. There is a relative increase in renal blood flow and glomerular filtration, so fluids and solids pass freely into the collecting tubules. Tubule maturation lags, however, making it difficult for the newborn to resorb substances and retain them in the body. The ability to concentrate or dilute urine is compromised. At the same time there is an increased solute load as feedings are begun. Both of these factors contribute to increased urine production. Over the first few postpartum days, kidney function improves. Approximately 66% of newborns void within the first 12 hours of life, 93% by 24 hours, and 99% by 48 hours. Normal urine output is 1.5 to 2.5 ml/kg/hr.

Water is also deposited into new tissues during growth and is lost through the skin, feces, and respirations. Insensible water loss is significant in the newborn. Approximately 35 ml/kg/day is lost—30% from respirations and 70% from the skin. The normal water requirement at birth is approximately 60 ml/kg/day. By the second week of life, with increased growth and urine production, water need increases to 120 to 150 ml/kg/day.

Metabolism of glucose changes after delivery. During fetal life glucose and insulin play the major roles in anabolism and energy production. In the third trimester the fetus stores glucose as glycogen. When the fetus experiences intrauterine growth restriction or fetal distress or when the neonate is preterm or postterm, there is a diminished supply of glycogen available for extrauterine metabolism. After birth, insulin activity decreases. Fat rather than glucose is the major substrate for energy production and anabolism (gluconeogenesis). Fatty acid levels rise rapidly within 3 hours after birth as a result of lipolysis. There is a physiologic nadir of blood glucose 1 to 1.5 hours after birth, but glucose levels stabilize in 3 to 4 hours. The mean glucose level in the newborn is 60 to 70 mg/dl. A drop below 40 mg/dl is cause for concern. Signs of hypoglycemia include jitteriness, lethargy, weak cry, apnea, limpness, refusal to feed, and cyanosis; however, hypoglycemia is often asymptomatic. Infants at risk for hypoglycemia include low-birth-weight infants, large infants (greater than 4000 g), and infants who experienced intolerance of labor. A glucose test strip is quick and convenient but not always an accurate reflection of glucose status. Venous stasis and polycythemia (hematocrit >55%) can cause falsely low glucose results. Properly warming the infant's heel before obtaining the specimen may help to avoid stasis. Anemia (hematocrit <35%) may cause falsely high results. In critical circumstances a venous puncture should be done to obtain both glucose and hematocrit levels.

Gastrointestinal Changes

At birth the infant's gut is sterile and functionally immature. Bowel sounds normally begin after approximately 30 minutes. Gut colonization during the first week after delivery is affected by environmental flora. After the first week, flora depends on method of feeding. Breast-feeding results in an acidic environment, favoring the growth of lactobacillus and bifidobacterium. Formula feeding produces a more alkaline environment where gram-negative enterobacteria thrive. Gut acidity deters invasion by pathogenic organisms. However, the mucosa is not an effective barrier against invading bacteria and other antigens until approximately 4 to 6 months of age. Breast milk contains immunoglobulin A, white cells, and complement, which help protect the infant from infection.

Hormones that control motility and digestive enzymes are present in decreased amounts in the newborn. Pancreatic secretion is minimal, and the infant relies on salivary and gastric secretions to aid digestion. Enzymes found in human milk help the newborn to digest. Colostrum contains three growth factors that produce rapid intestinal cell growth and increased protein and deoxyribonucleic acid content of intestinal mucosa. These beneficial changes are not seen in infants fed formula or water only.

The term newborn's stomach capacity is approximately 30 ml. During the first 2 weeks the infant takes in 30 to 60 ml every 2 to 4 hours. Because the cardiac sphincter is immature, 80% of normal infants regurgitate a small amount of their feedings. The normal newborn may lose approximately 10% to 15% of body weight over the first 3 days and then gain it back by 1 week of age. Thereafter average weight gain is 1 oz/day, and the infant grows approximately 1 inch in length per month.

IMMEDIATE CARE OF THE NORMAL NEWBORN

With an understanding of the physiologic changes occurring in the newborn, a rational approach to care is possible. The practitioner must avoid disrupting the newborn's own successful efforts to adapt to extrauterine life. The goal of care is to support transition, prevent potential complications, identify abnormalities, and intervene as necessary. The infant's condition is assessed immediately by observing color, tone, and respiratory effort. The first interventions center around clearing the infant's airway and facilitating initiation of respirations. Although suctioning immediately after birth is common practice, simply wiping secretions from the infant's face is equally effective. Potential advantages of suctioning are reduced aspiration of secretions and less chance of introducing infection to the respiratory tract. However, disadvantages include cardiac arrhythmias, laryngospasm, and pulmonary artery vasospasm. Respirations normally begin spontaneously. If not, gently rubbing the infant's back is particularly effective in stimulating respirations in the infant with good color and tone.

Immediately drying the infant and maintaining skin-to-skin contact with the mother aids thermoregulation (Gardner, 1979). Research indicates that skin-to-skin contact is preferable to the use of a warmer to maintain a neutral thermal environment for the normal newborn. Infants placed in skin-to-skin contact with their mothers have higher skin and rectal temperatures during the first 45 minutes after delivery when compared with those who have an initial period under the warmer (Fardig, 1980). Wet blankets should be replaced promptly with

Table 23-1 *APGAR Scoring*

	0 points	1 point	2 points
Color	Blue or pale	Acrocyanosis	Completely pink
Resp effort	None	Weak, irregular	Crying, regular
Muscle tone	Limp	Some flexion	Active, motion
Heart rate	Absent	<100	>100
Reflex irritability	None	Sneeze or grimace	Vigorous cry

warm dry ones. Drafts should be eliminated, and the infant's head should remain covered. Any surface in contact with the infant should be warmed.

The practitioner continues assessment by performing the APGAR scoring, physical examination, and gestational age determination. She or he assesses each infant with an APGAR score at 1 and 5 minutes. Using the APGAR system, the infant is rated 0 to 2 for each of the following categories: color, muscle tone, respiratory effort, heart rate, and reflex irritability (Table 23-1).

The 1-minute APGAR score is used to determine the need for resuscitation. Infants with a score less than 7 may need special intervention. Five-minute APGAR scores evaluate the infant's response to resuscitation. They are not predictive of later neurologic functioning. Infants with scores greater than 7 need only observation, warmth, and time to bond with parents.

Newborn Resuscitation

The birth attendant must be prepared for resuscitation at every birth. Approximately 6% of newborns need resuscitation and approximately 30% to 50% of these are unanticipated (Chance and Hanvey, 1987). The practitioner is obliged to have training and regular updates in resuscitation procedures. The Neonatal Advanced Life Support (NALS) course that is jointly offered by the American Heart Association and the American Academy of Pediatrics is highly recommended (Phone (800) AHA-USA1).

The first step to successful resuscitation is readiness. Before each birth, the birth attendant or nurse should check the suction apparatus. It should be confirmed that the pressure gauge is functioning and set at 100 mm Hg. Suction pressures should not exceed 200 mm Hg. A bulb syringe is usually available in delivery packs for use as necessary. A neonatal resuscitation bag with mask and pressure release valve should be connected to an oxygen supply and functioning properly. Oral infant airways sized 00 and 000 should be available. If using an oxygen tank, it should be opened so that a simple twist of the flow meter will begin the flow of oxygen. It should be determined that there is sufficient oxygen in the tank to last for 1 hour. A No. 8 French feeding tube is needed in case prolonged bag and mask ventilation is required.

There are two types of neonatal resuscitation bags: anesthesia and self-inflating. The bags have important differences that the practitioner must understand to properly choose and use equipment. The anesthesia bag is a closed system that does not admit any ambient air into the bag. The concentration of the oxygen that enters the bag is the same concentration delivered to the infant. An advantage of the anesthesia bag is its ability to deliver precise concentrations of oxygen. A disadvantage is that an intact bag and positive pressure of air flow are needed to inflate the bag. If the oxygen source malfunctions and there is no positive-pressure flow of air or if there is a puncture in the bag, it will not inflate, and it is useless. This is an important consideration in out-of-hospital settings.

The self-inflating bag draws ambient air into the bag in addition to air from the oxygen source. Thus it is more difficult to deliver high or very precise concentrations of oxygen. By adding a tail or reservoir to the end of the bag, the concentration of oxygen can be greatly increased and can approach 90% to 100% levels. The self-inflating bag will function even with no oxygen source, so that at least room air with 21% oxygen can be delivered in the event of a malfunctioning oxygen source.

Another critical difference between the two types of bags is important to consider when delivery of free flow of oxygen is needed. When using the anesthesia bag, it is important to remember that the oxygen flows out of the face mask, so this is the part to place near the infant's nose and mouth. With most self-inflating bags, there is a valve that prevents oxygen flow from the mask unless the bag is being squeezed. The tail of the bag must be placed near the infant's nose and mouth to deliver free-flow oxygen. Oxygen is usually cold and can quickly cause drops in the baby's temperature. Thus oxygen should be warmed and humidified if it is needed for any lengthy duration.

A prewarmed, firm surface, warm blankets, and a stethoscope are needed for effective resuscitation. A laryngoscope with No. 0 and 1 blades should be readily available. The functioning of batteries and bulb should be checked before each birth. Endotracheal tubes in sizes 2.5, 3, and 3.5 should be available. A meconium aspirator is ideal for suctioning after intubation. If suctioning with a catheter, it is important to make sure that it is narrow enough to fit through the endotracheal tube. A stylet, tape, and scissors are also helpful for intubation. Although use of resuscitation medications are beyond the scope of this text, it is important to have the following available: epinephrine (1:10,000), naloxone, volume expanders, sodium bicarbonate (5 mEq/10 ml), tubing, catheters, needles, syringes, and tape.

An understanding of the process of asphyxia is needed for rational decision-making. When a fetus/neonate is oxygen deprived, the first response is a series of rapid breathing movements, followed by a period of decreasing heart rate and no breathing efforts. This is called primary apnea. During primary apnea, most infants will respond to free flow oxygen and stimulation. If oxygen deprivation continues, there is a period of deep, gasping respiratory movements while the heart rate and blood pressure continue to fall. Respiratory efforts become progressively weaker until the infant takes a last gasp and secondary apnea ensues (Figure 23-3). Infants in secondary apnea are not likely to respond to stimulation and require positive-pressure ventilation (PPV). A short delay in oxygen delivery will result in long delays before spontaneous respirations begin, thus lengthening resuscitation times. Because the determination of whether the event is primary or secondary apnea can only be made retrospectively, the birth attendant needs to assume secondary apnea until proven otherwise. The pathophysiologic results of asphyxia are oxygen deprivation of tissues, carbon dioxide excess, and metabolic acidosis. The neurologic, renal, and gastrointestinal systems are particularly vulnerable to tissue damage from asphyxia. Time is of the essence for an infant in secondary apnea.

As the infant is born, the clinician assesses color, tone, and respiratory efforts immediately to decide whether to resuscitate. Consideration of the presence of risk factors such as infant size, gestational age, presence of meconium, maternal conditions that compromise placental circulation, or fetal distress during labor should be included in the immediate assessment. If resuscitation is needed, the clinician summons assistance and

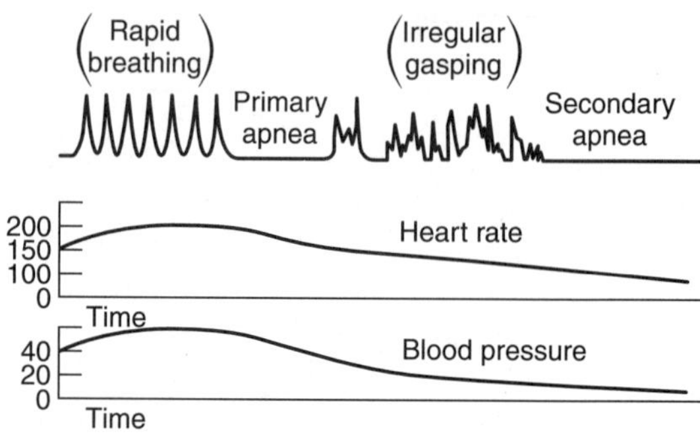

Figure 23-3 Breathing patterns preceding secondary apnea.

takes the infant to a warm flat surface with adequate lighting. The infant is quickly dried with warm towels, and wet towels are removed. When using an overhead warmer, it is best to attach a thermal probe to the infant's skin because often the resuscitator inadvertently blocks the overhead heat source and the infant cools off. Position the infant with his or her neck in a neutral position, avoiding hyperextension or flexion of the neck.

The airway is cleared with either a bulb syringe or a catheter attached to suction apparatus. It is important to suction the oropharynx before the nasopharynx to prevent aspiration of large amounts of debris in case the infant gasps. The clinician should avoid vigorous stimulation of the posterior pharynx since the stimulation elicits a vagal response. The catheter should be passed swiftly but smoothly and gently. Suctioning that is too vigorous traumatizes the airway, causing edema and occlusion.

When there has been thick or particulate meconium in the amniotic fluid, the birth attendant should suction the oropharynx, stomach, and nasopharynx before the birth of the shoulders. The oropharynx and stomach should be suctioned first because the stomach is the largest reservoir of meconium available for aspiration. The nasopharynx comprises very little volume. Immediately after birth, keep stimulation to an absolute minimum. Before the infant's first breath, a practitioner skilled in intubation should visualize the vocal cords and suction if meconium is seen.

After clearing the airway, respiratory effort is assessed. If it is weak or absent, the provider must consider whether the infant is in primary apnea and would respond to stimulation or in secondary apnea and needs PPV without further delay. The entire chain of events leading up to the birth should be reviewed. Heart rate, tone, color, reflex irritability, amniotic fluid, and the umbilical cord are assessed. If the heart rate is less than 100, PPV is indicated. If the rate is above 100, the pulse in the umbilical cord is strong, amniotic fluid is clear, and the cord is plump and healthy looking, stimulation and/or free flow oxygen may induce spontaneous respirations. If there is meconium staining, a weak cord pulsation, or limp, thin cord, the infant may not respond to stimulation. Appropriate forms of stimulation include rubbing the baby's back and flicking the soles of the feet. If stimulation and free flow oxygen do not induce spontaneous respirations, PPV is initiated. It is essential that the infant's face is dry and the appropriate-size mask is used to obtain a good seal around the nose and mouth.

A pressure gauge should be attached to the neonatal resuscitation bag. Pressures of 30 to 40 cm H_2O are needed for the initial breath, and approximately 15 to 20 cm H_2O are needed for subsequent breaths. Insufficient pressures will not open alveoli, and oxygen will not be delivered. Excessive pressures may result in pneumothorax. The resuscitator should watch for the chest rising and falling and have an assistant auscultate the lung fields to ensure that the lungs are being ventilated. If bagging is not aerating the lungs, the baby and mask placement should be repositioned. Inserting an oral airway may remedy the problem. If repeated attempts at bag and mask fail, intubation should be attempted by appropriately prepared personnel. The rate of bagging should be 40 breaths/min. If PPV is needed for longer than 2 minutes, an orogastric tube should be placed to prevent the stomach from filling with air and limiting diaphragmatic excursion.

After 15 to 30 seconds of ventilation, an assistant rechecks the heart rate. If the rate is 60 to 100 and increasing, ventilation is continued. If the heart rate is 60 to 100 and not increasing, adequacy of ventilations should be assessed, and monitoring the heart rate continues. Chest compressions should be initiated if the heart rate drops below 80 beats/min. If the initial heart rate is less than 60 beats/min, chest compressions should be initiated immediately. Compressions should be applied over the lower third of the sternum, avoiding the xiphoid process. Compress ½- to ¾-inch deep at a rate of 120/min. The infant's heart rate should be reevaluated after 30 seconds of compressions and frequently thereafter. Compressions should be continued until the infant spontaneously has a rate of 80 beats/min. Ventilation should be continued until the heart rate is above 100 and spontaneous respirations ensue. If compressions are not sufficient to revive the infant, intubation, umbilical artery catheterization, and medication administration may be necessary. These are procedures that are beyond the scope of this text and ideally left to persons who have many opportunities to practice these skills.

After successful resuscitation, the infant should be monitored for hypoglycemia, hypothermia, and signs of tissue damage. It is appropriate to observe the infant in a nursery setting. Complete documentation of resuscitation, particularly the timing of events, is critical to the subsequent care of the infant.

SUBSEQUENT CARE OF THE NORMAL NEWBORN

Infant Behavioral States

Subsequent care is based on an understanding of the neurobehavioral changes that occur in the newborn. Desmond, Rudolph, and Phitaksphraiwan (1966) were the first to describe the neurobehavioral transition of neonates. The normal, unsedated newborn experiences a period of reactivity immediately after birth that lasts approximately 30 minutes. The infant's eyes are open, and he or she is alert. The heart rate and respiratory rate are slightly increased. The infant's color is variable. Mucus, rales, and rhonchi may be present. The infant is easily startled and may have transient tremors. After the initial phase of reactivity, the infant enters a period of unresponsive sleep. This second phase may last from 20 minutes to 2 hours. The heart rate is decreased, and a systolic murmur is often heard. A third phase, which lasts from 2 to about 6 hours after delivery, is characterized by reactivity. Again, the infant is alert and responsive. Recent research by Ronca, Abel, and Alberts (1996) addresses the critical nature of the first period of reactivity. Multiple stimuli impact the infant before and after birth—proprioceptive stimulation from maternal movement, tactile stimulation during the birth, and environmental stimulation after birth (air, cold, cord occlusion). In response, human infants have a surge of catecholamines and a state of heightened stimulation. The authors assert that this alertness plays a key role in assisting the transition to extrauterine life by inducing specific behaviors necessary for survival. For example, tactile stimulation is particularly associated with the production and release of catecholamines, which in turn is associated with the onset of respirations. The arousal state also facilitates the early learning associated with feeding. It has been demonstrated that a newborn placed between its mother's breasts during the first phase of reactivity will locate the nipple without assistance.

Initiating Breast-feeding

Initiating breast-feeding during the first phase of reactivity optimizes chances of success. During the second stage of unresponsive sleep, breast-feeding attempts are likely to fail, undermining maternal confidence. Furthermore, early feeding decreases the risk of neonatal hypoglycemia, which may occur during the physiologic nadir of blood sugar at 1 to 1½ hours after birth. Delayed initiation of breast-feeding is associated with increased supplementation and shorter periods of breast-feeding (Hossain et al., 1995). Mothers who initiate breast-feeding within 2 hours after delivery are the most likely to exclusively breast-feed during the infant's first 11 weeks of life. Mothers who breast-fed within the first hour after delivery breast-fed considerably longer than mothers who delayed initiation of breast-feeding (de Chateau and Wiberg, 1977). Other trials consistently report higher breast-feeding rates at 13 months in women who were allowed to have early extra contact with their infants (Illingworth et al., 1952; Salariya, Easton, and Carter, 1978; Sousa et al., 1974; Taylor et al., 1985; Thomson, Hartsock, and Larson, 1979).

Normal infants are born with intact rooting and sucking reflexes. They are able to coordinate sucking and swallowing. Bursts of sucking are followed by brief pauses for swallowing. The infant must learn to suck long enough to stimulate the milk let-down and ejection processes in the mother. The birth attendant can assist the mother with positioning herself and her infant in a way that enhances breast-feeding efforts. It is important to teach the mother about the rooting reflex. If the corner of the infant's mouth is stroked, the infant will turn its head in that direction and open its mouth widely. When the roof of the infant's mouth is touched by the nipple, the infant will suck. Once the infant has latched on, it is important not to stroke the cheeks since this may re-elicit the rooting reflex and the infant will lose its grasp on the nipple. It is important to teach the mother that it takes some time to learn successful latching on. Otherwise mothers may misinterpret the normal learning phase as a problem with breast-feeding.

Parent-Infant Bonding

The first period of reactivity is also critical for the development of the parent-child relationship. Research demonstrates that early extra contact between mother and infant positively affects the relationship. Klaus and Kennell (1976) were the first to popularize the notion of a "sensitive period" soon after birth. They found that mothers who had extra contact with their infants soon after birth demonstrated more affectionate behaviors and expressed more concern for their infants at 1 month. Extra early contact is associated with more attentiveness by mothers during a standardized physical examination at 1 year (Taylor et al., 1985), and mothers with poor social supports who experience early contact with their infants demonstrate increased affectionate behaviors (Anisfield and Lipper, 1983). Early maternal infant contact is also associated with a decrease in child abuse, neglect, and failure to thrive (O'Connor et al., 1980). Conversely, several researchers have noted less affectionate behavior, feelings of incompetence, and lack of confidence in the mothers they studied who had limited early contact with their infants (Hales et al., 1977; Gomez-Pedro et al., 1984; Greenburg, Rosenberg, and Lind, 1973; Grossman, Thane, and Grossman, 1981; Kontos, 1978). Thus it is important to provide initial care to the infant without separating mother and child.

Vital Signs, Weight, and Medications

Ongoing assessment of the physiologic transition to extrauterine life is important. Research is lacking regarding the optimal frequency for obtaining vital signs. The first set is done within the first 30 minutes while the infant is still on the mother's abdomen. Thereafter, vital signs are obtained at least every 30 minutes until the neonate has remained stable for 2 hours (AAP and ACOG, 1997). Once stable, they can be obtained every 4 to 8 hours. The infant's color, muscle tone, and respiratory efforts are assessed at the same time.

The practitioner must obtain an accurate birth weight, administer newborn medications, and perform a thorough assessment of the infant. Timing is important. Infant feeding and bonding are the first priorities in the healthy neonate and must not be interrupted for the convenience of the care providers.

An accurate birth weight is important because it helps to identify potential health problems, provides a comparison for later assessment of the infant, and guides the provider in calculating appropriate medication dosages for the newborn. The weight can be delayed until after the first feeding for a normal term infant who appears grossly well nourished. Infants who fall below the tenth percentile for their cohort group are classified as small-for-gestational-age (SGA). Infants weighing less than 2500 g are classified as low-birth-weight, and infants weighing less than 1500 g are considered very low–birth-weight. Infants above the 90th percentile are classified large-for-gestational-age (LGA). Both LGA and SGA infants are at increased risk for selected neonatal problems and need closer monitoring. Box 23-1 lists the morbidities associated with each.

Vitamin K

It is the standard of practice to administer vitamin K during the first 2 hours of life to prevent hemorrhagic dis-

Box 23-1 *Morbidity Associated with LGA and SGA Infants*

Morbidity Associated with LGA Infants	Morbidity Associated with SGA Infants
Asphyxia	Asphyxia
Birth injury (fractured clavicle, brachial plexus injury, facial palsy)	Chromosomal anomalies, especially trisomies and Turner syndrome
Respiratory distress syndrome (infants of diabetic mothers)	Congenital malformations, especially CNS and skeletal systems
Transposition of great vessels	Congenital infections, especially rubella and CMV
Beckwith-Wiedemann syndrome	Substance withdrawal
Erythroblastosis fetalis	Meconium aspiration
Hyperinsulinism/hypoglycemia	Pulmonary hemorrhage
Polycythemia	Persistent pulmonary hypertension
Meconium aspiration	Hypothermia
	Hypoglycemia, hypocalcemia, hyponatremia
	Polycythemia
	Long term: poor growth, neurologic, and developmental delays

From DeWayne M., Pursley DM, Hohn P: Identifying the high-risk newborn. In Cloherty JP, Stark AR, editors: *Manual of neonatal care,* ed. 3, Boston, 1991, Little, Brown, pp. 95-101.

ease of the newborn (HDNB). Vitamin K is a co-factor in coagulation and is produced by bacteria in the gut. Until gut colonization is accomplished, the infant is at risk for bleeding. Because there is less vitamin K in breast milk than in formula, breast-fed infants are more likely to be affected. HDNB is classified as early, classic, or late. Early disease begins within 24 hours of the birth. Classic disease presents in the first 7 days, and late occurs 1 to 12 months after birth. Problems range from gastrointestinal bleeding and ecchymoses to intracranial hemorrhage. Estimates of the incidence of HDNB range from 0.25% to 1.7% (Oski and Naiman,1972; Brousson and Klein,1996). Infants at increased risk of HDNB include preterm infants and infants experiencing traumatic deliveries. Administration of 1 mg of vitamin K intramuscularly virtually eliminates the disease, with the incidence decreasing to 0.25/100,000 live births. The injection is administered via tuberculin syringe into the vastus lateralis muscle, taking care to aspirate before injection. In 1990 Golding, Paterson, and Kinlen raised the concern of pediatric cancer after intramuscular administration of vitamin K after their study found an association between vitamin K administration and increased chromatid exchanges in human placental lymphocytes in vitro. Sutor, Dagres, and Niederhoff (1995) corroborated the findings regarding extremely high dosage of vitamin K injections intramuscularly but found no correlation between oral vitamin K administration and pediatric cancer. Three subsequent studies (Ekelund, Finnstrom, and Gunnarskog, 1993; Klebanoff et al., 1993; Olsen, Hertz, and Blinkenberg, 1994) did not support the concern for pediatric cancer when normal intramuscular dosages were studied. However, the researchers point out that the numbers of pediatric cancers were so small overall that an association cannot absolutely be ruled out. Oral administration of vitamin K as a means of protecting the neonate from injection-related pain has been studied in Europe and Canada (O'Connor and Addeigo, 1986). The single oral dose does not prove to be a viable alternative. It is only protective for 4 weeks and does not sufficiently cover the period of greatest vulnerability for late onset HDNB, which occurs at 3 at 8 weeks. With no prophylaxis at all, the incidence of late hemorrhagic disease is 4.4 to 7.1/100,000. After a single oral dose of vitamin K, the risk is only decreased to 1.4 to 6.4/100,000. Almost all late hemolytic disease is seen in breast-fed infants. Motohara, Endo, and Matsuda (1986) found that giving two 5-mg oral doses, one at birth and one at 2 weeks, resulted in only 3.4% of infants with low vitamin K levels at 4 weeks. This is similar to the 5.5% of infants who had a vitamin K deficiency at 4 weeks after a 1-mg IM dose (Hathaway, Isarangkura, and Mahasandana, 1991). Henderson-Smart (1994) recommends 1-mg oral doses at birth, 3 to 5 days, and 4 weeks after delivery. Although repeated oral doses appear to be a viable alternative to intramuscular vitamin K, more study is needed to clarify dosages and timing.

Neonatal Ophthalmia Prophylaxis

Administration of an agent to prevent ophthalmia neonatorum is standard practice, even though controlled trials are lacking to support prophylactic treatment over clinical observation and treatment based on symptomatology. Instillation of 0.5% erythromycin ointment, ½ inch strip in each eye 1 to 2 hours after birth, is the most common practice because it is effective in treating both chlamydia and gonorrhea. Infections can also be caused by *Haemophilus influenzae, Staphylococcus aureus, Escherichia coli,* and *Pseudomonas* (Nsanze et al., 1996; Gao, 1993). Studies evaluating the effectiveness of prophylaxis using povidone iodine, 1% silver nitrate, erythromycin ointment, and tetracycline ointment have failed to provide evidence that one particular method is superior (Chen, 1992; Isenberg, Apt, and Wood, 1995). Findings suggest that more study is needed regarding the epidemiology of neonatal ophthalmia in different geographic locations and the effectiveness of different agents in preventing infection. Eye prophylaxis should be deferred until after the first period of reactivity when the neonate is awake and taking in the visual stimuli around him or her.

INITIAL NEONATAL ASSESSMENT

A thorough neonatal assessment includes history, physical examination, and gestational age assessment. Examination is normally deferred during the first phase of reactivity because it interferes with feeding and bonding and causes undue fatigue and stress. The infant may be relatively unresponsive during the second phase of reactivity. Thus the examination is best accomplished during the third phase, while the infant is quiet and alert.

It is important to review the maternal and infant medical records and interview the caregiver(s) to obtain a complete history. Categories include maternal and paternal family history, past obstetric history, history of this infant's gestation, social and community assessment, labor and delivery history, and neonatal history.

Family History

Family history should be obtained prenatally and reviewed before the newborn assessment. Box 23-2 lists conditions that may have genetic implications.

Past Obstetric History

The mother's past obstetric history for age, sex, and number of siblings should be reviewed. Family constellation has an impact on family adjustment. History of congenital anomalies, jaundice, or other perinatal morbidity/mortality should be noted since some conditions increase the risk of this infant also experiencing the complication. Current health of siblings should be elicited, and circumstances surrounding siblings who do not live in the household should be explored. Any history of postpartum depression or difficulty parenting should be identified, and referrals made as appropriate.

Box 23-2 *Conditions to Identify in Family History*

Cystic fibrosis
Phenylketonuria
Sickle cell disease
Metabolic disorders
Hemophilia
Polycystic kidney
Congenital anomalies
Perinatal deaths

Box 23-3 *Maternal Risk Factors Associated With Neonatal Problems*

Maternal Illnesses	Maternal Infections
Hypertension	Tuberculosis
Cardiac disease	Syphilis
Diabetes	Gonorrhea
Anemia	Chlamydia
Renal disease	Group B streptococcus
Asthma	Hepatitis B or C
Isoimmunization	Human immunodeficiency virus
Vaginal bleeding	Herpes
Affective disorders	Varicella
Substance use	

History of Current Infant's Gestation

Maternal blood type, Rh, and antibody screen should be identified to assess the risk of hemolytic disease for the infant. Maternal history of medical illnesses or infections that may have compromised the fetus should be identified. The timing and amount of any exposure to teratogens such as radiation, solvents, fumes, chemicals, or drugs should be noted. The results of fetal diagnostic tests should also be reviewed (Box 23-3).

Social/Environmental Assessment

Social environment and parenting ability greatly affect the health of the newborn. It is important to have an understanding of the family context into which the infant must integrate. The mother's age, language, and educational level may influence her ability to effectively communicate with her care providers. Identification of the people she considers her family and support is important when considering the cultural influence on childrearing practices. The number of people living in the home, the size and nature of the dwelling, and the relationships of the people to the mother should be reviewed, as well as the availability of food, cooking facilities, refrigeration, heat, water, electricity, bathroom facilities, and transportation. The home and community assessment should also identify dangers or potential dangers such as emotional, physical, or sexual violence. The presence of mental illness or substance abuse may compromise parenting. Ideally a home visit is done for every family during the postpartum period.

Labor and Birth History

The history of the labor and birth should be reviewed. The gestational age at time of birth, length of labor, fetal presentation, and route of delivery should be noted. Prolonged rupture of membranes, maternal fever, and foul amniotic fluid are significant risk factors for or predictors of neonatal infection. Meconium-stained amniotic fluid increases the risk for respiratory disease. Medications during labor such as analgesics, anesthetics, magnesium sulfate, and glucose may affect the newborn's behavior and metabolism. The infant's sex, birth weight, and APGAR scores are noted, as well as any resuscitation needed. Certain abnormalities of the placenta and a two-vessel cord are associated with increased incidence of neonatal anomalies. The amount and quality of time the infant spent with the parent(s) immediately after birth, as well as the quality of the attachment behaviors, are important to note.

Neonatal History

The history of the infant since birth should be reviewed, including patterns of feeding, voiding, stooling, sleeping, and crying. Vital signs, medications given to the newborn, and laboratory results such as blood type, hematocrit, glucose, cord pH, or arterial blood gases should be reviewed.

PHYSICAL EXAMINATION

The practitioner is encouraged to develop a system for physical examination and practice it consistently to prevent omissions. The order of the components of the examination should depend on infant behavior and comfort. For example, adequate assessment of the heart and lungs is not possible when the infant is crying. Likewise, examination of the eyes and superficial palpation of the abdomen are not done when the infant is crying. Thus these areas are often examined first before the baby is disturbed. The infant must be kept warm when exposed. Take time to warm hands and instruments. Practitioners' hands are the most common source of infectious pathogens and should be thoroughly washed before each infant contact. If they are present, parents should be involved in the physical examination since it is an excellent teaching opportunity.

General Appearance

The first step is to carefully observe the general appearance of the baby at rest. The examiner should note the tone, color, expression, and behavior. The healthy term neonate demonstrates adduction and flexion of the extremities. The infant's cry is strong and lusty. This initial assessment addresses the question, "Is this baby healthy or sick?" An infant who is able to nurse frequently and vigorously is most often healthy. If this is not the initial examination, the present weight should be compared to previous weights. The normal newborn may lose up to 10% of birth weight during the first few days of life, but should regain the weight by 2 weeks after delivery. Thereafter weight gain varies individually, but an average of 160 g/week is normal during the first months. Weight loss after the first week or failure to gain weight warrants further investigation.

Anthropomorphic Measurements

The infant's length is measured from tip of head to heel, making sure that the legs are fully extended. Length is then plotted on a growth chart, where it can be compared with weight to determine whether growth has been appropriate. Head circumference is obtained with the tape measure around the occiput, at the top of the ears, and at the top of the eyebrows. Chest circumference is measured at the nipple line. Normally the head circumference is slightly larger than the chest circumference. Head circumference should be compared to previous measures, bearing in mind that marked molding at birth may alter the measurements. Increasing head circumference may indicate increased intracranial pressure. Head and chest circumferences are also plotted on a growth chart to assess normalcy.

Temperature can be taken via the axilla or rectum or electronically via the ear. Rectal temperatures reflect the core body temperature but carry the risk of trauma. Axillary temperatures are normally 1° cooler than the core temperature: 36.5° to 37.5° C (97.7° to 99.5° F). A drop in temperature or temperature instability may indicate serious infection. Normally the infant's respiratory rate is 30 to 60 breaths/min, and the heart rate is 120 to 160 beats/min when at rest. Since the neonate's respirations and heart rate normally fluctuate as the infant responds to the variety of stimulation during the examination, the examiner should attempt to count the rates for a full minute.

Integument

Skin color, temperature, and texture should be assessed. Any normal skin variations should be noted and explained to the parents. The presence of vernix caseosa, a creamy white material composed of sebum and desquamated epithelium cells, is common in the skin folds and creases of term infants. Lanugo—fine hair over the back, forehead, and ears—is also common. Milia are tiny yellow or white papules commonly found on the chin and face, resulting from collections of sebaceous material in the skin. Erythema toxicum is characterized by areas of redness with small white or yellow papules superimposed. It usually presents during the first 24 to 48 hours and may last from a few hours to days. It is most common on the face, trunk, or extremities and often migrates to other areas of the body. Acrocyanosis is a blueness of the hands and feet caused by vasomotor immaturity within the first 48 hours. Mongolian spots are hyperpigmented areas most commonly found over the buttocks and back in dark-skinned babies. This pigmentation may continue to be apparent for up to 2 years. Telangiectasia, also known as simple nevi or "stork bites," are small red lesions that most often appear over the glabella, eyelids, and nape of the neck. They are dilated capillaries and usually disappear by age 2.

A port-wine nevus, or nevus flammeus, is a flat red or purple lesion usually located on the face. It is benign, but may affect the infant's appearance and usually does not resolve. A strawberry nevus is a raised, red capillary and endothelial cell lesion, usually located on the head and neck. It may alarm parents when it enlarges over the first 6 months before it gradually recedes over several years. Most often surgical removal is not necessary. Café-au-lait spots are light brown macular lesions that are benign when small. Larger (>3 cm) or multiple (>6) café-au-lait spots are associated with neurofibromatosis.

Central cyanosis is never normal and requires immediate medical evaluation. When petechiae are noted, the location and pattern usually gives a clue to their origin. The most common cause is traumatic birth or tight nuchal cord. Generalized petechiae are worrisome and may indicate serious neonatal infection. Plethora is a sign of elevated hematocrit. This is more serious when severe or when the infant is dehydrated. Both generalized petechiae and plethora require medical consultation.

Head

The infant's skull is made up of 13 bones, including two frontal bones, two parietal bones, and one occipital bone. The bones can often be felt overriding each other at birth, making fontanelles smaller or difficult to feel. By the first postpartum day, both fontanelles should be easily palpable and neither bulging nor retracting. A pulse may be felt over the fontanelles. The entire scalp should be palpated and inspected. Caput succedaneum is a common finding. It is swelling of the scalp due to the pressures of birth. Caput may cross suture lines, but cephalohematoma, another common finding, does not. Cephalohematoma is extravasation of blood between the periosteum and the skull. It may increase in size during the first days after delivery and then is gradually resorbed over several weeks. It does not cause intracranial pressure, but, if large, it can contribute to jaundice. Craniotabes is a small soft area on the skull. When depressed, it causes a snapping sensation similar to pressing on a ping-pong ball. Craniotabes usually disappears in days and is rarely associated with other abnormalities. Lesions from a scalp electrode and abrasions, lacerations, or bruising that occurred during the birth may be present. These should be documented and observed for possible infection.

The infant's face should be carefully inspected. Asymmetry of expression may indicate nerve palsy. A small degree of asymmetry may be a result of uterine positioning. Eyebrows, eyelashes, and a normal hairline should be present. A prominent or narrow flat forehead is suggestive of chromosomal anomaly. Micrognathia, or markedly small chin, is associated with Pierre Robin syndrome.

Placement of the eyes should be noted. Hypertelorism is associated with fetal alcohol syndrome and phenytoin exposure. Epicanthal folds, although normal in Asian infants, may be associated with chromosomal anomalies. Pupils should be equal and reactive to light. Presence of a red reflex indicates a normal cornea and lens. Absence may indicate cataract, retinoblastoma, or glaucoma. To elicit the red reflex, the examiner shines a light in the pupil, and a red/orange color is seen as a result of light reflecting back from the retina. The iris should be inspected for intactness. White spots on the iris, known as Brushfield's spots, are associated with trisomy 21 (Down syndrome). The sclera should be examined. Small hemorrhages are normal and should be discussed with parents. Redness of the conjunctiva may indicate infection. Intermittent nystagmus, or oscillation of the eyes, is normal and is caused neurologic immaturity. Continuous "nystagmus" may actually be seizure activity and should be investigated. Strabismus, or crossed eyes, is caused by uncoordinated eye muscles and usually resolves, although it should be documented and followed up. Setting sun sign, a downward gaze that allows visualization of the sclera above the iris, is ominous and indicates increased intracranial pressure.

The position, shape, and size of the ears should be closely inspected. The front and back of the ear should be assessed. Multiple skin tags or sinuses may indicate congenital anomalies of the ear and occasionally the urogenital tract. A Darwin tubercle is a small bump on the upper helix and is normal. Low-set ears are associated with chromosomal anomalies. The ears should attach at the point of a horizontal line drawn from the outer canthus of the eye. The cartilage should be firm and well developed. Preterm infants lack cartilage and full incurvation of the pinna. A large flabby ear may be associated with renal agenesis. Gross hearing should be intact. The infant should startle with loud noises and is capable of turning attention in the direction of a familiar voice.

The nose should be assessed for symmetry and patency. The nose should be midline, and the mucous membranes should be pink and moist. Neonates are nose breathers, and patency must be determined. The examiner should block each naris while the infant's mouth is closed to ensure that air flows freely through the opposite naris. Inability to note air passage, along with inability to pass a catheter through each nostril, may indicate choanal atresia.

The mouth should be assessed using inspection and palpation. The lips and their movement should be symmetric. The entire hard and soft palate and uvula for clefts should be inspected. This is best accomplished by shining a light in the mouth while the infant is crying. It is not sufficient to simply palpate the roof of the mouth, because some small clefts of the soft palate may be missed. Sucking blisters, Epstein pearls, and teeth are normal variations. Epstein pearls are small, round white growths of epithelial tissue that disappear spontaneously. Loose teeth present at birth ("natal teeth") are best removed to prevent aspiration. The frenulum should not be short or thickened since this may interfere with nursing and speech development. Occasionally cysts are noted under the tongue. They are usually benign and will resolve spontaneously. The infant should have a strong suck reflex. Profuse saliva and a large tongue are suggestive of chromosomal anomaly and require medical evaluation. Profuse saliva is also associated with tracheoesophageal fistula or atresia. Sores or plaques should be evaluated further.

The entire neck should be inspected and palpated. The infant should have full and symmetric range of motion. Masses may represent a cystic hygroma, which is cystic lymph tissue. It usually requires surgical intervention unless it is very small. Webbing is associated with Turner syndrome. A palpable thyroid is abnormal and needs further evaluation. The full length of the clavicles should be palpated, and crepitus indicates fracture.

Upper Extremities

The upper extremities are assessed for size and mobility. The sizes of each bone should be in proportion to the size of the rest of the limb and the body in general. Limbs should be symmetric. There should be 10 digits. The palm should be opened entirely to check for extra digits and palmar creases. A single simian crease is associated with trisomy 21. Syndactyly is the fusion or omission of digits, and polydactyly indicates extra digits. Fingernails should be present on each digit and in term infants; they may extend over the end of the fingers. The brachial pulses should be equal. The normal infant is born with a strong grasp reflex, and the upper extremities are flexed on each other with good tone when the infant is in the quiet alert state.

Thorax, Respiratory, and Cardiovascular Assessment

The infant's chest is assessed using inspection, palpation, and auscultation. The shape of the thorax should be assessed. Normally the anteroposterior diameter is equal to the transverse diameter. Depression or protrusion of the sternum warrants further investigation. The xiphoid process may be seen in normal neonates because of the thinness of the chest wall. Breast and nipple placement should be assessed. Supernumerary nipples are generally normal, may be more common in dark-skinned infants, and usually do not contain breast tissue. The size of the breast bud should be palpated. The term infant usually has greater than 5 mm of breast tissue. The breast bud may be enlarged or leaking fluid in the male or female infant. It is important to educate parents that this is a normal, transient effect of maternal estrogen. Widely spaced nipples are often noted in Turner syndrome.

The axilla should be palpated, and small nodes may be noted in some healthy neonates. Neonates who have been exposed to the human immunodeficiency virus (HIV) may have axillary lymphadenopathy.

Respirations should appear unlabored. There should be no intercostal, substernal, or suprasternal retractions or nasal flaring. During normal inspiration the abdomen may rise slightly before the chest rises. Movements should be symmetric and even. See-saw respirations are a sign of respiratory distress. During see-saw respirations, the abdomen rises while the chest is depressed or "pulled" inward.

Respirations should be auscultated anteriorly and posteriorly with the warmed diaphragm of the stethoscope. Because of the small chest cavity, breath sounds are bronchial, and transmitted upper airway sound may be noted. Respiratory rate should be determined, and the breath sounds of the upper, middle, and lower lung fields are evaluated. The right and left sides should be equal. The lower lobes are best heard over the infant's back. An area of decreased breath sounds may indicate a pneumothorax or blockage of the bronchi supporting that area. Louder breath sounds are heard over areas of consolidation such as atelectasis or a solid mass. Fine rales or crackles are most often normal during the first hour after delivery. Persistent rales, rhonchi, rubs, wheezes, grunting, and stridor need further investigation.

Auscultation of the heart is done by inching one's way across the chest in a Z pattern, beginning at the right sternal border in the second intercostal space and ending on the left chest at the point of maximum impulse near the left nipple. Both the diaphragm and the bell of the stethoscope should be used. The rate, rhythm, and any murmurs should be noted. A grade II systolic murmur in the first days of life is most often normal. Diastolic murmurs, rubs, thrills, and clicks need further investigation. The point of maximal impulse may be found more laterally (to the left) in the neonate than in the adult. This is normal and does not indicate pulmonary hypertension. The precordium may be active the first hours of life, but thereafter it should be quiet. Perfusion to the extremities should be evaluated. They should be warm and pink and have quick capillary refill. Peripheral edema is not normally seen, except in unusual birth presentations. The brachial and femoral pulse should be present but not bounding. By checking the right brachial and femoral pulses simultaneously, inequalities or lags may be noted, suggesting coarctation of the aorta. The blood pressure is not usually assessed in a normal newborn but is essential if the infant is ill.

Abdomen

The abdomen is assessed using inspection, auscultation, and both light and deep palpation. The examiner begins by inspecting the contour, size, and muscle tone of the abdomen. Any obvious masses must be investigated. The abdominal skin should be intact. Normally the abdomen is symmetric, soft, and rounded. It should not be protruding or sunken. Auscultation of all four quadrants with the bell of the stethoscope should identify bowel sounds. Bowel sounds appear as early as 15 minutes after birth. Normally, gurgling sounds are heard every 10 to 20 seconds. Either absent or hyperactive bowel sounds not associated with a recent feeding may be associated with obstruction or other pathology and require medical evaluation. Immediately after feeding, hyperactive bowel sounds may be normal. The entire abdomen is then lightly palpated systematically. The infant must be quiet and relaxed. Masses, increased or decreased tone, and painful areas should be noted. Palpation on the right side is used to identify the liver edge. Normally it is smooth, firm, and mobile. The examiner must palpate lightly and with exquisite attention, starting at the groin and moving upward. The liver margin is usually 1 to 2 cm below the ribs on the right side. The spleen may be palpable on the left, but it is mobile and difficult to distinguish. With initial palpation the spleen is often under the ribs and will not be felt. Although as many as 25% of infants have palpable spleens, palpation greater than 1 cm below the costal margin is abnormal. Light palpation should be continued systematically until the entire abdomen has been covered. A continuously distended bladder, usually felt below the umbilicus, is not normal. Deep palpation is necessary to locate the kidneys. The left kidney is usually easier to palpate because the right kidney is beneath the liver. One technique to palpate kidneys is to place four fingers behind the infant's back and wrap the thumb around the front, beneath the costal margin. Use the other hand to gently raise the infant from a lying to semi-sitting position as the palpating hand squeezes the fingers and thumb together. The kidney should feel like a small cherry sliding between the thumb and fingers as the infant's head is raised and lowered. Palpation of the abdomen is a skill that requires much practice. It generally disturbs the infant and should be done toward the end of the examination.

The umbilical cord is inspected, and the presence of three vessels should be determined. The cord begins to dry within several hours of birth and is usually shriveled and blackened by the second to third day of life. Foul odor, redness, or purulent discharge at the base of the cord is associated with infection.

Umbilical and inguinal hernias are common alterations. Umbilical hernias are caused by persistent separation of the recti muscles and are most common in black boys. They are most apparent when the infant cries. Parents should be educated that they will usually resolve by age 2 or 3. Inguinal hernias should be evaluated to see if the herniated contents can be reduced. Surgery may be necessary for large, persistent hernias or in the case of strangulation of herniated tissue. Many abdominal abnormalities may be first identified by a careful examination as outlined in preceding paragraphs. Any suspect examination findings should be further evaluated by a physician skilled in neonatal assessment. It is notable that many abdominal abnormalities are associated with anomalies of the urogenital tract.

Lower Extremities

The infant's hips should be evaluated for congenital dislocation using the Ortolani and Barlow techniques. With the infant's knee flexed, the examiner grasps the thigh with the thumb on the inner thigh and the fingers wrapped around the outside of the leg. The middle fingers are positioned directly over the infant's greater trochanters. The examiner then abducts the infant's hips while feeling for a clunk produced by the dislocated hip slipping back into the acetabulum. Normally the examiner should be able to abduct the infant's hips so that the knee is within 10 degrees of the examining surface. The infant's knees are then brought back together while outward pressure is applied on the infant's thighs to feel for a clunk, indicating that the hip has dislocated. Infants born in the breech position are at increased risk for congenital hip dislocation. The infant must be cooperative and not kicking for accurate results. If a dislocated hip escapes detection and remains uncorrected, the normal functioning of the legs is at risk. The length of the bones in the lower extremities should be evaluated for appropriateness in relation to the rest of the infant's body. Creases should be assessed to ensure symmetry. Incurvation of the calves and ankles may be normal. If the torsion can be gently reduced by the examiner, it is likely to be transient and related to the position in utero. Normally the extremities are flexed with good tone and full range of motion. Infants born in the breech presentation may have hyperextended knees and hyperflexed hips. Creases on the sole of the foot and number of digits should be assessed.

Genitalia

In the female infant the prominence of labia majora, minora, and clitoris should be noted. The vagina is inspected for patency by separating the labia and inspecting the introitus. Hymenal tags are common and generally resolve. There may be mucoid or slight bloody discharge noted 2 to 7 days of age. Parents should be advised that this is a normal, transient effect of maternal estrogen. The labia and inguinal areas should be palpated for masses. If urination is observed, it should be a steady stream running over the vulva. Decreased flow or a dribble should be investigated further.

The location of the urethral meatus should be noted in the male neonate. It should be directly at the tip of the penis. Hypospadias describes a ventrally located meatus. If slight, it may not cause dysfunction. If severe, it may need surgical correction. Epispadias describes the dorsally located meatus. It is more often associated with other anomalies and warrants investigation. The foreskin is normally adherent to the glans, and retraction should not be attempted. The scrotum may be edematous or enlarged. Hydrocele, fluid surrounding the testicle, is a common occurrence and usually resolves by 1 year of age. The examiner should determine the location of both testes. Undescended testes often spontaneously resolve but should be monitored over time. The flow of urine should be a strong, continuous stream. Erections are a normal occurrence. Parents should be advised that the size of the testes and scrotum at birth are not predictive of size as the infant matures. It is normal to note a small amount of orange-red coloration on the diaper of a male infant caused by passage of crystals in the urine as a result of lack of tubular resorption of solute.

Back

The patency of the anus should be determined, and passage of meconium confirms patency. The infant should be turned over so that the examiner can inspect the gluteal folds for symmetry. Asymmetric folds may indicate hip or limb abnormality. The buttocks should be separated and assessed for dimples and sinuses that may indicate spinal cord anomalies. The presence of a dimple with a tuft of hair is suspect. The spine should be palpated for masses. The presence and amount of lanugo should be noted. The infant's muscle tone can be assessed with ventral suspension. It is normal for the infant to hold head up only for a several seconds, but there should be good tone in the rest of the spinal muscles. Drooping or floppiness is not normal in the term infant.

Neurologic Assessment

A full neurologic assessment is not necessary in the normal term infant. Much of the assessment has already been done in the physical examination. Normally the infant moves through the following behavioral states in an orderly fashion: deep sleep, light sleep, quiet alert, active alert, and crying. The newborn is able to look toward a familiar voice when in the quiet alert phase, and should be startled by loud noises. The infant can distinguish smells as demonstrated by the preference for its own mother's milk absorbed on breast pads over pads from other mothers. The infant is normally in a flexed posture and has full and equal range of motion and strength. The cry is neither weak nor high pitched and shrill. The suck is strong and coordinated with the swallow. The grasp reflex of the fingers and toes is strong. The Moro reflex is intact and is elicited by supporting the infant in a sitting position and then rapidly moving her or him to a supine position. The normal newborn responds first by extending the arms with the fingers forming a C-shape and then flexing the arms again. The Babinski reflex is assessed by stroking the infant's foot from heel to little toe and then stroking toward the great toe. The normal response is for the infant to fan the toes. The stepping reflex is elicited by holding the infant upright and touching feet on a solid surface. The infant will raise and lower its feet in a walking pattern.

With the general physical assessment is complete, the gestational age assessment is done. Both the Dubowitz and the Ballard scales provide accurate gestational age assessment within a 2-week margin of error. The Ballard is described here because of its simplicity. There are six tests of neuromuscular maturity and signs of physical maturity that are assessed. Use the score sheet depicted in Figure 23-4. Mark the boxes that most closely correspond to the infant's behavior. Total the scores and note which gestational age most closely corresponds with the infant's score.

Guidance for neurologic scoring. When assessing posture, if there is a discrepancy between the upper and lower extremities, use the upper extremities unless there is a known injury of the upper extremities. When assessing the square window, gently flex the wrist on itself and note the angle formed by the ulna and the little finger. When eliciting arm recoil, flex the infant's arms at the elbows and hold them for at least 6 seconds. Then rapidly extend the elbow and let go of the infant's arms. Note the angle of the elbow when the arms are most flexed. When assessing the popliteal angle, make sure the hips remain on the mattress. Gently apply pressure on the infant's heel to extend the knee. Note the angle of the knee when you feel resistance. When assessing scarf sign, keep the infant's shoulders on the mattress. Grasp the infant's hands and gently guide the arm across the chest. Note the location of the infant's elbow in relation to the chest when resistance is felt. To assess heel to ear, grasp the infant's foot and raise it toward the ear until resistance is felt. Note the angle of the leg and how close the heel is to the head.

Choose the description of the skin, lanugo, and plantar creases that best corresponds to the infant. Palpate and measure the diameter of the breast bud. Do not pinch; rather, palpate them flat, noting where they begin and end in order to measure. Fold the pinna of the ear and then let go to assess ear cartilage. Observe the infant's genitalia and check the box that best describes the infant.

Once the gestational age is known, plot it on the length, weight, and head circumference graphs to assess if the infant is average-for-gestational-age, SGA, or LGA.

Once the physical and gestational age assessments are completed and the infant is found to be normal, the focus of care is maintaining and promoting optimal health. Educating and supporting parents in their role is key to this endeavor. It is critical to use language that the parents understand and to recognize cultural aspects of parenting that may influence parenting style and expectations.

Infant Feeding

Parents must be given accurate information regarding infant feeding choices in order to make informed decisions. Breast-feeding has several well-documented advantages over bottle feeding. Human milk contains whey proteins, which produce less curd in the stomach and are more easily absorbed than the proteins in formula. Fifty percent of the caloric content of breast milk is lipid-based. Although both human milk and cow's milk are low in iron, the iron in human milk is better absorbed by the infant. Human milk contains taurine, a neurotransmitter important for brain growth. It contains growth

Maturational Assessment of Gestational Age (New Ballard Score)

Name ____________ Date/time of birth ____________ Sex ____________
Hospital no. ____________ Date/time of exam ____________ Birth weight ____________
Race ____________ Age when examined ____________ Length ____________
Apgar score: 1 minute ________ 5 minutes ________ 10 minutes ________ Head circ. ____________
Examiner ____________

Neuromuscular Maturity

Neuromuscular maturity sign	Score -1	0	1	2	3	4	5	Record score here
Posture								
Square window (wrist)	>90¡	90¡	60¡	45¡	30¡	0¡		
Arm recoil		180¡	140¡-180¡	110¡-140¡	90¡-110¡	<90¡		
Popliteal angle	180¡	160¡	140¡	120¡	100¡	90¡	<90¡	
Scarf sign								
Heel to ear								

Total Neuromuscular Activity Score ______

Score:
Neuromuscular ____
Physical ________
Total ________

Maturity Rating

Score	Weeks
-10	20
-5	22
0	24
5	26
10	28
15	30
20	32
25	34
30	36
35	38
40	40
45	42
50	44

Gestational Age (weeks)
By dates ________
By ultrasound ______
By exam ________

Physical Maturity

Physical maturity sign	Score -1	0	1	2	3	4	5	Record score here
Skin	sticky friable transparent	gelatinous red translucent	smooth pink visible veins	superficial peeling and/or rash few veins	cracking pale areas rare veins	parchment deep cracking no vessels	leathery cracked wrinkled	
Lanugo	none	sparse	abundant	thinning	bald areas	mostly bald		
Plantar surface	heel-toe 40-50 mm: - 1 <40 mm: - 2	>50 mm no crease	faint red marks	anterior transverse crease only	creases anterior 2/3	creases over entire sole		
Breast	imperceptible	barely perceptible	flat areola no bud	stippled areola 1-2 mm bud	raised areola 3-4 mm bud	full areola 5-10 mm bud		
Eye/ear	lids fused loosely: -1 tightly: -2	lids open pinna flat stays folded	sl. curved pinna, soft; slow recoil	well-curved pinna, soft but ready recoil	formed and firm; instant recoil	thick cartilage ear stiff		
Genitals (male)	scrotum flat, smooth	scrotum empty faint rugae	testes in upper canal rare rugae	testes descending few rugae	testes down good rugae	testes pendulous deep rugae		
Genitals (female)	clitoris prominent & labia flat	prominent clitoris & small labia minora	prominent clitoris & enlarging minora	majora & minora equally prominent	majora large minora small	majora cover clitoris and minora		

Total Physical Maturity Score ______

Figure 23-4 Gestational age scoring system: neurologic and physical criteria (New Ballard Score). (From Ballard JL et al.: New Ballard score, expanded to included extremely premature infants, *J Pediatr* 119(3):418, 1991. Reprinted with permission.)

factors that promote gut maturity, and lipase, an enzyme that aids fat digestion. Human milk also contains many immunoglobulins that help to protect the infant during the first weeks of life. Breast-fed infants tend to have fewer food allergies than formula-fed infants. Breast milk is convenient, is always the right temperature, and carries no risk of contamination from impure water. Most often, nursing is emotionally satisfying to both mother and infant.

As discussed above, feeding should be initiated during the first period of reactivity. Data indicate that subsequent feedings should follow the infant's individual rhythm. Infants who regulate the frequency of their feeds themselves gain weight more quickly and breast-feed until older ages than infants who were fed according to a schedule. The infant nurses every 1 to 8 hours. Irregularity is the rule. Feeding is usually infrequent on the first postpartum day. The frequency rapidly increases between day 3 and 7 after delivery. Thereafter it may decrease slowly. During periods of rapid growth the frequency increases. Mothers should be reassured that these growth spurts are transient.

Limiting the length of feedings is discouraged unless absolutely necessary for specific maternal or neonatal medical reasons. During the first part of the feeding, the infant ingests foremilk, which is high in water content. By 7 to 10 minutes of nursing the infant ingests hindmilk, which contains more fat and vitamin K. Infants who are exclusively breast-fed and dark-skinned or who have minimal exposure to sunlight, may not produce sufficient vitamin D and should be supplemented with 400 IU daily. The infant regulates feeding according to his or her own needs. Slaven and Harvey (1981) found there to be no difference in nipple soreness or cracking between women who limited the number of minutes the infant nursed and those who did not. Supplementing should also be discouraged. Gray-Donald and colleagues (1985) noted that women who supplemented during the first week were five times more likely to stop breast-feeding. Women who supplemented during the second week were twice as likely to stop breast-feeding. The fact that the infant must wait for let-down to occur during breast-feeding but gets formula immediately from the bottle may be a factor in the infant's preference for the bottle. The nipples also are shaped differently; thus the infant may experience "nipple confusion." In some cultures it is important to administer teas or special foods to the infant. The caregiver should inquire in a respectful manner and learn the customs of the family's culture. These practices should be supported unless they are harmful, in which case the provider must identify and work with the important family members to find a workable substitution or compromise.

Burping is often not necessary when breast-feeding. However, if the infant swallows air, he or she may need to burp. It is helpful to exert very gentle pressure on the stomach by holding the infant upright against the body with his or her head on the shoulder. Alternately the infant may be laid down in a prone position across the lap. Very gentle patting or stroking over the infant's back with an upward motion facilitates burping. If the infant has not burped after several minutes, it is not necessary to continue the efforts. An infant may burp later. The cardiac sphincter in the newborn is immature, and, as a result, approximately 80% of infants "burp up" some of their feeding. Parents should be reassured that a couple of teaspoonfuls of regurgitated white fluid are normal. Large amounts, forceful vomiting, the presence of blood or bile, and changes in infant behavior are not normal. Parents should report poor feeding to the infant's health care provider since it is often the first sign of illness.

Breast-feeding mothers should be taught the proper process for expressing milk from the breast and storing it safely. Realistically, there are times women may have to miss a feeding or several feedings. Maternal illness, family responsibilities outside the home, and maternal employment outside the home are examples of situations in which offering breast milk from a bottle may be indicated. Breast milk can be expressed either manually or by using manual or electric commercial pumps. To manually express milk, the woman places her thumb on the upper part of the areola and her fingers along the lower edge. By exerting pressure first back toward the chest wall, then pressing toward the nipple, she will begin to express small amounts of milk. Once the let-down reflex occurs, the amount of milk expressed increases. The woman should be reassured that the amount of milk manually expressed is usually less than that taken in by the infant during a feeding and the lessor amount does not indicate decreased production. Women can be referred to local chapters of La Leche League or Nursing Mothers Council for information of breast pumps available in the community. Most hospitals with obstetrical services also offer resources for breast-feeding mothers who have delivered their babies in the facility.

Breast milk can be stored in a refrigerator for up to 72 hours. If longer storage is necessary, the breast milk can be frozen for as long as 3 months. Frozen milk can be defrosted by placing it in the refrigerator for several hours or by placing the container in warm water. Disposable bottle insert bags are convenient containers for the storage of breast milk.

Mothers who choose to formula feed must be supported in a nonjudgmental manner. With the increased attention to the benefits of breast-feeding, mothers who choose to use commercial formulas may think that they have to defend their decisions. Use of commercial formula preparations can be safe as long as the parents can properly prepare and store the formula. Commercial formulas are prepared using nonfat dry milk or soy preparations, and most manufacturers strive to make the combination of proteins, fats, carbohydrates, and minerals similar to those in human milk. Some formula preparations are ready to feed, whereas others are liquid concentrates or powders requiring dilution. A parent who dilutes a ready-to-feed preparation or gives a concentrate instead of ready-to-feed may inadvertently cause harm to the infant.

Initially 4 ounce bottles of formula are offered on demand. The infant usually takes ½ to 2 ounces every 2 to 4 hours during the first 2 weeks. Burping should be encouraged after every ounce. Parents should understand that propping bottles puts the infant at risk for aspiration, ear infection, and tooth decay. Any formula that has been at room temperature for 4 hours or longer should be discarded. Nipples should be cleaned in a dishwasher or boiled for 5 minutes. Vitamins or medications should not be added to bottles because the infant may not finish the entire bottle. Parents should understand that the infant should be offered only breast milk or formula for the first 4 to 6 months of age. The newborn is not capable of digesting other foods until the gastrointestinal tract is able to produce the digestive enzymes necessary for absorption and metabolism of the fats, proteins, and carbohydrates found in "solid" foods. Early introduction of solid supplements of food may also trigger allergic reactions and will interfere with the supply and demand balance necessary in breast-feeding.

Both breast milk and commercial formula preparations contain 20 kcal/ounce. Newborns require an estimated 115 kcal/kg of body weight for adequate growth and development. Therefore the average 7-pound newborn requires 18.3 ounces of breast milk or formula per day. Breast-fed babies meet this requirement by nursing 8 to 12 times in each 24-hour period. Bottle-fed babies feed 6 to 8 times per day and are able to go for longer periods between feedings because the formula preparation is less readily absorbed into the infant's system.

Hygiene

The newborn's skin is extremely susceptible to drying. In addition to causing discomfort, overbathing can cause diaper dermatitis and exacerbate cradle cap. During the first 24 to 48 hours the energy expenditure required by the newborn to maintain body temperature during and after a bath must be weighed against the benefit of a bath. The potential benefit of bathing is to prevent spread of infection from the infant to others by eliminating body fluids and secretions. Standard precautions should be practiced when handling a baby who is still wet from birth and before the initial bath, as well as when handling infant body fluids.

Preventing newborn infection is a challenge in the hospital setting. Rapid turnover of infants and staff expose the infant to many different hosts. The hospital environment has the potential to harbor numerous pathologic organisms. The most common organism infecting infants is *S. aureus,* a normal skin flora transmitted to infants by the hands of caregivers. Meberg and Shoyen (1985), in their study of bacterial colonization and neonatal infections, found that 91% of infants were colonized with *S. aureus,* 39% were colonized with *E. coli,* and 20% with group B streptococcus. The use of soap baths and Hibiscrub baths and treatment of the cord with benzine solution to prevent infections have been studied. Although the Hibiscrub resulted in lower colonization rates, none of the treatments resulted in fewer clinical infections. Rush (1986) found that colonization rates were more than doubled if infants spent less than 50% of their hospital stay with their mothers. Handwashing and rooming in are the first lines of defense against nosocomial infection.

If the mother is known to be infected with hepatitis B or HIV at the time of delivery, a bath may decrease vertical transmission. Because of this, standard precautions have incorporated routine bathing of infants in normal neonatal procedures. In general, however, research has not shown a decrease the number of infections when the infant is bathed. Certain antimicrobial agents can actually be harmful. For example, hexachlorophene was used routinely in the late 1960s until it was found to be neurotoxic. If the infant is dried immediately after birth, there is usually no need for a bath. Vernix is absorbed by the skin. If a bath is needed, it should be delayed until at least 4 to 6 hours after delivery, after the infant's temperature has stabilized.

Subsequent baths are appropriate two to three times a week. Soaps remove oil from the infant's skin, which is already very vulnerable to drying. A sponge bath is given until the umbilical cord has fallen off. Parents should be taught to cleanse the infant's eyes first, wiping from the inner to the outer canthus to prevent infection and blockage of the lacrimal duct. Often the infant has dacryostenosis, or blocked lacrimal ducts. A white or light yellow mucoid discharge presents. Parents should be shown how to gently milk the lacrimal duct upward and cleanse away discharge. Any purulent discharge or redness of the sclera and conjunctiva should be assessed by a care provider to rule out infection. The parents should be taught to use a different part of the cloth for each eye to prevent spread of infection from one eye to the other.

It is important to bathe the infant in a warm environment. Equipment, clothing, diaper, and towel should be assembled ahead of time; and the parts of the baby that are not being bathed should remain covered to maintain normal temperature. Shampooing need only be done once or twice a week. The use of perfumes, lotions, powders, and other chemicals that may cause skin rashes should be discouraged. In addition, use of powders may lead to respiratory problems in the infant.

When caring for the umbilical cord, the single most important action is to ensure sterility of the instrument used for cutting the cord. Neonatal tetanus has continued to be a problem internationally where sterile equipment for cutting the cord is not available. Various substances have been applied to the cord after delivery to prevent infection. Data indicate that application of triple dye to the cord is more effective in preventing infection than bathing with medicated soap. However, the use of triple dye is also associated with delayed separation of the cord. The diaper should be folded down so that the cord stump is open to the air, preventing urine and feces from soiling the cord. The cord should be inspected during diaper changes, and any exudate should be cleansed away with a clean cotton ball moistened with warm water. Further study is needed to assess the appropriateness of using alcohol alone, a common practice in many institutions. The cord normally shrivels and dries in the first couple days and then falls off in approximately 1 to 2 weeks. It is normal to have scant blood and mucus discharge from the base of the cord as it gradually loosens and detaches. Signs of infection such as foul odor, redness of the skin at the base of the cord, red streaks extending onto the abdomen, and purulent discharge should be reported to the infant's health care provider immediately.

Parents may question how often to change the infant's diaper. It should be changed several times a day when soiled. Before the milk comes in, the breast-fed infant should void and/or stool approximately five times per day. After the milk comes in, it is normal to have 8 to 10 wet or soiled diapers per day. Initially the meconium appears dark black or green and has the consistency of tar. Thereafter transitional stools gradually get lighter in color until they are yellow. Breast-fed babies may vary from having several stools a day to no stools for several days. The consistency is usually similar to mustard with curds. It may be quite loose, but there should be no water ring in the diaper. Formula-fed infants have stools that are similar in color but more formed. Often parents mistake normal stool patterns for constipation or diarrhea. Parents should be reminded to gently cleanse urine and feces from all creases—a process that can be difficult at times with copious amounts of stool.

Circumcision is the surgical removal of the foreskin, thereby exposing the glans of the penis. Routine circumcision remains controversial in the United States. Benefits are thought to include a decrease in urinary tract infections and cancer of the penis. However, both of these problems are rare in males. Risks include bleeding, infection, less-than-optimum cosmetic results, and genital mutilation. Couples in the United States may choose to circumcise their sons for religious or cultural reasons. The procedure can be done by obstetricians, pediatricians, and advanced practice nurses and midwives. Parents choosing the procedure for religious reasons may use a mohel or other specially trained individual.

If a male infant has been circumcised, the site should be checked with diaper changes for bleeding, swelling, redness, and pus. The area should be cleansed liberally with water. Parents should be counseled to expect a whitish granulation tissue to appear after the first day. They should not try to wipe it away. Some clinicians advocate putting a petroleum-based jelly (with or without antibiotic) on the incision area to prevent sticking to the diaper.

NORMAL NEWBORN BEHAVIOR

The newborn sleeps 16 to 18 hours a day, most often in 45-minute to 2-hour blocks of time. Irregularity is the rule. Trying to get the infant on a sleep schedule is not usually successful. Crying is a means of communication. Infants may cry as few as 5 minutes per day to as much as 2 hours per day, depending on individual temperament. The most common reasons for crying are hunger, discomfort from a soiled diaper, extremes in temperature, and overstimulation. Infants need to suck for nutrition, but they also have nonnutritive sucking needs. Even when they are not hungry, they still need to suck to comfort themselves. The health care provider should show parents how to comfort the infant by holding, swaddling, and offering a finger to suck. Studies show that rocking is soothing, especially if done with the infant in an upright position. There will be occasions when all efforts to calm the infant will fail. This is distressing to parents. They must be instructed that this can be normal and that remaining calm will help the situation. Taking a break and going back to the infant later is also helpful. A weak, shrill, or continuous cry should be reported to a health care professional.

Colic is a condition characterized by paroxysmal spasms of the gut. The infant may cry inconsolably, often at the same time each day. Stress and overstimulation exacerbates the situation, so altering schedules to decrease stimulation at the time of colic attacks is important. Placing the infant prone over a hot water bottle is usually soothing. Riding in a car may also calm the infant. It is critical that parents be provided emotional support to help them through this difficult stage. The primary caregiver must take breaks, as it is extremely stressful. The family can be reassured that colic usually subsides by 3 months of age.

JAUNDICE

One half to two thirds of all normal term infants appear jaundiced. To understand jaundice, it is important to review normal hematologic changes in the newborn. The normal red blood cell (RBC) count is 4.6 to 5.2 million/mm^3, and mean hematocrit is 50%. The shorter lifespan of the newborn's RBCs coupled with the relatively high number of RBCs means that the newborn infant needs to metabolize twice as many RBCs than later on in life. This is more difficult, considering the functional immaturity of the newborn's liver. Hemoglobin from destroyed RBCs is transformed to bilirubin. A liver enzyme, glucuronyl transferase, conjugates bilirubin, and it is then removed via the bile ducts and gut. If conjugated bilirubin remains in the gut too long, it can become unconjugated and resorbed into the enterohepatic circulation. Unconjugated or indirect bilirubin is fat soluble and has an affinity for fatty tissues. Conjugated or direct bilirubin is water soluble and is easily eliminated. Some bilirubin is eliminated by the skin. Light in the blue spectrum reacts with bilirubin deposits in the skin, where it is isomerized and excreted. Jaundice, the yellowing of skin tissues, is usually present when the total serum bilirubin level exceeds 7 mg/dl. This yellow discoloration of the skin is the result of the accumulation of unconjugated bilirubin in the tissues.

When large amounts of unconjugated bilirubin collect in central nervous system tissue, kernicterus can occur. The infant exhibits seizure activity, spasticity, and irreversible brain damage. Although kernicterus can occur in ill infants at lower bilirubin levels, most often the total bilirubin exceeds 20 mg/dl when kernicterus occurs. Before advances in our understanding of Rh and ABO incompatibility, many infants suffered kernicterus, but it is rare today.

Most jaundice is physiologic. Physiologic jaundice begins after the first 24 hours, with a peak at 2 to 3 days after delivery. The degree of jaundice begins to decline by the fifth day and then resolves by about 10 days. Total bilirubin levels rarely exceed 15 mg/dl in physiologic jaundice. Hyperbilirubinemia, the abnormally high level of bilirubin in the blood, is diagnosed when total bilirubin exceeds 12 mg/dl in the term formula-fed infant, 14 mg/dl in the breast-fed infant, and 15 mg/dl in the preterm infant. East Asian and Native American infants tend to have bilirubin levels that are higher than those of the general population.

Delayed feeding, dehydration, or constipation can increase jaundice by causing bilirubin to be delayed in the gut. Early and frequent feeding promotes the excretion of bilirubin. Certain medications may also exacerbate jaundice by competing with bilirubin for albumin-binding sites. Sulfonamides, furosemide, and salicylates are to be avoided for this reason. Free fatty acids also compete with bilirubin. Because conditions such as acidosis and hypothermia create free fatty acids, they may increase jaundice.

Approximately 2% of breast-fed infants experience breast milk jaundice. Early breast milk jaundice begins 2 to 4 days after delivery and is related to decreased caloric intake, delayed timing of first feeding, and infrequent (<8 feeds/24 hours) feedings during the first 3 days of life. Late breast milk jaundice begins on day 4 to 7, peaks on day 10 to 15, and persists for 3 to 4 weeks. It is suggested that components of the breast milk are the etiology of late breast milk jaundice. The enzyme glucuronidase, the hormone pregnanediol, and nonesterified free fatty acids found in breast milk are thought to interfere with glucuronyl transferase. Bilirubin levels may exceed 20 mg/dl, but kernicterus does not occur. If pathologic causes of jaundice are ruled out, it is not necessary to interrupt nursing. If in doubt, interruption of breast-feeding for 24 to 48 hours will cause a dramatic decrease in bilirubin levels, thus confirming the diagnosis of breast milk jaundice.

Bilirubin may be measured directly in the serum. It is also measured by transcutaneous bilirubinometry with 86% sensitivity. Carboxyhemoglobin is a product of heme catabolism and can be measured with chromatography. Alternatively, pulmonary excretion of carbon monoxide can be measured in the infant's expired breath. These methods are not available to most practitioners but may be in the near future. An icterometer is a simple tool for gross screening. Different shades of yellow are compared to the color of blanched skin on the newborn for an estimation of jaundice. Generally the farther down the body the jaundice extends, the higher the bilirubin level.

If excessive bilirubin levels are noted, there are choices for treatment. Phototherapy (exposing the infant to ultraviolet light to accelerate metabolism of bilirubin by the skin) is one option. Phototherapy can be used in the hospital nursery or in the home. High-intensity fluorescent lighting oxidizes unconjugated bilirubin in the skin, making it water soluble and able to be excreted in bile and urine. Traditional phototherapy lights require protection of the infant's eyes using a mask. Phototherapy lights can cause insensible water loss and diarrhea, increasing the risk of dehydration. Frequent breast milk or formula feedings are indicated to maintain hydration. There is no evidence to support the use of dextrose water supplementation to decrease bilirubin levels. Use of traditional phototherapy lights results in separation of the infant from his or her mother. More recently, BiliBlanket have been developed as a way to provide phototherapy without the danger of the high-intensity lights and allow the infant to remain in close contact with the mother. The system uses a fiberoptic blanket or vest that receives energy from a halogen light source. The blanket is wrapped around the infant's trunk, and then the baby is dressed in shirt, diapers, and baby blanket. Treatment with the BiliBlanket does not carry the risk of dehydration that traditional phototherapy has.

In severe cases of hyperbilirubinemia, exchange transfusion is a lifesaving treatment option. Other treatments that are under investigation include the use of metalloporphyrins, which inhibit heme catabolism and therefore limit bilirubin production. Tin, zinc, and chromium metalloporphyrins may be used.

Risk factors for pathologic jaundice are listed in Box 23-4. Preventive measures include encouraging early and frequent feedings and promptly identifying and correcting dehydration and constipation.

Jaundice within the first 24 hours is never normal and needs immediate evaluation. Cord bilirubin should be 3 mg /dl or less. Physician consultation is necessary when jaundice is identified within the first 24 hours of birth. If jaundice presents after 24 hours, the provider should evaluate the infant for risk factors. Determination of the bilirubin level will guide management. The American Academy of Pediatrics recommends phototherapy if total bilirubin exceeds 15 mg/dl for the 1-day-old infant, >18 mg/dl for the 2-day-old infant, and >20 for the 3-day-old infant. There is room for clinical judgment because, as noted above, the otherwise normal breast-fed infant may have levels greater than 20 mg/dl without deleterious effects.

Box 23-4 *Risk Factors for Pathologic Jaundice*

Isoimmune hemolytic disease
G6PD disease
Red blood cell membrane defects
Prematurity
Maternal diabetes
Polycythemia
Sequestered blood
Infection
Ethnicity (Japanese, Korean, Chinese, some Native American)
Acidosis
Hypothermia
Medications

A rational approach to the jaundiced infant is needed. One must avoid inappropriate phototherapy of the infant with physiologic jaundice yet intervene promptly to prevent kernicterus in the ill infant. Some clinicians have criticized the current recommendations of the American Academy of Pediatrics as leading to unnecessary testing and treatment in jaundiced term infants. Since most jaundiced term infants have no underlying pathology and the recommended laboratory tests lack sensitivity and specificity, it has been proposed that the only blood tests that are necessary are determination of the infant's and mother's blood type and Rh and a direct Coombs' test to determine whether hemolytic disease is present. In the absence of hemolytic disease, it is suggested that term infants may not require close evaluation of jaundice, a change in practice that would decrease the costs of testing and treatment but not have a negative impact on the infant's health (Newman and Maisels, 1992).

Parents of infants with physiologic jaundice require education and reassurance regarding the normalcy of their child. As with any newborn, they should report signs of dehydration, poor feeding, temperature instability, or changes in behavior (either lethargy or irritability).

SUBSEQUENT CHECKUPS

The infant born at home or discharged from the hospital within 24 hours needs evaluation by a health care professional by 3 days after delivery. A history and physical examination is performed as described in preceding paragraphs. Parent-infant bonding is assessed. When possible, the infant's care provider should observe breast-feeding to identify any problems or potential problems. The infant may have lost 10% of its birth weight but should be well hydrated and voiding and stooling normally. A gross screening for hearing is done by noting a startle or crying response to a loud noise. Alternately the examiner may notice the infant attending to a familiar voice. Full audiometric screening before 3 months of age is recommended for the following high-risk infants: (AAP/ACOG Guidelines, 1997)

- Severe hyperbilirubinemia requiring exchange transfusion
- Family history of hereditary sensorineural hearing loss
- Birth weight less than 1500 g
- Low APGAR (0 to 4 at 1 minute, 0 to 6 at 5 minutes)
- Ototoxic medications (e.g., aminoglycosides)
- Perinatal infection
- Presence of any anomaly associated with hearing loss
- Mechanical ventilation longer than 5 days

Metabolic screening should be obtained once feeding is well established. Screening too early may cause false-negative results because toxic metabolites may not yet be detectable. Testing for phenylketonuria and hypothyroidism is required in every state. Inclusion of the following additional tests varies state by state: biotinidase deficiency, congenital adrenal hyperplasia, galactosemia, homocystinuria, branch-chained ketoaciduria (maple syrup urine disease), tyrosinemia, and sickle cell disease (Heid, Preston, and Wheeler, 1993). The incidence of these diseases in the population served should dictate which tests are indicated. To obtain a specimen, the infant's heel should be warmed, cleansed with alcohol, and punctured on the lateral aspect of the heel. The circles on the filter paper test card must be completely saturated with the infant's blood. Having an assistant hold the infant in an upright position makes sample collection quicker.

The next well-baby visit should be at 2 weeks of age. Again, an interval history is obtained and a physical examination is performed. The infant should have regained birth weight by this point. Continued anticipatory guidance regarding infant development should be offered to the family.

Box 23-5 *Infant Safety Education*

Place infant on the back or side for sleeping.
Do not prop bottles.
Ensure that crib slats are less than 2⅜ inches apart, mattress fits snugly, and crib sides are always up.
Don't leave infant unattended with siblings or pets.
Don't place anything around the infant's neck.
Tie drapery and window shade cords out of reach of infant.
Never leave infant unattended on a high surface or in the bath.
Always test bath water temperature and keep water heater temperature at low setting.
Avoid heating formula in the microwave.
Keep plastic bags and small/sharp objects away from infant.
Provide a smoke-free environment.
Use sunblock/hats.
Avoid honey and Karo syrup (botulism).
Do not shake the infant.
Always use an infant car seat when traveling in an automobile and position it in the back seat facing backward.

The infant should be assessed 8 weeks after delivery with a history and physical examination. Anticipatory guidance is given regarding infant care, development, and safety. A checklist for client education regarding infant care and safety is a helpful tool in the infant's chart. Accidents are a primary cause of postneonatal morbidity and mortality. During the first 4 months, suffocation, falls, burns, and motor vehicle accidents are the most common accidents. Parents should be encouraged to take infant cardiopulmonary resuscitation classes and choose baby-sitters who know the skill. Box 23-5 contains an infant safety education checklist.

IMMUNIZATIONS

Immunization of newborns is a public health initiative to attempt to eradicate hepatitis. Although hepatitis vaccines are highly effective, the duration of immunity is unknown. The vaccine and immunoglobulin (hepatitis B immunoglobulin 0.5 ml intramuscularly) are absolutely indicated for the infant born of the mother who has active hepatitis or is a chronic carrier. When parents test negative for hepatitis B or the mother has immunity because of immunization, the parents should be counseled regarding the increased incidence of hepatitis B and the benefits and risks of the vaccine. If parents choose the vaccine, the first dose is administered the first day after birth, with repeat doses at 8 weeks and 6 months. Dosages are 10 μg intramuscularly for Energix-B and 10 μg intramuscularly for Recombivax.

At 8 weeks after delivery, inactivated polio vaccine (IPV) injection or oral polio vaccine (OPV), diphtheria, pertussis, tetanus (DTAP), and hemophilus influenza type B vaccines are recommended. The DTAP contains diphtheria and tetanus toxoids, as well as acillnear pertussis antigen. This newer vaccine is much safer than the previous DPT, which contained whole cell pertussis vaccine. It rarely has any side effects and is even more effective in protecting against pertussis. The dosage is 0.5 mg given intramuscularly.

HIB vaccines contain purified bacterial protein of *Haemophilus influenzae B.* Current preparations available for infants include HbOC, PRP-T, and PRP-OMP. The dosage is 0.5 ml intramuscularly. Common side effects are low-grade fever and local pain. No major side effects are known.

The OPV contains live polio virus. Rare cases of polio have occurred in vaccinees and close contacts (1 in 6.4 million doses). The use of vaccination has completely eradicated wild polio in the United States. The AAP and CDC advocate the use of IPV, an inactivated trivalent polio vaccine for all doses. OPV should be used only in specific situations (e.g., when parents will not consent to injections but will consent to oral administration).

Some parents choose not to immunize their children because extremely rare vaccine reactions involving long-term sequelae are reported in the literature. Parents must be educated regarding the benefits and risks of each vaccine both for their own child and for the community at large. Declining vaccines has very real consequences from a public health perspective. The incidence of fatal and crippling diseases that have been virtually eradicated by the use of vaccines would again begin to rise if herd immunity is lost. If the parent declines an immunization(s) after all information has been given in a comprehensible manner, the decision must be respected.

References

American Academy of Pediatrics and American College of Obstetricians and Gynecologists: *Guidelines for perinatal care,* ed 4, Elk Grove Village, Ill, 1997, American Academy of Pediatrics.

Anisfield E, Lipper E: Early contact, social support and mother-infant bonding, *Pèdiatrics* 72:79-83, 1983.

Brousson MA, Klein MC: Controversies surrounding the administration of vitamin K to newborns: a review, *Can Med Assoc J* 154(3):307-315, 1996.

Chance GW, Hanvey L: Neonatal resuscitation in Canadian hospitals, *Can Med Assoc J* 136:601-606, 1987.

Chen JY: Prophylaxis of ophthalmia neonatorum: comparison of silver nitrate, tetracycline, erythromycin and no prophylaxis, *Pediatr Infect Dis J* 11(12):1026-1030, 1992.

de Chateau P, Wiberg B: Long-term effect on mother-infant behavior of extra contact during the first hour postpartum, *Acta Paediatr Scand* 66:137-143, 145-151, 1977.

Desmond M, Rudolph A, Phitaksphraiwan P: The transitional care nursery: a mechanism for preventive medicine in the newborn, *Pediatr Clin North Am* 13:656, 1966.

Ekelund H, Finnstrom O, Gunnarskog J: Administration of vitamin K to newborn infants and childhood cancer, *Br Med J* 307:89-91, 1993.

Fardig JA: A comparison of skin-to-skin contact and radiant heaters in promoting neonatal thermoregulation, *J Nurse Midwifery* 25(1):19-28, 1980.

Gao YN: Bacterial condition of the lower genital tract of pregnant women and neonatal infection, *Chinese J Obstet Gynecol* 28(12):717-719, 759, 1993.

Gardner S: The mother as incubator after delivery, *JOGNN* 8(3):174-176, 1979.

Golding J, Paterson M, Kinlen LJ: Factors associated with childhood cancer in a national cohort study, *Br J Cancer* 62(2):304-308, 1990.

Gomez-Pedro J et al: Influence of early mother-infant contact on dyadic behaviour during the first month of life, *Dev Med Child Neurol* 26:657-664, 1984.

Gray-Donald K et al: Effect of formula supplementation on the duration of breast-feeding: a controlled clinical trial, *Pediatrics* 75(3):514-518, 1985.

Greenburg M, Rosenberg I, Lind J: First mothers rooming-in with their newborns: its impact upon the mother, *Am J Orthopsychiatry* 43:783-788, 1973.

Grossman K, Thane K, Grossman KE: Maternal tactual contact of the newborn after various postpartum conditions of mother-infant contact, *Dev Psychol* 17:158-169, 1981.

Hales DJ et al: Defining the limits of the maternal sensitive period, *Dev Med Child Neurol* 19:454-461, 1977.

Hathaway WE, Isarangkura PB, Mahasandana C: Comparison of oral and parenteral vitamin K prophylaxis for the prevention of late hemorrhagic disease of the newborn, *J Pediatr* 119:461-464, 1991.

Heid PL, Preston RN, Wheeler JS: Discharge considerations and process. In Seidel HM, Rosenstein BJ, Pathak AP, editors: *Primary care of the newborn,* St Louis, 1993, Mosby, pp 447-457.

Henderson-Smart D: Vitamin K and childhood cancer, *Med J Aust* 160(2):91, 1994.

Hossain MM et al: The timing of breastfeeding initiation and its correlates in a cohort of rural Egyptian infants, *J Trop Pediatr* 41(6):354-359, 1995.

Illingworth RS et al: Self-demand feeding in a maternity unit, *Lancet* 1:683-687, 1952.

Isenberg SJ, Apt L, Wood M: A controlled trial of povidone-iodine as prophylaxis against ophthalmia neonatorum, *N Engl J Med* 332(9):562-566, 1995.

Klaus MH, Kennell JH: *Maternal-infant bonding: the impact of early separation or loss on family development,* St Louis, 1976, Mosby.

Klebanoff MA et al: The risk of childhood cancer after neonatal exposure to vitamin K, *N Engl J Med* 329(13):905-908, 1993.

Kontos D: A study of the effects of extended mother-infant contact on maternal behavior at one and three months, *Birth Fam J* 5:133-140, 1978.

Meberg A, Shoyen R: Bacterial colonization and neonatal infections, *Acta Paediatr Scand* 74:366-371, 1985.

Motohara K, Endo F, Matsuda I: Vitamin K deficiency in breastfed infants at one month of age, *J Pediatr Gastroenterol Nutr* 5:931-933, 1986.

Newman TB, Maisels MJ: Evaluation and treatment of jaundice in the term newborn: a kinder, gentler approach, *Pediatrics* 89(5 Pt 1):809-818, 1992.

Nsanze H et al: Ophthalmia neonatorum in United Arab Emirates, *Ann Trop Paediatr* 1:27-32, 1996.

O'Connor ME, Addeigo JE: Use of oral Vitamin K to prevent hemorrhagic disease of the newborn infant, *J Pediatr* 108(4):616-619, 1986.

O'Connor S et al: Reduced incidence of parenting inadequacy following rooming-in, *Pediatrics* 66:176-182, 1980.

Olsen JH, Hertz H, Blinkenberg K: Vitamin K regimens and incidence of childhood cancer in Denmark, *Br J Med* 308:895-896, 1994.

Oski FA, Naiman JL: *Hematologic problems in the newborn,* Philadelphia, 1972, WB Saunders, pp 236-272.

Ronca AE, Abel RA, Alberts JR: Perinatal stimulation and adaptation of the neonate, *Acta Paediatr Suppl* 416:8-15, 1996.

Rush J: Does routine newborn bathing reduce *Staphylococcus aureus* colonization rates? A randomized controlled trial, *Birth* 13(3):176-180, 1986.

Salariya EM, Easton PM, Carter JI.: Duration of breastfeeding after early initiation and frequent feeding, *Lancet* 2:1141-1143, 1978.

Slaven S, Harvey D: Unlimited sucking time improves breastfeeding, *Lancet* 1(8216):392-393, 1981.

Sousa PLR et al: Attachment and lactation. Pediatria XIV, vol 3, XIV Int Gogr Pediat, Buenos Aires, 1974, Editorial Medica Panamericana SA, pp 136-138.

Sutor A, Dagres N, Niederhoff N: Late form of vitamin K deficiency bleeding in Germany, *Klinische Padiatri* 207(3):89-97, 1995.

Taylor PM et al: Effects of extra-early mother-infant contact, *Acta Pediatr Scand* 316(suppl):3-14, 1985.

Thomson ME, Hartsock TG, Larson C: The importance of immediate postnatal contact: its effect on breastfeeding, *Can Fam Physician* 25:1374-1378, 1979.

Chapter 24

Fourth Trimester

Maureen Wolfe CNM, MSN

The postpartum period has been defined in medical literature as 6 weeks following the birth. However, historically and culturally the definition of the postpartum period (puerperium) has been influenced by the beliefs and values surrounding the childbearing process and maternal role. As childbearing increasingly became a biomedical event in the United States, childbirth became treated more like a surgical procedure. Not surprisingly, the completion of the process was determined by the 6-week follow-up visit with the obstetrician. Although many of the physical and physiologic changes that occur in the transition to the nonpregnant state are complete by 6 weeks after delivery, many others continue for several more weeks or months. In addition, the psychosocial and emotional transition that occurs with the addition of the new infant into the family and community is not a process that fits neatly into a 6-week time frame. In viewing pregnancy and childbirth as a healthy phenomenon for most women, the postpartum period must be reconceptualized as a period in which the woman's individual needs are central. The woman's own health and her family and community relationships and resources then become central in determining the care that is appropriate for her experience. This chapter reviews the physical, physiologic and psychosocial changes that occur in the postpartum period, as well as care processes that can be offered by the health care professional to facilitate the woman's maternal role adoption.

PHYSICAL CHANGES IN THE FOURTH TRIMESTER

Reproductive System

Ovarian function and return of ovulation is influenced by breast-feeding. Lactational amenorrhea has been well documented (Labbok et al., 1997; Visness et al., 1997), and recent work has established the validity of the contraceptive effect of this physiologic response to breast-feeding. Visness et al. (1997) followed bleeding patterns and levels of estrogen and pregnanediol on primiparous and multiparous women who were fully breast-feeding and found that median return of ovulation for women without bleeding between 6 and 8 weeks after delivery was 269 days. Women who experienced vaginal bleeding between 6 and 8 weeks after delivery had a median of 224 days. This differs from the previously estimated mean period of time to ovulation of 190 days (Bowes, 1996). Nonlactating women experience a mean time to ovulation of 70 days, although ovulation as early as 27 days after delivery has been documented (Bowes, 1996). Research suggests that younger women resume ovarian function faster than older women (Moran et al., 1994).

Little research has been done on bleeding patterns during the postpartum period, yet texts traditionally have noted that the length of lochial discharge is about 2 weeks. One recent investigation has found that median duration of lochia in one population was 27 days, with a range of 5 to 90 days (Visness, Kennedy, and Ramos, 1997), which was consistent with one earlier study (Oppenheimer et al., 1986). Guidelines for the use of lactational amenorrhea as a contraceptive method consider lochial discharge up to 8 weeks after delivery in breast-feeding women normal and not associated with return to menstruation (Labbok, Cooney, and Coly, 1994). Maternal age, parity, infant birth weight, breast-feeding frequency, and level of supplementation are not associated with the length of lochial discharge (Visness, Kennedy, and Ramos, 1997).

Visness and colleagues (1997) found that women who experienced the "6-week bleed," a bleeding episode distinct from the lochia, resumed menses approximately 5 weeks earlier than those who did not experience the late postpartum bleed. As many as 46% of women experience the 6-week bleed. Women who fully breast-feed and who do not have the late postpartum bleeding episode have a median time to first menses of 33 weeks (Visness et al., 1997). Nonlactating women experience first menses 6 to 10 weeks after delivery. In both lactating and nonlactating women, the first menses is almost always anovulatory. Moran et al. found that 61% of women ovulate during the second menstrual cycle after delivery, 93% during the third cycle, and 100% during the fourth cycle (Moran et al., 1994).

In nonlactating women prolactin levels fall by the third week after delivery, and estrogen levels begin to rise after the first postpartum week. By about 3 weeks after delivery, estrogen levels are at follicular phase levels. Pituitary release of follicle-stimulating hormone (FSH) and luteinizing hormone (LH) under the stimulation of gonadotropin-releasing hormone usually resumes 4 to 6 weeks after delivery. The presence of human chorionic gonadotropin and prolactin during the first 2 weeks after delivery is thought to be influential in the suppression of the pituitary-hypothalamic function.

In lactating women prolactin remains elevated throughout the 6-week period after delivery. Since FSH levels are similar in both lactating and nonlactating women, it is theorized that prolactin inhibits the ovary's response to FSH, thereby inhibiting ovulation.

Involution of the reproductive organs continues for 6 to 8 weeks after delivery. By postpartum day 5 the uterine fundus is usually 4 to 5 cm below the umbilicus. By postpartum day 10 the uterus has become a pelvic organ and usually is not palpable abdominally. However, there is considerable variability in the pattern of involution experienced by healthy women (Cluett, Alexander, and Pickering, 1997). By 6 weeks after delivery the uterus returns to the nonpregnant state, weighing 60 to 80 g. Internal measurements at that time average 6.1 cm from fundus to the internal os, with a transverse diameter of 6.3 cm (Willms et al., 1995). By 6 months after delivery, the fundus-to-internal os diameter decreases to an average of 5 cm (Willms et al., 1995). Contractions of the uterus as it involutes may be noted by the woman for about 1 week after delivery. Regeneration of the endometrium is usually complete by 2 to 3 weeks after delivery, and completion of healing of the placental site is expected by 6 to 7 weeks after delivery.

The cervix continues to close through the first week after delivery. Return to the usual nonpregnant size, shape, and consistency occurs through the first month following birth. The normal regeneration of cervical squamous epithelium contributes to regression of abnormal antepartal cytologic findings in many women who experience vaginal birth. Women experiencing cesarean birth do not appear to have this regression (Ahdoot et al., 1998). Vaginal tone in the first week after delivery remains lax, and the walls are edematous and smooth. Edema and mucosal congestion decrease by the third week, when rugae reappear. The vaginal muscles increase in tone and decrease the internal dimensions over the 6- to 8-week period after delivery. Research suggests that the use of muscle exercises involving voluntary contracting of the pelvic muscles (Kegel's exercise) may increase vaginal tone after delivery and reduce the incidence of urinary stress incontinence (Sampselle et al., 1998). However, research findings have been limited by small samples, lack of ability to be certain of adherence to the intervention, and the fact that participants in the control groups may also practice vaginal muscle exercises on their own.

Other System Changes

Most of the cardiac changes in pregnancy revert to their nonpregnant status within the first few days after delivery. Elimination of the increased extracellular fluid decreases the increased cardiac load present in pregnancy. Cardiac output returns to the prepregnant level as the increased fluid volume is eliminated. By 6 weeks after delivery, cardiovascular indices should return to prepregnant values.

Decreases in intraabdominal pressure following delivery and progesterone production lead to rapid return of the pregnancy-induced changes in the respiratory tract. Tidal volume decreases, and residual volume increases almost immediately after delivery. Expiratory reserve volume increases to prepregnant level slowly and may not reach it until 2 to 3 months after delivery. Most other changes return to normal during the first month after the birth.

The renal system responds to the cardiovascular changes and fluid shifts with natriuresis and diuresis from the second to the fifth days after delivery. Complete fluid and electrolyte balance should be achieved by 3 weeks after delivery. Excretion of calcium, phosphate, vitamins, glucose, and other solutes should reach prepregnant levels by the end of the first week. Plasma renin activity and angiotensin II levels remain elevated for 2 weeks. Renal blood flow, glomerular filtration rate, plasma creatinine, and blood urea nitrogen return to the woman's usual levels by 6 weeks after delivery (Blackburn and Loper, 1992). Pregnancy-induced dilation of the renal pelves and ureters may continue for up to 12 weeks after delivery. Stress incontinence may continue to be a problem for some women, most likely because of permanent changes in sphincter tone (Meyer et al., 1998).

Gastrointestinal tone returns to normal as progesterone levels decrease following the birth. Resumption of the woman's normal bowel habits is expected by 2 weeks after delivery. Women who experience forceps-assisted deliveries and those who have anal sphincter damage during the birth are at increased risk for flatus and fecal incontinence and urgency (Meyer et al., 1998). Women experience an immediate weight loss of about 12 pounds following the birth, with little further loss during the first week. By 6 weeks after delivery, 28% of women return to their prepregnant weight.

The hyperpigmentation of the skin that occurs during the pregnancy under the influence of estrogens and, to a lesser degree, progesterone may fade during the postpartum period. Fading is most pronounced in fair-skinned women, and women with darker skin may notice little change. Striae fade following the birth but continue to be noticeable as whitish bands of variable consistency. Vascular changes (spider nevi and capillary hemangiomas) do not recede after birth. The decreased hair loss in pregnancy under the stimulation of estrogen is reversed when estrogen levels drop, leading to an increase in hair loss during the postpartum period. During pregnancy the anagen (growth) phase of the hair follicles is prolonged, resulting in a decrease in the rate of hair growth and in the normal loss of hair as the follicle goes through the telogen phase. Normally about 15% to 20% of the hair fibers are in the telogen phase, whereas in pregnancy less than 10% of hair fibers are in the phase for shedding. After delivery the excess anagen follicles mature, and from 4 to 20 weeks after delivery 30% to 35% of the hair fibers enter the telogen phase and are shed (Blackburn and Loper, 1992).

The neuromuscular and sensory systems undergo profound changes during the postpartum period. As fluid balance is restored, ocular and otolaryngeal changes that occurred under the hormonal influence of pregnancy recede. Nasal and sinus congestion is relieved in the first few days after delivery. Alterations in fluid and electrolyte balance may lead to frontal and bilateral headaches in the first postpartum week (Blackburn and Loper, 1992).

The estrogen-induced changes in thyroxine-binding globulin, thyroxine, and triiodothyronine reverse slowly and may not return to the woman's prepregnant normal level until 6 to 12 weeks after delivery. The increased size of the thyroid regresses to the woman's norm by 12 weeks after delivery.

Nutritional Needs

During the first 2 weeks after delivery, nutritional guidance focuses on physical healing and stabilization following the birth and establishment of lactation. During the latter part of the postpartum period, the focus shifts to maintenance of an adequate milk supply, healthful weight loss strategies, and maintenance of good nutrition when return to work or school is necessary (Institute of Medicine, 1992).

All women, regardless of lactation status, should be encouraged to continue a healthy diet similar to the one recommended in pregnancy. Data collection necessary to develop an appropriate nutritional plan includes review of the pregnancy and delivery to identify problems or potential problems, identification of medications routinely taken, review of a typical day's intake, and establishment of social and cultural factors that influence dietary choices and preparation. Generally women who are not lactating can be counseled to achieve an intake of 1800 kcal daily. Nonlactating women can be counseled that, by limiting their caloric intake to slightly less than their usual intake, they will most likely lose 1 to 2 pounds per week.

Lactating women have additional nutritional needs. Daily caloric intake should be at least 1800 kcal, although some sources recommend as much as 2700 kcal/day (American Academy of Pediatrics and American College of Obstetricians and Gynecologists, 1997; Institute of Medicine, 1992). In general, lactation requires approximately 500 kcal above the woman's normal prepregnant intake. It seems reasonable to counsel that the lower level recommended is appropriate during the first postpartum week when the woman is less active, but calories should be added as the woman increases her activity. There is an increased need for fluids, so women should be instructed to drink enough fluids to prevent thirst (Institute of Medicine, 1992). During the first postpartum week women can be encouraged to drink 3000 ml per 24 hours (Simpson and Creehan, 1996). Consuming excess fluid is associated with decreased milk production in some women. Lactating women should eliminate or limit beverages containing caffeine, alcohol, and food that contains sugar substitutes. Women at risk for nutritional deficiencies should continue taking a multiple vitamin while lactating. One source notes that breast-feeding women can lose 2 pounds per month without affecting lactation (American Academy of Pediatrics and American College of Obstetricians and Gynecologists, 1997).

Women who gain 25 to 35 pounds during pregnancy are likely to return to prepregnant weight by 6 months after delivery (Schauberger, Rooney, and Brimer, 1992). Schauberger et al. (1992) found no difference in weight loss when comparing breast-feeding and non-breast-feeding women, and found that women who experienced higher weight gain in pregnancy lost more weight after delivery. Multiparous women lost less weight during the postpartum period, but it was not possible to determine the relationship with age and other variables that might have confounded results. In addition to weight gain in pregnancy, prepregnant weight, race, and exercise have also been associated with postpartum weight loss (Boardley et al., 1992) (Research Box 24-1).

Maintenance of Lactation

The average rate of milk production for breast-feeding mothers who are not supplementing at 2 to 3 months after delivery is 700 to 800 ml/24 hours. However, it is clear that milk production adjusts to meet demand, and production of over 2 L/24 hr has been identified (Daly and Hartmann, 1995a). Frequency of suckling and volume of milk taken at each feeding both contribute to milk production in the early weeks of breast-feeding. Once lactation has been established, frequency of feed-

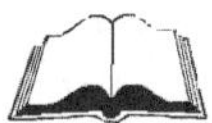

Research Box 24-1

Walker LO, Freeland-Graves J: Lifestyle factors related to postpartum weight gain and body image in bottle- and breast-feeding women, *JOGNN* 27(2):151-160, 1998.

Background

Women commonly express concerns about weight retention and body image after giving birth. Obesity is a significant health problem in the United States, and it is estimated that one third of women are overweight. Numerous studies have identified weight retention following pregnancy, and weight gains of 11 to 15 pounds or more are associated with health problems, including coronary artery disease and hypertension. Because of the psychologic aspects of postpartum adjustment, the postpartum period may be a critical period for achieving appropriate weight for height and preventing problems associated with obesity.

Research Question

(1) Do bottle- and breast-feeding women differ on postpartum weight gain, body image attitudes, or lifestyle? (2) Within feeding-method groups, are weight gain and body image attitudes related to lifestyle factors such as aerobic exercise, fat intake habits, smoking, overall lifestyle, and self-regulation? (3) Within feeding method groups, do women with higher and lower postpartum weight gains differ on lifestyle factors?

Methods

This study used a cross-sectional design to recruit a diverse sample of postpartum women. An eight-page questionnaire was mailed to 513 new mothers whose names were published in newspaper birth announcements. Items on the questionnaire included anthropometric variables (e.g., height and weight), reproductive variables (e.g., parity, mode of delivery), social and demographic variables, and body image and exercise measures. Five instruments with documented validity and reliability were used to measure dissatisfaction with body, level of aerobic exercise, dietary habits, overall lifestyle, and skill in managing distress. Appropriate statistical analyses were done based on the level of measurement of the data items.

Sample

The breast-feeding and bottle-feeding groups were similar in parity, family income, ethnicity, maternal age, time since delivery, gestational weight gain, and prepregnant body mass index. The women in the breast-feeding group were more likely to have some

ing is not strongly correlated with volume produced (Daly and Hartmann, 1995a). Research to measure milk production has identified that there is considerable within-day variation in the amount of milk consumed by breast-fed infants and the pattern of suckling frequency. Daly and Hartmann (1995b) used the findings from their extensive research on milk synthesis and transfer to propose a model of short-term control of milk synthesis that can be summarized as follows:

- The breast assesses the need of the infant by measuring the amount removed against the amount it can hold (emptying).
- Milk synthesis is directed by the degree of emptying, and the rate of synthesis is reset with each breast-feeding experience.
- Mothers with large storage capacities in their breasts have greater flexibility in feeding intervals. Mothers with limited storage capacity by necessity need to feed more frequently to meet infant demand (Daly and Hartmann, 1995b).

Breast engorgement is frequently referred to in the literature and in perinatal textbooks, but there is no definitive definition of the condition. One theory of the etiology of engorgement is that alveoli distention compresses the milk ducts, resulting in obstruction of the transfer of milk from the ducts to the infant. Obstruction leads to further distention, and ultimately secondary vascular and lymphatic stasis is experienced. Another popular theory is that the increase in blood and lymph circulation when milk is first synthesized causes swelling in the areola that may interfere with infant latch-on. This results in incomplete emptying of the collecting ductules, with further distention and obstruction. Increased vascularity can progress to the level at which the whole breast is firm and tender (Lawrence, 1994). Consistent in both these theories is the distention of the collecting system in the breasts. Research studies have found decreased problems with engorgement when mothers are encouraged to nurse immediately, frequently, and on demand, without restriction in sucking time.

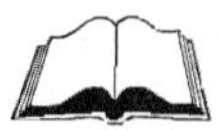

Research Box 24-1—cont'd

college and be married to the father of the baby. Women were excluded from the study if they had health conditions that might influence weight, if they were younger than 18 years of age, and if they had multiple gestation. Adjusted response rate for the mailed survey was 52%.

Results

Method of infant feeding was not associated with significant differences in postpartum weight gain or body image dissatisfaction. Gestational weight gain was significantly associated with postpartum weight gain in both groups. Breast-feeding mothers had instrument scores that indicated generally healthier lifestyle and lower fat intake. In the bottle-feeding group, higher postpartum weight gains were associated with less vigorous exercise patterns and higher fat intake. These associations were not present in the breast-feeding group.

Clinical Application

Results of this study contradict the commonly held belief that breast-feeding is associated with greater weight loss in the early postpartum period. Although there was no difference found in weight retention when comparing breast-feeding and bottle-feeding mothers, there were differing effects of lifestyle behaviors on weight retention. In bottle-feeding women, higher postpartum weight gains were associated with less vigorous exercise and higher fat intake than lower weight gains. This difference was not found in the breast-feeding group. The authors note that there is no clear explanation for the lack of association between lifestyle behaviors and weight gain in breast-feeding women. They propose that higher prolactin levels may stimulate appetite, thereby delaying mobilization of fat stores, and that vigorous exercise in the postpartum period may not result in weight loss in breast-feeding women because of decreases in other areas of activity and increased caloric intake. Limitations of this study include the response rate of approximately 50%, the overrepresentation of white women, and the use of self-reported data.

Clinicians can use the findings from the study when counseling women regarding postpartum weight loss/retention. Bottle-feeding women can specifically be counseled regarding the positive effects of aerobic exercise and lower fat intake. Further research on the influence of lifestyle behaviors in breast-feeding women is necessary to understand the associations among behaviors and weight loss/retention.

Hill and Humenick (1994) conducted the first longitudinal study to determine the incidence and characteristics of breast engorgement during the first 2 weeks after delivery. Ninety-five percent of the women indicated at least beginning feelings of tenderness in the breasts, and 78% indicated firmness and tenderness of the breasts. Their findings suggest that women breast-feeding for the first time tend to experience a peak of engorgement at 3 to 6 days after delivery, with women breast-feeding for a second time experiencing the peak a little earlier. Although this peak is consistent for the aggregate, some individual women experienced multiple peaks or sustained engorgement through the 14-day period of data collection (Humenick, Hill, and Anderson, 1994).

EMOTIONAL, PSYCHOSOCIAL, AND CULTURAL ASPECTS OF THE FOURTH TRIMESTER

Fatigue is probably the most common complaint offered by new mothers. Recovery from the birth, adjustment to sleep pattern disturbances, pain, and anxiety all contribute to the experience of fatigue for the first 6 to 8 weeks after delivery. Gardner (1991), in her study of 35 married white women who delivered vaginally, found that women were mildly fatigued, with demonstrable improvement by 6 weeks after delivery. Other studies have found that moderate levels of fatigue were reported, with peak levels between 2 and 6 weeks after delivery (Wambach, 1998). Wambach found that breast-feeding mothers experience moderate levels of fatigue, with a peak at 3 weeks after delivery, a significant drop at 6 weeks, and further drop in levels of fatigue at 9 weeks after delivery. Fatigue is associated with breast-feeding problems, maternal medical complications, depression, stress, and infant difficulties. The association between maternal age and fatigue is conflicting in the literature. Wambach found that older mothers reported higher levels of fatigue, whereas Gardner found that younger mothers reported higher levels. Another research team compared sleep patterns of postpartum women to those of nonpostpartum women (Swain et al., 1997). Findings suggest that, although postpartum women experience more awakenings at night, they were able to attain similar total weekly sleep hours using naps and later arising.

Women experiencing a first birth have the added stressors of concern about ability to care for the infant and role transition. Women experiencing second or subsequent births usually are much more confident in their maternal role, although differences in infant temperament and needs may cause concerns. Fatigue and the stressors of early parenting are associated with postpartum "blues," described as "feelings of sadness, fear, anger, or anxiety occurring about 3 days after childbirth and usually fading within 1 to 2 weeks" (American College of Obstetricians and Gynecologists, 1995). It is estimated that 70% to 80% of women experience the blues after delivery. Women experiencing the blues may cry unexpectedly, have trouble sleeping, not feel like eating, and question their ability to take care of their infants. These feelings subside spontaneously within the first week or two after delivery. A few women progress to true depression (see Chapter 27). It is thought that the dramatic decrease in estrogen, progesterone, and thyroid hormones may contribute to this condition.

Maternal role attainment continues during the first months following birth. Mercer (1985) found that the process of maternal role attainment begins in pregnancy and extends for up to 10 months after the birth. She found that about 85% of her sample had achieved role internalization by 9 months after delivery.

Virtually all cultures have certain beliefs and practices surrounding the postpartum period. Chinese women understand the importance of "doing the month" (Holroyd et al., 1996). Fijian women refer to the practice as "sitting the month" (Becker, 1998). Women in Kenya have a 7-day period of seclusion during which they must rest with their infants. During the culturally specified time period, women are relieved of their usual house-

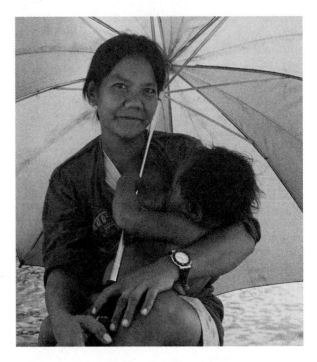

(Courtesy Caroline E. Brown.)

hold responsibilities. One international survey of over 200 societies found that about half of the societies expected women to resume work 2 weeks following the birth, and the others deferred work for at least 1 month.

Jambunathan (1995) found that Hmong women believe that the mother should rest for 1 month. Participants in her study noted that the postpartum mother is "not allowed to do much at all, only eat and take care of the child" (p. 340). During the first month after delivery, the husband contributes to household responsibilities. Fijians expect that women will rest for several months after the birth and that mothers will not resume heavy physical labor until infant weaning at about 1 year of age (Becker, 1998).

Many cultural groups, including Asian, Latino, and Native American women, believe the postpartum period to be a "cold" state; thus the woman needs to eat and dress in a manner that fosters warmth. Several studies of cultural aspects of postpartum care note that women need to be protected from drafts or breezes because they chill the woman. Traditional Hmong women believe that the use of warm clothing, including a head covering and shoes and socks, protects women during the month after the birth (Jambunathan, 1995). Women may bathe, but only with warm water. Rural Korean women are kept inside, isolated from those outside the family, for 3 days, and are specifically protected from "the wind" (Sich, 1981). Women are covered in thick blankets, even when it is warm outside. Even if they are uncomfortable with this practice, traditional women will still hold to it in order to not upset their mothers-in-law. Similar practices have been observed in Taiwan.

Chicken is the food of choice for Hmong women; duck, pork, and beef are not recommended. Vegetables are believed to make one sick and cause coughing; thus they are not consumed during the first month after delivery (Jambunathan, 1995).

Sexual intercourse is forbidden for the first month in Hmong communities. It is thought that the "blood from the pregnancy" needs to be drained and resumption of sexual

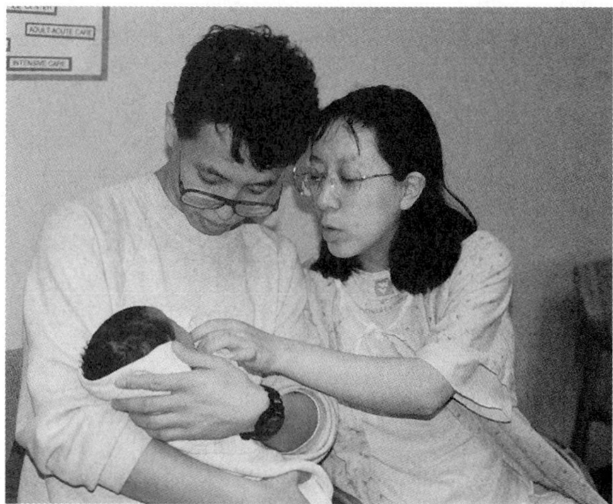

(Courtesy Caroline E. Brown.)

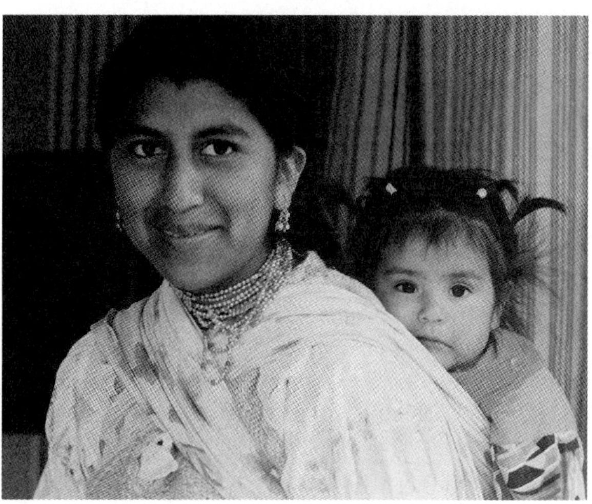

(Courtesy Caroline E. Brown.)

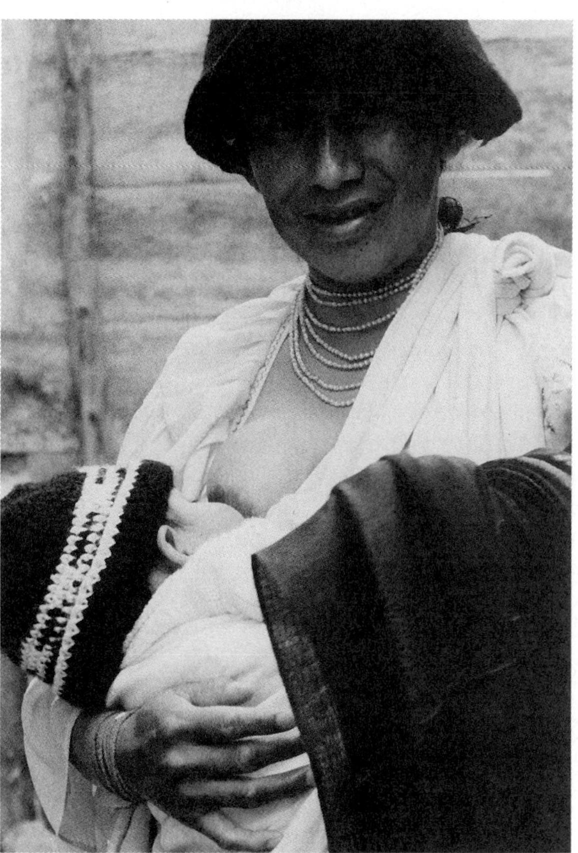

(Courtesy Caroline E. Brown.)

activity before 1 month after delivery decreases the chance of future healthy pregnancies (Jambunathan, 1995).

Although it is easy to think that average American women don't follow distinct cultural practices during the postpartum period, one must consider that the usual care of mothers reflects much about American beliefs about childbearing. Length of stay in the hospital is determined by third-party payers rather than by maternal and infant need. Care, for the most part, is delivered by physicians—one for the woman (the obstetrician) and one for the infant (the pediatrician or family practice physician). The provider counsels her that she should not experience any sexual activity ("pelvic rest") for 6 weeks, demonstrating a reliance on the medical model that does not recognize the normal variation in healing time. Women are routinely seen for their postpartum examinations at 4 to 6 weeks after delivery, and the examination centers around the physical examination of the breasts and pelvis. State disability programs and employer benefits are often the determining factors regarding when women return to the paid work force. The more one examines the practices surrounding the postpartum period in America, the more it becomes clear that beliefs and decision making have moved from the woman and her supportive others to "experts" in the health care system.

Adoption of a midwifery model of care during the postpartum period puts the woman in the center of planning and implementing care and support. The provider who practices in this model recognizes that women differ in their needs, and care practices are adjusted to meet those needs. A woman with minimal social support may need to see the provider frequently during the first few weeks to facilitate the transition to maternal role attainment. Likewise, a woman whose husband and mother or mother-in-law will be present for several weeks to assume household responsibilities so that she can care for herself and her infant may need minimal contact with the provider until 6 to 8 weeks after delivery. Although routines are often efficient, they may not be effective for meeting needs identified by the woman herself. The provider practicing in the midwifery model maintains her or his role as advocate for each individual woman to ensure that care delivery is safe, effective, and culturally sensitive.

SEXUALITY DURING THE POSTPARTUM PERIOD

The process of maternal and paternal role attainment affects not only the bonds formed between the infant and parents, but also the relationship between the couple. These emotional and psychosocial aspects of the parents' relationship, as well as the physical and physiologic changes of pregnancy and birth, influence the couple's desire, expectation, and initiation of sexual activity.

American obstetric texts have historically either ignored sexuality in pregnancy and the postpartum period or proposed arbitrary coital restrictions from 6 weeks before the expected date of delivery to 6 weeks following the birth. These proscriptions are based more on subtle societal beliefs about the pregnant woman's or new mother's asexuality than on scientific rationale. Cultures are quite varied in the expectations of reestablishment of sexual relations. Some support resumption within weeks of the birth, whereas others may forbid relations until weaning 2 to 3 years after the birth (Reamy and White, 1987). Anthropologists have contributed to the body of knowledge about sexuality in the childbearing year more than medical researchers.

Little research has explored the area of sexuality during the postpartum period. Byrd and colleagues (1998) found that the mean time for resumption of sexual intercourse was 7.3 weeks after delivery, but there was wide variability in the time of resumption. Nineteen percent of women had resumed intercourse within the first month after birth, and 19% did not resume activity until at least 4 months after the birth. Breast-feeding mothers reported decreased sexual activity and satisfaction when compared to nonbreast-feeding mothers. In addition, the male partners of nonbreast-feeding women reported higher levels of satisfaction with the sexual relationship than those of breast-feeding women.

The only other recent study found in the medical literature cited by the U.S. Library of Medicine explored the relationships among mood, sexuality, breast-feeding, and weaning in women who were still breast-feeding at 6 months after delivery (Forster et al., 1994). Participants reported a mean monthly frequency of intercourse of eight times before pregnancy (SD = 4, range 2-16), four times during pregnancy (SD = 4, range 1-16), and three times during the month preceding the interview (SD = 2, range 0-7). The mean time for resumption of intercourse following the birth was 2 months (SD = 1, range 0-6). Following weaning, participants reported a significant increase in frequency of intercourse with no change in sexual responsiveness and frequency of orgasm. In addition, findings suggest that cessation of breast-feeding is associated with decrease in fatigue and improvement in general mood.

Previous work has suggested that breast-feeding women experience sensual and sexual feelings while nursing, and these feelings may influence their interest in sexual activity with their partners. The prospective survey conducted by Byrd and colleagues (1998) suggests distinct differences in sexual satisfaction and satisfaction with the relationship when comparing lactating and nonlactating women and their partners. These differences appear to be influenced by the hormonal differences between lactating and nonlactating women, the ability of nursing to meet the needs for intimate touch in lactating women, and the fatigue experienced by breast-feeding women, since they are responsible for all of the infant feeding.

Discussion of issues surrounding sexuality in the postpartum period should ideally begin in the prenatal period. The provider should approach these discussions with sensitivity toward cultural expectations and personal beliefs held by the woman and her partner. In general, before discharge from the facility in which the birth occurred, the provider should review the factors that should be considered before resuming intercourse and should again guide discussion of the couple's feelings about resuming sexual activity during the first postpartum visit. Couples should be assured that sexual expression following childbirth is a normal, healthy response in the relationship and that they should keep in mind that sexual expression is not limited to only intercourse. Intimacy has a wide range of expression, and the couple can be encouraged to be creative in maintaining their emotional and physical bonds during this period of transition.

MANAGEMENT OF THE FOURTH TRIMESTER

Breast-Feeding Support

The health care professional plays a significant role in supporting the new mother with her breast-feeding efforts. In addition to providing counseling and guidance during prenatal visits and in the immediate postpartum period, the clinician should provide the mother with phone contacts to nursing mother support groups and resources in the community. Women should be encouraged to call the provider with any questions or concerns surrounding breast-feeding.

Preventing or diminishing of the discomfort of engorgement is enhanced by frequent breast-feeding around the clock (Hill and Humenick, 1994). Mothers should be encouraged to keep their infants with them so that true "on demand" feeding can be achieved. Encouraging the mother to allow the infant to be fed by others at night so that she can rest interferes with the establishment and maintenance of lactation. Frequent suckling prevents stasis and distention of the collecting ducts and should be encouraged unless there are maternal or infant medical complications that prevent nursing.

Numerous home remedies have been suggested for the relief of engorgement. A well-fitted bra provides support for the increased weight of the breasts and may decrease discomfort. Application of cold compresses or packs have been recommended based on the fact that the cold temperature causes vasoconstriction and local blockage of neurotransmission of pain.

Recently several researchers have investigated the folk remedy of placing chilled green cabbage leaves on the breasts to decrease the pain and fullness of engorgement. Nikodem and colleagues, using a randomized control design, found that the group using chilled cabbage leaves tended to report less engorgement and had a higher rate of exclusive breast-feeding at 6 weeks after delivery but not at the level of significance (Nikodem, 1993). These study findings are limited by the small sample size. Roberts (1995) compared the use of chilled cabbage leaves with chilled gelpacks and found that both decreased pain to a similar degree but that mothers preferred the use of cabbage leaves. Roberts, Reiter, and Schuster (1998) compared the difference in relief using chilled vs. nonchilled cabbage leaves and found no difference in treatment effects. It has been suggested that cabbage leaves contain a chemical that is absorbed into the skin to decrease the tenderness of engorgement, yet no studies have been able to identify any specific agent. Cold tea bags are also recommended in some communities, but no studies have evaluated the effectiveness of this approach.

Warm compresses should be discouraged since they may increase the swelling because of vasodilation. However, standing under a warm shower and manually expressing milk may be helpful in preparing the nipples for suckling. Herbalists have also suggested that short (3- to 5-minute) application of warm Comfrey leaves may alleviate pain in sore nipples, reduce the pain of engorged breasts, and help milk flow through the ducts (Weed, 1986). Comfrey has been shown to have an anti-inflammatory action and to promote healing of tissue (Weiner and Weiner, 1994). Parsley, with its antibacterial and antifungal action, can also be used effectively in warm compresses, particularly when there has been trauma to the nipple (Weed, 1986; Weiner and Weiner, 1994). Acetaminophen or ibuprofen taken 30 minutes before nursing may decrease the nipple pain to facilitate relaxation so let-down is more efficient.

Women should be prepared for the increased suckling that occurs when infants need to increase the production of milk. These periods of increased nursing appear to correspond to typical times of growth during infancy. Commonly infants increase suckling at 2 to 3 weeks after the birth, and unless women are prepared for this, they may feel that they have "lost" their milk. Reassurance that the increased suckling is usually limited to 24 to 36 hours is appropriate.

Counseling Regarding Self-Care

The clinician should provide counseling that is sensitive to the woman's cultural beliefs surrounding the postpartum period. In general, the following areas should be addressed.

Nutrition. Breast-feeding women should be encouraged to continue a diet similar to that which they followed during pregnancy. Lactation requires an additional 500 kcal above the woman's normal caloric needs. All women, regardless of infant feeding status, should be encouraged to maintain adequate hydration to facilitate the cardiovascular and renal changes in the first week after delivery. A complete diet history will identify deficiencies or risks for deficiencies in protein, vitamins, and minerals. Women who are not lactating and who are particularly interested in weight loss can be counseled to decrease calories, particularly through decreasing fats in the diet.

Activity and rest. Mothers should be encouraged to rest as much as possible during the first week after delivery. Naps and maintaining quiet activity while awake should be encouraged. When possible, women should have others available to help with the usual household responsibilities. Research has suggested that the effects of sleep disturbances are most evident during the first week after delivery, so counseling should stress the wisdom in not doing anything beyond caring for self and baby during that time.

Women who are interested in establishing an exercise regime during the postpartum period can be counseled to begin slowly and pay attention to the body's response. Until 6 weeks after delivery simple stretches and muscle toning exercises are appropriate (Figure 24-1). Gilleard and Brown (1996) found that the ability to stabilize the pelvis against resistance is decreased for at least 8 weeks after delivery, resulting in the recommendation that abdominal exercises that increase pressure against the pelvic structures be avoided. Most women develop diastasis recti, a splitting of the rectus abdominis muscle, during or following pregnancy. The diastasis can be evaluated when the women is lying flat on her back. As she raises her head, bringing her chin to her chest, the separation can be palpated midline from the xiphoid to the symphysis. The degree of separation is noted in fingerbreadths. Women can be instructed to guard the diastasis with their hands when they begin exercises to tone the abdominal musculature and can be counseled that, although exercise may not entirely eliminate the separation, it will decrease the degree of separation and strengthen the muscles of the abdominal wall.

Hygiene. Women should be counseled that bathing is safe during the postpartum period and that good hygiene enhances physical well-being. When cultural proscriptions surround bathing, the clinician can gently explore the woman's beliefs and determine strategies that are acceptable to her and her family. Using a "peribottle" or squeeze bottle to direct a flow of warm water over the perineum from front to back can be continued until laceration or episiotomy repairs feel healed. Breast-feeding women should be counseled to avoid soaps on the nipples since their drying effect may increase the chance of nipple trauma.

Contraceptive options. Similar to other postpartum counseling, contraceptive counseling ideally begins in the prenatal period. The provider should discuss the woman's plans for future fertility and provide her with information that will help her make a decision that is in concert with her personal beliefs and needs. Exploration of experience with previous contraceptive use provides an historical perspective on what has been satisfactory and what has been less than satisfactory.

Hatcher and colleagues (1999) suggest that the provider consider the following when engaging in contraceptive counseling:

- Be aware of one's own biases.
- Recognize that each method has both advantages and disadvantages.
- Recognize the importance of both effectiveness and safety of the method for a given patient.
- Consider the need for protection against sexually transmitted infections (STIs)/human immunodeficiency virus (HIV).
- Recognize the importance of convenience and ability to use the method correctly.
- Consider the necessity of partner negotiation for consistent usage.

The following is a summary of factors to consider for recommendation of use of each method during the postpartum period (Grimes and Wallach, 1997; Hatcher et al., 1997; Hatcher, Zieman, and Watt, 1998; Hatcher et al., 1999). The reader is referred to a family planning text for further information about management of each

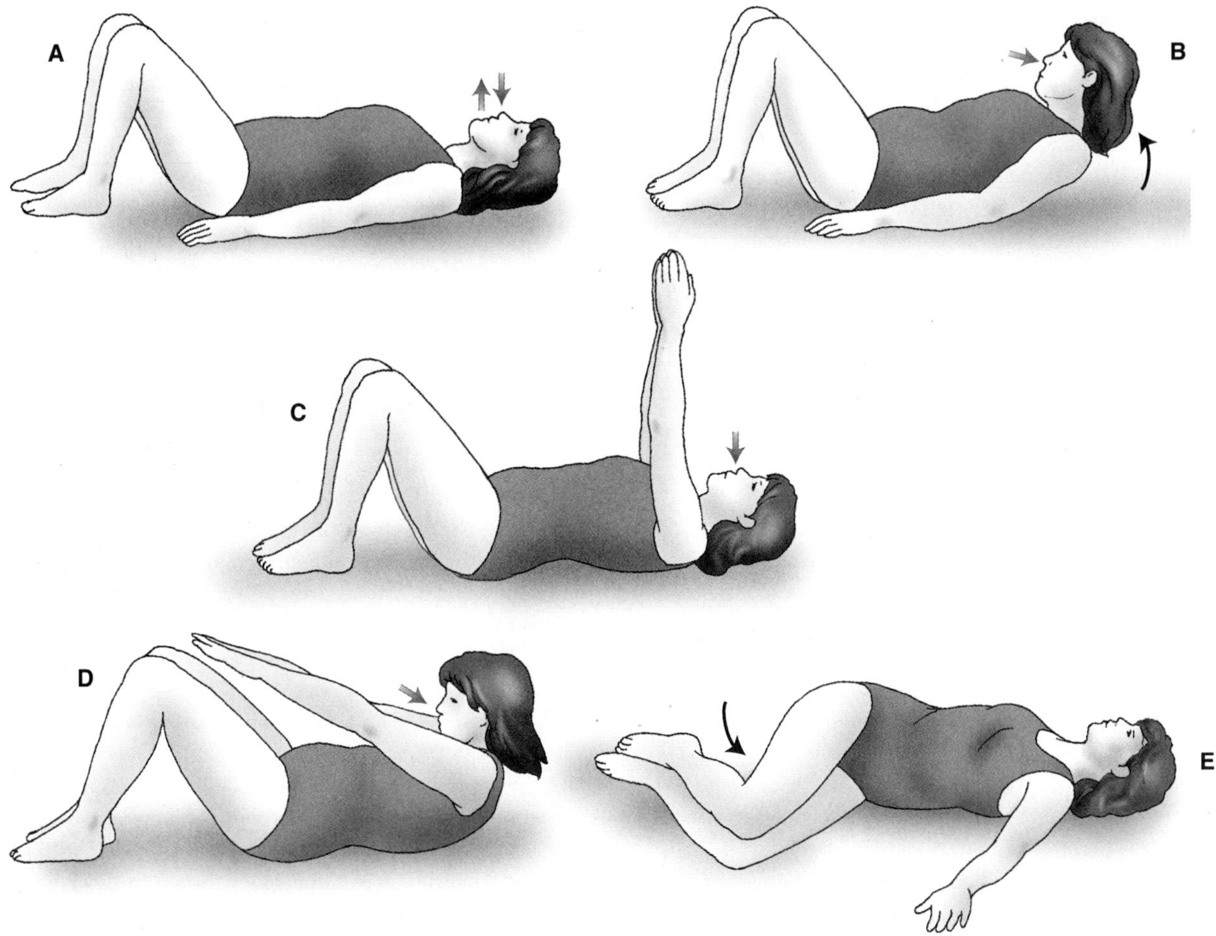

Figure 24-1 Postpartum exercises. A, Abdominal: Lying supine with the knees bent or with a pillow under the knees, the woman takes a deep chest breath through the nose while keeping the ribs still. This will expand the abdominal wall. She then exhales through the mouth, tightening her abdominal muscles voluntarily. B, Abdominal: Lying supine with the knees bent, the woman inhales through the nose while lifting her chin to her chest. During exhalation, she lowers her head back to the neutral position and relaxes. C, Abdominal: Lying supine with the knees bent, the woman extends her arms out so that they are perpendicular to her torso. As she inhales, she raises her arms slowly until her hands meet above her chest. She returns her arms to the resting position during exhalation. D, Abdominal: Lying supine with the knees bent, the woman lifts her head and shoulders and reaches for her knees with her hands. As she raises her head, she inhales. She then returns to the resting position while exhaling. E, Abdominal, Buttock, and Thigh Stretching: Lying supine with knees and hips flexed, the woman extends her arms so they are perpendicular to the torso. Throughout the exercise, the shoulders should stay stationary. She then rolls both knees to one side, touching the floor, then returning to the resting position. She repeats the exercise, rolling the knees to the opposite side. As flexibility increases, she can roll one knee at a time, bringing the knee over the opposite knee.

method since the management goes beyond the scope of this text.

Abstinence Abstinence is practiced by many cultures as a means to protect the mother from closely spaced pregnancies and facilitate her return to a healthy non-pregnant state. Couples using this method in the postpartum period are usually practicing secondary abstinence, which is the state in which previous sexual activity has been their norm, but the decision is made to abstain for a given period of time.

Mechanism of action Since there is no deposit of semen in or near the vagina, fertilization is not possible.

Issues in the postpartum period This is commonly accepted as a normal response to the postpartum period, usually for 6 to 8 weeks after the birth.

Effectiveness Data are not available to determine the typical user failure rate in the first year.

Advantages There is no possibility of hormonal side effects experienced with other pharmacologic approaches. It can be practiced at any time, and there is no need for a provider examination or to obtain materials for use. Many religious groups endorse the use of this method. Abstinence decreases the risk of STIs.
Disadvantages The method requires firm commitment and self-control on the part of both partners. Power or force may be used to force a woman to comply with her partner's sexual wishes.
Side effects/complications Partner discord may result if a woman's partner does not support this approach.
Ideal candidates Couples in mature, committed relationships are most likely to be successful with this method.

Fertility Awareness Methods

Mechanism of action The woman is taught to determine when ovulation occurs to then either abstain from intercourse at the time of fertility or use other methods to prevent conception. Several methods can be used to determine days in which the risk of pregnancy are high, and women often combine methods to increase effectiveness.

1. *Calendar method.* The women records her menstrual cycles for at least 6 months, then determines the earliest day of the fertile period by identifying the shortest cycle and subtracting 14 from the number of days in that cycle. This assumes that ovulation occurs 14 days before the onset of menses. She then determines the latest day of fertility by identifying the longest cycle and subtracting 14 days. Assuming that sperm are capable of fertilizing the ovum for 2 to 3 days, 3 days are subtracted from the first day of possible fertility determined by the shortest cycle.

   Example: Your client's shortest cycle is 25 days. Subtract 14 days, then subtract another 3 days for sperm viability. Her earliest day of possible fertility is day 9 of her cycle. Her longest cycle is 30 days. Subtract 14 days, giving you day 16 as her last day of possible fertility. During days 9 through 16 she either abstains or uses another barrier method to prevent pregnancy.

2. *Ovulation method.* Women follow their cyclic cervical mucus changes with their fingers to identify the changes that occur immediately before ovulation. From menses until preovulation cervical mucus is scant, but in the preovulation phase the mucus changes to cloudy, yellowish-white color with sticky consistency. At the time of ovulation, the mucus becomes clear and very thin and watery. Once the mucus becomes scant again, it is assumed that she is no longer fertile. Abstinence or use of another barrier method should be used during the period of thinned cervical mucus (usually about 4 days).
3. *Basal body temperature method (BBT).* This method uses the usual rise of basal body temperature of 0.4° to 0.8° F that occurs with ovulation to identify the most fertile period. The fertile period is defined as the first drop or elevation through 3 consecutive days of elevation of temperature.
4. *Symptothermal method.* This combines at least two methods, usually cervical mucus and BBT. Some women also learn to assess cervical consistency and dilation of the cervical os to further identify the period of fertility.

Issues in the postpartum period Breast-feeding, because of its effect on vaginal secretions and cervical mucus, may make it more difficult for a woman to identify signs of ovulation. Women may want to consider further protection with a barrier method until the infant is weaned.
Effectiveness The typical failure rate in the first year averages 25% for all methods of fertility awareness.
Advantages This method empowers the woman to be more aware of her own physiology. There are no side effects as with pharmacologic methods. Couples who are in mature and committed relationships can work cooperatively to control fertility.
Disadvantages Women with irregular periods may have a more difficult time determining periods of fertility. During the period of data gathering to determine the woman's normal cycles, there must be commitment to either abstinence or reliable use of a barrier method that does not interfere with the signs of ovulation. The method requires full commitment from both partners.
Side effects/complications There are no known complications.
Ideal candidates Couples who are highly motivated to first document the woman's experience with cycles and possibly experience extensive periods of abstinence are ideal candidates. Couples who face religious proscriptions against other methods benefit from this method.

Lactational Amenorrhea (LAM) Several large international studies have validated the use of LAM as a temporary method of contraception for women who are fully breast-feeding, women whose menses have not returned, and women whose infants are younger than 6 months old.

Mechanism of action Infant suckling stimulates the hypothalamic-pituitary axis to release prolactin, which inhibits ovulation.

Issues in the postpartum period This method can be used up to six months after delivery. The method cannot be used effectively if the infant is greater than 6 months of age, if menses has returned, if other food has been introduced into the infant's diet and frequency of nursing has been decreased. LAM is also not appropriate if the woman is using medication or recreational drugs that are contraindicated during breast-feeding, or if the woman is HIV positive.

Effectiveness Typical-use failure rate during 6 months of use is 2%.

Advantages Breast-feeding is the best food substance for infants. Breast-feeding is usually a pleasurable experience for the woman and her infant, it facilitates maternal-infant attachment, and it protects against certain infections in the newborn. In addition, breast-feeding facilitates uterine involution, decreases postpartum blood loss, and may offer a protective effect against ovarian and premenopausal cancer of the breast in the woman.

Disadvantages Frequent breast-feeding may be difficult for some women. If the woman is HIV positive, there is a 14% to 29% risk of infant infection with exposure to breast milk.

Side effects/complications The woman may experience sore nipples, tenderness of the breast, and mastitis. These complications decrease after the first few weeks of lactation.

Ideal candidates Women who are committed to fully breast-feeding and those who breast-feed for a minimum of 6 months are the best candidates for this method.

Withdrawal (Coitus Interruptus) Withdrawal is still practiced in some cultures even though the limitations of the method are well recognized.

Mechanism of action The male withdraws the penis from the vagina before ejaculation. This eliminates or significantly decreases the chance that sperm are deposited in the vagina near the cervix.

Issues in the postpartum period The method may be used in the postpartum period.

Effectiveness Typical-use failure rate in the first year of use is 19%.

Advantages There are no hormonal side effects, the method is readily available, and it does not require abstinence.

Disadvantages The method requires the male's full cooperation and ability to withdraw immediately before ejaculation. This may decrease the pleasure of orgasm for both the man and the woman. Withdrawal does not provide any protection against STIs. Sperm may be present in preejaculatory secretions.

Side effects/complications Couples may experience frustration with the lack of opportunity to complete sexual expression with intercourse.

Ideal candidates Couples in committed, mature, monogamous relationships who can accept the higher risk of pregnancy are good candidates for this method. In addition, couples without religious beliefs that proscribe withdrawal will be more successful with this method.

Barrier Methods: Condoms (Male)

Mechanism of action Sheaths made of latex, polyurethane, or natural membranes are placed over the penis before ejaculation to prevent sperm from being deposited in the vagina.

Issues in the postpartum period Condoms may be used effectively in the postpartum period. The use of condoms lubricated with spermicides may increase pleasure by overcoming the dryness associated with breast-feeding.

Effectiveness Typical-use failure rate in the first year is 14%. Breakage occurs in less than 1 in 100 uses with experienced users.

Advantages There are no hormonal side effects. Men may take longer to reach orgasm during intercourse, thereby increasing pleasure for some couples. The method offers protection against most STIs and decreases the risk of human papilloma virus (HPV)-induced cervical changes. Condoms are readily available and are usually relatively inexpensive.

Disadvantages Partners must be comfortable with putting the condom on the penis, and the placement of the condom may interrupt sexual activity. Purchasing condoms may be embarrassing for some individuals, and negotiating partner use of condoms may be difficult for some women. Some oil-based lubricants may decrease the strength of latex condoms.

Side effects/complications Allergic reactions to latex may develop.

Ideal candidates Couples with the commitment to use the method with every sexual encounter are ideal candidates. Couples who desire reduction of risk of infection (including pregnant and postpartum women) and couples who desire a longer plateau phase of sexual excitement are also good candidates.

Barrier Methods: Condoms (Female)

Mechanism of action The female condom is a polyurethane tube, 15 cm long and 7 cm wide. A flexible inner ring at the closed end gets placed as deeply in the vagina as possible, and a larger outer ring remains external. This mechanical barrier prevents passage of sperm to the cervix.

Issues in the postpartum period The method may be used in the postpartum period.

Effectiveness Typical-use failure in the first year of use is 21%.

Advantages The woman using this method has control over its use. Because she puts it in place, she is sure it is being used. It can be inserted up to 8 hours before intercourse. It decreases the risk of STIs and may decrease the risk of HPV-induced cervical changes. All lubricants can be used safely with the female condom.

Disadvantages Some women may have difficulty inserting the condom. The penis needs to be manually inserted into the condom for best results, and this may be unacceptable for some couples, and the presence of the condoms may decrease pleasure for either or both partners. Movement of the polyurethane in the vagina may cause noise before or during intercourse.

Side effects/complications Frequent use of female condoms may lead to vaginal flora changes, increased urinary tract infections (UTIs), and vaginitis.

Ideal candidates Women who need to have control of protection against both pregnancy and infection are good candidates for this method.

Spermicides (Foam, Suppositories, Film, Cream, Jelly)

Mechanism of action The most common spermicides found in the United States are nonoxynol-9 and octoxynol-9, and they are prepared in vaginal creams, gels, foams, films, suppositories, and tablets. They provide a certain amount of mechanical barrier to the sperm but are more effective with their ability to alter sperm flagella and bodies, thereby reducing motility. In addition, these chemicals affect the fructolytic activity in the sperm and interfere with necessary nourishment.

Issues in the postpartum period These agents can be used in the postpartum period. The lubrication provided by the agents may increase pleasure for lactating women by overcoming the physiologic dryness experienced by most breast-feeding women.

Effectiveness Typical-use failure rate in the first year averages 26%. When combined with other methods, effectiveness for contraception increases.

Advantages The agents are readily available in clinics and pharmacies, and they require no professional visit or instruction in use. Most are easy to insert. The chemicals have been shown to have antimicrobial properties that may decrease the risk of STIs. They carry no hormonal side effects.

Disadvantages Some women may be uncomfortable inserting the agents, and women may find them "messy." Used alone, they have a relatively high failure rate.

Side effects/complications Sensitivity to the chemicals may cause irritation. Vaginal mucosa irritation may lead to increased risk of STIs because of creation of portals of entry for organisms.

Ideal candidates Women who can negotiate spermicide use with another barrier method are ideal candidates for this method.

Diaphragm

Mechanism of action The latex, dome-shaped device comes in sizes from 60 to 90 mm diameter to maximize proper fit. The four types of diaphragms available in the United States are the flat spring, coil spring, arcing spring, and wide seal. The device acts as a mechanical barrier to sperm entry into the cervix and provides a chemical barrier through the use of spermicide against the cervix.

Issues in the postpartum period Involution of the vagina must be complete to effectively fit the device.

Effectiveness Typical-use failure rate in the first year is 20%.

Advantages The use of this method is under the control of the woman, it may be placed up to 6 hours before intercourse, and it can be used during lactation. The diaphragm decreases the risk of STIs, cervical dysplasia, and pelvic inflammatory disease (PID). It does not carry any hormone-related side effects.

Disadvantages Placement may be difficult or unpleasant for some women. The device requires professional fitting and brief training in use. Women with pelvic relaxation may not be able to be fit effectively. The failure rate is relatively high.

Side effects/complications Use of the device may alter vaginal flora, particularly increasing coliform counts. This increases the risks of vaginitis and UTIs. Improperly fitting a diaphragm that is too large may lead to vaginal mucosa erosion. Leaving the device in the vagina for a prolonged period of time may increase the risk of toxic shock syndrome. Latex allergy may develop in some individuals.

Ideal candidates Women who are motivated to use the device with every act of intercourse and women who can tolerate the relatively higher failure rate are good candidates for this method.

Cervical Cap

Mechanism of action This small, dome-shaped latex device comes in four sizes to form a tight fit over the cervix. A groove on the inner rim creates suction that keeps it in place. The cap provides both a mechanical barrier against sperm entering the cervix and a chemical barrier through the use of spermicide inside the cap.
Issues in the postpartum period The cap cannot be used until the cervix has completed involution—usually 6 to 8 weeks.
Effectiveness Typical-use failure rate in the first year is 20% for nulliparous women and 40% in parous women.
Advantages Use of this method can be controlled by the woman, and the cap can be inserted up to 6 hours before intercourse and left in place for multiple acts of intercourse for up to 48 hours. There are no hormone-related side effects. The cap may decrease the risk of PID.
Disadvantages The method has a relatively high failure rate. It may be difficult for some women to place, and partners may not like feeling the cap in place. There is an increased risk for cervical dysplasia secondary to the erosion and inflammation that may result from use. Professional fitting and a repeat Pap smear after 3 months of use are recommended. Women with irregularly shaped cervixes or women with known cervical lesions are not candidates for use.
Side effects/complications Cervical erosion and abnormal cervical cytology may develop with use. Change in vaginal flora, particularly increased coliform counts, may lead to increased UTIs. Latex allergy may develop.
Ideal candidates Women committed to use of the cap with every intercourse and those who have no problems inserting and removing the device are the best candidates for the method. The high failure rate is associated with difficulties using the device and poor fit. Women with smooth cervical anatomy are likely to have better fit of the device.

Oral Contraceptives (Combined)

Mechanism of action Combined oral contraceptives (COCs) suppress ovulation in 90% to 95% of cycles. In addition, the pills cause thickening of the cervical mucus, and continued use leads to poor development of the endometrium, leading to inhibition of implantation. COCs with an estrogen component less than 50 μg contain ethinyl estradiol. Numerous progestins are used to complement the estrogen component. Almost all COCs available in the United States use 21 active pills followed by 7 placebo pills. COCs can be monophasic—using the same dosage throughout the cycle—or multiphasic—using varying dosages as the cycle progresses.
Issues in the postpartum period The use of COCs in breast-feeding women is controversial. The World Health Organization (WHO) advises that COCs never be used during the first 6 weeks after delivery in lactating women and used from 6 weeks to 6 months after delivery in lactating women only if there are no other appropriate and acceptable methods. However, many clinicians support the use of COCs once lactation has been established, usually at 6 weeks after delivery. Use of COCs may change the composition of breast milk, and the estrogen component may decrease the quantity of milk produced. Ingestion of hormones in breast milk may lead to hormonal side effects in the infant.
Effectiveness Typical-use failure rate in the first year of use is 5%.
Advantages COCs have been found to decrease dysmenorrhea, ovulatory pain, and actual menstrual blood loss. The method may enhance satisfaction with sexual activity because of decreased fear of pregnancy. Manipulation of the pill-free interval can decrease the number of cycles per year or alter the onset of menses. Use of COCs is an effective approach to the problems of irregular periods, heavy menses, and dysfunctional uterine bleeding. The facts that the use of the method is not associated with sexual activity and that COCs are highly effective when taken correctly increase satisfaction for couples. Use of COCs is associated with decreased risk of ovarian and endometrial cancer. COCs may improve acne and hirsutism, and there is evidence that the method may decrease the occurrence of osteoporosis and rheumatoid arthritis.
Disadvantages Women may experience vaginal spotting during the first few cycles and may develop amenorrhea. This method increases the risk of adenocarcinoma of the cervix, although some experts believe that the increase may be the result of confounding variables. COCs provide no protection against STIs; thus concurrent use of condoms is recommended for women at risk for infections. Certain drugs may decrease the effectiveness of COCs, and COCs may alter the effect of some drugs.
Side effects/complications Women may experience nausea, breast tenderness, increased breast size, weight gain secondary to increased appetite, and headaches when using COCs. Some women experience hypertension. There is a slightly increased risk for deep vein thrombosis in women using COCs. Contraindications for COCs are age 35 years or older and smoking, moderate to severe hypertension, undiagnosed vaginal bleeding,

diabetes with vascular involvement, deep vein thrombosis, ischemic heart disease, history of stroke, migraine headaches with auras, current or past history of breast cancer, active viral hepatitis, mild or severe cirrhosis, major surgery with immobilization within the past month, history of cholestasis with OC, and family history of thrombosis.

Ideal candidates Women who desire the advantages of COCs and who can remember to take a pill at the same time each day are the ideal candidates for the method.

Oral Contraceptives (Progestin-Only)

Mechanism of action Progestin-only pills (POPs) suppress ovulation in about 50% of cycles, thicken cervical mucus, and lead to thin endometrium, which inhibits implantation.

Issues in the postpartum period The WHO and the International Planned Parenthood Federation recommend initiating POPs at 6 weeks after delivery; however, the National Medical Committee of Planned Parenthood Federation of America considers initiation immediately after delivery to be appropriate. Infants who are breast-fed have a daily intake of synthetic steroids through breast milk as follows: norethindrone, 100 to 200 ng; levonorgestrel, 40 to 140 ng. There are no known adverse effects in the infant when exposed to these levels of progestins.

Effectiveness Typical-use failure rate in the first year is 5%.

Advantages Use of POPs is associated with decreased dysmenorrhea, ovulatory pain, and menstrual blood loss. Similar to COCs, the method may offer protection against ovarian and endometrial cancer. POPs can be used by lactating women and by women who have had problems with the estrogen component of COCs. POPs can also be used by women with a history of thrombophlebitis, smokers, and women over age 35.

Disadvantages Menstrual disorders associated with use of POPs include spotting in the first few cycles, missed menses, scant flow during menses, and breakthrough bleeding.

Side effects/complications Use of POPs may increase depression, anxiety, fatigue, and appetite.

Ideal candidates Lactating women and women who have contraindications to the estrogen component of the COCs are ideal candidates.

Injectable Progestins (DMPA)

Mechanism of action Depo-medroxyprogesterone acetate (DMPA) inhibits the LH and FSH surge, thereby suppressing ovulation. DMPA also thickens the cervical mucus and decreases the thickness of the endometrium. DMPA, 150 mg, is administered intramuscularly every 12 weeks.

Issues in the postpartum period The WHO and Planned Parenthood Federation recommend initiating DMPA after 6 weeks postpartum. The National Medical Committee of the Planned Parenthood Federation of America considers it safe and appropriate to initiate DMPA immediately after delivery. In the first week following injection, breast-fed infants receive10 μg of DMPA daily through breast milk. The exposure decreases over the next 11 weeks, and by the twelfth week after injection the intake is 0.3 μg daily. Exposure to DMPA has not been associated with adverse effects to the infant.

Effectiveness Typical-use failure rate in the first year is 0.3%.

Advantages Use of DMPA is associated with decreased dysmenorrhea, ovulatory pain, and menstrual blood loss. The method may enhance satisfaction with sexual activity because of decreased fear of pregnancy. Amenorrhea is experienced by 50% of users after 1 year's use. There is a theoretic decrease in risk of ovarian and endometrial cancer. The couple does not have to initiate any protection against pregnancy at the time of intercourse, and the woman does not need to remember to take pills on a daily basis. DMPA can be used by women who cannot use estrogen-containing preparations and can be used with lactation.

Disadvantages The method does not offer protection against STIs. Many women are disturbed by the irregular bleeding generated by the method. DMPA is associated with increased appetite and weight gain. Women experience an average of 10 months' delay in return of ovulation following the last injection, so the method is not ideal for someone desiring relatively closely spaced pregnancies.

Side effects/complications Persistent weight gain, severe depression, and severe allergic reactions are rare complications.

Ideal candidates Women who cannot use estrogen yet desire a highly effective contraceptive are ideal candidates for this method. In addition, women who fear discovery of their contraceptive use are good candidates.

Norplant

Mechanism of action Norplant is comprised of six soft plastic capsules containing levonorgestrel, 36 mg, in each capsule. The capsules are surgically implanted into the inner aspect of the woman's upper arm. Release of the progestin leads to thickening of the cervical mucus and inhibition of ovulation. Over time the endometrium becomes atrophic.

Issues in the postpartum period The WHO and Planned Parenthood Federation recommend initiating Norplant after 6 weeks postpartum. The National Medical Committee of the Planned Parenthood Federation of America considers it safe and appropriate to initiate this method immediately after delivery. Breast-fed infants receive 25 to 300 ng of progestin daily when this method is used, and this exposure has not been shown to be associated with any infant growth or health problems.

Effectiveness Typical-use failure rate in the first year is 0.05%.

Advantages Use of Norplant is associated with decreased cramping, ovulatory pain, and menstrual blood loss. The method may enhance satisfaction with sexual activity because of decreased fear of pregnancy. There is evidence that the risk of ovarian and endometrial cancer is decreased for users. Norplant is a highly effective long-term method and may be used by women for whom there are contraindications to estrogen.

Disadvantages Irregular bleeding patterns may be unsatisfactory for many women. The method does not offer protection against STIs. Breast tenderness and weight gain are common in users. The capsules may be visible under the skin, which would be cosmetically unacceptable for some women. Local discomfort, especially the first few days after insertion, may be experienced. Removal requires surgical intervention, and adhesion formation may make removal difficult.

Side effects/complications Amenorrhea is a common problem for users. Ovarian enlargement secondary to unruptured follicles stimulated by FSH may occur. Inflammation or infection at the site of insertion is a risk. Difficult removal may lead to unacceptable scarring and/or nerve damage.

Ideal candidates Women who desire long-term contraception that is highly effective and who are at low risk for STIs are ideal candidates. When women are at risk for STIs, condoms should be used with each intercourse.

Intrauterine Device (IUD)

Mechanism of action The T-shaped polyethylene device is wrapped in copper, and double strings hang from the vertical limb of the device. The mechanism of actions are thought to be a mechanical and chemical alteration in the uterus that decreases the proportion of sperm that reach the oviduct and ovum, chemical action on the sperm that decreases the ability to penetrate the egg, and alteration of the endometrium that decreases the chance of implantation should fertilization occur.

The T-shaped IUD that has progesterone embedded in the vertical limb releases 65 μg of progesterone per day. In addition to the mechanisms noted for the copper device, the progesterone IUD causes thicker cervical mucus, which inhibits sperm migration into the uterus. It also alters uterotubal fluid in a way that inhibits sperm migration and suppresses endometrium development, preventing implantation.

Issues in the postpartum period In the United States insertion of an IUD should be deferred until uterine involution is complete since the uterine contractions that occur during involution may increase the risk of perforation and expulsion. However, many international family planning programs insert the IUD between delivery and 48 hours after delivery without increase in expulsion or perforation.

Effectiveness Typical-use failure rate in the first year of use is 0.8% for the copper device and 2% for the progesterone device. The copper device is approved for effectiveness for 10 years, but it is probably effective for 12 years. The progesterone device must be replaced annually.

Advantages The IUD is a highly effective method for long-term contraception, yet it is easily reversible. The woman does not need to initiate use at the time of intercourse. Lactating women may use the device effectively. The method may enhance satisfaction with sexual activity because of decreased fear of pregnancy. The strings need to be checked only once per month, and the cost over time is relatively low.

Disadvantages Women may experience increased spotting or heavier menses and increased dysmenorrhea with the copper IUD. Eleven percent of women using this device have it removed in the first year because of bleeding problems. Use of the progesterone IUD may decrease blood loss and dysmenorrhea. Some women may find checking the strings difficult or unpleasant. The device offers no protection against STIs, and the WHO discourages use in women at increased risk for HIV infection.

Side effects/complications Risk of PID is increased in the first month following insertion. There are risks of pain with insertion, uterine perforation, and allergy to copper. If women become pregnant with the IUD in place, they are at risk for spontaneous abortion and severe pelvic infections. Women using the progesterone IUD are at risk for development of ovarian follicular cysts caused by hormonally induced unruptured follicles. These cysts may be extremely painful and require further evaluation.

Ideal candidates Parous women desiring long-term contraception who are at low risk for STIs (e.g., monogamous relationship) are the ideal candidates for this method.

Voluntary Female Sterilization (Tubal Ligation)

Mechanism of action Surgical interruption of the fallopian tubes inhibits the ability of the sperm to fertilize the ovum.

Issues in the postpartum period Tubal ligation (TL) may be done any time in the postpartum period.

Effectiveness Typical-use failure rates vary by the type of procedure used. In general, cumulative 10-year failure rates range from 0.8% to 3.7%. Two-year failure rate is 0.7%.

Advantages TL is permanent and highly effective. The method may enhance satisfaction with sexual activity because of decreased fear of pregnancy. Although it is a surgical procedure, it can be done in an outpatient facility.

Disadvantages There may be some changes in menstrual patterns during the first few months following the procedure. The method does not offer protection against STIs.

Side effects/complications Surgical risks include infection, wound separation, hemorrhage, damage to other organs, and death (usually related to anesthetic complications). If fertilization occurs, there is a higher risk for ectopic implantation. Menstrual disorders may continue in the long term.

Ideal candidates Women who are mature and sure that they want no more children are ideal candidates. Although reversal is possible, women should recognize that successful pregnancy following reversal is not common. Women who have medical problems that make pregnancy a risk to their health and well-being are also good candidates.

Voluntary Male Sterilization

Mechanism of action Interruption of the vas deferens prevents passage of sperm in the seminal fluid. Cutting and/or cauterizing are the commonly used means of interrupting the vas.

Issues in the postpartum period None

Effectiveness Typical-use failure rate is estimated to be 0.1%.

Advantages Since this is a male method, there are no advantages to the woman, except that the male takes an active role in contraception and the effectiveness enhances satisfaction with sexual activity because of the decreased fear of pregnancy.

Disadvantages One or both partners may regret the decision later. Alternate contraception is needed for the first 20 ejaculations following the procedure. The method does not offer any protection against STIs.

Side effects/complications Surgical complications include bleeding, infection, and pain. There is a weak increase in risk of prostate cancer in men who have undergone the procedure.

Ideal candidates Men who desire permanent contraception and who are at low risk for STIs are ideal candidates. Men at risk for STIs should continue to use condoms at each intercourse.

References

Ahdoot D et al: The effect of route of delivery on regression of abnormal cervical cytologic findings in the postpartum period, *Am J Obstet Gynecol* 178(6):1116-1120, 1998.

American Academy of Pediatrics, and American College of Obstetricians and Gynecologists: *Guidelines for perinatal care,* ed 4, 1997, Elk Grove Village, Ill, American Academy of Pediatrics.

American College of Obstetricians and Gynecologists: *Postpartum depression,* Washington, DC, 1995, American College of Obstetricians and Gynecologists.

Becker AE: Postpartum illness in Fiji: a sociosomatic perspective, *Psychosom Med* 60(4):431-438, 1998.

Blackburn ST, Loper DL: *Maternal, fetal, and neonatal physiology :a clinical perspective,* Philadelphia, 1992, WB Saunders.

Boardley DJ et al: The relationship between diet, activity, and other factors, and postpartum weight change by race, *Obstet Gynecol* 86(5):834-838, 1992.

Bowes WA: Postpartum care. In Gabbe SG, Niebyl JR, Simpson JL, editors: *Obstetrics—normal and problem pregnancies,* ed 3, New York, 1996, Churchill Livingstone.

Byrd JE et al: Sexuality during pregnancy and the year postpartum, *J Fam Pract* 47(4):305-308, 1998.

Cluett ER, Alexander J, Pickering RM: What is the normal pattern of uterine involution? An investigation of postpartum uterine involution measured by the distance between the symphysis pubis and the uterine fundus using a paper tape measure, *Midwifery* 13(1):9-16, 1997.

Crowell MK, Hill PD, Humenick SS: Relationship between obstetric analgesia and time of effective breastfeeding, *J Nurse Midwifery* 39:150-155, 1994.

Daly SEJ, Hartmann PE: Infant demand and milk supply. Part 1. Infant demand and milk production in lactating women, *J Hum Lactation* 11(1):21-26, 1995a.

Daly SEJ, Hartmann PE: Infant demand and milk supply. Part 2. The short-term control of milk synthesis in lactating women, *J Hum Lactation* 11(1):27-37, 1995b.

Forster C et al: Psychological and sexual changes after the cessation of breastfeeding. *Obstet Gynecol* 84(5):872-876, 1994.

Gardner DL: Fatigue in postpartum women, *Appl Nurs Res* 4(2):57-62, 1991.

Gilleard WL, Brown JM: Structure and function of the abdominal muscles in primigravida subjects during pregnancy and the immediate postbirth period, *Phys Ther* 76(7):750-762, 1996.

Grimes DA, Wallach M, editors: *Modern contraception—updates from the contraception report,* Totowa, NJ, 1997, Emron.

Hatcher RA, Zieman M, Watt AP: *Managing contraception,* Tiger, Ga, 1998, Bridging the Gap Foundation.

Hatcher RA et al: *The essentials of contraceptive technology,* Baltimore, 1997, Johns Hopkins University School of Public Health, Population Information Program.

Hatcher RA et al: *A pocket guide to managing contraception,* Tiger, Ga, 1999, Bridging the Gap Foundation.

Hill PD, Humenick SS: The occurrence of breast engorgement, *J Hum Lactation* 10(2):79-86, 1994.

Holroyd E et al: "Doing the month": an exploration of postpartum practices in Chinese women, *Health Care Women Int* 18:301-313, 1996.

Humenick SS, Hill PD, Anderson MA: Breast engorgement: patterns and selected outcomes, *J Hum Lactation* 10(2):87-93, 1994.

Institute of Medicine: *Nutrition during pregnancy and lactation—an implementation guide,* Washington, DC, 1992, National Academy of Sciences.

Jambunathan J: Hmong cultural practices and beliefs: the postpartum period, *Clin Nurs Res* 4(3):335-345, 1995.

Labbok M, Cooney K, Coly S: *Guidelines: breastfeeding, family planning, and the lactational amenorrhea method—LAM,* Washington, DC, 1994, Institute for Reproductive Health.

Labbok MH et al: Multicenter study of the lactational amenorrhea method (LAM). I. Efficacy, duration, and implications for clinical application, *Contraception* 55(6):327-336, 1997.

Lawrence RA: *Breastfeeding—a guide for the medical profession,* ed 4, St Louis, 1994, Mosby.

Mercer RT: The process of maternal role attainment over the first year, *Nurs Res* 34:198-204, 1985.

Meyer S et al: The effects of birth on urinary continence mechanisms and other pelvic-floor characteristics, *Obstet Gynecol* 92(4):613-618, 1998.

Moran C et al: Recovery of ovarian function after childbirth, lactation and sexual activity with relation to age of women, *Contraception* 50(5):401-407, 1994.

Nikodem VC: Do cabbage leaves prevent breast engorgement? A randomized, controlled study, *Birth* 20(2):61-64, 1993.

Oppenheimer LW et al: The duration of lochia, *Br J Obstet Gynaecol* 93:754-757, 1986.

Reamy KJ, White SE: Sexuality in the puerperium: a review, *Arch Sexual Behav* 16(2):165-186, 1987.

Roberts KL: A comparison of chilled cabbage leaves and chilled gelpacks in reducing breast engorgement, *J Hum Lactation* 11(1):17-20, 1995.

Roberts KL, Reiter M, Schuster D: Effects of cabbage leaf extract on breast engorgement. *J Hum Lactation* 14(3):231-236, 1998.

Sampselle CM et al: Effect of pelvic muscle exercise on transient incontinence during pregnancy and after birth, *Obstet Gynecol* 91(3):406-412, 1998.

Schauberger CW, Rooney BL, Brimer LM: Factors that influence weight loss in the puerperium, *Obstet Gynecol* 79(3): 424-429, 1992.

Sich D: Traditional concepts and customs on pregnancy, birth and postpartum period in rural Korea, *Soc Sci Med* 15B(1):65-69, 1981.

Simpson KR, Creehan PA, editors: *AWHONN perinatal nursing,* Philadelphia, 1996, JB Lippincott.

Swain AM et al: A prospective study of sleep, mood and cognitive function in postpartum women and nonpostpartum women, *Obstet Gynecol* 90(3):381-386, 1997.

Visness CM, Kennedy KI, Ramos R: The duration and character of postpartum bleeding among breast-feeding women, *Obstet Gynecol* 89(2):159-163, 1997.

Visness CM et al: Fertility of fully breastfeeding women in the early postpartum period, *Obstet Gynecol* 89(2):164-167, 1997.

Wambach KA: Maternal fatigue in breastfeeding primiparae during the first nine weeks postpartum, *J Hum Lactation* 14(3):219-229, 1998.

Weed SS: *The wise woman herbal childbearing year,* Woodstock, NY, 1986, Ash Tree Publishing.

Weiner MA, Weiner JA: *Herbs that heal,* Mill Valley, Calif, 1994, Quantum Books.

Willms AB et al: Anatomic changes in the pelvis after uncomplicated vaginal delivery: evaluation with serial MR imaging, *Radiology* 195(1):91-94, 1995.

Unit IV

Collaborative Care of Complications During Pregnancy

Chapter 25

Medical Complications During Pregnancy

Community-based care requires that the clinician provide ongoing screening for problems or potential problems that may have an impact on perinatal outcome. When deviations from normal are identified, the clinician must determine whether clinical management can continue to be provided independently, whether consultation and/or collaboration is appropriate, or whether referral to an obstetric specialist is indicated. State regulations, professional organization policies and position statements, and the relationship between the midwife and other members of the perinatal health care team all must be considered when determining the appropriate level of management. Decisions regarding level of care must be made in collaboration with the woman and her family in a way that respects the cultural values and beliefs held in the family and community.

CARDIOVASCULAR SYSTEM PROBLEMS

Anemia

Anemia is the general term used for deficiency in the quantity or quality of red blood cells (RBCs), with a resulting decrease in the oxygen-carrying capacity of the blood (Sweet, 1997). Anemia is not a specific diagnosis but rather an indication of an underlying disorder. Anemia is commonly defined as a lower-than-normal hemoglobin (Hgb) concentration or a lower-than-normal concentration of RBCs in the blood (Engstrom and Sittler, 1994). The Centers for Disease Control and Prevention (1998b) has adjusted the definition to take into account the normal physiologic dilution of the vascular system in pregnancy, as well as the influence of smoking and altitude on RBC quantity and quality (Table 25-1). Anemias can be acquired or hereditary, with acquired iron deficiency anemia the most common found in pregnancy.

Acquired anemias

Iron Deficiency Anemia

Pathology Iron requirements in pregnancy are significantly increased as a result of the increased maternal and fetal needs. It is estimated that maternal need throughout a term pregnancy averages 1000 mg of elemental iron—300 mg for fetal and placental development and 500 mg for expansion of maternal Hgb mass. About 200 mg is lost through urinary, bowel, and skin excretion. Another way to consider the pregnant woman's iron needs is the recognition that her demand for iron is approximately 5 mg of elemental iron per day during the second and third trimester. The estimated need for pregnancy exceeds the maternal iron stores in

Table 25-1 *Recommended Cut-offs for Iron-Deficiency Anemia in Pregnancy and Adjustments Suggested for Smokers and Women Residing at High Altitudes*

	Hemoglobin concentration (g/dl)	Hematocrit (%)
Trimester		
First	1.0	33.0
Second	10.5	32.0
Third	11.0	33.0
Cigarette smoking	Decrease Hgb by g/dl to adjust for usual increase in Hgb in smokers	Decrease Hct by % points to adjust for usual increase in Hct in smokers
0.5-<1 pack per day	0.3	1.0
1-<2 packs per day	0.5	1.5
>2 packs per day	0.7	2.0
Altitude (feet)	Decrease Hgb by g/dl to make laboratory finding comparable to the distribution found at sea level	Decrease Hct by % points to make laboratory finding comparable to the distribution to the distribution found at sea level
5,000-5,999	0.5	1.5
7,000-7,999	1.0	3.0
10,000-10,999	2.0	6.0

From Centers for Disease Control and Prevention: Recommendation to prevent and control iron deficiency in the United States, *MMWR* 47 (RR-3):1-29, 1998.

Hgb, Hemoglobin; *Hct,* hematocrit.

Example: A pregnant woman in second trimester has a Hgb/Hct of 11.0/33%. This is a normal finding. However, if she smokes 1.5 packs of cigarettes per day, she would be at the cut-off point for anemia since one needs to decrease the laboratory finding by 0.5 g/dL and 1.5 percentage points respectively. Her Hgb/Hct level should be considered to be 10.5/31.5. Additionally, if she lives at 7,000 feet altitude, a further reduction is necessary to make the lab findings comparable with the standard at sea level. Her adjusted Hgb is 9.5 g/dL and adjusted Hct is 28.5%. These adjusted levels require further evaluation and intervention.

most American women; therefore increased intake through dietary sources and supplementation is necessary to meet the demand.

It has been suggested that iron deficiency anemia has declined in the United States over the past few decades, most likely a result of increased iron fortification of flour and cereals, availability of iron-rich food, availability of vitamins with iron and folic acid, and availability of supplementation programs such as the Women, Infants, and Children Program (Scholl and Hediger, 1994). The prevalence of anemia in low-income women in the United States has remained stable since 1979, with studies estimating prevalence of 9%, 14%, and 37% in the first, second, and third trimesters, respectively (CDC, 1998b). Other authors have estimated the prevalence of anemia in pregnancy from <5% in white women to 12% to 15% in black women (Beard, 1994). However, the distribution of Hgb and hematocrit (Hct) values in American blacks suggest lower levels, even when samples are controlled for income; Asian Americans and Native American women have distributions similar to those of white women. Care should be taken in comparing populations since these findings suggest that there may be normal racial differences in RBC quantity and composition.

It is well accepted that certain factors are associated with increased risk for iron deficiency anemia: periods of rapid growth (e.g., young adolescent age), poor nutrition, closely spaced pregnancies, multiple gestation, history of heavy menstrual bleeding, recent use of an intrauterine device, gastrointestinal tract blood loss (including that caused by parasites), and low income.

Iron deficiency can occur rapidly or slowly over time. Iron storage depends on the intake of dietary iron, and absorption of dietary iron depends on the quality of food iron (heme or nonheme iron) and any enhancers or inhibitors of absorption ingested along with the iron-containing food. The absorption of heme iron, found in meat, poultry, and fish, is not affected by enhancers or inhibitors. Absorption of nonheme iron, found in grain, cereals, fruits and vegetables, increases in pregnancy (Barrett, 1994), but the absorption of nonheme iron is more variable because of the effect of other dietary factors. For example, it is well documented that vitamin C enhances the absorption of iron, whereas calcium inhibits absorption. Iron absorption increases when an individual is iron deficient, particularly if the depletion has been more rapid (as in anemia secondary to acute blood loss).

Iron deficiency has been associated with urinary tract infections (UTIs), preterm delivery, low birth weight, preeclampsia, perinatal mortality, and increased ratio of placental weight to birth weight. However, these associations are also found with other types of anemia and are often confounded by additional risk factors, including extremes in maternal age, low socioeconomic status, and smoking. Studies have illustrated that the association with perinatal problems holds for anemia identified before the third trimester, but, when anemia develops late in pregnancy, there is no significant difference in outcomes (Scholl and Hediger, 1994).

Signs and symptoms Most women experiencing iron deficiency anemia are asymptomatic. Those who present with symptoms may complain of fatigue, lack of energy, or light-headedness. Women with severe anemia may also experience dyspnea and palpitations. Physical examination may identify pale mucous membranes. In severe cases of iron deficiency anemia, angular stomatitis (erosion at the corners of the mouth), cracking of the lips, glossitis, and brittle nails may be noted.

Screening/diagnosis Diagnosis is often made as a presumptive diagnosis because of the recognition that iron deficiency is the most common type of anemia in many of the populations receiving prenatal care. Results from venipuncture are most accurate, although screening through fingersticks is acceptable to monitor response to supplementation. Peripheral blood smear shows characteristic microcytic, hypochromic RBCs.

Hgb and Hct are the most common laboratory tests used to screen for iron deficiency anemia. When comparing the two, Hgb is more sensitive in estimating the iron contained in cells, since Hct is more likely to be influenced by changes in fluid balance, including dehydration. The tests are relatively cheap and readily available in most clinical settings. When iron therapy is initiated based on the presumptive diagnosis of iron deficiency anemia, Hgb and Hct that increase by 1 g/dl and 3%, respectively, after 1 month of treatment, are considered a confirmation of the diagnosis.

A more definitive test for diagnosing iron deficiency anemia is serum ferritin because, apart from iron deficiency, other causes of anemia in pregnancy are not characterized by low ferritin levels. For this reason, serum ferritin <15 μg/L should be considered diagnostic of iron deficiency anemia. Individuals who are iron deficient also have low transferrin saturation (<16%) and high erythrocyte protoporphyrin concentrations (>30 μg/dl) (Beard, 1994).

RBC characteristics are also commonly used for screening for anemias. Since iron deficiency anemia is characterized by microcytic, hypochromic cells, a mean cell volume (MCV) of less than 80 fl, particularly when associated with a low Hgb, is considered suggestive of anemia. When other causes of microcytic anemia are ruled out (lead poisoning, infection, chronic inflammatory disease, thalassemia minor), a presumptive diagnosis of iron deficiency anemia can be made.

Management—community-based All women should be screened for anemia at the first prenatal visit. If the Hgb is <11 g/dl, supplementation with a multiple vitamin with iron and folic acid is suggested. Women with poor dietary intake, closely spaced pregnancies, or other risk factors for iron depletion may benefit from further iron supplementation. Box 25-1 identifies common iron preparations available for supplementation and the amount of elemental iron that is provided.

Box 25-1 *Common Iron Preparations for Supplementation*

Percentage of Elemental Iron Present

Ferrous sulfate (hydrated): 20%
Ferrous sulfate (desiccated): 30%
Ferrous gluconate: 11%
Ferrous fumarate: 33%

The optimal dose of iron supplementation is controversial. Excessively high doses of iron may lead to gastrointestinal distress and constipation. The Institute of Medicine (IOM) (1992) recommends supplementation of 30 mg of elemental iron/day after the twelfth week of gestation for women who are at risk for developing anemia during the pregnancy, and the Centers for Disease Control and Prevention (CDC) (1998b) recommends starting 30 mg of elemental iron/day at the first prenatal visit. Once a diagnosis of iron deficiency anemia is made, supplementation with 60 to 120 mg of elemental iron is recommended in addition to a multiple vitamin with low-dose iron (30 mg elemental iron) (IOM, 1992). When a woman has difficulty swallowing iron tablets, chewable or liquid preparations can be recommended.

Response to supplementation is rapid, particularly for women with severe deficiency. An increase in the reticulocyte count to >2% can be seen after 10 to 14 days of treatment. Once the increased production of RBCs occurs, Hct rises 1 to 2 percentage points per week until stores are no longer depleted. Most clinicians evaluate response to iron at the next prenatal visit after starting supplementation (in 1 month, if early in pregnancy). If no improvement is seen, it should first be determined whether the woman is taking the supplements as instructed. If she has been taking supplements correctly with no improvement in Hct, other causes of anemia should be explored. Once Hgb, Hct, and serum ferritin levels have reached normal levels, iron supplementation can be reduced to the low dose of 30 mg of elemental iron/per day.

Nutrition education and counseling should provide the woman with an understanding of the increased iron needs in pregnancy. Foods high in iron include organ meats, red meat, fish, egg yolks, whole grains and enriched breads and cereals, dark green leafy vegetables, legumes, apricots, and prunes. Blackstrap molasses can be ingested by the tablespoon or used as an additive to other food. Women can be instructed to take iron with a vitamin C–containing food or beverage to increase absorption.

Counseling points should include:

- Nausea and diarrhea may occur with the initiation of iron supplementation and usually resolve spontaneously. If these side effects continue, the health care provider should be notified.
- Iron supplementation causes darkening of the stools.
- Constipation is a common side effect. Dietary measures to prevent constipation should be reviewed.
- Iron, like other medications, can be harmful if ingested in large quantities. For that reason, iron supplements should be kept out of the reach of children to prevent accidental overdosage.

It should be remembered that one of the conditions associated with iron deficiency anemia is pica. Pica is the purposeful ingestion of nonfood items, including but not limited to laundry starch, clay, ice, and ashes. The exact relationship between pica and anemia has not been determined. One theory proposes that the ingested minerals may bind with the dietary iron, preventing absorption through the gut. Studies have shown that correction of anemia leads to a decrease in nonfood cravings.

Management-referral Hgb electrophoresis should be obtained to rule out alpha or beta thalassemia when women are not responsive to iron supplementation. Women who are unresponsive to iron supplementation without documented thalassemia should be referred to a physician with expertise in hematologic problems.

Implications for the fetus When maternal sickle cell trait or disease is identified, screening of the baby's father is recommended. Genetic counseling should be offered so that parents understand the probability of the fetus carrying the sickling gene. Since anemia is associated with preterm labor and low birth weight, women experiencing anemia should be counseled regarding signs and symptoms of preterm labor. In cases of severe anemia, ultrasound examination for serial growth of the fetus should be considered.

Implications for labor and delivery Women who are severely anemic are at increased risk for postpartum hemorrhage, and, should hemorrhage occur, they have no stores to meet the need for increased RBC production. Therefore, when a woman is experiencing severe anemia, the midwife should consider having immediate access for intravenous fluid replacement. In most institutions administration of intravenous fluids throughout the labor is the norm for these women, but the placement of a saline lock is a reasonable alternative to a continuous infusion.

Implications for postpartum and neonatal care Women who have been diagnosed with iron deficiency anemia during pregnancy or those with risk factors for iron deficiency anemia should continue their iron supplementation through the postpartum period. Laboratory screening for anemia should be done 4 to 6 weeks after delivery with continued treatment if the anemia persists. When a woman has been severely anemic throughout the pregnancy, the neonate's health care provider should be notified so that the infant's iron stores can be assessed at 6 to 9 months of age. Full-term infants usually have sufficient iron stores from the pregnancy to meet their demand for iron for 4 to 6 months. Because of this, depleted iron stores usually do not develop until the second half of the first year of life. Preterm and low-birth-weight infants commonly have depleted stores and can only meet their demand for iron for 2 to 3 months after birth. Primary prevention for iron deficiency anemia in infants includes recommending exclusive breast-feeding for 4 to 6 months after birth, using iron supplementation when breast-feeding is stopped, and recommending iron supplementation for low-birth-weight and preterm infants.

Megaloblastic Anemia

Pathology Most megaloblastic anemia found in the United States is a result of folic acid deficiency. Folate requirements increase dramatically in pregnancy, and deficiency can develop in women who do not ingest animal protein or green leafy vegetables. Deficiency of folic acid leads to the formation of megaloblasts (large red cells) by the bone marrow. Factors that increase the risk of folic acid deficiency include poor nutrition, closely spaced pregnancies, multiple gestation, anticoagulant therapy, long-term use of sulfonamides or anticonvulsives, and heavy alcohol use. The association between folate deficiency and neural tube defects has been well documented.

Megaloblastic anemia may also be caused by vitamin B_{12} deficiency, but this is a rare condition in healthy women of childbearing age. Vitamin B_{12} requires intrinsic factor (IF), a protein that is made in the cells of the stomach, to be absorbed in the distal ileum. When IF is not available, usually because of autoimmune-mediated anti-IF antibodies, pernicious anemia results. Disease or surgical resection of the distal ileum also prevents the absorption of B_{12}-IF.

Signs and symptoms Most women with megaloblastic anemia are asymptomatic. Identification of risk factors, particularly heavy alcohol use, may assist the clinician in identifying the cause of the anemia. Severe anemia may be associated with fatigue, and vitamin B_{12} deficiency may be associated with neurologic symptoms, including lower extremities loss of proprioception and loss of sense of smell (Andreoli et al., 1997).

Screening/diagnosis A presumptive diagnosis can be made through peripheral blood smear findings of macrocytic RBCs, hypersegmented neutrophils, and, in severe cases, poikilocytosis. An erythrocyte folate level of less than 150 ng/ml is diagnostic of folate deficiency. A serum folate level of less than 4 ng/ml is suggestive of deficiency but influenced by the increase in plasma volume as pregnancy progresses. Elevated formiminoglutamic acid may also aid in diagnosis. Below-normal vitamin B_{12} levels, along with the presence of anti-IF antibodies, is diagnostic of pernicious anemia.

Management—community-based Nutritional counseling stressing foods high in folic acid should be provided. Foods high in folic acid include green leafy vegetables, asparagus, dried beans and legumes, eggs, fish, organ meats, nuts, whole grains, and yeast.

Prenatal vitamins with 0.4 mg of folic acid are the recommended supplement for preconception and pregnancy. Multiple vitamins with less than 1 mg of folic acid may be purchased without a prescription. Doses of 1 mg of folic acid or greater are available by prescription only. In severe cases of folic acid deficiency, an additional 0.4 to 0.8 mg per day may be added. Pernicious anemia is treated using parenteral vitamin B_{12}.

Management—referral Women who are unresponsive to folic acid supplementation and those who have pernicious anemia should be referred to a physician with expertise in hematologic problems.

Implications for the fetus When folate deficiency is identified, maternal serum alpha-fetoprotein (triple marker screen) findings should be obtained, and an ultrasound examination to identify neural tube and abdominal wall defects should be offered. In cases of severe anemia, assessment of fetal growth using serial ultrasound examinations is warranted.

Implications for labor and delivery Implications for labor and delivery are the same as those noted for iron deficiency anemia.

Implications for postpartum and neonatal care Implications for postpartum care are the same as those noted for iron deficiency anemia.

Hereditary anemias

Sickle Cell Hemoglobinopathies

Pathology Sickle cell anemia (SS), sickle cell-Hgb C disease (SC), and sickle cell-B-thalassemia (S-B-thalassemia) continue to be conditions associated with an increase in maternal and perinatal mortality and morbidity. In addition, women with the sickle cell trait (AS) experience increased morbidity because of UTIs and concurrent iron and folate deficiency anemias. Sickle cell trait is the most common type of hemoglobinopathy, occurring in 1 out of 12 black individuals or those of Mediterranean descent. Because of the prevalence of sickle cell trait and the fact that there has been an increase in multi-racial individuals, clinics in communities with diverse populations are commonly screening all patients for hemoglobinopathies.

Normal adult HgbA contains two alpha chains and two beta chains. Two variations of Hgb may be present in normal adults. HgbF, the primary Hgb during fetal life, may persist into adulthood at a proportion of $<1\%$ of the total Hgb in the individual. A common variation of HgbA is $HgbA_2$, which may comprise up to 4% of normal Hgb.

HgbS differs from normal adult gb by a minor change in 2 of the 574 amino acids in Hgb. The resulting change dramatically decreases the oxygen-carrying capacity and survival period for RBCs. Sickle-shaped cells are easily hemolyzed, leading to shortened lifespan of RBCs and chronic anemia. The increased RBC production in response to the shortened lifespan may lead to folic acid deficiency. When the sickle cell patient is stressed by hypoxia or acidosis, the sickling of HbS cells increases, causing capillary and arteriole obstruction. The patient experiences severe pain at the points of intravascular sickling. Repeated or extensive sickling leads to necrosis and organ damage. Vasoocclusive crises increase in pregnancy. In addition to sickling, the cellular changes increase viscosity of the blood, resulting in decreased perfusion and hypoxia. The decreased perfusion is particularly pronounced when the Hct is greater than 30%.

Signs and symptoms Signs and symptoms are similar to those of other anemias and depend on the severity of the anemia. In severe cases the patient may complain of fatigue, dyspnea, and palpitations; and mucous membranes may be pale.

Screening/diagnosis A sickle cell screening test (Sickledex) identifies individuals for whom diagnostic testing is warranted. Hgb electrophoresis identifies the type and proportion of Hgb present. Because of the severity of HbSS disease, it is diagnosed in childhood, and women with HbSS disease continue to be under medical management during their childbearing years. Asymptomatic and mild forms of the disease may be initially diagnosed during a first pregnancy assessment. Table 25-2 summarizes laboratory findings in sickle cell hemoglobinopathies.

Since folic acid deficiency is associated with HbS, folate status should also be assessed during pregnancy.

Management—community-based Women with HbSS or HbSC disease are at high risk for maternal and fetal complications and should be referred to a perinatologist at a high-risk perinatal center for care.

Although some sources call for universal screening of all childbearing women, at the least screening for sickle hemoglobinopathies should be done at the first prenatal visit for black women and women of Mediterranean descent if no previous testing results are available. Community-based care of women with mild anemias and sickle trait includes screening for infections, education regarding maintenance of health, and genetic counseling.

Because sickle cell trait is associated with increased risk for UTIs, trait patients should have urine cultures to rule out asymptomatic disease each trimester. Women with a history of UTI in the current pregnancy and those with history of UTIs in previous pregnancies should have monthly urine cultures. When UTI is diagnosed, treatment with an appropriate antibiotic is in order. Suppression therapy should be considered for recurrent infections.

Management—referral Women who are HbSS or HbSC and those whose anemia worsens or who develop associated medical problems should be referred to a physician skilled in caring for pregnant women with hemoglobinopathies.

Thalassemias

Pathology Thalassemias are genetically determined hematologic disorders characterized by an impaired rate of production of one or more of the peptide chains found in globin (Gant and Cunningham, 1993). The two major forms of thalassemia involve the impaired production of alpha peptide chains (alpha-thalassemia) and beta peptide chains (beta-thalassemia).

Homozygous beta-thalassemia (thalassemia major, Cooley's anemia) is usually diagnosed in early childhood when the child fails to thrive. The affected genes are not able to produce Hgb, and the resulting severe anemia requires transfusions beginning early in child-

Table 25-2 *Laboratory Values in Sickle Cell Hemoglobinopathies*

			Hgb (%)			Av. Hgb	
	S	**A**	**A2**	**F**	**C**	**(g/dl)**	**Severity**
SS	80-90	0	<3.5	1-15	0	7.5-8.5	Marked
$S\text{-}B^0$	80-95	0	>3.5	1-15	0	8.0-9.0	Marked
$S\text{-}B^+$	70-90	10-25	>3.5	1-15	0	8.5-10	Moderate
AS	25-40	60-75	<3.5	1-15	0	Normal	Asymptomatic
SC	50	0	<3.5	1-3	50	8.5-12	Mild to moderate

Hgb, Hemoglobin; *SS*, sickle cell disease; *$S\text{-}B^0$*, $S\text{-}B^0$ thalassemia (silent); *$S\text{-}B^+$*, $S\text{-}B^+$ thalassemia; *AS*, sickle cell trait; *SC*, SC disease.

hood. Individuals with this form of thalassemia may survive to the childbearing years, although conception is rare. Alpha-thalassemia major results from four defective alpha genes and produces hydrops fetalis and incompatibility with extrauterine life.

Thalassemia minor involves affected alpha or beta chains in a heterozygous individual and is characterized by mild hypochromic, microcytic anemia. Thalassemia is most common in individuals of Mediterranean or Asian descent.

Signs and symptoms Mild forms of the anemias are often asymptomatic. A screening complete blood count (CBC) often shows Hct of 30% to 35% and reticulocyte counts elevated to 10% to 20%.

Screening/diagnosis Further investigation for thalassemia trait should be done when mean corpuscular Hgb is <27 pg (Rogers, Phelan, and Bain, 1995). Alternately, MCV <80 can be used as an indicator for the need for further testing. A definitive diagnosis is made with Hgb electrophoresis. Alpha-thalassemia is essentially a diagnosis of exclusion of other hemoglobinopathies since diagnosis can only be made definitively through deoxyribonucleic acid (DNA) analysis.

Management—community-based Individuals with thalassemia minor can be managed effectively through pregnancy by monitoring of the anemia and referral for further evaluation when severe anemia is identified. Since iron stores are overloaded in thalassemia, iron supplementation is not appropriate. Folic acid supplementation is recommended to support the increased bone marrow production of RBCs.

Once thalassemia is identified, couples should be offered genetic counseling to understand the risk to their children.

Management—referral All cases of thalassemia with severe anemia should be referred to a perinatologist for management.

Implications for the fetus Since the fetus can be a carrier of abnormal Hgb, genetic counseling should be done so that parents can make rational decisions about management of the pregnancy. In cases of moderate-to-severe anemia, monitoring of fetal growth through serial ultrasound examinations may be indicated.

Implications for labor and delivery Midwives can provide intrapartum care independently for women with mild-to-moderate anemia related to hemoglobinopathies according to their practice guidelines. Because of the increased risks associated with anemia, a saline-lock or continuous intravenous infusion may be indicated.

Implications for postpartum and neonatal care Women with hemoglobinopathies should be offered further counseling for fertility planning. The World Health Organization reports that the progestin-only oral contraceptives, depo-medroxyprogesterone acetate, progestin implants, condoms, spermicides, diaphragm, cervical cap, and fertility awareness methods of contraception are safe with hemoglobinopathies, but women choosing methods with lower effectiveness rates need to consider the increased risk of a pregnancy that may result in maternal or fetal/neonatal problems (Hatcher et al., 1999). Women choosing combined oral contraceptives or the intrauterine device may need more frequent follow-up to rule out associated side effects that may exacerbate anemia. The pediatric provider for the neonate should be alerted to any hemoglobinopathy in the parents to most effectively evaluate the infant's status.

Hypertensive Disorders

Classification of hypertensive disorders in pregnancy. Terminology used to categorize hypertension in pregnancy is not uniform and is confusing with diagnoses and definitions that change periodically. The American College of Obstetricians and Gynecologists (ACOG) has suggested that the clinician consider two distinct types of hypertensive disorders in pregnancy—chronic hypertension and pregnancy-induced hypertension (PIH) (ACOG, 1996). Chronic hypertension is apparent before 20 weeks' gestation (except in cases of gestational trophoblastic disease when early hypertension may also be present) and may co-exist with the pathologic changes present in PIH. PIH is a multiorgan disorder that may result in not only hypertension, but also proteinuria, thrombocytopenia, mild renal dysfunction, occasional liver dysfunction, and neurologic disturbance, including seizures. PIH is often categorized as preeclampsia without proteinuria; preeclampsia with proteinuria; eclampsia; and *H*emolysis, *E*levated *L*iver enzymes, and *L*ow *P*latelet count (HELLP) syndrome. An additional category of transient hypertension is also recognized. Hypertension in pregnancy is associated with maternal and fetal/neonatal morbidity and mortality. The extent of morbidity and mortality is relative to the degree of pathologic alterations in the maternal system.

The diagnosis of hypertension is made using one of two definitions. The classic definition of hypertension is a blood pressure (BP) greater than or equal to 140/90 on two separate occasions at least 6 hours apart. Since healthy young women may often have BP as low as 90/60, a second definition for PIH is an increase of systolic BP greater than 30 mm Hg over the woman's baseline or an increase of diastolic BP greater than 15 mm Hg over her baseline after 20 weeks' gestation.

Preeclampsia/Eclampsia

Pathology Numerous theories regarding the genesis of preeclampsia have been proposed, but currently there is no clear explanation of the cause of the disorder. Abnormal immune response, genetic predisposition, nutritional excess or deficiency, endocrine disorders, and renal disorders have all been suggested as contributing to the development of preeclampsia. Most sources agree that the cause of preeclampsia is multifactorial. Risk factors for preeclampsia are listed in Box 25-2. It must be remembered that these risk factors are often co-variables (e.g., black women are at higher risk for chronic hypertension).

Vasospasm is most likely at the foundation of the disease process. As vasospasm continues, damage to the vessel walls occurs, resulting in passage of platelets and fibrin into the subendothelial layer of the vessel wall. It is well recognized that women who develop preeclampsia have a sensitivity to angiotensin II, which is thought to be a primary contributor to the vasospasm process. The vasoconstriction also contributes to damage to the RBCs as they pass through the decreased diameter of the vessels. Vasospasm eventually leads to local tissue hypoxia in numerous organ systems, including the placenta, liver, lungs, brain, and retinas. Cerebral vasospasm contributes to the symptoms of headache and visual disturbances and may progress to cerebrovascular accident (stroke).

Vasospasm in the kidney system contributes to decreased renal blood flow. The renal system develops glomerular endothelial cell swelling, glomerular capillary lumens constrict, and glomerular filtration further decreases. Because filtration decreases, serum blood urea nitrogen, creatinine, and sodium increase; and urine output decreases. Sodium retention further contributes to the sensitivity to angiotensin II and increased extracellular fluid volume. In severe cases, vasospasm and arterial thrombus formation can lead to necrosis of the renal cortex.

Development of generalized edema occurs because of the vessel wall damage and the retention of fluid secondary to decreased glomerular filtration. As fluid shifts from the intravascular to the extravascular space, hypovolemia and hemoconcentration develop. This in turn puts a demand on the heart as pressoreceptors in major organs provide feedback to increase cardiac output. Research on cardiac output in preeclampsia has been conflicting. Some investigators have noted decreased cardiac output associated with increased peripheral vascular resistance, whereas others have found that some women with preeclampsia actually have increased cardiac output and decreased peripheral resistance until the disease becomes severe (Bosio et al., 1999). Using a longitudinal model to follow hemodynamics in pregnancies complicated with hypertension, the authors confirmed increased cardiac output and decreased peripheral resistance in the latent phase of preeclampsia, with "cross-over" to low cardiac output and increased peripheral resistance when clinical disease presents. Conversely, women with gestational hypertension and no preeclamptic alterations maintained high cardiac output and vasodilation.

Liver dysfunction in preeclampsia can range from mild enzyme changes to hepatic edema, subcapsular edema, or hemorrhage. The severe changes may present as upper right quadrant pain. As hepatic edema represents a degree of generalized edema that includes cerebral edema, the right upper quadrant pain often is associated with a degree of cerebral edema that results in seizure activity (eclampsia).

The vessel wall damage and leakage of blood products into the extravascular space eventually leads to a consumptive coagulopathy similar to disseminated intravascular coagulation. The mechanisms of the thrombocytopenia seen in preeclampsia are not well understood. One theory is that the endothelial damage is associated with platelet aggregation and destruction. Disruption of the normal clotting mechanisms may lead to hemorrhage and death.

Some women experiencing preeclampsia progress to development of HELLP syndrome, which is associated with rapid progression of the pathologic process and resulting adverse maternal and fetal outcomes. Women

Box 25-2 *Risk Factors for Preeclampsia*

- Nulliparity
- Maternal age older than 35 years
- Maternal age younger than 18 years
- Family history of pregnancy-induced hypertension (PIH)
- History of PIH in a previous pregnancy
- First pregnancy with a new father of the baby
- Chronic hypertension
- Chronic renal disease
- Antiphosholipid syndrome
- Diabetes mellitus
- Multiple gestation
- Black race
- Fetal hydrops

who develop HELLP syndrome probably represent a subset of individuals who have more severe endothelial dysfunction, and it is thought that this predisposition may be genetic in nature.

Besides the indirect effect of decreased maternal perfusion on the fetus, the vasospasm process also directly affects the placenta. Placental lesions that are a result of infarcts further decrease perfusion to the fetus, leading to intrauterine growth restriction (IUGR) and hypoxia.

Complications associated with severe preeclampsia include placental abruption, acute renal failure, retinal detachment, cardiac failure, cerebral hemorrhage, fetal growth restriction, and maternal and fetal death.

Signs and symptoms Mild preeclampsia (diastolic BP <110 mm Hg) is often asymptomatic. The first suggestion of the development of the disease is a finding of increased BP during a prenatal visit. Proteinuria and edema are the two other classic findings in preeclampsia. However, proteinuria is a late finding. When protein excretion is found to be greater than 1+ on a routine screening using a reagent strip or greater than 0.3 g in a 24-hour urine collection, a diagnosis of preeclampsia is strengthened. Although edema is consistent with the disease process, it is difficult to differentiate normal edema in pregnancy from early edema associated with preeclampsia. Any sudden weight gain of more than 2 pounds per week in the second half of pregnancy that is unexplained by dietary intake should be considered a sign of edema until proven otherwise.

Screening/diagnosis Screening for preeclampsia is done at every prenatal visit by obtaining the maternal BP and testing for urinary protein. Sources, including the Expert Panel on the Content of Prenatal Care (1989), suggest that BP and testing for urinary protein at every prenatal visit, may not be essential nor cost effective for women without risk factors for the disease.

Diagnosis is confirmed using laboratory examinations that also establish the severity of the disease. Common laboratory tests used in assessment of the problem are summarized in Table 25-3.

Management—community-based Mild preeclampsia can be managed collaboratively in the community with the obstetric consultant according to practice guidelines. Baseline laboratory studies should be obtained in women at increased risk for preeclampsia. In cases in which the diastolic BP is below 100 mm Hg, in which there is proteinuria equal to or less than 1+ on a random urine screen, and in which serum markers remain in the normal range for pregnancy, it is appropriate to offer home care. Women who are determined to be candidates

Table 25-3 *Laboratory Tests Used to Evaluate Hypertension in Pregnancy*

Test	Change consistent with preeclampsia	Rationale
Hemoglobin and hematocrit	Increased	Reflects hemoconcentration; in severe cases, may have decrease in values when hemolysis occurs
Platelet count	Decreased	<100,000 consistent with severe disease
Serum creatinine	Increased above 0.6 mg/dl	Mild increase noted in mild disease; rising levels, coupled with oliguria, indicate severe disease
Serum uric acid	Increased above 6 mg/dl	Increasing levels reflect severity of renal compromise
Aspartate aminotransferase, formerly serum glutamate oxaloacetate transaminase	Increased above 25 U/L	Increase reflects hepatic insult consistent with severe disease
Alanine aminotransferase, formerly serum glutamate pyruvate transaminase	Increased above 30 U/L	Increase reflects hepatic insult consistent with severe disease
Fibrinogen	Decreased below 175 mg/dl	Decrease is consistent with DIC
Fibrin split products	Increased above 2.5 μg/dl	Increase is consistent with DIC
D-dimer screen	Increased above 0.5 μg/dl	Increase is consistent with DIC

DIC, Disseminated intravascular coagulation.

for home care should be instructed to continue a sound pregnancy diet with adequate fluids. Modified bed rest in the left lateral position improves uterine and renal perfusion. Improved renal perfusion should lead to increased urinary output and decrease in BP. Women should be taught to monitor fetal activity and to report any decrease in fetal movement to the health care provider. When possible, home monitoring of the BP can be offered. Women can also be taught to test for urinary protein using reagent testing strips and counseled to contact the provider if they note two separate findings of >2+ on a clean-catch specimen. Women should notify the provider immediately with increase in BP, increase in generalized edema, headache, visual disturbances, or epigastric pain. Fetal assessment, including nonstress testing twice per week and monitoring fetal growth with serial ultrasound examinations every 2 weeks, should be initiated.

Management—referral Women whose BPs increase during conservative treatment of mild preeclampsia, whose laboratory values indicate disease progression, and who demonstrate signs of severe preeclampsia should be referred to an obstetrician skilled in managing the disease. Hospitalization with possible early delivery of the fetus can be expected in severe cases.

Medical management of preeclampsia includes administration of magnesium sulfate to prevent seizures. A loading bolus of 4 g over 20 minutes is usually administered, followed by continuous infusion of 2 to 3 g/hr. Serum magnesium levels should be determined to confirm levels in the therapeutic range (4 to 8 mg/dl). Signs of magnesium toxicity include loss of deep tendon reflexes, respiratory rate of less than 12 breaths/minute, and urinary output of less than 30 ml/hr. Magnesium toxicity is reversed using calcium gluconate (1 g intravenously [IV] over 1 minute). Antihypertensive agents may also be prescribed in severe cases of preeclampsia. However, care must be taken to not decrease BP too dramatically, since decreased uteroplacental perfusion may be further impaired by lowering the BP.

Implications for the fetus Because of the pathologic changes in the placenta, the fetus is at risk for restricted growth and hypoxemia. Serial ultrasound studies of growth, nonstress tests (NSTs), biophysical profiles, and Doppler flow studies have all been suggested for fetal assessment in preeclampsia.

Implications for labor and delivery Medical management of preeclampsia in the intrapartum period is indicated. In some midwifery practices, co-management of mild preeclampsia is possible, with the midwife supporting the woman through labor and birth while the obstetrician makes clinical decisions regarding the medical management of the preeclampsia.

Implications for postpartum and neonatal care Women with preeclampsia usually experience a return to normotension in the first week after delivery. Rarely women who were normotensive in pregnancy develop postpartum preeclampsia or eclampsia.

Chronic Hypertension Chronic hypertension is thought to be present in 2% to 5% of pregnancies. Mild-to-moderate hypertension in pregnancy does not increase maternal risk but is associated with fetal IUGR and fetal death. Women who have chronic hypertension and smoke during pregnancy have a 90% increased risk of placental abruption (Ananth, Smulian, and Vintzileos, 1999).

Pathology Risk factors for chronic hypertension include age over 35 years, family history of hypertension, black race, alcohol abuse, and underlying renal or cardiovascular pathology. A primary contributor to hypertension is atherosclerosis.

Signs and symptoms Chronic hypertension is often asymptomatic. Individuals with hypertension may have had progression of the disease to the point of end-organ disease in the heart, brain, and kidneys. In these cases, signs and symptoms would be consistent with the degree of organ involvement, including coronary artery disease, congestive heart failure, cerebrovascular disease, and renal disease.

Screening/diagnosis Often chronic hypertension has been diagnosed before pregnancy, and the woman is already on a regimen that includes antihypertensive medication. Hypertension identified during prenatal care before 20 weeks should be considered chronic hypertension unless gestational trophoblastic disease is present.

Management—community-based Women who have well-controlled hypertension can be managed during pregnancy by the community provider in consultation with the obstetrician or primary care provider. Alpha-methyldopa, labetalol hydrochloride, and atenolol are hypertensive agents considered to be safe in pregnancy. Angiotensin-converting enzyme (ACE) inhibitors are contraindicated in pregnancy because of their association with fetal hypocalvaria, renal failure, oligohydramnios, and fetal and neonatal death (ACOG, 1996). Women planning pregnancy should have their medications adjusted before conception, and women who have pregnancy diagnosed while using ACE inhibitors should be switched to an acceptable antihypertensive agent immediately. A change in antihypertensive agent should also be considered when a woman has been maintained with beta-blocking agents since these medications are associated with increased risk for IUGR. Diuretics should not be used as first-line drugs in pregnancy since decreased plasma volume is associated with fetal morbidity.

Since women with chronic hypertension are at risk for superimposed preeclampsia, baseline preeclampsia laboratory studies should be done in late second trimester and repeated if BPs increase late in pregnancy. Superimposed preeclampsia is defined as an increase of 30 mm Hg systolic and/or 15 mm Hg diastolic BP, new-onset proteinuria, or altered laboratory values suggestive of preeclampsia. It is estimated that the incidence of superimposed preeclampsia in women with chronic hypertension is 20% to 25%.

Management—referral Women with uncontrolled or severe hypertension should be referred to a perinatologist for management during pregnancy.

Implications for the fetus Since chronic hypertension is associated with decreased uteroplacental perfusion, fetal growth should be monitored using serial ultrasound examinations. NSTs and biophysical profiles twice weekly after 28 weeks are also indicated.

Implications for labor and delivery Continued monitoring of the BP during labor with treatment for preeclampsia as noted in previous paragraphs is indicated.

Implications for postpartum and neonatal care Women with chronic hypertension should be referred back to their primary care providers for continued management of their hypertension.

Mitral Valve Prolapse

Pathology Mitral valve prolapse (MVP) is estimated to occur in 6% of the population and may occur in 12% to 17% of women of childbearing age. Prevalence in women peaks in 20- to 29-year-olds and is the lowest in 50- to 59-year-olds. Although there has been much written about MVP in general, there is limited knowledge about the effect pregnancy-induced cardiovascular changes have on MVP. MVP can be a primary disease function or a secondary pathology associated with connective tissue disorders or decreased left ventricle size (Cowles and Gonik, 1990). In addition, MVP can be a temporary occurrence triggered by dehydration or tachycardia (Dajani et al., 1997). The usual anatomic abnormality found in MVP is enlargement of one or both mitral leaflets, most commonly the posterior leaflet. The chordae are redundant and can be absent or ruptured (Cowles and Gonik, 1990). Conditions associated with the diagnosis of MVP are noted in Box 25-3. Auscultatory and echocardiographic findings may occur independently of each other. In the Framingham Heart Study, only 15% of individuals with MVP diagnosed on echocardiogram had auscultatory findings (Savage, Garrison, and Devereux, 1983).

The normal cardiovascular changes in pregnancy may actually improve the cardiovascular status in a woman with MVP. Increased left ventricular end-diastolic volume with realignment of the mitral valve complex may decrease the distinct auscultatory findings associated with MVP. Decreased peripheral vascular resistance also may decrease the murmur. Almost two thirds of the pregnant patients with MVP followed through pregnancy and at 6 weeks after delivery may show no echocardiographic evidence of MVP during the pregnancy (Rayburn et al., 1987). The few studies that have assessed the outcomes of pregnancy in women with MVP have found no significant difference in spontaneous abortion, preterm labor, length of labor, low birth weight, neonatal mortality, cesarean section, and antenatal hospitalization (Rayburn et al., 1987).

It is now believed that, when normal mitral valves prolapse without leaking, the risk of endocarditis is not increased above that of the normal population. In addition, normal valves with normal motions but minimal leaks are not associated with increased risk of endocarditis. Individuals with prolapsed and leaking valves as evidenced by audible clicks and murmurs or by Doppler studies are at increased risk for endocarditis and should be treated with prophylactic antibiotics when undergoing invasive procedures (Dajani et al., 1997).

Signs and symptoms Most pregnant women with MVP are asymptomatic. However, some women may experience an increase in palpitations, arrhythmias, and chest pain, particularly with physical exertion.

Screening/diagnosis Diagnosis can be made by auscultation of the heart, angiography, and echocardiography. The classic finding on auscultation is the midsystolic click and late systolic regurgitation murmur. The systolic click is best heard at the cardiac apex. The murmur most likely indicates some degree of mitral insufficiency. Since heart sounds are dynamic in nature, repeated examinations may be needed to identify the click or murmur. Rapid change of position from sitting to standing may make the click and murmur easier to detect.

Echocardiogram findings of buckling of the leaflets or holosystolic prolapse are considered diagnostic. Although angiography can identify prolapse, it is rarely used as a routine diagnostic study.

Management—community-based When there is history of MVP, records of any previous cardiac evaluations

Box 25-3 *Conditions That May Have an Association with Mitral Valve Prolapse*

Connective Tissue Disorders

Marfan's syndrome
Osteogenesis imperfecta
Rheumatoid arthritis

Cardiac Disorders

Congenital heart disease
Bicuspid aortic valve
Septal defects
Tetralogy of Fallot
Patent ductus arteriosis
Ebstein's anomaly
Electrocardiogram abnormalities
- Atrioventricular nodal dysfunction
- Wolff-Parkinson-White syndrome
- Idiopathic QT prolongation

Endomyocardial fibrosis
Cardiomyopathy
Atherosclerotic coronary disease

Hematologic Disorders

Platelet hypercoagulability
von-Willebrand syndrome
Sickle cell diease

Metabolic and Neuroendocrine Disorders

Migraine
Hyperthyroidism
Hypercatecholamine disorders

Psychiatric Disorders

Agoraphobia
Anorexia nervosa
Anxiety disorders

Genetic Disorders

Klinefelder's syndrome
Fragile X syndrome
Turner's syndrome

Miscellaneous Disorders

Muscular dystrophy
Irritable bowel syndrome
Primary pulmonary hypertension

Adapted from Cowles T, Gonik B: Mitral valve prolapse in pregnancy, *Semin Perinatol* 14(1):34-41, 1990.

should be obtained. If no previous cardiac workup has been done, referral for a basic cardiac evaluation to determine whether there is regurgitation is indicated. In the absence of moderate-to-severe mitral insufficiency, it is appropriate to manage care in the community setting. If palpitations and/or chest pain occur, a referral to a cardiologist for complete cardiac workup, including electrocardiogram and echocardiogram should be made. Although cardiac symptoms usually lessen in pregnancy, some women who experience chest pain, palpitations, or arrhythmias may be candidates for beta-adrenergic blockers.

The American Heart Association recommends that since bacteremia rarely is associated with uncomplicated vaginal delivery or cesarean section, antibiotic prophylaxis for normal vaginal birth or cesarean section is not warranted (Dajani et al., 1997). The Committee on Rheumatic Fever and Infective Endocarditis of the American Heart Association (AHA) recommends antibiotic prophylaxis only for patients with MVP complicated by regurgitation. Box 25-4 summarizes the American Heart Association's recommendations for antibiotic prophylaxis in individuals with increased risk for bacterial endocarditis.

Management–referral Women with documented cardiac compromise should be referred to a maternal-fetal medicine specialist for management of care.

Implications for the fetus In MVP with no cardiac compromise, there are no implications for the fetus. When cardiac compromise is present, fetal status is influenced by the woman's general cardiac status.

Implications for labor and delivery When women have been diagnosed with MVP with regurgitation, antibiotic prophylaxis should be considered during intrapartal care.

Implications for postpartum and neonatal care Women with MVP with regurgitation should be referred to their primary care providers for continuing care.

Box 25-4 *AHA Recommendations for Antibiotic Prophylaxis for GI/GU Procedures*

High-Risk Patients

Ampicillin, 2 g IM or IV, plus gentamycin, 1.5 mg/kg (not to exceed 120 mg), within 30 minutes of procedure; 6 hours later, ampicillin, 1 g IM or IV, or amoxicillin, 1 g PO

High-Risk Patients Allergic to Ampicillin

Vancomycin, 1 g IV over 1-2 hours, plus gentamycin, 1.5 mg/kg IV or IM (not to exceed 120 mg)

Moderate-Risk Patients

Amoxicillin 2 g PO 1 hour before procedure or ampicillin 2 g IM/IV within 30 minutes of procedure

Moderate-Risk Patients Allergic to Ampicillin

Vancomycin, 1 g IV over 1-2 hours; complete infusion within 30 minutes of procedure

From Dajani AS et al: Prevention of bacterial endocarditis: recommendations by the American Heart Association, *JAMA* 277(22):1794-1801, 1997.

RESPIRATORY TRACT PROBLEMS

Asthma

Pathology It is estimated that approximately 1% to 4% of pregnancies are complicated by asthma (Clark et al., 1993). During the last decade, prevalence, morbidity, and mortality of asthma have increased, perhaps because of air pollution, reduction of indoor air quality, and the increase in exposure to new chemicals in everyday life. Asthma is a chronic inflammatory disorder of the airways characterized by denudation of airway epithelium, collagen deposition beneath the basement membrane of the airway, edema, mast cell activation, and inflammatory cell infiltration (National Heart, Lung and Blood Institute, 1997). Airway inflammation is associated with bronchoconstriction, bronchial edema, and bronchial mucus plugging, leading to arterial hypoxemia. Decreased CO_2 is a major reflection of disease severity, but retention of CO_2 can occur in 15% to 20% of severe asthmatics as a result of hypoventilation. Asthma can be categorized as mild intermittent, mild persistent, moderate persistent, and severe persistent.

Because of increased plasma cortisol and histaminase in pregnancy, some patients experience improvement in their status, especially in first trimester. When worsening occurs, it does so after the fourth month of pregnancy, with the most compromise noted during third trimester.

Asthma has been associated with increased risk for preterm birth, low birth weight, neonatal mortality, hyperemesis gravidarum, vaginal bleeding, and preeclampsia. Data suggest that poor asthma control may be the most important factor in poor outcomes in pregnancy complicated by asthma. Women with severe asthma before conception are more likely to experience further problems during pregnancy.

Signs and symptoms Symptoms include shortness of breath; feeling of "tightness" in the chest; wheezing; and complaint of worsening of symptoms at night, with exertion, or with exposure to known irritants.

Screening/diagnosis Screening may be accomplished through thorough history-taking. Reports of frequent "bronchitis," frequent episodes of shortness of breath associated with cold or respiratory irritants, and strong family history of asthma are suggestive of the disease.

The diagnosis is made when the patient experiences episodic dyspnea with wheezing. General physical assessment may reveal acute distress, shortness of breath, cyanosis, or lethargy. Inspection of the chest may reveal increased respiratory rate and intercostal retractions. Auscultation of the lungs reveals bilateral wheezing or rhonchi. Rales may be heard but are usually associated with other pulmonary pathology. The expiratory phase of respirations is prolonged. Pulmonary studies may be normal in milder forms of the disease but may be helpful in monitoring the severity of the disease.

Management—community-based Women with mild intermittent and mild persistent asthma that is well controlled by pharmacologic therapy may be managed in community-based settings in collaboration with the woman's primary care provider. Asthma management includes reduction of environmental triggers, pharmacologic therapy, and patient education. Recommended pharmacologic agents are noted in Table 25-4. Women with mild asthma can be reassured that mild asthma is usually well controlled in pregnancy with only rare problems encountered by the fetus/neonate. Fetal assessment by serial ultrasounds for growth and NSTs may be reassuring in the third trimester.

Patient education should include recognition of common triggers, correct use of inhalers and other medications, and signs of worsening of the disease. A plan for immediate treatment of attacks should be made in collaboration with the primary care physician.

Table 25-4 *Drugs and Dosages for Asthma Treatment in Pregnancy*

Drug class	Specific drug	Dosage
Antiinflammatory	Cromolyn sodium	2 puffs 4 times per day, or 2 sprays in each nostril 2-4 times per day
	Beclomethasone	2-5 puffs 2-4 times per day, or 2 sprays in each nostril 2 times per day
	Prednisone	Burst for active symptoms: 40 mg/day, single or divided dose for 1 week, then taper for 1 week
Bronchodilator	Inhaled $beta_2$-agonist	2 puffs every 4 hrs as needed
	Theophylline	Oral: dose to reach serum concentration of 8-12 μg/ml
Antihistamine	Chlorpheniramine	4 mg PO up to 4 times per day; 8-12 mg sustained release twice per day
	Tripelennamine	25-50 mg PO up to 4 times per day; 100 mg sustained release twice per day
Decongestant	Pseudoephedrine	60 mg PO up to 4 times per day; 120 mg sustained release twice per day
	Oxymetazoline	Intranasal spray or drops up to 5 times per day
Cough	Guaifenesin	2 tsp PO 4 times per day
	Dextromethorphan	2 tsp PO 4 times per day

Adapted from Clark SL et al.: Asthma in pregnancy, *Obstet Gynecol* 82:1036-1040, 1993.

Management—referral Women with moderate persistent to severe persistent asthma are best managed with a team that includes a maternal-fetal medicine specialist, an internal medicine and/or allergy specialist, and a nurse specialist to monitor the patient between medical visits. Management includes having the woman take twice-daily peak expiratory flow rate measurements at home with a peak flow meter. Personal best peak expiratory flow rates should be determined for the individual; expected range is 380 to 550 L/min. These findings are used for adjusting therapy as needed.

Moderate persistent asthma is defined as symptoms that are poorly regulated by episodic administration of a β_2-agonist. Frequent exacerbations is defined as greater than three asthma attacks per week. Inhaled antiinflammatory agents are the treatment of choice for moderate persistent asthma. Combinations of bronchodilators, cromolyn sodium, or inhaled corticosteroids are usually prescribed with moderate persistent and severe persistent asthma.

Implications for the fetus Early and serial ultrasound studies are recommended to follow fetal growth when women are diagnosed with moderate persistent and severe persistent asthma. NSTs or biophysical profiles in the third trimester further monitor fetal status. The mother can also monitor fetal status by doing daily kick counts in the third trimester.

Implications for labor and delivery The pharmacologic regimen for a woman with asthma should be continued in the intrapartum period. Since pain may trigger bronchospasm, a plan for pain management should be discussed with the woman and the obstetrician and anesthesiologist consultants before labor. Demerol and morphine are not recommended for pain control since they may induce bronchospasm. Further, prostaglandin (PG) F_{2a} (Hemabate, Protin/15M, Carboprost) is not recommended for control of postpartum hemorrhage since it can induce bronchospasm. PGE_2 (dinoprostone) can be used with women who are diagnosed with asthma.

Implications for postpartum and neonatal care Women who live with asthma should be referred to their primary care providers for ongoing management of this chronic condition.

URINARY TRACT PROBLEMS

Urinary Tract Infection

Pathology Anatomic and physiologic changes in pregnancy increase the risk of UTI. Factors that predispose pregnant women to UTI include progesterone-induced decrease in ureteral motility leading to distention and urinary stasis; compression of the ureters at the pelvic rim; alteration of the ureteral-vesicular junction; and altered renal clearance of glucose creating a supportive medium for bacterial growth. Asymptomatic bacteriuria occurs in approximately 5% to 10% of childbearing women. If asymptomatic disease is not treated appropriately, 25% to 40% of affected women will develop pyelonephritis.

Lower tract infection can ascend rapidly, causing pyelonephritis, which in turn can lead to gram-negative septic shock. In severe cases of pyelonephritis, the kidney may develop nephric and perinephric abscesses, and spread of bacterial "seeds" to other organs may occur. Pregnant women with pyelonephritis can develop a syndrome that involves bacterial infiltration of the lungs, resulting in a condition similar to adult respiratory distress syndrome.

The causative organisms most often associated with UTIs in pregnancy are *Escherichia coli, Proteus mirabilis, Klebsiella pneumoniae,* a variety of *Citrobacter* and *Enterobacter* species, and group B beta hemolytic streptococci. *E.coli* accounts for approximately 95% of infections when infections are associated with procedures (e.g., catheterization) and treatment of resistant organisms are excluded. Nonpathologic organisms that may be identified on urine cultures include alpha-hemolytic *Streptococcus, Staphylococcus epidermidis,* and *Lactobacillus.*

UTIs in pregnancy are associated with low birth weight, preterm labor and birth, hypertension/preeclampsia, maternal anemia, and amnionitis.

Signs and symptoms Symptoms of cystitis include dysuria caused by inflammation of the bladder wall and urethra and urinary urgency and incontinence caused by irritability of the detrusor muscle. Suprapubic tenderness and flank discomfort may be present. The sediment in spun urine contains many polymorphonuclear leukocytes, bacteria, and blood.

Signs and symptoms of pyelonephritis include generalized malaise, fever and chills, severe flank pain, tachycardia, and hypotension if significant septicemia has developed. Nausea and vomiting may be present.

Screening/diagnosis Diagnosis of UTI is made when a clean-catch midstream urine culture is reported to be >100,000 colonies/ml of a single uropathogen. Any pathogen grown from a catheterized specimen is considered diagnostic of UTI, even if the colony count is less than 100,000. Colony counts of less than 100,000 with mixed flora and colony counts of greater than 100,000 colonies of nonpathologic organisms are most likely contaminated specimens.

UTI is suspected when urine reagent strip tests show positive leukocyte esterase, positive nitrites, positive blood, and/or positive protein. When reagent strip tests for leukocytes, nitrites, protein, and blood are negative, there is over a 99% chance of negative culture. When a positive nitrite test is identified, there is a greater than 90% chance for positive urine culture (Etherington and James, 1993).

Presumptive diagnosis of cystitis is made when the woman presents with complaints of dysuria and urgency and a urine microanalysis that indicates many white blood cells (WBCs) and bacteria. Diagnosis of pyelonephritis is made when the patient presents with fever and severe flank pain and urine microanalysis indicates many WBCs and bacteria.

Management—community-based When a diagnosis of asymptomatic bacteriuria is made, a 7- to 10-day course of a broad-spectrum antibiotic selected by culture results should be ordered. Antibiotics that produce high urinary levels and limited systemic effects (e.g., nitrofurantoin) are preferred for lower tract infections. Recent studies on the use of single-dose antibiotics suggest that, for the pregnant woman without significant history of urinary problems, single-dose amoxicillin (3 g) produces cures in about 80% of cases. Single-dose trimethoprim/sulfamethoxazole (TMP-SMZ) (2 double-strength or 4 single-strength) produces cures in greater than 80% of cases (Vercaigne and Zhanel, 1994), but TMP/SMZ is not recommended in first trimester. Single-dose sulfisoxazole (2 g) or nitrofurantoin (200 mg) may also be effective. Counseling regarding the effects of UTI on pregnancy, use of medication, and necessity of test of cure should be done.

When a presumptive diagnosis of cystitis is made, antibiotic selection is based on knowledge of the usual effectiveness of the drug with common urinary pathogens since culture results are usually pending. Common pharmacologic regimens are noted in Box 25-5. Once culture results are obtained, antibiotic therapy can be changed if necessary. In addition to the counseling done with asymptomatic bacteriuria, women with cystitis should be counseled regarding additional comfort measures. For

Box 25-5 *Common Antibiotic Regimens for Lower Tract Infection in Pregnancy (Asymptomatic bacteriuria, Acute cystitis)*

Trimethoprim-sulfamethoxazole	160 mg/800 mg PO BID × 3 days, *or*
Amoxicillin	500 mg PO TID × 3 days

example, if there is significant urethral involvement, warm sitz baths may provide comfort. The woman should further be instructed to contact the provider if she develops a fever or if an existing fever is not improved after 48 hours of therapy, if she develops flank pain, if she is not feeling better in 48 hours, or if she generally feels as if she is becoming more severely ill. Test of cure should be planned following completion of treatment.

There is controversy over whether all patients with pyelonephritis need in-hospital management or whether out-patient care may be effective. Patients who are severely ill should be hospitalized for intravenous antibiotic therapy. Ampicillin (1 g IV q6h and gentamycin (2 mg/kg IV q8h) is commonly used because of the coverage of common urinary pathogens *(E. coli, Proteus* sp., *Klebsiella-Enterobacter* sp., *Pseudomonas aeruginosa,* and *Enterococcus).* Ceftriaxone (1 g IV q24h) or cefotaxime (1 IV q8h) can be used when there are contraindications to aminoglycoside therapy (McCormack et al., 1996).

Patients who are mildly to moderately ill with UTI and who are reliable and compliant may be treated orally. Common oral treatment includes TMP-SMZ (160 mg/800 mg PO BID) (McCormack et al., 1996). Ciprofloxacin, a common oral agent for treatment of pyelonephritis, is contraindicated in pregnancy.

When patients experience recurrent urinary infections, suppression therapy may be considered. Common therapies include nitrofurantoin (50 to 100 mg PO HS) and TMP-SMZ (40 to 200 mg PO HS or after intercourse if infections are associated with sexual activity).

Management—referral Patients with pyelonephritis should be referred to an obstetrician or primary care physician for management. When the patient is seriously ill with upper tract infection, consultation and possible referral to a maternal-fetal medicine specialist is recommended.

Implications for the fetus Since UTI is associated with preterm labor and birth, women should be educated regarding signs and symptoms of preterm labor. No specific fetal assessment is necessary in uncomplicated UTIs in pregnancy. Sulfa drugs are contraindicated in late pregnancy because of their association with neonatal kernicterus.

Implications for labor and delivery There are no implications for labor and delivery.

Implications for postpartum and neonatal care Women with recurrent UTIs in pregnancy, women needing suppression therapy, and women with pyelonephritis in pregnancy should be referred to their primary care physicians for ongoing management and assessment.

ENDOCRINE PROBLEMS

Gestational Diabetes (Glucose Intolerance in Pregnancy)

Pathology Gestational diabetes mellitus (GDM) is defined as "carbohydrate intolerance of variable severity with onset or first recognition in pregnancy" (Garner et al., 1997, p. 190). Although this definition is not accepted by all experts in the field, it has been endorsed by the Second International Workshop-Conference on Gestational Diabetes Mellitus and reaffirmed at the Third International Workshop-Conference. It is estimated that 0.15% to 12.3% of pregnant women are diagnosed with gestational diabetes. Risk factors include maternal age over 35, previous GDM, previous infant >4000 g, previous unexplained fetal losses, family history of diabetes in first-degree relatives, obesity, and previous birth of a child with a congenital anomaly. GDM is associated with glycosuria and polyhydramnios.

GDM may be associated with increased maternal and neonatal morbidity. Macrosomia with its associated complications of prolonged or arrested labor, forceps or vacuum delivery, shoulder dystocia, and cesarean section is more common in women with GDM, even with good blood glucose control (Avery and Rossi, 1994). However, Spellacy and colleagues (1985) found that only 5.1% of infants with birth weights more than 4500 g were born to mothers with abnormal glucose tolerance tests. In their sample, 44% of macrosomic infants were born to mothers weighing more than 90 kg, and 10.8% were greater than 42 weeks' gestation. These findings suggest that obesity and postdates pregnancy may be more closely associated with macrosomia than GDM.

Normal physiologic changes in pregnancy serve to maintain a fairly constant level of nutrients to the fetus. Increased levels of estrogen and progesterone in early pregnancy stimulate insulin secretion through the stimulation of beta-cell hyperplasia in the pancreas. This effect, coupled with decreased production of hepatic glucose, increased peripheral glucose use, and tissue storage of glycogen leads to a decrease in fasting blood glucose levels. Lower fasting glucose levels result in lower fasting insulin levels, leading to fat catabolism to meet metabolic needs. During the second half of pregnancy, insulin resistance occurs as a result of human placental lactogen, prolactin, cortisol, and glucagon. Postprandial blood glucose levels become increased. The fetus maintains blood glucose levels about 10 to 20 mg/dl below the maternal levels, facilitating transfer of glucose through the placental system. Even with these changes, most women are able to maintain blood glucose in the normal range. However, some women demonstrate an inability to meet the demands created by the increased insulin resistance and are identified as having GDM.

Hunter and Keirse (Chalmers, Enkin, and Keirse, 1989) argue that the studies used to define the problem of gestational diabetes and evaluate the effect of treatment either with diet or insulin have numerous methodologic flaws and therefore do not support treating the condition as pathology. Several studies have illustrated that individuals with abnormal 3-hour glucose tolerance tests have normal results when the test is repeated up to 70% of the time. It has been argued that the increased risk of perinatal morbidity and mortality has been overstated since research findings suggesting improved outcomes with treatment of the condition have lacked appropriate controls for comparison. It is important to consider that treating gestational diabetes as pathology if it truly is not pathologic has the potential for causing harm. A woman diagnosed with this disease carries a diagnosis that exposes her to numerous tests and interventions that have not been proven beneficial for women with normal glucose control. Conversely, a negative glucose tolerance may falsely lead the woman and her clinician to believe that the risk that led to the testing has been removed.

Current ACOG guidelines recommend selective screening for GDM based on the presence of maternal risk factors for patients younger than 30 years of age (ACOG, 1994a). The American Diabetes Association (ADA) recommends screening based on risk status. Low-risk status is defined meeting the following characteristics and requires no testing:

- Age less than 25 years
- Weight normal before pregnancy
- Member of an ethnic group with a low prevalence of GDM
- No known diabetes in first-degree relatives
- No history of abnormal glucose tolerance
- No history of poor obstetric outcome

High-risk status is defined as meeting one of the following characteristics:

- Marked obesity
- Personal history of GDM
- Glycosuria
- Strong family history of diabetes

Women with high risk factor(s) should have glucose testing as soon as possible in the pregnancy, and, if they screen normoglycemic, they should be rescreened at 24 to 28 weeks' gestation. Women with average risk (e.g., age greater than 25 years) should be screened at 24 to 28 weeks' gestation (American Diabetes Association, 2000).

Even with these recommendations that do not support universal screening, most obstetricians advocate screening all pregnant women for GDM (Khine, Winklestein, and Copel, 1999).

Signs and symptoms Although most women with GDM are asymptomatic, some may experience excessive weight gain and glucosuria.

Screening/diagnosis Most clinical sites use the two-step approach to screening for GDM. An initial screen measuring plasma or serum glucose 1-hour after a 50-g glucose load is administered, and it is recommended that women with 1-hour blood glucose level greater than or equal to 140 mg/dl have a 3-hour oral glucose tolerance test (GTT) using 100 g of glucose. Two or more plasma concentrations greater than the following cut-offs are considered diagnostic of GDM:

- Fasting: 95 mg/dl
- 1 hour: 180 mg/dl
- 2 hour: 155 mg/dl
- 3 hour: 140 mg/dl

In communities with a high prevalence of GDM and with limited access to care (e.g., some Native American groups, southwest Latino groups), a one-step approach using only the 3-hour 100-g oral glucose tolerance test can be used.

Early screening is recommended for women at high risk for GDM (history of gestational diabetes in previous pregnancy, obesity, strong family history of diabetes, history of repeated fetal losses). Random blood glucose of greater than 200 mg/dl or fasting blood glucose of greater than 126 mg/dl is highly suggestive of diabetes and precludes the need for a full glucose tolerance test. Women with a normal second trimester screen and/or normal 3-hour GTT who exhibit persistent glucosuria unrelated to recent intake, suspected macrosomia, or polyhydramnios should be rescreened later in the third trimester.

Management—community-based Treatment for GDM is appropriate at the community level of care. Treatment includes dietary management and monitoring of blood glucose levels. A small proportion of women may need insulin therapy. Fetal assessment is also a component of the management plan.

Women diagnosed with GDM should be referred to a dietitian or nutritionist for counseling and creation of a diet plan. The ADA recommends a low-fat (<30% total kcal) and high–complex carbohydrate (50% to 60% total kcal) diet. Intake should be spread over three meals and one to two snacks. Caloric intake of 2000 to 2400 kcal/day is recommended for women with normal prepregnant body weight. Obese women usually do well with an intake of 1500 to 1800 kcal/day.

In general, women should be counseled to avoid simple sugars and instructed to read nutritional labels to understand ingredients in prepared foods. Dietary recommendations should allow for cultural variation in foods and personal preferences.

Home glucose monitoring is the preferred method for daily periodic measurements of glucose levels. There is currently no national standard of frequency for glucose monitoring. Hollingsworth and Ney (1992) recommend testing four times per day—fasting and 1- or 2-hour postprandial evaluations—for 2 weeks or until dietary control is assured. Testing then may be reduced to 1 to 2 days per week as long as normal glucose levels are maintained. Most sources recommend maintaining the fasting blood glucose at less than 105 mg/dl, 1-hour postprandial glucose at less than 140 mg/dl, and 2-hour postprandial glucose at less than 120 mg/dl. Dietary adjustment is made accordingly when deviations from normal are identified.

Monitoring urinary ketones is also recommended as a means to ensure that food intake is adequate. Monitoring urinary glucose is not recommended since it is not a sensitive indicator of metabolic status.

Many experts recommend ongoing management by a multidisciplinary team of health care professionals.

Management—referral Women with type I diabetes (insulin-dependent) and women who cannot control blood glucose with diet alone should be referred to a center with a multidisciplinary team who can meet the needs of the diabetic woman.

Implications for the fetus Although antepartum fetal assessment is recommended in pregnancies complicated by GDM, there have been no adequate epidemiologic studies to definitively establish the type or frequency of testing. Some experts recommend daily fetal movement counts alone when blood glucose levels are well controlled by diet (Landon and Gabbe, 1993). Others recommend weekly NSTs from 32 weeks' gestation until delivery. The ADA (2000) recommends fetal assessment during the last 4 to 8 weeks of gestation when fasting blood glucose levels are greater than 105 mg/dl.

Implications for labor and delivery Labor and delivery management when women have experienced diet-controlled GDM is no different than the supportive care given to women who are not diabetic. Midwives should do a careful assessment of estimated fetal weight and watch for risk factors for shoulder dystocia.

Implications for postpartum and neonatal care Macrosomic neonates should be evaluated for hypoglycemia.

Women who have experienced GDM should be reassessed at 6 weeks after delivery. A diagnosis of diabetes mellitus is made if she has symptoms of diabetes and a random blood glucose of >200 mg/dl, fasting blood glucose of >126 mg/dl, or a 2-hour level of >200 mg/dl on a 3-hour oral glucose tolerance test (ADA, 2000). If glucose levels are normal, reassessment should be done at least every 3 years, since there is evidence that women diagnosed with GDM may be at increased risk for developing diabetes mellitus.

Types I and II Diabetes In Pregnancy

Pathology Pregestational diabetes is associated with fetal anomalies and early pregnancy loss. These fetal outcomes are associated with poorly controlled diabetes, resulting in maternal ketoacidosis. Women with type I diabetes are at increased risk for delivering a small-for-gestational-age infant because of the vascular involvement that leads to decreased uteroplacental perfusion. Women with type II diabetes are at increased risk for delivery of a macrosomic infant, especially if they are obese. Women with diabetes are also at increased risk for hypertensive disorders of pregnancy and infections. UTIs can be a particular problem.

In type I diabetes the beta cells in the islets of Langerhans in the pancreas fail to produce insulin. Therefore exogenous insulin is needed for glucose metabolism. In type II diabetes there is an increased demand for insulin, and the beta cells are unable to meet the demand. Type II diabetes in association with obesity is common, since the body cannot meet the needs of the carbohydrate-rich diet common in obesity.

The normal physiologic changes of pregnancy make control of preexisting diabetes more difficult. Nausea and vomiting of the first trimester puts the diabetic woman at risk for hypoglycemia and insulin shock. Ketoacidosis associated with fat metabolism to meet energy needs can lead to fetal mortality. Changes in caloric requirements for pregnancy and alterations of insulin effectiveness at the cellular level resulting from hormonal effects of pregnancy in the second and third trimesters make alterations in dietary intake and insulin dosage necessary.

Signs and symptoms The classic signs and symptoms of uncontrolled diabetes include polyuria, polydipsia, nocturia, and weight loss—all common in the first trimester of pregnancy. More often, particularly in type II diabetes, the condition is asymptomatic.

Screening/diagnosis In an asymptomatic patient a fasting blood glucose of >140 mg/dl on two separate occasions is diagnostic. Hgb A_{1c} of >7% is also diagnostic.

Management—community-based Women with preexisting diabetes in pregnancy can be cared for in the community only if there is a multidisciplinary team that can address the many needs during pregnancy. Team members include a physician skilled in diabetes management, an obstetrician or perinatologist, a registered nurse case manager, and a nutritionist. Close monitoring of blood glucose levels and adjustment of insulin dosage are necessary as the pregnancy progresses.

Management—referral Women with poorly controlled diabetes should be referred to a perinatologist for management during pregnancy.

Implications for the fetus Because of the potential problems associated with hyperglycemia, hypoglycemia, and maternal vascular compromise, a management plan for fetal assessment is necessary. Serial ultrasound examinations to assess fetal growth are recommended. Weekly NSTs or biophysical profiles are recommended during the third trimester. Since lung maturation can be delayed, tests for fetal maturity are usually indicated if induction of labor or elective cesarean section is planned.

Implications for labor and delivery Blood glucose levels must be closely monitored during the intrapartum period. Most intrapartum policies recommend hourly evaluations of glucose. If macrosomia is suspected, cesarean section may be considered.

Implications for postpartum and neonatal care Since a term infant of a diabetic mother may lack lung maturity, nursery facilities that can support an immature infant should be available. This may require transfer of care to a tertiary care center if the community facility does not have adequate nursery support.

Immediately after delivery, some women require no insulin for 24 to 48 hours. Frequent monitoring of blood glucose provides the data necessary for insulin dosing. The woman should be referred back to her primary care provider for ongoing monitoring of her diabetes. The importance of preconception planning for future pregnancies should be stressed.

PERINATAL INFECTIONS (IN ALPHABETIC ORDER)

Bacterial Vaginosis

Pathology Bacterial vaginosis (BV) occurs when the normal H_2O_2-producing *Lactobacillus* in the vagina is replaced by an overgrowth of anaerobic bacteria *(Bacteroides, Mobiluncus), Gardnerella vaginalis,* and *Mycoplasma hominis.* The cause of the alteration in vaginal flora is not well understood. Although BV is associated with sexual activity, it is not considered exclusively an STI (CDC, 1998a).

BV is associated with postpartum and postcesarean endometritis, PID, and vaginal cuff cellulitis following surgical procedures and invasive diagnostic procedures. Further study is necessary to determine the effectiveness of treating asymptomatic women before invasive procedures. BV has been associated with premature rupture of membranes, preterm labor, and preterm birth.

Signs and symptoms Foul-smelling vaginal discharge is the most common symptom noted. However, half of all women with clinically diagnosed BV are asymptomatic.

Screening/diagnosis The CDC (1998a) recommends that diagnosis of BV be made when three of the following four criteria are met:

- Homogeneous, white, noninflammatory discharge that adheres to the vaginal walls
- Presence of clue cells on microscopic examination
- pH of vaginal fluid of >4.5
- Fishy odor of vaginal discharge before or after addition of 10% KOH (whiff test)

Vaginal cultures are not of value in diagnosing BV.

Management—community-based Data suggest that treatment of BV in pregnancy may decrease the incidence of premature rupture of membrane and preterm birth. During the first trimester, symptomatic women can be treated with clindamycin cream 2%, one applicator (5 g) hs for 7 nights. Topical therapy is preferred since it has less systemic effect, thereby reducing exposure of the fetus to the medication. After the first trimester the preferred treatment is metronidazole, 500 mg PO BID for 7 days. Oral metronidazole has been found to achieve cure rates of 95% for the 7-day regimen. Partners do not need to be treated.

Management—referral Referral for specialist care is usually not indicated for BV.

Implications for the fetus There are no implications for the fetus.

Implications for labor and delivery There are no implications for labor and delivery.

Implications for postpartum and neonatal care There are no implications for postpartum and neonatal care.

Chancroid

Pathology Chancroid is endemic in selected areas of the United States, and an estimated 10% of patients infected with chancroid will be coinfected with syphilis or herpes simplex virus (CDC, 1998a).

Signs and symptoms Chancroid usually presents as painful genital ulcers and inguinal lymphadenopathy.

Screening/diagnosis Diagnosis is usual made as a probable diagnosis since identification of *Haemophilus ducreyi* has poor sensitivity using currently available culture media. A probable diagnosis is made if the following criteria are met:

- The individual has one or more painful genital ulcers.
- There is no evidence of *Treponema pallidum* infection using dark-field examination or serologic tests for syphilis.
- Regional lymphadenopathy is present when a diagnostic test for herpes simplex is negative.

Management—community-based The recommended treatment for chancroid is azithromycin (1 g PO in a single dose), although the safety of the drug has not been established in pregnancy. Alternately, ceftriaxone (250 mg intramuscularly [IM] in a single dose) can be used. Patients should be examined 3 to 7 days after treatment; if treatment was successful, there should be marked improvement.

Management—referral There is no indication for referral to other sources.

Implications for the fetus The effect of the disease on the fetus is not clear.

Implications for labor and delivery Suspicious lesions identified in labor and delivery without treatment may be infections. Consultation with a physician skilled in infectious disease management may be indicated, and antibiotic treatment may be prescribed.

Implications for postpartum and neonatal care If not treated previously, women should be treated in the postpartum period.

Chlamydia trachomatis

Pathology Chlamydial genital infections occur frequently in adolescents and young adults; currently *Chlamydia* is the most prevalent sexually transmitted disease in the United States. Chlamydiae are similar to viruses in that they can only grow intracellularly and in tissue cultures. Almost all chlamydiae invade only columnar epithelial cells. Left untreated, genital infection leads to salpingitis, with resultant infertility, risk of ectopic pregnancy, and chronic pelvic pain. *Chlamydia trachomatis* is also associated with preterm labor and birth and chlamydial conjunctivitis and pneumonia in the newborn.

Signs and symptoms Most women are asymptomatic until the disease progresses to salpingitis or significant cervicitis. Symptoms may include pelvic pain and mucopurulent vaginal (cervical) discharge. Physical examination may reveal normal pelvic findings or may identify cervical discharge, cervical motion tenderness, and adnexal tenderness.

Screening/diagnosis All pregnant women should be screened for chlamydial infection at the first prenatal visit. Women at increased risk for infection (multiple partners, new partner, history of other sexually transmitted infections (STIs) should be screened again during the third trimester. Screening can be done through the use of direct fluorescent antibody tests and immunoassays. Direct tissue culture provides a definitive diagnosis. Nucleic acid amplification tests (polymerase chain reaction, ligase chain reaction) hold promise for screening with a more sensitive test.

Management—community-based Treatment of *Chlamydia* is appropriately done at the community level. Since doxycycline and ofloxacin are contraindicated in pregnancy, the following regimen may be instituted:

- Erythromycin base 500 mg PO four times a day for 7 days, *or*
- Amoxicillin 500 mg PO three times a day for 7 days, *or*
- Erythromycin base 250 mg PO four times a day for 14 days, *or*
- Erythromycin ethylsuccinate 800 mg PO four times a day for 7 days, *or*
- Erythromycin ethylsuccinate 400 mg PO four times a day for 14 days, *or*
- Azithromycin 1 g PO in a single dose (CDC, 1998a)

The safety and efficacy of azithromycin has not been established in pregnancy. Since none of these drug regimens are highly efficacious and since the frequent gastrointestinal side effects associated with erythromycin may lead a woman to stop treatment, repeat testing should be done 3 weeks after completion of treatment. Chlamydial culture testing less than 3 weeks after completion of treatment may lead to false-negative results because of small numbers of organisms. Testing using nonculture techniques may lead to false-positive results less than 3 weeks after treatment because of continued shedding of dead organisms.

Patient education should include emphasis on the importance of completing the medication, the possible side effects of erythromycin, and the importance of partner treatment. Women should be counseled to refrain from sexual activity until partners have completed treatment and confirmed cure through repeat testing. Safer sex behaviors, including condom use, should be reviewed.

Management—referral Referral for specialist care is usually not indicated for chlamydial infections.

Implications for the fetus Transmission of the organism usually occurs during the birth process. Untreated infection is associated with premature rupture of membranes and preterm labor.

Implications for labor and delivery There are no specific interventions needed in intrapartum care.

Implications for postpartum and neonatal care Pediatric personnel should be notified of the maternal history of *Chlamydia* infection when there has not been documentation of a cure or when there is increased risk of reinfection. Potentially infected infants should be evaluated for chlamydial conjunctivitis and pneumonia.

Women at increased risk for reinfection should be encouraged to establish a plan for repeat screening on a regular basis. In addition, natural history of the disease, route of infection, and practices that can decrease the risk of infection should be discussed with the woman in the postpartum period.

Gonorrhea

Pathology *Neisseria gonorrhea* is an intracellular gram-negative diplococcus that can infect the cervix, fallopian tubes, urethra, rectum, and mouth. The organism thrives in the columnar and transitional epithelium of the cervix. Left untreated, the infection leads to salpingitis, tubo-ovarian abscess, and pelvic abscess. The tubal and pelvic involvement puts the woman at increased risk for infertility, ectopic pregnancy, and chronic pelvic pain. Less often, the disease progresses to a systemic infection that may include tenosynovitis, dermatitis, purulent arthritis, endocarditis, and meningitis.

Transmission to the neonate during birth leads to ophthalmia neonatorum (gonorrheal conjunctivitis). Incubation period is usually 2 to 5 days.

Signs and symptoms The infection is usually asymptomatic in women until it spreads to the Bartholin glands and the fallopian tubes. Occasionally the woman may complain of a mucopurulent vaginal discharge, dysuria, or rectal discharge. Symptoms are most often caused by concurrent infections such as *Chlamydia* or *Trichomonas.*

Screening/diagnosis Diagnosis is made through culture of the endocervix or urethra. The specimen needs to be put into suitable media immediately since it is sensitive to heat and drying. Definitive diagnosis is made through the use of selective media culture with specific carbohydrate fermentation testing. Presumptive diagnosis can be made by Gram stain, which identifies intracellular gram-negative diplococci. Identification of oxydase-positive gram-negative diplococci on selective culture media may also constitute a presumptive diagnosis.

Women at increased risk for STIs should be rescreened in third trimester.

Management—community-based It is appropriate to treat uncomplicated gonococcal infections in community-based sites. Recommended treatment in pregnancy include:

- Ceftriaxone 125 mg IM in a single dose, *or*
- Cefixime 400 mg PO in a single dose
- If cephalosporins not tolerated, spectinomycin 2 g IM

Since the cure rates with the single-dose regimens are high and there is no concern about noncompliance or taking medication improperly, it is not necessary for patients to return specifically for a test of cure. However, screening in the third trimester is recommended to rule out reinfection.

Co-infection with *Chlamydia trachomatis* is common. Therefore patients should be treated presumptively with erythromycin:

- Erythromycin base, 250 mg PO QID × 14 days, *or*
- Erythromycin ethylsuccinate, 800 mg PO qid × 7 days, *or*
- Erythromycin ethylsuccinate, 400 mg PO qid × 14 days
- If erythromycin not tolerated, amoxicillin 500 mg PO tid × 7 to 10 days

Partner notification is necessary for all partners exposed within 60 days of diagnosis. If patient has not had any sexual partners in prior 60 days, notification of last partner is necessary.

Management—referral Patients with disseminated disease should be referred to an appropriate perinatal center.

Implications for the fetus Once the membranes have adhered to the decidua in pregnancy, ascending infection is inhibited. However, when there is premature rupture of membranes, the fetus is exposed and may become infected.

Implications for labor and delivery There are no specific implications for intrapartum care.

Implications for postpartum and neonatal care When gonorrhea treatment has been inadequate and when there is an increased risk of reinfection, consideration of prophylactic antibiotic prophylaxis using one of the recommended treatment regimens to prevent postpartum endometritis should be discussed with the obstetric consultant.

Group B Streptococcus

Pathology Group B streptococcus (GBS) has received much attention because it has been found to cause more perinatal morbidity and mortality than any other organism (Greenspoon, Wilcox, and Kirschbaum, 1991).

Early-onset disease occurs in utero or within the first week of life. It is associated with neonatal pneumonia, shock, and stillbirth. Incidence is 1 to 3 infected infants per 1000 live births to colonized mothers, and neonatal mortality in infected infants is estimated to be 10% to 20% (Gigante et al., 1995; Katz, 1993). Approximately 80% of GBS infection is early-onset disease. Early-onset disease is thought to begin while the infant is still in utero, and it is presumed that the fetus becomes infected through aspirating or swallowing GBS that is present in the amniotic fluid.

Late-onset disease occurs from 1 week to 4 months after birth. Although the mortality rate is lower than in early-onset disease, long-term sequelae may be dramatic. The organism most often causes meningitis that leads to long-term neurologic impairment in 50% of affected infants. Transmission of GBS in late-onset disease is less understood than early onset transmission. Nosocomial and community-acquired infections have been proposed as contributing to development of late-onset disease.

GBS colonizes in the gastrointestinal tract of 15% to 35% of the population. Colonization is sometimes spread to the genital and urinary tracts. Colonization in the genital tract of healthy women is estimated to be 6% to 25%. Vaginal colonization is intermittent, whereas anorectal colonization is more constant. Significant variation by race/ethnicity has been noted, with one multisite study finding 13.7% of whites positive for GBS, 21.2% of blacks positive, and 20.9% of Hispanics positive (Regan, Klebanoff, and Nugent, 1991).

Probably the most significant factor in determining risk of infant colonization is the degree of colonization in the mother. Women with heavy colonization and colonization from more than one site have higher rates of transmission to the newborn and preterm delivery. Women with light colonization have been found to have similar risk as those without GBS colonization (Allen, Navas, and King, 1993; Regan, Klebanoff MA, and Nugent RP, 1991). GBS UTIs are associated with heavy colonization in the mother. Women with GBS bacteruria are at increased risk for preterm labor and for giving birth to infants who develop GBS disease. For this reason it is recommended that any woman with GBS bacteriuria be treated with antibiotics, regardless of colony count.

Signs and symptoms Women who are GBS carriers are usually asymptomatic. Women with GBS bacteriuria may experience similar symptoms as any individual with a UTI.

Screening/diagnosis One of the difficulties in identifying the prevalence of the disease is that GBS can colonize intermittently in the genital tract. Periodic cultures taken in pregnancy have documented the transient status. Definitive diagnosis is made through cultures that identify presence of GBS. Cultures are best done where colonization is more likely—the anorectal and distal vaginal areas. Cervical and urethral cultures are not as accurate in identifying the presence of the organism.

Management—community-based Clinicians need to develop a policy regarding screening for GBS consistent with one of the nationally promulgated sets of guidelines. GBS screening is now often included in the routine cervical-vaginal cultures done at the first prenatal visit. However, as noted above, cervical cultures may not identify all of the women who are colonized. Routine third trimester distal vaginal and anorectal cultures may be used to identify women who would benefit from intrapartum antibiotic therapy.

Women who are identified as GBS-positive should receive verbal and written information about GBS and the policies of the practice for management during the intrapartum period. Women can be referred to the health care provider planned for the newborn to receive further information on management during the neonatal period.

Management—referral Referral for specialist care is usually not indicated for women colonized with group B streptococcus.

Implications for the fetus The fetus of a heavily colonized woman is at increased risk for development of early-onset disease. Therefore a plan should be made for antibiotic prophylaxis in labor to prevent ascending infection to the fetus.

Implications for labor and delivery All women with a history of GBS bacteriuria during pregnancy or a previous infant infected with GBS should receive intrapartal antibiotic prophylaxis. For women without these risk factors, two approaches to early-onset GBS disease in the neonate are accepted:

1. *Antepartal screening.* Pregnant women should be offered screening at 35 to 37 weeks' gestation for anogenital colonization. Women who screened positive should received antibiotic prophylaxis in labor. The CDC recommends administration of intravenous penicillin G (5 million U for a loading dose, then 2.5 million U every 4 hours) since penicillin G has a narrow spectrum and is less likely to select for antibiotic-resistant organisms (CDC, 1996). An alternate approach is the use of ampicillin (2-g loading dose, then a 1 g every 4 hours). When women are allergic to penicillin, clindamycin or erythromycin can be used, although their efficacy in preventing perinatal group B streptococcal infection in the neonate has not been determined.

When women screen negative, they do not need prophylaxis at term unless they develop signs of infection in labor, including maternal fever, uterine tenderness, or fetal tachycardia. Rupture of membranes longer than 18 hours alone is not an indication for antibiotic prophylaxis when there is a known negative culture in the late third trimester.

2. *Treatment by the presence of risk factors.* When GBS status is not known, the decision to administer antibiotics in the intrapartal period is determined by the presence of risk factors. Risk factors include preterm labor, rupture of membranes longer than 18 hours, fever, or other signs of infection.

   The relatively low sensitivity of rapid screen tests to identify GBS colonization at the onset of labor continues to be a concern. Therefore rapid screen tests should not be considered as an alternate to screening by culture until new tests demonstrate acceptable sensitivity and specificity.

Implications for postpartum and neonatal care Postpartum and neonatal care pediatric providers and institutional policies vary in their approaches to the care of the infant born to a woman with known GBS colonization or suspected colonization based on risk factors. The American Academy of Pediatrics (1997) has issued *Revised Guidelines for the Prevention of Early-Onset Group B Streptococcal Infection,* which recommends the following approaches for neonatal care.

All neonates with signs of infection should have a full septic evaluation and initiation of antibiotic therapy. Ampicillin and gentamycin are recommended because of their broad-spectrum coverage. The duration of therapy is determined by the initial CBC, the blood culture, and the clinical course of the infant. When the laboratory results indicate that infection is not present, antibiotics can be stopped at 48 to 72 hours following initiation of treatment (American Academy of Pediatrics, 1997).

Asymptomatic infants less than 35 weeks' gestation can receive expectant care for 48 hours. If the pediatric provider's findings are equivocal, however, antibiotic therapy is recommended since preterm infants have a tenfold to 15-fold increased risk for early-onset disease. Asymptomatic infants who are older than 35 weeks' gestation and whose mothers received at least two doses of penicillin G or ampicillin before delivery can receive routine newborn care with observation for 48 hours. Most infants who develop early-onset GBS disease develop symptoms by 48 hours of age. If less than two doses of antibiotics were administered during labor, infants should have limited evaluation and observation (American Academy of Pediatrics, 1997). In most institutions a combination of CBC, blood cultures and C-reactive protein determination is used to identify those infants who may benefit from antibiotic therapy.

Women who are colonized with GBS are at increased risk for endometritis in the postpartum period. However, guidelines do not recommend universal antibiotic therapy at this time.

Hepatitis A Virus

Pathology Hepatitus A virus causes approximately one third of all cases of acute hepatitis in the United States. The infection is transmitted through fecal-oral contamination. Community epidemics are frequently caused by food and water contamination. The incubation period for the virus is 15 to 50 days, with a mean of 28 to 30 days. The highest concentration of viral load is in feces; it can also be found in blood. It is not usually carried in urine or other body fluids. Once an individual has been infected, she or he maintains immunity to further outbreaks. Hepatitis A virus does not produce a carrier state.

Signs/symptoms Individuals who become infected with hepatitis A virus experience the usual hepatitis symptoms of malaise, fatigue, nausea, weakness, low-grade fever, and right upper quadrant or epigastric pain. Signs of infection include jaundice, upper abdominal tenderness, and hepatomegaly. Some infected individuals do not develop jaundice. Typically the urine becomes dark (bilirubinuria), and stools become light-colored.

Screening/diagnosis In addition to the classical symptoms of flu-type syndrome and jaundice, laboratory findings help in determining the definitive diagnosis. Elevated serum alanine aminotransferase, aspartate aminotransferase, and bilirubin are expected. In severe cases coagulation abnormalities may be present. Identification of IgM antibodies to hepatitis A virus confirm the diagnosis. IgG antibodies are present several months after the infection.

Management—community-based Treatment is primarily supportive. Maintenance of fluid balance and nutrition should be monitored. A low-fat, high-carbohydrate diet is usually tolerated. Alcohol should be avoided. The woman's primary care provider is the usual manager of care, although midwives can co-manage according to practice guidelines. Householders should be offered the inactivated-virus vaccine.

Pregnant women living in or planning travel to areas in which hepatitis is endemic should be offered the vaccine, and women who have had intimate contact with an individual diagnosed with hepatitis A should be offered immune serum globulin (ISG). Screening for antibodies is not necessary before administration of ISG.

Management—referral Women should be referred for physician-directed care and hospitalization when patients exhibit signs of encephalopathy, coagulopathy, or severe debilitation.

Implications for the fetus Fetal status is associated with the severity of the maternal disease. When severe disease is experienced, resulting in maternal debilitation, fetal assessment of growth may be indicated.

Implications for labor and delivery There are no specific implications for labor and delivery.

Implications for postpartum and neonatal care There are no specific implications for postpartum and neonatal care.

Hepatitis B Virus

Pathology Hepatitis B is a virus that can be transmitted through blood, saliva, vaginal secretions, and semen. It is estimated that sexual transmission accounts for one third to two thirds of the 200,000 to 300,000 new hepatitis B (HBV) cases annually in the United States. Eighty-five to ninety percent of infected individuals experience complete resolution of the disease and develop protective antibodies. About 6% to 10% of those infected as adults become carriers and are at risk for developing cirrhosis and hepatocellular carcinoma. These carriers continue to have elevated levels of hepatitis B surface antigen (HBsAG), and about one third of the carriers experience continued viral replication and persistent positive HBeAG. HBV transmission to the newborn occurs in 10% to 85% of infected women. Risk of transmission to the infant is associated with the mother's HBe antigen status. Women who are seropositive for both HBsAG and HBeAG have a high risk of transmission to their neonates. Most transmission occurs during the birth process. However, 10% to 15% of transmission occurs transplacentally, through breast milk, or through close contact between the infant and the infected individual.

Passive immunity can be stimulated with hepatitis B immune globulin (HBIG). HBIG is recommended for all individuals at risk for exposure (CDC, 1991). Hepatitis B vaccine given as a series of three injections is available in the United States.

Signs and symptoms Acute viral hepatitis begins with a prodromal phase during which the individual may experience malaise, fatigue, anorexia, nausea, vomiting, myalgia, and headache. Individuals infected with HBV may also experience arthritis and urticaria, suggesting a flu-type syndrome (Andreoli et al., 1997). The prodromal period lasts for several days and is followed by development of jaundice and loss of stool color. The jaundice phase of the disease may last from several days to weeks. Jaundice may not be apparent; therefore the individual may not seek treatment.

Physical examination reveals tenderness and enlargement of the liver; about 20% of patients also exhibit splenomegaly. Laboratory findings include elevated alanine transaminase and aspartate transaminase, elevated serum bilirubin, and mildly elevated serum alkaline phosphatase.

Screening/diagnosis All pregnant women should be screened for hepatitis B. Definitive diagnosis of the status of infection is made through assessment of serologic markers listed in Table 25-5.

Table 25-5 *Serologic Markers for Hepatitis B Virus*

Marker	Definition	Significance
HBsAg	HBV surface antigen	Positive in most cases of acute or chronic infection
HBeAg	e antigen; core antigen	Transiently positive in acute HBV; may persist in chronic infection; reflects presence of viral replication and high infectivity
Anti-HBe	Antibody to e antigen	Transiently positive in convalescence; may be positive in chronic HBV Usually indicates low infectivity
Anti-HBc (IgM or IgG)	Antibody to core antigen	Positive in all acute and chronic cases; reliable marker of infection, past or present IgM anti-HBc reflects active trial replication; not protective
Anti-HBs	Antibody to surface antigen	Positive in late convalescence in most acute cases; confers immunity

Adapted from Andreoli TE et al: *Cecil essentials of medicine,* ed 4, Philadelphia, 1997, WB Saunders, p. 332.

Management—community-based There is no specific treatment for acute HBV. The individual's medical care should be managed by her primary care physician. Supportive therapy, including rest, hydration, and maintenance of a low-fat, high-carbohydrate diet is common. Liver function tests should be done either by the primary care physician or the obstetric provider when the woman is identified with chronic disease.

Patients should be counseled regarding the possibility of transmission to sexual partners and to their infants. Partners should be referred for evaluation of status and possible vaccination. Vaccination of the newborn is recommended, and the newborn's health care provider should be notified of the mother's HBV status to ensure that the proper regimen is followed.

Management—referral Women with acute-onset disease should be referred to a perinatologist for management of the pregnancy.

Implications for the fetus No specific guidelines have been promulgated for fetal assessment during pregnancy.

Implications for labor and delivery Standard precautions should be maintained throughout intrapartal care. There are no additional recommendations for HBV-infected women during labor and delivery.

Implications for postpartum and neonatal care The CDC (1991) has recommended that all neonates be immunized against HBV. The immunization should be initiated within the first few days of birth. A second dose is given 1 month later, followed by a third dose 6 months after the initial dose. The recommendation for universal screening of all infants, even when the mother screens negative, remains controversial. Some pediatric providers argue that, since the risk for HBV infection is low until the individual initiates sexual activity or other risky behaviors such as intravenous drug use, immunization of infants is not necessary.

When the mother of a neonate has screened positive for HBV, the infant should receive hepatitis B immunoglobulin for passive immunity, in addition to the vaccine series.

Women who received hepatitis B vaccine during pregnancy should be rescreened in the postpartum period to determine seroprotective response to the vaccine. Evidence suggests that pregnant women who are obese, of advanced maternal age, and smoke may have decreased immune response (Ingardia et al., 1999)

Herpes Simplex Virus-1

Pathology Herpes genitalis is caused by the herpes simplex virus and transmitted by direct contact. Seventy to ninety-five percent of genital herpes is caused by herpes simplex type 2 (HSV-2). Clinical recurrences are less frequent in herpes simplex type 1 (HSV-1). Identification of the type of virus may be helpful in counseling the individual regarding natural history of the disease and methods to decrease the risk of transmission of the virus to others.

Primary herpes is characterized by painful genital lesions, inguinal lymphadenopathy, and viral symptoms, including fever, malaise, and headache. However, some infected individuals have very mild infections and are not aware that they can transmit the virus to others. The incubation period averages 6 days, and about 70% of women who are exposed will contract the disease. Incidence is highest in adolescents, women who began sexual activity at an early age, and women with multiple sexual partners. Recurrences tend to be milder and resolve more rapidly.

Signs and symptoms Women experiencing a primary outbreak present with complaints of extremely painful lesions, burning in the vulvar area, urinary frequency and burning, fever, headache, and malaise. Physical examination reveals vesicles that may have opened, leaving tender ulcers or crusted healing lesions. Lymph nodes may be enlarged and tender. Lesions in a primary infection in a seronegative woman may be present for up to 30 days.

Women experiencing a recurrence complain of lesions of varying tenderness. Recurrent outbreaks usually clear in about 7 days.

Screening/diagnosis Presumptive diagnosis can be made through inspection and findings of cellular changes on cytologic smears. Definitive diagnosis is made through viral cultures.

Management—community-based Herpes simplex types 1 and 2 are appropriately managed at the community level. Acyclovir and valacyclovir have been shown to decrease the duration of viral shedding, pain, itching, and time required for crusting and healing of lesions (McCormack et al., 1996). Although recent studies suggest the safety of these drugs in pregnancy, their use in the perinatal period remains controversial. The manufacturer, Glaxo-Wellcome, Inc., in cooperation with the CDC, maintains a registry to assess the use and effects of these two antiviral agents in pregnancy. Women who use either of these drugs in pregnancy should register with the registry at (800) 722-9292, extension 38465 (CDC, 1998a).

The CDC recommends that a primary case of HSV should be treated with acyclovir, 400 mg PO three times a day for 7 to 10 days, or acyclovir, 200 mg PO five times a day for 7 to 10 days. Recurrent outbreaks can be treated with acyclovir, 400 mg PO three times a day for

5 days, or acyclovir, 200 mg PO five times a day for 5 days. Another recommended regimen is acyclovir, 800 mg PO twice daily for 5 days. Routine daily administration of acyclovir for suppression is not currently recommended in pregnancy (CDC, 1998a).

Patient education should include discussion of the natural history of the disease, including the expectation of recurrent outbreaks. To decrease transmission of the infection, patients should be encouraged to refrain from sexual activity when lesions or prodromal symptoms are experienced. Condoms should be recommended for all sexual activity with uninfected partners. Infected individuals should be counseled that transmission of the infection can also occur when she or he is asymptomatic, particularly in the first year of the infection. Dietary efforts to support the immune system can be encouraged. Comfort measures that can be used during outbreaks include sitz baths, oral analgesics, and topical viscous xylocaine.

Patient education should prepare the woman for the management of labor and delivery when lesions are present. Cesarean section is recommended for prodromal symptoms or presence of active lesions at the time of labor.

Referral Referral to a perinatal specialist is not usually indicated.

Implications for the fetus The risk of transmission of HSV to the neonate is highest when women develop a primary outbreak near the time of delivery and least in women who have a history of recurrent outbreaks near term. There is also decreased risk for transmission when the primary outbreak is in the first trimester. Since the results of viral cultures do not predict shedding, routine cultures in late pregnancy are not recommended (CDC, 1998a).

Implications for labor and delivery All women who present for labor evaluation should be questioned regarding history of or symptoms of HSV. Close inspection should be done to identify suspicious lesions. Women who have a history of herpes can deliver vaginally as long as there are no lesions present or no prodromal symptoms at the time of labor. Women with lesions or prodromal symptoms should be delivered by cesarean section. However, women need to understand that surgical deliver does not completely eliminate the risk of transmission to the neonate (CDC, 1998a).

Implications for postpartum and neonatal care Pediatric providers should be notified when there is a maternal history of herpes, when there has been a primary outbreak near term, and when there are lesions of prodromal symptoms at the time of labor. Infants exposed to lesions during birth or those exposed to a primary outbreak near the delivery date can be cultured to determine HSV status. Infants with evidence of neonatal HSV should be evaluated and treated with acyclovir (CDC, 1998a).

Human Immunodeficiency Virus

Pathology Human immunodeficiency virus (HIV) is a retrovirus that has an affinity for the CD4 molecule of the T helper lymphocytes that protect against intracellular organisms, including viruses, fungi, parasites, and malignancies. T lymphocytes are responsible for cell-mediated immunity. Other lymphocytes, B lymphocytes, are responsible for producing antibodies specific to invading antigens. This process is the development of humoral immunity. Healthy, normally functioning CD4 cells are needed for the coordinated response to antigens that must be mounted by the B lymphocytes. When HIV enters CD4 cells, it effectively incapacitates the immune system, which is essential for coordinating the immune response against viruses.

In 2 to 8 weeks after the initial exposure, 20% to 60% of individuals infected with the virus develop a mononucleosis-type syndrome. During the acute retroviral syndrome, antibodies are not usually detected, but culture can identify HIV in the blood. Following the acute phase, infected individuals enter an asymptomatic phase. During this asymptomatic period there is abundant viral replication, leading to a high viral load; over 1 billion new virions may be produced daily (Andreoli et al., 1997). After several weeks humoral immunity develops, and the viral load decreases. It is at this point that serum antibodies can be detected. An equilibrium between HIV and CD4 cells may be maintained for several years, but eventually circulating CD4 cells decline, and plasma viral load increases. As the disease progresses, functional impairment of the remaining lymphocytes also occurs (Andreoli et al., 1997). When CD4 counts decrease to under 200 cells per mm^3, infected individuals are at risk for developing multiple opportunistic infections. HIV infection eventually leads to acquired immunodeficiency syndrome (AIDS) in most individuals.

HIV is detectable in greater than 95% of infected individuals within 6 months of infection (CDC, 1998a). Women at highest risk are those who are intravenous drug users or partners of intravenous drug users and women with multiple partners.

Transplacental transmission of the HIV antibody occurs during pregnancy, with passively acquired antibodies in the newborn falling to undetectable levels by 15 months of age (CDC, 1998a).

Signs and symptoms About 20% to 60% of individuals infected with HIV experience symptoms of a viral syndrome during the first few weeks after exposure. Symptoms may include erythematous maculopapular rash, arthralgia, lymphadenopathy, pharyngitis, night sweats, fever, and weight loss. Misdiagnosis of mononucleosis may be made. Symptoms resolve spontaneously, and the length of time before development of symptoms of AIDS varies significantly among individuals.

HIV infection should be suspected in women experiencing the following problems:

- New onset or frequent *Candida* vaginitis
- Recurrent HSV outbreaks
- Cervical dysplasia/neoplasia, usually a result of impaired defense against human papillomavirus (HPV)

Screening/diagnosis All pregnant women should be offered HIV screening at the initial prenatal visit. Health providers skilled in pretest and posttest counseling must be available at sites to ensure appropriate counseling and consent. Informed consent must be obtained before testing. Screening is done with an enzyme-linked immunosorbent assay or a rapid assay, with positive results followed by a more specific test such as the Western blot or an immunofluorescence assay. Confirmation indicates that the individual is infected with HIV and is able to infect others.

Management—community-based Women who are diagnosed as HIV-infected should be counseled regarding pregnancy options. Prenatal and abortion services should be available on-site or through referral to a site accessible to the woman. Pregnant women who are infected with HIV should receive the same prenatal services as those who are not infected.

Antiviral and prophylactic antibiotic therapy for HIV positive women during pregnancy has been found to maintain the health of the woman and decrease perinatal transmission to the infant. Approximately 25% to 30% of infants born to untreated HIV-infected mothers will be infected. When treatment with zidovudine is carried out in pregnancy and during labor and delivery, the rate of perinatal transmission drops to about 8% (CDC, 1998a). Prophylactic regimens can decrease the risk of serious opportunistic infections.

Community-based treatment of HIV-positive women is possible when there is a multi-disciplinary team available to follow the woman's progress. Midwives may be members of the health care team, and research suggests that midwifery care is associated with increased continuity (De Ferrari et al., 1993). Treatment regimens are beyond the scope of this text; the clinician providing perinatal services to HIV-infected women should refer to the infectious disease literature for the most current therapies. Current therapy recommendations can also be found on the CDC web page: www.cdc.gov/hiv/treatment.htm.

Management—referral All women with diagnosis of HIV disease should be referred to a center that can offer a multidisciplinary approach to care.

Implications for the fetus As noted previously, the fetus is at risk for viral transmission from the mother, and antiviral treatment is recommended to decrease transmission. There is a theoretic risk of vertical transmission of the infection during invasive procedures, including amniocentesis, chorionic villi sampling, and percutaneous umbilical blood sampling.

Implications for labor and delivery Transmission of the virus occurs when the infant is directly exposed to maternal body fluids. Therefore the midwife must develop a plan to decrease the exposure. Procedures that increase exposure include use of the fetal scalp electrode, amniotomy, and episiotomy. Women who deliver vaginally and who have not been treated with zidovudine during the pregnancy have a 25% risk of transmission of the virus to the neonate. When both the woman and her neonate are treated with zidovudine, the risk of transmission drops to 5% to 8% during vaginal birth. The risk of transmission in treated mother-baby pairs decreases further to 2% if elective cesarean section is the mode of delivery. For this reason, ACOG has recommended that all infected women be offered the option of elective cesarean delivery (ACOG, 1999). The exact mechanism of transmission remains unclear, but maternal-fetal transfusion during uterine contractions and exposure to maternal cervical-vaginal secretions and blood have been proposed as possible factors.

Implications for postpartum and neonatal care Women should be referred back to their primary care providers for ongoing treatment after delivery. Neonates whose mothers are HIV positive should receive zidovudine for the first 6 weeks after birth. All neonates whose mothers are infected have circulating maternal anti-HIV antibodies for up to 6 months. Diagnosis of neonatal infection can be achieved by using sensitive plasma HIV ribonucleic acid assays or identifying circulating HIV p24 antigen (Andreoli et al., 1997).

Human Papillomavirus Infection

Pathology Genital warts are most often caused by HPV types 6 or 11. Other types (16, 18, 31, 33, 35) may also be present (CDC, 1998a). The virus infects squamous epithelium, producing distinct lesions known as genital warts or condylomata acuminata. Flat lesions (flat condyloma) may be found on the cervix. HPV is associated with cervical dysplasia and carcinoma and can cause laryngeal papillomatosis in the newborn. There is no therapy that has been shown to eliminate HPV.

Randomized control studies have shown that current treatments are 22% to 94% effective in eliminating external warts and that recurrence rates are at least 25% within 3 months of treatment. Studies suggest that treatment is more effective if the warts are small and if they have been present for less than 1 year. Recurrences of warts most likely result from reactivation of subclinical infection rather than through reinfection from a sexual partner. Failure to treat genital warts may result in no change in status, growth in size, and number of warts or spontaneous resolution.

Genital warts tend to increase in size in pregnancy and may rarely produce soft-tissue obstruction in the birth canal or form friable lesions that lacerate easily and bleed profusely.

Signs and symptoms Women may present with complaints of "bumps" in the vaginal area. Vaginal and cervical warts and subclinical infections may be asymptomatic.

Screening/diagnosis Presumptive diagnosis is made based on inspection of the genital area. Genital warts have a characteristic raised, rough appearance—so-called "cauliflower appearance." The lesions may appear as distinct individual growths or large, multi-lesion areas. Any part of the vulva or perianal area may be affected. Flat condylomata may be visualized on the cervix or vaginal walls and may be detected using an application of 3% acetic acid. Presumptive diagnosis of flat condylomata can be made through cytologic findings consistent with koilocytosis and dysplasia. Definitive diagnosis is made through DNA identification of the virus.

Management—community-based Most cases of HPV diagnosed during pregnancy can be managed in the community setting. Management depends on the extent of the infection and the patient's preference.

Simple external genital and perianal warts, vaginal warts: Trichloracetic acid (TCA) 80% to 90% applied directly to the warts weekly up to six applications may be the initial treatment in the community setting. Cryotherapy with liquid nitrogen or cryoprobe is also safe in pregnancy but requires special equipment that may not be available in all sites. Efficacy of cryotherapy is estimated to be 63% to 88% (CDC, 1998a). Efficacy of TCA was estimated to be 81% in the one randomized control study to date.

Partners with obvious warts can be referred for treatment. There is no need to treat subclinical infection in partners. Counseling for the woman and her partner should include explanation of the course of the infection and discussion of condom use to protect uninfected sexual partners. Women with HPV infection should be counseled regarding the importance of regular Pap smears, although the literature offers conflicting advice regarding the ideal frequency of testing. Most sources recommend Pap smears every 3 to 6 months when dysplasia is identified and every 6 months to 1 year once dysplasia has been eliminated.

Women with dysplasia identified on Pap smear or with visual changes on cervical and vaginal mucosa should be referred for colposcopy. Because of the increased vascularity of the cervix, biopsies are usually not recommended during pregnancy. A plan for postpartum follow-up of these positive findings must be made.

Management—referral Women with cervical warts or frequent recurrences should be referred to a physician skilled in treating HPV.

Implications for the fetus There are not specific implications for the fetus.

Implications for labor and delivery When large lesions are present in the perivaginal area, care to protect the area from lacerations should be taken. Consultation with an obstetrician is indicated for large lesions since the option of cesarean delivery may be considered.

Implications for postpartum and neonatal care Women with HPV lesions should have a plan for treatment made during the postpartum period. A plan for serial Pap smears should also be made.

Pediatric providers should be notified of the mother's HPV status so that the infant can be evaluated for laryngeal papillomatosis.

Syphilis

Pathology Syphilis is caused by *T. pallidum,* a spirochete that enters the body through the mucous membranes or a break in the skin and is spread via the bloodstream. The disease progresses through four stages: primary, secondary, latent, and tertiary. Neurosyphilis, the development of neurologic infection, can occur at any time during the natural history of the disease. Soft tissue granuloma lesions (gumma) occur during the tertiary stage and can affect the liver, brain, heart, bone, and skin. Cardiovascular lesions that develop in the tertiary stage include aortic valve disease, aortic aneurysms, and coronary artery disease.

Syphilis is easily transmitted to the fetus through the placenta. Untreated syphilis is associated with spontaneous abortion, intrauterine fetal demise, neonatal death, and congenital syphilis. Up to 80% of pregnant women with untreated syphilis experience perinatal mortality or morbidity.

Signs and symptoms Primary-stage syphilis produces symptoms within 9 to 90 days from exposure. The primary lesion (chancre) usually develops at the site of inoculation. It is most often on the genitals but may also appear on the lip, tongue, mouth, fingers, eyelids, nipple, or other skin or mucous membrane surface. At first it may appear as a small pimple, it then develops into a papula, and it finally ulcerates. The lesion is usually painless and is highly contagious. Very soon after infection, the organism invades the lymphatic system, and the regional lymph glands become large, firm, and nontender. Once the organism is in the bloodstream (4 to 8 weeks after infection), antibodies can be detected by serologic tests.

Signs and symptoms of secondary syphilis occur 6 to 10 weeks after the primary chancre and may be so mild that the individual may regard them as a mild viral infection. There may be low-grade fever, sore throat, laryngitis, and general malaise. Shallow painless ulcers form on mucous membranes in the mouth, nose, and genitals. The lesions are highly contagious. A mild papular rash develops on the palms and soles of the feet and may be present on the shoulders, chest, back, abdomen, and arms. It is pale pink at the onset; the color progresses to a copper color, and the rash may extend to the rest of the body. No itching or irritation is noted. Women may develop condylomata lata on the vulva or perineum. These flat, moist, wartlike lesions are highly contagious. They are not to be confused with condylomata caused by HPV.

Latent syphilis (infection between the symptomatic outbreaks) can be identified through serologic testing. Latent syphilis during the first year following a known exposure and infection is termed early latent syphilis. Individuals infected for greater than 1 year are said to have late latent syphilis; others have latent syphilis of unknown duration.

Tertiary-stage syphilis develops any time after 2 years from the initial infection. A tertiary lesion (gummatous syphilis) may form anywhere on the body. Blood vessels, especially the aorta, may be affected by inflammation or aneurysm. Cerebral and spinal cord vessels may be affected leading to paralysis or tabes dorsalis.

Screening/diagnosis Diagnosis is made through identification of the organism on dark-field microscope examination or through direct fluorescent antibody testing. Screening is done with nonspecific serologic tests. The Venereal Disease Research Laboratory (VDRL) or rapid plasma reagin (RPR) identifies any treponemal disease, and false-positive results may be found after recent viral infection or in lupus. Nontreponemal tests are reported quantitatively, and a fourfold change in titer is considered necessary to assume clinically significant difference between serial tests (CDC, 1998a). Nontreponemal tests usually return to nonreactive after treatment, although some individuals continue to maintain low titers for the remainder of their lives. The titers of nontreponemal tests correlate well with disease activity, so it is common to obtain serial results to assess response to treatment.

Specific diagnostic tests include the microhemagglutination assay for antibody to *T. pallidum* (MATP) or the fluorescent treponemal antibody (FTA) absorption test. Presumptive diagnosis is made through positive findings on both a nonspecific test and a treponemal test.

Management—community-based All women should be screened for syphilis at the first prenatal visit. Women at increased risk for exposure—those with multiple sex partners, history of STIs, or living in a community with a high prevalence of syphilis—should be rescreened during the third trimester.

Penicillin is the drug of choice for maternal treatment, treatment of established fetal infection, and prevention of transmission to the fetus. Parenteral penicillin G is the only drug with documented efficacy in pregnancy. Regimens depend on the stage of the disease (Box 25-6).

Serologic titers should be followed monthly to document decrease in titers and effectiveness of treatment. All women diagnosed with syphilis should have screening for HIV and other STIs. Partner notification is necessary, with treatment based on individual diagnosis and duration of infection.

Management—referral A perinatologist or obstetrician skilled in infectious disease should be consulted to develop an appropriate plan of care. The woman should be referred to a perinatologist when signs of fetal syphilis, including hepatomegaly and hydrops, are identified by ultrasound examination.

Implications for the fetus Because of the risk of transmission to the fetus, fetal assessment using ultrasound examination, NSTs, and biophysical profiles should be considered.

Implications for labor and delivery Serology status and treatment adequacy must be reported to perinatal staff to plan for neonatal assessment and postpartum follow-up.

Implications for postpartum and neonatal care Following treatment, VDRL or RPR titers should be followed monthly until they are nonreactive. Infants ex-

Box 25-6 *Recommended Treatment Regimens for Syphilis in Pregnancy*

Primary Syphilis

Benzathine penicillin G, 2.4 million U IM in a single dose. If allergic to penicillin, consider desensitization since doxycycline and tetracycline are contraindicated in pregnancy. Some authorities recommend a second dose of benzathine penicillin G, 2.4 million U IM, 1 week following the initial treatment.

Secondary Syphilis

Benzathine penicillin G, 2.4 million U IM in a single dose. If allergic to penicillin, consider desensitization since doxycycline and tetracycline are contraindicated in pregnancy. Some authorities recommend a second dose of benzathine penicillin G, 2.4 million U IM, 1 week following the initial treatment.

Early Latent Syphilis

Benzathine penicillin G, 2.4 million U IM in a single dose. If allergic to penicillin, consider desensitization since doxycycline and tetracycline are contraindicated in pregnancy.

Late Latent Syphilis

Benzathine penicillin G, 7.2 million U total, administered in three doses of 2.4 million U IM each at weekly intervals. If allergic to penicillin, consider desensitization since doxycycline and tetracycline are contraindicated in pregnancy.

Latent Syphilis of Unknown Duration

Same as Late Latent Syphilis

Tertiary Syphilis

Benzathine penicillin G, 7.2 million U total, administered in three doses of 2.4 million U IM each at weekly intervals. If allergic to penicillin, consider desensitization since doxycycline and tetracycline are contraindicated in pregnancy.

Neurosyphilis

2-24 million U aqueous crystalline penicillin G daily, administered as 2-4 million U IV q4h for 10-14 days. If allergic to penicillin, consider desensitization.

From Centers for Disease Control and Prevention: 1998 Guidelines for treatment of sexually transmitted diseases, *MMWR* 47(RR-1):1-118, 1998a.

posed during pregnancy should receive full evaluation by a pediatric provider skilled in infectious disease.

Trichomoniasis Infection

Pathology Trichomoniasis is caused by *T. vaginalis,* a protozoan. Recent studies have found an association between trichomoniasis and premature rupture of membranes and preterm delivery (Cotch et al., 1997).

Signs and symptoms Although trichomoniasis may be asymptomatic in women, most pregnant women present with a complaint of yellow-green or gray, foul-smelling discharge. Many women also experience severe vulvar irritation.

Screening/diagnosis Pelvic examination may reveal irritation of the vulva and vaginal mucosa. Petechiae and hemorrhagic spots caused by increased vascularity and thinning of the vaginal epithelium may be noted. Vaginal discharge may be profuse.

Wet mount examination of the discharge using normal saline reveals mobile flagellated trichomonads. Numerous leukocytes and epithelial cells are also common.

Management—community-based Metronidazole is the drug of choice for trichomoniasis. Many sources consider metronidazole to be contraindicated in the first trimester. Patients may be treated after the first trimester with metronidazole, 2 g in a single dose. Partners should be treated at the same time. Oral metronidazole results in cure in 90% to 95% of cases. Metronidazole gel is not recommended for treatment of trichomoniasis since it does not provide the therapeutic levels to eradicate infection in the perivaginal and urethral glands (CDC, 1998a).

Management—referral Referral for specialty care is usually not indicated for trichomonal infections.

Vulvovaginal Candidiasis

Pathology Vulvovaginal candidiasis (VVC) is most often caused by *Candida albicans,* although it can also be caused by other *Candida* species, *Torulopsis* species, or other fungi (CDC, 1998a). Hormonally induced changes in the genital tract in pregnancy increase the incidence of the infection during pregnancy. Besides the obvious discomfort caused by the infection, untreated VVC leads to friable vulvar and vaginal tissues that lacerate easily during the birth. VVC can be transferred to the fetus during delivery, leading to fungal infection of the mouth (thrush) or intractable diaper rash in the newborn. VVC infection can also be transmitted to the breasts.

Signs and symptoms Symptoms include severe itching, burning with urination, and itching or burning associated with intercourse. The woman may also complain of the characteristic thick, white vaginal discharge, often accompanied by a "yeastlike" odor.

Screening/diagnosis Pelvic examination reveals erythema of the vestibule and labia minora, erythema of the labia majora or external affected area, and white vaginal discharge. Occasionally the clinician notes abrasions caused by scratching the area and signs of a superimposed infection. Wet preparation of the secretions for microscopic examination reveals budding yeast and filaments (pseudohypha, mycelia). Use of 10% KOH solution in the wet mount improves visualization of the yeast by eradicating cellular material that might otherwise obscure the field. Acidity of the vagina is decreased slightly (pH <4.5).

Cultures are rarely needed for diagnosis, although general cervical cultures done for screening and Pap smears may identify *Candida.*

Management—community-based. CDC recommendations for topical therapies are listed in Box 25-7. Because of the changes in the vaginal mucosa and rugae in pregnancy, 7-day treatments are more effective in eliminating the infection.

Counseling should include reassurance that VVC is not an STI, and women should be educated about the course of the disease. Use of the cream or suppositories should be discussed, and the importance of completing treatment should be stressed. Patients should be counseled that the recommended topical agents are oil-based and may weaken latex condoms.

Comfort measures that may alleviate the itching and burning include warm sitz baths with careful drying after bathing. A hair dryer set on low provides an effective means to dry the vulva. Application of the prescribed cream externally may decrease itching. Pelvic rest appears to aid healing.

Recurrent VVC infections (greater than three annually) may indicate other predisposing conditions. Risk factors for recurrent VVC include broad-spectrum antibiotic use, corticosteroid use, diabetes mellitus, immunosuppression, and HIV infection. Screening and follow-up should be done accordingly.

Management—referral If workup for recurrent VVC identifies diabetes, immunosuppression, or HIV infection, referrals to the appropriate medical specialists are indicated.

Implications for the fetus There are no specific implications for the fetus.

Box 25-7 ***Topical Therapies for VVC in Pregnancy***

Butoconazole 2% cream 5 g intravaginally for 3 days, *or*
Clotrimazole 1% cream 5 g intravaginally daily for 7-14 days, *or*
Clotrimazole 100 mg suppository intravaginally daily for 7 days, *or*
Clotrimazole 100 mg suppository, two intravaginally daily for 3 days, *or*
Clotrimazole 500 mg suppository, one intravaginally as a single dose, *or*
Miconazole 2% cream 5 g intravaginally daily for 7days, *or*
Miconazole 200 mg suppository, one intravaginally daily for 3 days, *or*
Miconazole 100 mg suppository, one suppository daily for 7 days, *or*
Terconazole 0.4% cream 5 g intravaginally daily for 7 days, *or*
Terconazole 0.8% cream 5 g intravaginally daily for 3 days, *or*
Terconazole 80 mg suppository, one suppository qd × 3

From Centers for Disease Control and Prevention: 1998 Guidelines for treatment of sexually transmitted diseases, *MMWR* 47(RR-1):1-118, 1998a.

Implications for labor and delivery VVC at the onset of labor is associated with inflammation of vaginal tissues, with resulting risk of lacerations during the birth process.

Implications for postpartum and neonatal care Women with VVC in the perinatal period should be instructed to maintain meticulous hygiene to decrease transmission to the nipples or to the neonate. The postpartum lochial discharge may decrease symptoms and lead to spontaneous resolution. Infants of mothers with VVC should be evaluated for fungal infections in the mouth and in the diaper region.

ECTOPARASITIC INFECTIONS

Pediculosis Pubis (Pubic Lice)

Pathology Pubic lice *(phthirus pubis)* are tiny criblike parasites that infest the pubic and perianal hair. They can also be found in the hair of the axilla, trunk, and thighs. Adult lice are 1 to 2 mm long and have slender forelegs; the second and third pairs of legs are stouter and have claws. They can be identified using a magnifying glass or put on a slide to be identified under the microscope. Nits are oval, white, translucent eggs that are attached to hair, usually close to the skin. When evaluated under the microscope, the immature louse inside the nit can be observed.

Signs and symptoms Infected women usually present with a complaint of itching in the anogenital area. She may also present for evaluation after her partner or other householder(s) have been diagnosed with lice.

Screening/diagnosis Diagnosis is made through direct observation of the adult lice or nits in the pubic area.

Management—community-based Pregnant women can be treated with permethrin 1% cream (Nix) or pyrethrin with piperonyl butoxide (RID or A200 Pyrinate). Both are applied to the affected area, then washed off after 10 minutes. Both preparations are available without a prescription. Infected individuals should be reevaluated 1 week after treatment, and retreatment is necessary if lice or nits are found. All sexual partners within 1 month of diagnosis should be treated (CDC, 1998a).

Live lice can live off the host for up to 48 hours, and nits can be shed and hatch in 7 to 10 days. Therefore it is recommended that all bedding, towels, and clothing be washed in hot water and dried in a hot dryer. Carpets, upholstered furniture, and mattresses should be vacuumed. Fumigation of the living area is not necessary.

Management—referral There is no indication for referral.

Implications for the fetus There are no implications for the fetus.

Implications for labor and delivery When infestation is noted in the intrapartal period, a plan for treatment after delivery should be made. The labor room needs to be decontaminated before admission of any other patients.

Implications for postpartum and neonatal care Nursing mothers can be treated with permethrin 1% cream rinse or pyrethrin with piperonyl butoxide. Women who are not breast-feeding can alternately use Lindane 1% shampoo, which is the least expensive therapy.

Scabies

Pathology Scabies is a parasitic infestation caused by the mite, *Sarcoptes scabiei*. The impregnated female mite burrows into the stratum corneum of the epidermis to bury her eggs. A resulting inflammatory response causes intense itching. The first time a person is infected with scabies, sensitization and inflammation may take several weeks to develop. Subsequent infections develop symptoms within 24 hours of transmission. Scabies can be transmitted sexually. The lesions are generally found interdigitally on the hands but can also be found in the axillar, antecubital, popliteal, and inguinal areas.

Signs and symptoms Infected individuals usually present with the complaint of severe itching.

Screening/diagnosis Diagnosis is made by identifying the classical signs of burrowing. Occasionally the mite can be retrieved by scraping the area, then identified under the microscope.

Management—community-based Pregnant women can be treated with permethrin 5% cream, which is applied to the affected areas, then washed off in 8 to 14 hours (CDC, 1998a). Some experts recommend retreatment 1 week after the initial treatment. All sexual partners and householders with close contact to the infected individual should be treated. Bedding and clothing should be decontaminated using hot wash and dry cycles. Infected women should be counseled that the itching may continue for several weeks, even when the mites have been effectively eliminated.

Management—referral There are no indications for referral.

Implications for the fetus There are no implications for the fetus.

Implications for labor and delivery If infestation is noted during the intrapartal period, a plan for treatment after delivery should be made. The labor room needs to be decontaminated before admission of any other patients.

Implications for postpartum and neonatal care Nursing mothers can be treated with permethrin. Women who are not breast-feeding can alternately use Lindane 1% lotion or cream.

SUBSTANCE ABUSE

Pathology Substance abuse in pregnancy is considered to be a major perinatal problem and is associated with increased maternal and neonatal morbidity and mortality. The actual prevalence of substance abuse in pregnancy is difficult to determine, but some studies have indicated that 15% to 20% of women in some communities abuse alcohol or drugs (Chasnoff, Landress, and Barrett, 1990). Although certain substances may be more commonly used in specific communities, abuse crosses all socioeconomic groups. Substance abuse in pregnancy is associated with late or inconsistent prenatal care, STIs, poor nutrition, and violence. In addition, characteristics of the abuse may predispose women to other risks. For example, women using intravenous drugs are at increased risk for HIV and hepatitis B and C, as well as other systemic infections.

1. *Tobacco.* The association between tobacco use and low birth weight has been well documented. Smoking is also associated with preterm labor and birth, spontaneous abortion, placental abruption, and premature rupture of membranes. Vasoconstriction caused by nicotine contributes to these adverse outcomes, but the contribution of other factors, including the many chemicals in tobacco, are not well understood. There is evidence that quitting smoking by 16 weeks' gestation may ameliorate the adverse effects (MacArthur and Knox, 1988). Chewing tobacco produces some of the same adverse effects.
2. *Alcohol.* The effects of fetal alcohol syndrome (FAS) have been well documented in the literature. FAS is characterized by growth restriction, facial anomalies, and central nervous system (CNS) dysfunction (ACOG, 1994b). Skeletal abnormalities and cardiac defects are also common in FAS. Ethanol crosses the placenta by simple diffusion, and it easily crosses the blood-brain barrier of the fetus. It is thought that the effects are caused by direct toxicity, although other metabolites may also influence outcome.

   The dose response for alcohol is not well understood. Although it is known that women who are moderate-to-heavy drinkers (more than two glasses of wine, two mixed drinks, or two beers per day) have an increased risk for adverse outcomes, the development of FAS is highly variable. In addition, FAS has been identified in women who are not moderate-to-heavy drinkers. It appears that the most dramatic effects occur with exposure in the early first trimester.
3. *Marijuana.* Marijuana (cannabis sativa) use in pregnancy is associated with maternal tachycardia, hypotension, and respiratory disease. No specific fetal/neonatal outcomes of use in pregnancy have been isolated, in part because marijuana use is often combined with use of other substances.
4. *Cocaine.* Cocaine is a CNS stimulant that can be taken orally, IV, subcutaneously, and through inhalation. It is readily absorbed across all mucous membranes. In addition to euphoria, the drug produces vasoconstriction, tachycardia, and local anesthesia. "Crack" cocaine, an inexpensive, easily manufactured form of the drug, is extremely addictive (ACOG, 1994b). The vasoconstriction produced can result in malignant hypertension, cardiac ischemia, cerebral infarction, spontaneous abortion, intrauterine fetal death, and placental abruption. Cocaine use is also associated with premature rupture of membranes, preterm labor and birth, intrauterine growth retardation, meconium-stained amniotic fluid, and in utero fetal cerebral infarction. Microcephaly, limb defects, and genitourinary anomalies have been observed with perinatal cocaine use and theoretically could be the result of vasoconstriction during the prenatal period. However, since cocaine, like marijuana, is commonly used with other substances, it is difficult to confirm that these outcomes are specific to cocaine.
5. *Opiates.* Opiate (narcotic) use in pregnancy is associated with stillbirth, IUGR, prematurity, and neonatal mortality. Maternal withdrawal during pregnancy is associated with fetal distress and fetal death. Neonates whose mothers used narcotics during pregnancy must go through a potentially fatal narcotic withdrawal syndrome. The withdrawal is also experienced by infants whose mothers were on methadone maintenance. Since many opiates are injected IV, women who abuse this category of drugs are at increased risk for HIV and hepatitis and systemic infections, including endocarditis and cellulitis.
6. *Amphetamines.* Amphetamines are stimulants that have effects similar to those of cocaine. The use of crystal methamphetamine ("ice," "blue ice") has been associated with decreased fetal head circumference and increased incidence of placental abruption, IUGR, and intrauterine fetal death (ACOG, 1994b). It is thought that these effects may be related to the vasoconstriction caused by the amphetamines. Amphetamine use in pregnancy is also associated with poor nutrition and poor weight gain.
7. *Hallucinogens.* There is little known about the effect of hallucinogens on pregnancy. Although it was once thought that lysergic acid diethylamide (LSD) caused chromosomal damage, more recent research has found no evidence of that claim.

Signs and symptoms. Signs of substance abuse vary, depending on the effect of the agent. Lack of prenatal care and missed appointments are common when women are using illegal substances. Emergency room visits for related problems, including violence, may be identified. Behavioral attributes, including sedation, inebriation, euphoria, and agitation may be present. Physical examination may identify excoriated nasal mucous membranes (cocaine), needle tracks (injectable opiates and cocaine), dilated or constricted pupils, malnutrition, tachycardia, or hypertension.

Screening/diagnosis All women should be screened for substance use at the initial prenatal visit. Thorough history-taking identifies medical or social conditions associated with substance use. For example, frequent nosebleeds may indicate cocaine-induced nasal septal inflammation. The clinician should directly ask about substance use, using the terminology that is common in the community. Interviewing should go from least threatening (smoking and over-the-counter drug use) to most threatening (intravenous opiate use). Women should be reassured that all women are screened, not just specific individuals having certain characteristics. The "T-ACE" questionnaire to screen for alcohol abuse is illustrated in Box 25-8.

Urine testing for toxicology can identify recent drug use. Increased renal blood flow and clearance in pregnancy may clear drugs and their metabolites more quickly than in the nonpregnant state. Opiates and their metabolites may be found in urine for up to 72 hours after use in nonpregnant women, but during pregnancy they may be cleared by 36 to 48 hours. State laws and regulations vary regarding the collection of urine for drug screens, and toxicology screens may not be possible without the woman's permission.

Management—community-based. Women who are identified as smokers should be offered information on smoking cessation programs in the community. Health insurance plans increasingly cover the costs of enrollment in smoking cessation programs. At each prenatal visit the clinician should explore the level of smoking and provide positive feedback when the woman has been able to decrease the number of cigarettes smoked each day or the amount of tobacco chewed in a day.

Box 25-8 *T-ACE Questions for Alcohol Abuse Screening*

T: How many drinks does it take to make you feel high? (**T**olerance)
A: Have people **A**nnoyed you by criticizing your drinking?
C: Have you felt you ought to **C**ut Down on your drinking?
E: Have you ever had a drink first thing in the morning to steady your nerves or get rid of a hangover (**E**ye Opener)?

From Sokol RJ, Martier SS, Ager JW: The T-ACE questions: practical prenatal detection of risk-drinking [see comments], *Am J Obstet Gynecol* 160(4):863-868; discussion 868-870, 1989.

Women who abuse alcohol and other drugs can be referred to 12-step programs in the community. Alcoholics Anonymous and Narcotics Anonymous have been found to be highly effective in supporting activities that keep the individual clean and sober.

Since substance abusers often have to address a variety of psychosocial issues, including the need for income maintenance, assistance with child care, coordination of other medical services, and social support. In addition, many women in recovery face homelessness, legal problems, and threats of violence. For these reasons the use of a multidisciplinary team provides the most comprehensive approach to meeting the woman's health and social needs.

Management—referral Referral for extended medical and chemical dependency services are indicated based on the clinician's assessment of the woman and her resources. Unfortunately, most communities do not have sufficient placements for pregnant women who want to go into treatment for their addiction(s), and it is rare to find placements for women with children.

Implications for the fetus As noted previously, substance abuse has direct and indirect effects on the fetus. Fetal assessment often includes serial ultrasound examinations to assess growth, NSTs, and biophysical profiles.

Implications for labor and delivery When a woman has a history of drug or alcohol use, pain management is a challenge. Consultation with the obstetrician and anesthesiologist is indicated to create a plan that will result in appropriate pain relief based on the woman's individual needs.

Implications for postpartum and neonatal care When drug and alcohol use have been a problem during pregnancy, the pediatric staff should be informed so that a plan to support the neonate can be made. When withdrawal is expected, delivery in a level III hospital is preferred so that the neonate has the full complement of pediatric specialists necessary for recovery.

When there is a risk that drug and/or alcohol use will continue in the postpartum period, breast-feeding may be contraindicated. Alcohol, cocaine, heroin, methadone, diazepam, marijuana, and phencyclidine (PCP) all pass readily into breast milk, and their use is a contraindication to nursing. The midwife must also recognize that women who are experiencing substance abuse are also at increased risk for other behaviors that would put the infant at risk. Co-variables, including multiple partners and participation in sex trade, use of needles, and unsafe sexual practices all increase the risk of HIV and other infections. HIV is present in human milk and can be transmitted to the infant with breast-feeding. It is essential that the midwife discuss the potential for continued abuse, the resources available, and the social support for raising the infant with the woman to assess whether the home situation is safe for the infant. Referral to social services is indicated, and in some states or localities infants may be put in foster care until the mother completes recovery.

References

Allen UD, Navas L, King SM: Effectiveness of intrapartum penicillin prophylaxis in preventing early-onset group B streptococcal infection: results of a meta-analysis, *Can Med Assoc J* 149(11):1659-1665, 1993.

American College of Obstetricians and Gynecologists: *Management of diabetes in pregnancy* (Technical Bulletin 200), Washington, DC, 1994a, American College of Obstetricians and Gynecologists.

American College of Obstetricians and Gynecologists: Substance Abuse in Pregnancy (Technical Bulletin 195), Washington, DC, 1994b, American College of Obstetricians and Gynecologists.

American College of Obstetricians and Gynecologists: *Hypertension in pregnancy* (Technical Bulletin 219), Washington, DC, 1996, American College of Obstetricians and Gynecologists.

American College of Obstetricians and Gynecologists, Committee on Obstetrical Practice: *Scheduled cesarean delivery and the prevention of vertical transmission of HIV infection* (Committee Opinion), Washington, DC, 1999, American College of Obstetricians and Gynecologists.

American Academy of Pediatrics: *Revised guidelines for prevention of early-onset group B streptococcal (GBS) infection,* Chicago, 1997, American Academy of Pediatrics.

American Diabetes Association: *Gestational diabetes mellitus* (Clinical Practice Recommendation), New York, 2000, American Diabetes Association.

Ananth CV, Smulian JC, Vintzileos AM: Incidence of placental abruption in relation to cigarette smoking and hypertensive disorders during pregnancy: a meta-analysis of observational studies, *Obstet Gynecol* 93(4):622-628, 1999.

Andreoli TE et al: *Cecil essentials of medicine,* ed 4, Philadelphia, 1997, WB Saunders,

Avery MD, Rossi MA: Gestational diabetes, *J Nurse Midwifery* 39(2 suppl):9S-19S, 1994.

Barrett JFR: Absorption of non-heme iron from food during normal pregnancy, *Br Med J* 309:79-82, 1994.

Beard JL: Iron deficiency: assessment during pregnancy and its importance in pregnant adolescents, *Am J Clin Nutr* 59(suppl):502S-510S, 1994.

Bosio PM et al: Maternal central hemodynamics in hypertensive disorders of pregnancy, *Obstet Gynecol* 94(6):978-984, 1999.

Centers for Disease Control and Prevention: Hepatitis B virus: a comprehensive strategy for eliminating transmission in the United States through universal childhood vaccination: recommendations of the Immunization Practices Advisory Committee, *MMWR* 40((RR-13)):1-25, 1991.

Centers for Disease Control and Prevention: Prevention of perinatal group B streptococcal disease: a public health perspective, *MMWR* 45((RR-7):1-24, 1996.

Centers for Disease Control and Prevention: 1998 Guidelines for treatment of sexually transmitted diseases, *MMWR* 47(RR-1):1-118, 1998a.

Centers for Disease Control and Prevention: Recommendations to prevent and control iron deficiency in the United States, *MMWR* 47(RR-3):1-29, 1998b.

Chalmers I, Enkin M, Keirse M J, editors:. *Effective care in pregnancy and childbirth,* New York, 1989, Oxford University Press.

Chasnoff IJ, Landress HJ, Barrett ME:. The prevalence of illicit drug or alcohol use during pregnancy and discrepancies in mandatory reporting in Pinellas County, Florida, *N Engl J Med* 322(17):1202-1206, 1990.

Clark SL et al: Asthma in pregnancy, *Obstet Gynecol* 82(6):1036-1040, 1993.

Cotch MF et al: Trichomonas vaginalis associated with low birth weight and preterm delivery. The Vaginal Infections and Prematurity Study Group [see comments], *Sex Transm Dis* 24(6):353-360, 1997.

Cowles T, Gonik B: Mitral valve prolapse in pregnancy, *Semin Perinatol* 14(1):34-41, 1990.

Dajani AS et al: Prevention of bacterial endocarditis: recommendations by the American Heart Association, *JAMA* 277(22):1794-1801, 1997.

De Ferrari E et al:. Nurse-midwifery management of women with human immunodeficiency virus disease, *J Nurse Midwifery* 38(2):86-96, 1993.

Engstrom JL, Sittler CP: Nurse-midwifery management of iron-deficiency anemia during pregnancy, *J Nurse Midwifery* 39(2 suppl):S20- S34, 1994.

Etherington IJ, James DK: Reagent strip testing of antenatal urine specimens for infection, *Br J Obstet Gynecol* 100:806-808, 1993.

Expert Panel on the Content of Prenatal Care: *Caring for our future: the content of prenatal care,* Washington, DC, 1989, US Public Health Service, Department of Health and Human Services.

Gant NF, Cunningham FG: *Basic gynecology and obstetrics,* ed 1, Norwalk, Conn, 1993, Appleton & Lange.

Garner P et al: A randomized controlled trial of strict glycemic control and tertiary level obstetric care versus routine obstetric care in the management of gestational diabetes: a pilot study, *Am J Obstet Gynecol* 177(1):190-195, 1997.

Gigante J et al: Universal screening for group B streptococcus: Recommendations and obstetricians' practice decisions, *Obstet Gynecol* 85(3):440-443, 1995.

Greenspoon JS, Wilcox JG, Kirschbaum TH: Group B streptococcus: the effectiveness of screening and chemoprophylaxis, *Obstet Gynecol Surv* 46(8):499-508, 1991.

Hatcher RA et al: *Managing contraception,* Tiger, Ga, 1999, Bridging the Gap Foundation.

Hollingsworth DR, Ney DM:. Caloric restriction in pregnant diabetic women: a review of maternal obesity, glucose and insulin relationships as investigated at the University of California, San Diego, *J Am Coll Nutr* 11(3):251-258, 1992.

Ingardia, CJ et al: Hepatitis B vaccination in pregnancy: factors influencing efficacy, *Obstet Gynecol* 93(6):983-986, 1999.

Institute of Medicine: *Nutrition during pregnancy and lactation: an implementation guide,* Washington DC, 1992, National Academy Press.

Katz VL: Management of group B streptococcal disease in pregnancy, *Clin Obstet Gynecol* 36(4):832-841, 1993.

Khine ML, Winklestein A, Copel JA: Selective screening for gestational diabetes mellitus in adolescent pregnancies, *Obstet Gynecol* 93(5):738-742, 1999.

Landon MB, Gabbe SG: Fetal surveillance in the pregnancy complicated by diabetes mellitus, *Clin Perinatol* 20(3):549-560, 1993.

MacArthur C, Knox EG: Smoking in pregnancy: effects of stopping at different stages. *Br J Obstet Gynaecol* 95(6): 551-555, 1988.

McCormack J et al, editors: *Drug therapy decision making guide,* Philadelphia, 1996, WB Saunders.

National Heart, Lung and Blood Institute: Guidelines for the diagnosis and management of asthma (97-4051), Washington, DC, 1997, National Institutes of Health.

Rayburn WF et al:. Mitral valve prolapse: Echocardiographic changes during pregnancy, *J Reprod Med* 32(3):185-187, 1987.

Regan JA, Klebanoff MA, Nugent RP: The epidemiology of group B streptococcal colonization in pregnancy: vaginal infections and prematurity study group, *Obstet Gynecol* 77(4):604-610, 1991.

Regan JA: Colonization with group B streptococci in pregnancy and adverse outcome, VIP Study Group [see comments], *Am J Obstet Gynecol* 174(4):1354-1360, 1996.

Rogers M, Phelan L, Bain B: Screening criteria for beta thalassemia trait in pregnant women, *J Clin Pathol* 48(11): 1054-1056, 1995.

Savage D, Garrison R, Devereux R: Mitral valve prolapse in the general population. I. Epidemiologic features: the Framingham Study, *Am Heart J* 106:571, 1983.

Scholl TO, Hediger ML: Anemia and iron-deficiency anemia: compilation of data on pregnancy outcome, *Am J Clin Nutr* 59(suppl):492S-501S, 1994.

Spellacy WN et al: Macrosomia—maternal characteristics and infant complications, *Obstet Gynecol* 66(2):158-161, 1985.

Sweet BR: *Mayes' midwifery: a textbook for midwives,* ed 12, London, 1997, Baillière Tindall.

Vercaigne LM, Zhanel GG: Recommended treatment for urinary tract infection in pregnancy, *Ann Pharmacother* 28(2):248-251, 1994.

Chapter 26

Obstetric Complications in the Prenatal Period

BLEEDING IN PREGNANCY

Spontaneous Abortion

Etiology/pathology. Spontaneous abortion (miscarriage) is the termination of pregnancy before the period of viability of the fetus or before 20 weeks' gestation or birth weight of 500 g. The incidence of spontaneous abortion is estimated to be between 30% to 40% of conceptions. Spontaneous abortion can be a result of abnormal development of the products of conception, or maternal anatomic or physiologic factors that inhibit the support of the pregnancy. It is estimated that more than 80% of spontaneous abortions occur in the first trimester and that 50% to 60% are caused by chromosomal abnormalities (Cunningham et al., 1997). Pregnancies aborted because of chromosomal abnormalities are more likely to terminate before 8 weeks' gestation.

Spontaneous abortion is usually further described as follows:

- Threatened abortion: Bleeding or spotting with no cervical change
- Inevitable abortion: Bleeding and cramping with cervical dilation
- Complete abortion: Bleeding and complete expulsion of the products of conception
- Missed abortion: Cessation of development or death of the fetus with retention of the dead products of conception

Habitual abortion (recurrent abortion) is defined as three or more consecutive spontaneous abortions. Factors associated with habitual abortion are summarized in Box 26-1.

Signs and symptoms

Threatened Abortion Threatened abortion is defined as any vaginal bleeding or spotting before 20 weeks' gestation. The bleeding may vary from scant spotting to bleeding similar to a light menses, may be light pink to dark red, and may be accompanied by cramping. Cramping may be rhythmic or a constant dull ache. About 20% to 25% of women experience spotting in early pregnancy, and approximately half go on to abort (Cunningham et al., 1997). The prognosis for continuation of the pregnancy is poor when both bleeding and cramping are present. Ultrasound findings that demonstrate a well-formed gestational ring with echoes from the embryo imply that the pregnancy is most likely healthy. Lack of embryo echoes implies probable death of the tissue or inaccurate dating.

Box 26-1 *Factors Associated with Habitual Abortion*

Maternal

Uterine anomalies: Uterine adhesions, uterine malformations, fibroids, incompetent cervix
Infectious agents: *Listeria, Ureaplasma, Mycoplasma*
Environmental toxins: Lead, arsenic, benzene, anesthetic gases, radiation
Alcohol, tobacco, drugs
Endocrine problems: Progesterone deficiency, thyroid, diabetes
Autoimmune disease

Fetal

Nonrecurring aneuploid abnormality

Inevitable Abortion Bleeding may start as spotting and progress to heavy bleeding, or it may start as heavier bleeding. Cramping is usually present, and the woman may notice passage of tissue. The woman may notice gross rupture of the membranes if gestational age is 12 weeks or more. Pelvic examination may reveal cervical dilation and bulging membranes or products of conception at the os.

Missed Abortion The first symptom of missed abortion may be a sudden cessation of signs of pregnancy, including cessation of nausea and vomiting and breast tenderness. Spotting, particularly of dark brown color, may be noticed. Most women experiencing missed abortion eventually spontaneously abort. Lack of uterine growth or decrease in uterine size, as well as lack of documentation of fetal heart motion, are signs of missed abortion.

Screening and diagnosis. Screening is done at each prenatal visit when the clinician asks whether the woman has experienced any spotting or bleeding (Box 26-2). Diagnosis is made when the following findings are noted.

Threatened Abortion
- Spotting with no cervical change
- Fetal heart motion present if greater than 6 weeks' gestation
- Serum beta human chorionic gonadotropin (hCG) in normal range for gestational age

Box 26-2 *Data Collection for Bleeding in Early Pregnancy*

Historical

Menstrual history and diagnosis of pregnancy
Previous bleeding in current pregnancy
Bleeding characteristics—color, amount
Presence or absence of cramping
Activity associated with onset of bleeding or cramping
Recent sexual activity
History of threatened or complete abortion in previous pregnancies
History of medical diagnoses the increase risk of abortion

Physical

Temperature, pulse, blood pressure
Abdominal examination for tenderness, rigidity
Fundal height (after 12 weeks)
Fetal heart tones per doptone (after 10 weeks)
Costovertebral angle tenderness or suprapubic tenderness
Speculum examination for blood in vagina and visual inspection of cervix
Bimanual examination to assess cervical status, uterine size, adnexa
Rectal inspection and examination (optional) to identify hemorrhoids or fissures

Laboratory/Special Studies

Urine pregnancy test
Serum beta human chorionic gonadotropin—qualitative or quantitative
Pelvic/abdominal ultrasound findings
Complete blood count or hematocrit/hemoglobin

Inevitable Abortion
- Spotting, cramping, and/or rupture of membranes
- Cervical dilation
- Absent fetal heart motion

Complete Abortion
- Passage of products of conception
- No products of conception identified on ultrasound examination
- Uterus firm
- Falling hCG levels

Missed Abortion

- Spotting may be present
- Lack of uterine growth on serial examinations
- Absence of fetal heart motion
- "Empty sac" noted on ultrasound or fetal tissue without signs of viability

Management—community-based

Threatened Abortion After discussing findings with the patient, the clinician and patient develop a plan to monitor the pregnancy to assess whether it is viable. During first trimester serial quantitative serum hCG levels done 48 hours apart that show a doubling in values suggest normal growth of the fetus. Lack of the expected increase in hCG raises the suspicion of a non-viable pregnancy. Lower than expected levels reflect the possibility of abortion, ectopic pregnancy, or inaccurate dating. Further history taking, review of early serial uterine sizing, and ultrasound are appropriate approaches to assessing accurate dating. If the initial prenatal laboratory studies have not been done in the past month, a baseline complete blood count (CBC) and determination of blood type and Rh should be obtained.

Threatened abortion is usually managed in the ambulatory setting with counseling addressing the stress experienced by the woman when the viability of the pregnancy is threatened. Although bed rest has traditionally been recommended as treatment for threatened abortion, research has shown no association between bed rest and outcome of the pregnancy for this condition (Goldenberg et al., 1994). The clinician should discuss with the woman that she may want to limit activity for psychologic reasons but that there is no evidence that level of activity is associated with outcome of the pregnancy. The patient should be instructed to contact the provider immediately if she experiences increased bleeding, cramping, or fever.

Inevitable and Complete Abortion When inevitable abortion is diagnosed, the woman should be given the options to either await spontaneous evacuation of the uterus or to have surgical evacuation. Before 10 weeks' gestation, the fetus and placenta are usually expelled together with normal uterine contracting and involution. For that reason, conservative management without surgical intervention, even after the passage of products of conception, is appropriate. Ultrasound examination to confirm lack of retained products and appropriately sized uterus for gestation may be helpful in making the decision to manage conservatively. After 10 weeks' gestation, bleeding may be profuse, especially if placental tissue remains partially separated from the uterine wall. Dilation of the cervix and surgical evacuation of the uterus are appropriate to prevent excessive blood loss. Non-physician providers should consult with an appropriate physician skilled in surgical evacuation of the uterus when inevitable abortion or complete abortion after 10 weeks is diagnosed. Patients who are more than 6 weeks' gestation and Rh negative should receive Rh_o D immunoglobulin to prevent sensitization.

Missed Abortion If the gestational age is less than 12 weeks, the patient should be given the options of either awaiting spontaneous expulsion of the products of conception or surgical intervention to evacuate the uterus. For psychologic reasons, many women desire termination of the pregnancy as soon as possible. The non-physician provider should refer the patient to a physician skilled in surgical termination of the pregnancy if the patient desires. If the patient chooses to await spontaneous abortion, she should be counseled to contact the provider when she experiences bleeding, cramping, and probable complete abortion. She should be evaluated in the outpatient setting after the abortion to assess whether the abortion is complete or whether further intervention is appropriate.

Prolonged retention of the products of conception may occasionally stimulate coagulation defects, particularly if the pregnancy has progressed into the second trimester. For this reason, baseline coagulation studies are usually obtained when missed abortion is diagnosed.

Postabortion follow-up. Patients should be counseled to contact the provider if she experiences fever, continued bright red bleeding, or increased or continued pelvic pain. A 2-week postabortion examination should be scheduled to assess the physical status of the woman and to offer support and counseling regarding the loss of the pregnancy. Unless there are complications such as infection or severe hemorrhage, physical findings include progressive normal involution of the uterus to non-pregnant size and minimal bleeding. Patient education should include discussion of the fact that the woman may ovulate as early as 2 weeks after the abortion. Contraceptive options should be reviewed. Counseling regarding normal grieving patterns, and allowing time before conceiving again should be covered. Investigators have noted that almost all women experiencing spontaneous miscarriage experience grief, even when the pregnancy was unplanned (Zaccardi, Abbott, and Koziol-McLain, 1993). In some cases, it may be helpful to refer the patient to a support group.

Management—referral. Referral to a physician for management of inevitable abortion and missed abortion is expected. However, collaborative care is possible in some settings, depending on practice guidelines. In collaborative care the physician provides the medical and surgical care related to the termination, while the midwife continues to offer the supportive care to the woman. Referral to an obstetrician skilled in maternal-fetal medicine should be considered in cases of habitual abortion. The couple should also be offered the option of genetic counseling in cases of habitual abortion.

Implications for the current pregnancy. First-trimester bleeding is associated with increased risk for preterm delivery and low birth weight (Williams et al., 1991). However, there are no current recommendations for screening or interventions apart from usual prenatal care procedures.

Ectopic Pregnancy

Etiology/pathology. Ectopic pregnancy occurs when the blastocyst implants in any site other than the endometrium of the uterine cavity. Sites of implantation in ectopic pregnancy include the fallopian tube (tubal), ovary, cervix, or abdominal organs (Figure 26-1). Almost 98% of ectopic pregnancies are tubal implantations. Implantation in the tube can occur in the ampulla, the isthmus, the interstitial part of the tube, or the fimbria. Strong risk factors for ectopic pregnancy include previous ectopic pregnancy, documented tubal pathology, and in utero diethylstilbestrol (DES) exposure. Lesser risk factors include previous pelvic inflammatory disease, infertility, more than one lifetime sexual partner, and previous sexually transmitted diseases (STIs) (Ankum et al., 1996).

Extrauterine implantation only rarely continues to the point of viability. Implantation in the tube eventually results in rupture, and the timing of the rupture depends on the ability of the tubal wall to stretch with the growing conceptus. As the trophoblastic cells proliferate, their hormonal production stimulates endometrial growth. Early gestation uterine changes also occur. The cervix and isthmus soften, and uterine size increases. However, because the tube does not have the structures to continue supporting the placental development, hormone levels do not reach the levels necessary to maintain the decidual tissue. Low hCG levels lead to endometrial degeneration and vaginal bleeding. Bleeding also occurs at the site of implantation as the trophoblasts penetrate the tubal wall and surrounding arteries.

When implantation has occurred in the isthmus of the tube, rupture usually occurs by 6 weeks' gestation. Implantation in the ampulla results in rupture after 6 weeks. Rupture of an interstitial implantation in the segment of tube that penetrates the uterine wall has grave implications, since the rupture does not occur until 9 to 16 weeks' gestation when hemorrhage from the branches of the uter-

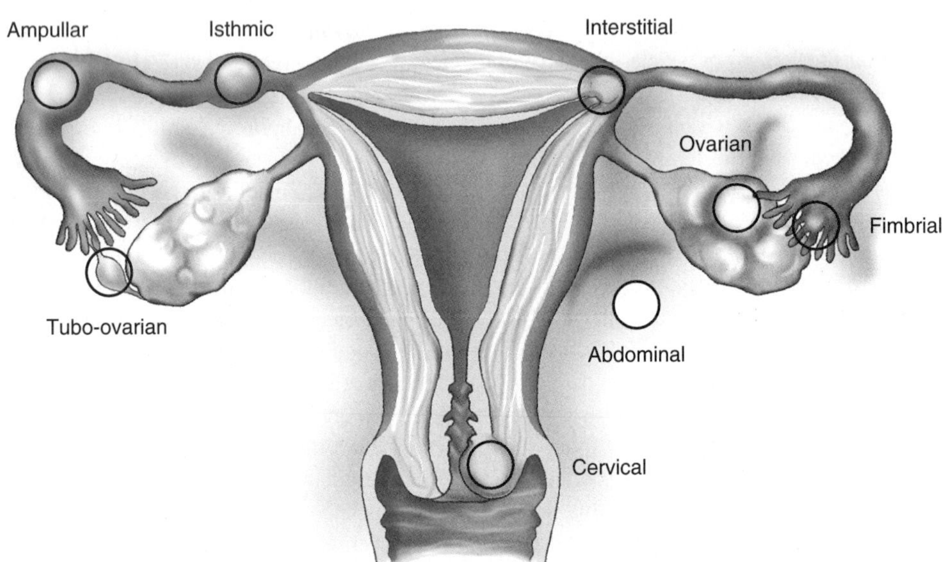

Figure 26-1 Sites of implantation of ectopic pregnancies. In order of frequency of occurrence: ampulla, isthmus, interstitium, fimbria, tubo-ovarian ligament, ovary, abdominal cavity, and cervix (external os).

ine and ovarian arteries leads to rapid vascular collapse (Cunningham et al., 1997).

Ectopic pregnancy continues to be a significant perinatal problem in the United States, even with improved diagnostic and treatment techniques. The incidence of ectopic pregnancy has increased dramatically in the last three decades, and it is estimated that extrauterine implantation occurs in about 20 per 1000 pregnancies. Since medical treatment of ectopic pregnancy may be managed in a physician's office rather than a hospital or clinic, ectopic pregnancy estimates may be affected by underreporting. Ectopic pregnancy accounts for 9% of maternal pregnancy-related deaths and is the primary cause of death in the first trimester (Centers for Disease Control and Prevention, 1995). Early diagnosis, particularly diagnosis before rupture, decreases maternal mortality and morbidity.

Signs and symptoms. Vaginal spotting when pregnancy has been previously diagnosed is a common early sign of ectopic pregnancy. When pregnancy has not been identified, the woman may mistake the classic vaginal bleeding in ectopic pregnancy as an unusual menstrual period. The most frequent symptom is abdominal or pelvic pain, often unilateral on the side of implantation. During physical examination the clinician may note pain with abdominal palpation and cervical motion tenderness. Uterine size smaller than expected for gestational age is consistent with ectopic pregnancy.

Screening and diagnosis. Transvaginal ultrasound can establish ectopic pregnancy vs. intrauterine pregnancy in 75% of cases in which women present with complaints of vaginal bleeding and pelvic pain (Kaplan et al., 1996). An intrauterine gestational sac can usually be seen when the hCG level is between 1000 and 2000 mIU/ml (ACOG, 1998a). Detection of an intrauterine gestational sac is usually considered an exclusion of ectopic pregnancy as a diagnosis. Rarely, multiple gestation pregnancy can result in both intrauterine and ectopic implantations. Identification of a ectopic gestational sac is diagnostic of the condition. Sensitivity of transvaginal ultrasound to identifying ectopic pregnancy ranges from 20.1% to 84%; specificity ranges from 98.9% to 100% (ACOG, 1998a).

Serial beta hCG levels have been a traditional way to screen for ectopic pregnancy. Eighty-five percent of normal pregnancies demonstrate a 66% increase in beta hCG levels every 48 hours in early pregnancy. Failure to see "doubling" of hCG level every 48 hours is suggestive of ectopic pregnancy or nonviable intrauterine pregnancy. Sensitivity to detect ectopic pregnancy using serial beta hCG testing is 36%; specificity is 63% to 71% (ACOG, 1998a).

Some clinicians also assess serum progesterone levels when assessing for ectopic pregnancy. Viable intrauterine pregnancy is probable with serum progesterone levels greater than 25 ng/ml, although 2% of ectopic pregnancies occur with this normal progesterone value (ACOG, 1998a; Gabbe, Niebyl, and Simpson, 1999). A serum progesterone level of less than 5 ng/ml indicates a nonviable pregnancy, although one cannot determine if the diagnosis is spontaneous abortion or ectopic pregnancy.

Management—community-based. Management at the community level includes screening and initiation of special studies to establish the diagnosis of ectopic pregnancy. The midwife should order an ultrasound for localization of the gestational sac. When ultrasound examination is not readily available, serial beta hCG levels done 48 hours apart aid in the diagnosis. Women at increased risk for ectopic pregnancy should be counseled to seek emergency treatment for any pelvic pain experienced.

Management—referral. When ectopic pregnancy is diagnosed or strongly suspected, referral to an obstetrician is indicated. Women with early diagnosis of ectopic pregnancy may be candidates for medical management rather than surgical intervention. Medical management is associated with decreased morbidity and increased preservation of tubal function. Methotrexate, a folic acid antagonist, inhibits the synthesis of deoxyribonucleic acid and cell replication. Criteria for management and contraindications to using methotrexate are summarized in Box 26-3. Side effects to methotrexate include gastric problems (nausea, vomiting, diarrhea, stomatitis), dizziness, pneumonitis, neutropenia, and alopecia. Mild pelvic pain of limited duration (24 to 48 hours) is usually experienced during the tubal abortion (ACOG, 1998a). Abdominal pain that increases in severity indicates tubal rupture. Successful treatment is determined by decreasing hCG levels by at least 15% between days 4 and 7 following treatment.

When there are contraindications to medical management or when medical management fails, surgical intervention is necessary.

Implications for future pregnancies. Because the same risk factors may be present in future pregnancies, women experiencing an ectopic pregnancy are at increased risk for future ectopic pregnancies. These women should be counseled regarding use of effective contraception to prevent unplanned pregnancies and en-

Box 26-3 *Medical Management of Ectopic Pregnancy*

Criteria for Use of Methotrexate

Absolute Indications:
Hemodynamically stable—no signs of bleeding or hemoperitoneum
Nonlaparoscopic diagnosis
Patient desires future fertility
Patient is able to return for follow-up care
Relative Indications:
Unruptured mass less than 3.5 cm in diameter
No fetal heart activity noted
Beta human chorionic gonadotropin less than 6,000-15,000 mIU/ml

Contraindications for Use of Methotrexate

Absolute Contraindications:
Breast-feeding
Immunodeficiency
Alcoholism, alcoholic liver disease, or chronic liver disease
Preexisting blood dyscrasias
Active pulmonary disease
Peptic ulcer disease
Hepatic, renal, or hematologic dysfunction
Known sensitivity to methotrexate
Relative Contraindications:
Gestational sac greater than 3.5 cm in diameter
Embryonic cardiac motion

Adapted from ACOG: *Medical management of tubal pregnancy (Practice Bulletin 3)*, Washington, DC, 1998a, American College of Obstetricians and Gynecologists.

couraged to seek early confirmation of pregnancy should pregnancy be suspected.

Gestational Trophoblastic Disease

Etiology/pathology. Gestational trophoblastic disease (GTD) occurs when normal cell differentiation in the blastocyst ceases and trophoblastic cells proliferate. The proliferation of the trophoblasts results in elevated levels of hCG. Complete hydatidiform mole occurs when the ovum is devoid of chromosomes and the sperm replicates its own chromosomes into an abnormal zygote. The chorionic villi develop into vesicles that resemble bunches of grapes. In partial mole there are excess chromosomes—23X from the ovum and 46XX or 46XY from duplicate sperm chromosomes. Some fetal tissue and/or amnion may develop in addition to the vesicles, and rarely a normal twin may develop along with the molar tissue. Hydatidiform mole occurs in 1/500 to 1/1000 pregnancies. Advanced maternal age is a risk factor for GTD; women over age 45 have a relative risk of 10, whereas women over age 50 have a relative risk of over 500 (Cunningham et al., 1997; Gabbe, Niebyl, and Simpson, 1999). Women with one previous molar pregnancy have a 1% to 2% risk of GTD in subsequent pregnancies, and those with two previous molar pregnancies have a 25% risk of a third. Approximately 20% of women with GTD develop gestational trophoblastic neoplasm, which can progress to choriocarcinoma, a rapidly metastasizing malignancy.

Signs and symptoms. Most women with GTD experience dark brown spotting by late first trimester. Hyperemesis gravidarum and pregnancy-induced hypertension before 20 weeks' gestation are associated with GTD. Women may report the passage of vesicles vaginally as the pregnancy progresses into the second trimester.

Physical examination identifies uterine size greater than expected for dates and lack of fetal heart tones. Serum hCG is elevated for gestational age, and plasma thyroxine may be elevated. Anemia may be present secondary to bleeding and poor nutritional intake. Ultrasound examination of the uterus identifies the classic pattern of the growing vesicles.

Screening and diagnosis. Women experiencing signs of GTD should have ultrasonic examination to diagnose the condition. Many women are diagnosed at the time of routine ultrasound screening or ultrasound examination to determine viability when there are signs of spontaneous abortion.

Management—community-based. When GTD is suspected, the midwife should order a diagnostic ultrasound examination. When the diagnosis is made, referral to an obstetrician is indicated.

Management—referral. Because the treatment of GTD is surgical evacuation of the uterus and follow-up to rule out or treat choriocarcinoma, medical management is expected. Typically the complete evaluation before evacuation of the uterus includes chest x-ray, thyroid studies if the pulse is greater than 100 beats/min, CBC with differential and platelets, prothrombin time, partial thromboplastin time, blood type, and antibody screen. If metastasis is found, oncologic treatment is initiated. If metastasis is not diagnosed, weekly serum hCG levels are done until they are in normal non-pregnant range, followed by monthly serum hCG levels for 6 months. hCG levels are then followed every 2 to 3 months for 1 year. Because a new pregnancy would cause a rise in hCG unrelated to the GTD, women should be counseled to avoid pregnancy for at least 1 year. GTD is not a contraindication for any of the current contraceptive methods, and women should be encouraged to consider one of the methods that are highly effective. If the woman has religious beliefs opposing contraception, she can be reassured that pregnancy prevention is recommended to protect her life through close monitoring of her health status and that counseling with clergy or a member of the hospital ethics committee is available to help her clarify the issues surrounding this diagnosis.

If hCG levels rise or plateau, chest x-ray is repeated to determine whether there has been metastasis to the lungs. Treatment depends on findings. When a woman does not desire future pregnancies, hysterectomy may be performed.

In some clinical settings the midwife may work collaboratively with the obstetrician during the postpartum monitoring. Following the diagnosis of GTD, the woman and her partner may experience grief related to the lost pregnancy, as well as anxiety related to the potential development of cancer. Although the midwife can certainly provide ongoing support through the follow-up period, referral for counseling may be offered to further help the couple through the experience.

Implications for future pregnancies. Women who experience GTD should be counseled to seek confirmation of pregnancy as soon as pregnancy is suspected. Because of the increased risk for GTD in a future pregnancy, first trimester ultrasound is used to assess the embryologic development.

Placenta Previa

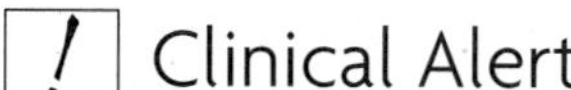

Safety Warning

All vaginal bleeding during the second half of pregnancy must be considered placenta previa until proven otherwise. Digital examination of the cervix can cause severe hemorrhage, with death of mother and infant.

Etiology/pathology. Placenta previa is the implantation of the placenta over or adjacent to the internal cervical os. The incidence of placenta previa is estimated to be 1 in 200 pregnancies. Incidence increases with increasing maternal age and increased parity. Other factors associated with placenta previa include history of lower uterine scar, history of puerperal endometritis, multiple gestation, and erythroblastosis. Three classifications of placenta previa have been identified:

Total Placenta Previa The placenta totally covers the internal cervical os.

Partial Placenta Previa The placenta partially covers the internal cervical os.

Marginal Placenta Previa The edge of the placental is adjacent to the edge of the internal cervical os. In addition, most ultrasonographerswill document low-lying placenta, in which the placenta lies in the lower uterine segment with its edge near but not adjacent to the internal cervical os. In addition, most ultrasonographers document low-lying placenta, in which the placenta lies in the lower uterine segment with its edge near but not adjacent to the internal cervical os.

The degree of placenta previa may vary with the degree of cervical dilation. As the cervix dilates, a low-lying previa may become a partial previa because the dilating cervix exposes the edge of the placenta. Conversely, a complete previa may become partial as the cervix dilates beyond the edge of the placenta.

When the placenta is covering the internal os and implanted in the lower uterine segment, the placental attachments tear as the os dilates. Hemorrhage from the uterine vessels occurs, and, because of poor contractibility of the myometrial fibers of the lower uterine segment, normal control of blood loss in not accomplished. Approximately 90% of patients with placenta previa experience some bleeding in pregnancy, and 10% to 25% of patients develop hypovolemic shock secondary to the acute blood loss. Bleeding commonly develops in the third trimester when the lower uterine segment develops and placenta attachment may be disrupted.

With increased use of ultrasound in early gestation, placenta previa or low-lying placenta is being diagnosed in second trimester. However, it must be kept in mind that normal placental growth and development, as well as the normal growth of the uterus, anatomically causes the placenta to appear to be close to the os when, it fact, as the lower segment of the uterus develops, it becomes clear that no previa is present.

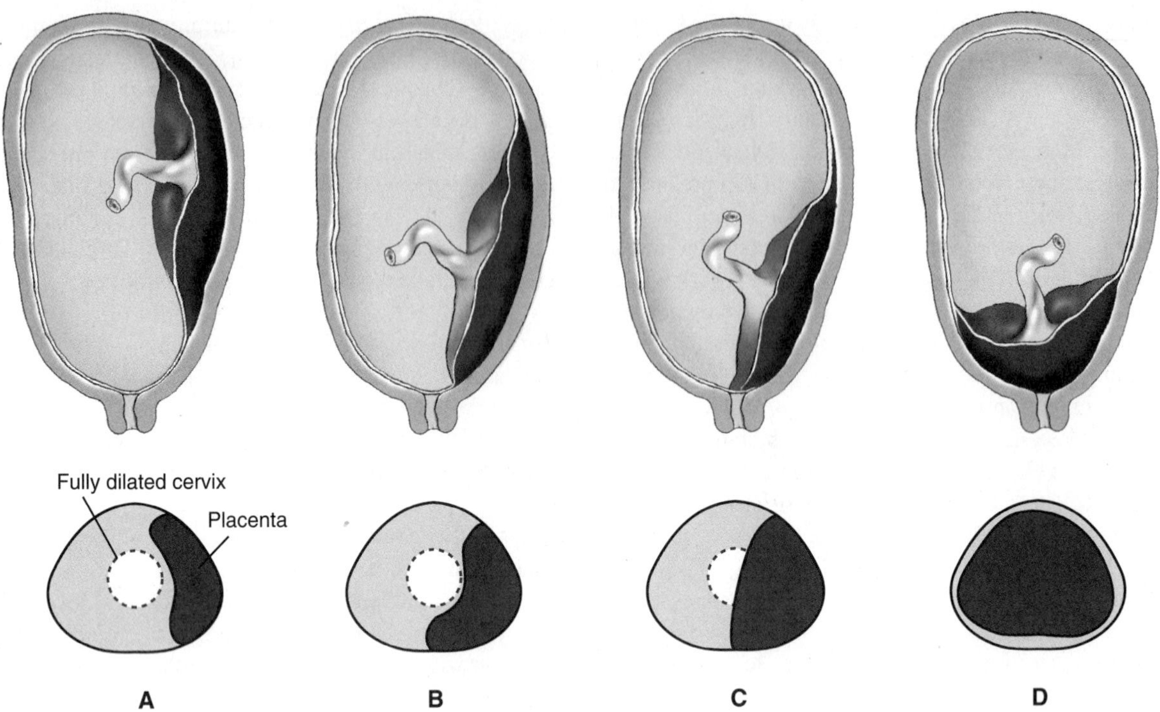

Figure 26-2 Classification of placenta implantation. **A,** Normal implantation; **B,** low implantation; **C,** partial placenta previa; **D,** total placenta previa.

Signs and symptoms. The classic sign of placenta previa is painless vaginal bleeding from second trimester until term. The bleeding is usually unrelated to activity and may occur while the woman is sleeping. The initial bleeding may be slight, but, as the pregnancy progresses, there is greater chance of hemorrhage. The earlier in pregnancy that bleeding occurs, the more serious the previa (Knuppel and Drukker, 1993). Fifty percent of patients with complete placenta previa experience episodic bleeding before 30 weeks' gestation.

Screening and diagnosis. Placenta previa should be suspected with any painless vaginal bleeding. It should also be suspected in a primigravida at term presenting with an unengaged vertex. Definitive diagnosis is made using sonography, which can identify placenta previa with 98% accuracy (Cunningham et al., 1997). False-positive results on ultrasound examination may occur with bladder distention.

Management—community-based

Management of Placenta Previa Before Term

When placenta previa is suspected because of vaginal bleeding, the patient should be hospitalized for a full evaluation. Baseline blood work for CBC and type and crossmatch for type and Rh should be obtained. When there is no bleeding, fetal heart tones should be assessed every shift, and nonstress tests (NSTs) should be done weekly. When bleeding occurs, continuous fetal monitoring is warranted to determine whether there are any abnormal fetal heart patterns indicating stress.

There is controversy regarding whether a woman with documented placenta previa who is stable needs to be hospitalized to ensure rapid intervention should she develop vaginal bleeding. Clearly there are financial as well as social costs associated with hospitalization for a period of time that could span weeks. For this reason, when a woman demonstrates understanding of her condition and has strong family support, reliable transportation, and the ability to get to a hospital in 20 to 30 minutes, outpatient management may be considered. Bed rest should be maintained, and assessment of fetal growth and maternal status can be accomplished through home visits by a home health nurse skilled in perinatal care or a midwife. Fetal assessment should be done every 3 to 4 weeks.

When a woman does not have good family support and does not have a way to be transported to a hospital immediately should bleeding occur, hospitalization may be the safest option.

Expectant management is appropriate until any of the following:

- Spontaneous labor occurs.
- The fetus is determined to be mature, through accurate dating parameters or appropriate lecithin/sphingomyelin ratio.
- There is fetal demise.
- An intrauterine infection is diagnosed.
- Spontaneous rupture of membranes occurs.
- Bleeding increases to a point where the woman's hemodynamic status is compromised (Knuppel and Drukker, 1993).

A woman who has experienced bleeding associated with placenta previa should have her hemoglobin and/or hematocrit evaluated to ensure that it remains above 10 g/dl and 30%. In some cases, blood replacement may be indicated to provide reserve in the case of severe hemorrhage. Women who are Rh negative should also have Kleihauer-Betke test to identify fetal-maternal transfusion.

Management of Placenta Previa at Term When it is determined that the fetus is mature, planned cesarean section should be the route of delivery in the case of total or partial placenta previa. Vaginal birth may be planned for a marginal placenta previa with no bleeding, as long as the facility for the site of birth is equipped to proceed to immediate cesarean section and manage severe hemorrhage should heavy bleeding occur. There is controversy regarding the recommended site of birth for women with known low-lying placentas. There is theoretic increased risk of postpartum hemorrhage as a result of the decreased ability of the myometrial fibers of the lower uterine segment to contract and retract to control bleeding after the delivery of the placenta. For this reason, some clinicians think that the safest place for birth is the hospital. However, birth centers that have immediate access to intravenous therapy, pharmacologic agents to promote uterine contractions, and readily available transport to a hospital setting are able to provide the same care and intervention that would be available in the hospital for an immediate postpartum hemorrhage.

The clinician caring for a woman with placenta previa must anticipate hemorrhage. For that reason a large-bore intravenous catheter should be in place, and medical consultants should be readily available in case of severe hemorrhage. A baseline CBC, type and Rh, and type and hold clot should be ordered. In cases of complete placenta previa, the patient may be given the option of having family members blood bank units in her name before term. In most cases, the patient is referred to an obstetrician for management. However, in some practice settings, the midwife may be able to collaborate in the care of a woman experiencing vaginal birth with a marginal placenta previa.

Management—referral. All patients with known complete placenta previa should be managed by a physician skilled in cesarean section and management of hemorrhage. The facility should have 24-hour availability of blood products, as well as availability of rapid response of anesthesia for emergency cesarean sections. If conservative management is in place for preterm gestations, the facility should have a level III nursery for care of the preterm infant.

When partial or marginal placenta previa with no bleeding is identified, the midwife should consult with the obstetrician. Collaborative care may be possible in some settings, depending on practice guidelines.

Implications for future pregnancies. Previous cesarean delivery increases the risk for placenta previa. In women with one previous cesarean delivery, there is a 1% to 4% risk of previa; with four or more cesareans deliveries, the risk increases to 10% (Gabbe, Niebyl, and Simpson, 1999).

Placental Abruption

Etiology/pathology. Placental abruption (abruptio placentae, ablatio placentae, accidental hemorrhage) is the premature separation of a normally implanted placenta from the uterine wall, resulting in retroplacental bleeding after the twentieth week of gestation and before the fetus is delivered. In approximately 80% of cases, there is vaginal bleeding (external hemorrhage); in the remainder the bleeding is concealed (concealed hemorrhage). Box 26-4 indicates the most common classification system for placental abruption. It is estimated that abruption occurs in 1 out of 150 to 1 out of 250 pregnancies. The incidence of grade 3 abruption is 1 in 500 pregnancies. Incidence of abruption is increased with higher parity, previous abruption, and drug use (e.g., cocaine).

Placental abruption can be partial or complete. In partial abruption the fetus has a chance of survival if the abruption involves less than 50% of the placental surface. Fetal demise is inevitable in complete abruption.

Predisposing factors for abruption include abdominal trauma, short umbilical cord, polyhydramnios, sudden decompression of the uterus, fibroids, uterine anomalies, circumvallate placenta, and hypertensive disorders. Maternal hypertension is strongly associated with grade 3 abruption, with 40% to 50% of cases having hyperten-

Box 26-4 *Classification of Placenta Abruption*

Grade 0

Asymptomatic. Diagnosed after delivery by noting small retroplacental clot. Rupture of a marginal sinus is included in this category.

Grade 1

Vaginal bleeding. Uterine tenderness and tetany may be present. No signs of maternal shock or abnormal fetal heart patterns.

Grade 2

External vaginal bleeding may or may not be present. Uterine tenderness and tetany are present. No signs of maternal shock. Abnormal fetal heart pattern present.

Grade 3

External vaginal bleeding may or may not be present. Marked uterine tetany. Persistent abdominal pain. Maternal shock. Fetal demise.

sive disorders. Maternal motor vehicle accidents and battering are the two most common sources of blunt trauma to the abdomen.

Marginal placental abruption involves the intervillous space and veins at the edge of the placenta and are typically less serious than abruptions occurring in the central part of the placenta. Central abruption can involve arteries leading to greater blood loss because of the increased pressure in the vessels.

When blood extravasates into the uterine muscle, a red to purple discoloration of the serosal surface is produced (Couvelaire uterus). When the placenta is implanted on the anterior wall of the uterus, the discoloration may be noted through the skin. It was once thought that this development would lead to atony and require hysterectomy to save the mother's life. However, with current suturing techniques and use of oxytocin, hysterectomy is rarely necessary.

Signs and symptoms. The signs and symptoms vary, depending on the extent of the abruption. Common findings include vaginal bleeding, uterine tenderness, back pain, fetal distress, uterine hypertonus, and fetal demise. The classic signs are vaginal bleeding and uterine tetany (the "boardlike abdomen"). Approximately 80% of women experiencing placental abruption present with the complaint of vaginal bleeding.

Screening/diagnosis. In classic cases the presenting signs of vaginal bleeding and rigid uterine tone lead to presumptive diagnosis with confirmation by ultrasound examination. Ultrasound can identify subchorionic, retroplacental, and preplacental (between the placenta and the amniotic fluid) bleeding. Retroplacental hematomas have a worse prognosis for fetal survival (>50% fetal mortality) than subchorionic hemorrhages (10% fetal mortality) (Gabbe, Niebyl, and Simpson, 1999). In mild cases, the diagnosis is often one of exclusion after ruling out placenta previa and other causes for vaginal bleeding. Diagnosis can also be made after the delivery with discovery of an adherent retroplacental clot.

Management—community-based. Management depends on the condition of the woman and the fetus. If bleeding is mild and there is no sign of fetal distress, observation is warranted as long as the facility has the ability to provide immediate intervention if necessary. Preparation for possible worsening of the maternal and/or fetal status includes establishing an intravenous line with a large-bore catheter and obtaining baseline blood work (type and Rh, antibody screen, CBC with platelets, and disseminated intravascular coagulation [DIC] or coagulation panel). A Kleihauer-Betke test should be done on Rh-negative women to identify fetal-maternal hemorrhage. Continuous fetal monitoring is warranted since further separation of the placenta can occur at any time leading to fetal distress or demise. If the hospital facilities cannot ensure availability of medical specialists who can manage both the obstetric complications and possible coagulation abnormalities, immediate transfer to a referral facility is indicated.

If there is maternal bleeding significant enough to cause hypovolemia or if there is an abnormal fetal heart rate pattern, immediate delivery is necessary. If vaginal delivery is not imminent, cesarean section should be performed. If there has been a fetal demise, vaginal delivery is preferred unless the woman's condition is unstable as a result of severe blood loss or there are other obstetric contraindications to vaginal delivery.

Management—referral. Consultation and/or referral to a high-risk perinatal center is recommended for all cases of suspected placental abruption. The management skills of a team that includes specialists in maternal-fetal medicine, hematology, and vascular surgery may be needed if the abruption is severe. When abruption occurs before term, even a grade 1 abruption can stimulate uterine activity, thereby placing the fetus at risk for preterm birth. Management usually includes tocolysis using magnesium sulfate, as long as there is no evidence of fetal compromise. Close monitoring of fetal status is essential. In addition, close monitoring of maternal hemodynamics is necessary. Hematocrit should be maintained above 30% and urinary output of 60ml/hour should be maintained. Since abruption is associated with DIC, serial plasma fibrinogen and platelets are monitored.

Implications for future pregnancies. When there has been significant blood loss, women should be counseled regarding the association of closely spaced pregnancies and anemia. Postpartum follow-up of hemoglobin and hematocrit should be done, and continued iron supplementation should be recommended when anemia is identified. When risk factors for placental abruption, including hypertension and drug abuse, are present in future pregnancies, women should be counseled to seek care immediately with vaginal bleeding or uterine irritability.

INCOMPETENT CERVIX

Etiology/pathology. Incompetent cervix traditionally has been described as painless dilation of the cervix without uterine contractions in second trimester, usually between 14 and 20 weeks' gestation. Often the dilation is accompanied by spontaneous rupture of the membranes. Factors associated with incompetent cervix include congenital structural abnormalities of the cervix (including those associated with intrauterine exposure to DES), cone biopsy, and cervical trauma.

Signs and symptoms. The woman with incompetent cervix may present with complaint of pelvic pressure and/or rupture of membranes. Pelvic examination reveals cervical dilation, often with bulging membranes.

Screening/diagnosis. Screening for women at risk for early fetal loss secondary to incompetent cervix begins with collection of complete family, gynecologic, and obstetric history. Family history includes an exploration regarding whether the woman's mother took DES when pregnant. Gynecologic history includes identification of any procedures associated with cervical trauma, including dilation and curettage and cone biopsy. Obstetric history includes identification of previous second trimester losses and cervical trauma during previous births. Diagnosis is made with a history of second trimester losses associated with cervical dilation without labor.

Management—community-based. Midwifery management at the community level includes screening and diagnosis, with referral to an obstetrician when incompetent cervix is suspected. Women with a history of cervical trauma but no previous second trimester loss can be followed at the community level with vaginal examinations every 2 weeks starting at 12 weeks' gestation and continuing until third trimester, with referral to an obstetrician when cervical change is noted. Cervical length can also be followed using transvaginal ultrasound. Short cervical length—less than 25 mm—and funneling are associated with preterm birth, often within 2 weeks of the examination (Andrews et al., 2000).

Management—referral. Women with documented cervical incompetence may be candidates for prophylactic cerclage of the cervix. The McDonald and modified Shirodkar techniques use a "purse-string" suture that is placed in the middle or upper third of the cervix and removed before delivery. The cerclage is usually placed between 10 and 14 weeks' gestation. Contraindications to cerclage placement include dilation greater than 3 cm, ruptured membranes, vaginal bleeding, chorioamnionitis, fetal anomaly incompatible with life, and fetal demise. Once the cerclage is in place, women are counseled to avoid intercourse, heavy lifting, and standing for more than 90 minutes at a time.

Occasionally a cerclage will be placed when there are premature cervical changes including dilation or funneling (effacement at the internal os) noted on ultrasound examination.

Although there have been no randomized control studies to establish the effectiveness of cerclage placement, there are data that suggests that the procedure decreases the risk of preterm birth (Gabbe, Niebyl, and Simpson, 1999).

PRETERM LABOR

Etiology/pathology. Preterm labor is defined as cervical effacement and dilation between 20 and 37 weeks' gestation. The association between preterm birth and perinatal mortality and morbidity has been recognized for decades. Birth reporting in the early twentieth century estimated that 7% of infants were "premature." Although progress has been made in neonatal care provisions that decrease mortality and severe morbidity in these small infants, there has not been a decrease in the incidence of preterm birth. Estimates for preterm birth in the United States range from 4% to 16% of pregnancies (Macones, Berlin, and Berlin, 1995). There is evidence that the incidence may be increasing, especially in populations vulnerable to poor outcomes in pregnancy.

Approximately 25% of early births are indicated because of medical or obstetric complications in the mother or fetus. Factors associated with these indicated preterm births include acute or chronic hypertension, diabetes, placenta previa, and intrauterine growth restriction (IUGR) (Gabbe, Niebyl, and Simpson, 1999). About half of the remaining mothers who deliver preterm infants have risk factors associated with preterm birth. The remaining women have no risk factors before the onset of preterm labor. Preterm birth is associated with increased infant mortality rates, increased hospitalization rates during the first year of life, and increased rates of neurologic problems such as cerebral palsy, seizure disorders, and mental retardation.

Identification of the causative factor in preterm labor continues to elude researchers. Studies have identified changes in uterine contractility patterns in the 24 hours before onset of preterm labor experiences, but there has been no progress in identifying factors that can predict those patterns that will progress to preterm birth (Bentley et al., 1990; Iams, Johnson, and Parker, 1994; Morrison, 1990). Consequently, the clinician is faced with the dilemma of not being able to judge which preterm labor events will progress to preterm delivery. Since the 1960s interventions to decrease the incidence of preterm labor have been explored. The development of preterm-birth programs that advocate patient education regarding early recognition of contractions, frequent clinical assessment for high-risk women, and use of pharmacologic agents to decrease uterine contractility have been explored in numerous studies. Unfortunately, assessment of the effectiveness of these approaches is limited by methodologic problems that include non-reproducibility across populations and difficulty in determining appropriate outcome measures. For example, some preterm labors that seem to be progressing toward a preterm birth may stop spontaneously. In addition, some labors seem to respond to interventions, and contractions cease, yet the woman progresses to preterm birth within 24 to 48 hours. A recent meta-analysis found that preterm birth prevention education programs have little effect on reducing preterm birth and may increase morbidity by overdiagnosis of preterm labor with resulting tocolytic intervention (Hueston et al., 1995).

Retrospective review of cases of preterm birth have identified the following risk factors:

- History of previous preterm birth
- History of hypertension, renal disease, or diabetes mellitus
- Generalized infections, particularly viral
- Uterine abnormalities
- Bleeding in pregnancy
- Urinary tract infections
- Genital infections, particularly bacterial vaginosis, chlamydia, and group B streptococcus
- Multiple pregnancy
- Polyhydramnios
- Fetal anomalies
- Rh disease
- Intrauterine fetal demise
- Substance use, particularly cocaine
- High social stress

Formal risk scoring systems have used these risk factors and others to identify women at increased risk for preterm labor. All of the published scoring systems have poor sensitivity, with rates that tend to be in the 40th to the 50th percentile. Positive predictive rates range from 12% to 50% (Creasy, Gummer, and Liggins, 1980; Edenfield et al., 1995; Fedrick and Anderson, 1976; Main et al., 1987; Owen et al., 1990). The effect of home uterine monitoring remains controversial. Criticism of the use of this technology to identify early signs of preterm labor includes the apparent overdiagnosis of preterm labor, with the resulting inappropriate use of further testing and intervention.

Identification of fetal fibronectin (fFN) in cervical and vaginal secretions has been used to identify impending preterm labor, but its use is limited by its high false-positive rate. fFN is an extracellular protein secreted by the trophoblasts and serves to anchor the fetus, placenta, and membranes to the uterus. It is normally found in amniotic fluid and vaginal secretions from early pregnancy through 22 weeks' gestation. Presence of fFN after 22 weeks indicates some disruption in the membranes or placental site, including changes caused by infection. Use of fFN and ultrasound determination of cervical length have been evaluated,and, although there are associations between presence of fFN and shortened crevices and development of preterm labor, there are limitations to the predictive ability of these screening tests (Khan et al., 1999; Yost et al., 1999). Cessation of fetal breathing movements within 24 hours of labor has also been studied, but the necessity of ultrasound technology and skilled technicians limits its use as a screening tool in large populations.

Success in preventing preterm birth rests in identifying preterm labor before significant cervical change. Numerous studies have evaluated the ability of women to identify uterine contractions and the impact of patient education programs that teach self-palpation of contractions. Studies comparing the ability of women to identify contractions that are documented on a home uterine monitoring device suggest that women may identify only 10% to 20% of contractions (Brustman et al., 1990). However, no determination has been made of the significance of all contractile activity picked up by the monitors. It stands to reason that an unknown proportion of the contractility reported by the monitors is normal activity not associated with preterm labor and birth. Patient education programs that attempt to increase the woman's ability to identify preterm labor contractions have not been shown to improve early diagnosis rates or perinatal outcomes. Hueston and colleagues (1995) in their meta-analysis of the six randomized control trials identified in the literature concluded that "preterm-birth prevention programs for women at high risk do not appear to be an effective means of reducing preterm births or increasing the rate of newborn survival" (p. 710).

Prophylactic use of pharmacologic agents to relax the myometrium has been explored. Keirse, Grant, and King (in Chalmers, Enkin, and Keirse, 1989) conclude:

> There is no evidence that prophylactic use of oral betamimetic agents does more good than harm. Because long-term treatment with these agents cannot be assumed to be free from adverse effects on the baby, they should currently not be used outside the context of controlled trials. There is some evidence, however, that oral maintenance treatment after inhibition of active preterm labor reduces the frequency of recurrent preterm labor (p. 736).

Signs and symptoms. Symptoms of preterm labor include cramping or rhythmic contractions (with or without pain), backache, pelvic pressure, intestinal cramping and/or diarrhea, and increased vaginal discharge. It is important for the clinician to recognize that the presenting symptoms are often much more subtle than those associated with active labor at term. Signs include palpable uterine contractions, change in cervical position, effacement, and dilation. Spontaneous rupture of membranes and/or bloody show may accompany preterm labor.

Screening/diagnosis. Screening begins with the collection of historical data that are known risk factors for preterm labor. Frequent cervical examinations may be done to identify early, painless cervical changes when women have risk factors for preterm labor. Softening of the cervix and effacement are more predictive of preterm birth than dilation. Diagnosis is made through the identification of contractions occurring more frequently than six to eight per hour and cervical change identified by vaginal examination, ideally by the same examiner. In some centers, serial ultrasound examination of the cervix and lower uterine segment are done to determine any symptomless change. Cervical length of greater than 30 mm by transvaginal ultrasound examination suggests that significant effacement has not occurred (Gabbe, Niebyl, and Simpson, 1999).

Management—community-based. The primary role of the clinician in community-based practice is identification of preterm labor or probable preterm labor. The clinician then refers the patient to an obstetrician skilled in management of preterm labor. In some settings, midwives can collaboratively manage preterm labor with the obstetric consultant. When the fetus is very immature or the woman has multiple risk factors for delivery of a very immature infant, referral to a perinatologist in a tertiary care setting is indicated.

When a woman has a history of previous preterm labor and birth, the midwife should assess for urinary tract infection and vaginal or cervical infections at each visit. She should be counseled to use condoms to protect against STDs and to prevent direct contact with semen, which is rich in prostaglandins. Avoidance of heavy lifting, standing, or other work-related stressors is usually recommended, although there is no research that assesses the effectiveness of these restrictions.

The secondary role of the midwife is follow-up care for patients in whom successful cessation of acute preterm labor has been accomplished. Patients should be seen weekly for a review of possible preterm labor signs and symptoms, cervical evaluation, and review of the presence of any medication side effects. Common pharmacologic agents used in the outpatient treatment of preterm labor prevention are identified in Table 26-1. However, meta-analyses have found that oral tocolytic therapy after suppression of acute episodes of preterm labor result in no decrease in preterm birth, no increase of interval from acute episode of preterm labor and birth, and no reduction in the incidence of recurrent preterm labor (Macones, Berlin, and Berlin, 1995). When signs of preterm labor are identified, referral back to the obstetrician is expected.

Patient education regarding side effects and signs of decreased efficacy of the drug should be reviewed at each visit. Patients using terbutaline should be counseled to call the health care provider if they experience dizziness, palpitations, chest pain, or difficulty breathing. Patients using nifedipine should be counseled to limit caffeine intake since it may inhibit action of calcium channel blocking agents. All patients treated for preterm

Table 26-1 *Common Pharmacologic Agents Used in Out-Patient Preterm Labor Prevention*

Drug	Dosage (PO)	Maternal side effects	Fetal side effects
Terbutaline (Brethine)	2.5 mg q4-6h, or 5 mg q6-8h	Tachycardia, decreased blood pressure, arrhythmias, facial flushing, sweating, shortness of breath, pulmonary edema, tremors, headache, hyperglycemia	Increased fetal heart rate, cardiac arrhythmia, hypoxia, increased serum glucose
Calcium channel blockers (Nifedipine)	10-20 mg q4-6h	Facial flushing Mild hypotension Tachycardia, headache, nausea	None reported
Prostaglandin synthetase inhibitors (indomethacin)	25 mg q4-6h	Nausea, vomiting, dyspepsia	Premature closure of the ductus arteriosus, decreased glomerular filtration rate, oligohydramnios

labor prevention should be counseled to contact the clinician if they experience increase in contractions or rupture of membranes.

Management—referral. Initial treatment of preterm labor in the hospital includes hydration, bed rest, and administration of pharmacologic agents that relax the myometrium. It is thought that hydration inhibits the release of the antidiuretic hormone released when hydration is not adequate. In addition, hydration may increase uteroplacental perfusion, thereby decreasing uterine irritability. Bed rest decreases the pressure of the presenting part on the cervix and increases uteroplacental perfusion.

The most commonly used drugs are currently magnesium sulfate, beta-adrenergic agonists (ritodrine, terbutaline), prostaglandin synthesis inhibitors (indomethacin), and calcium channel blockers (nifedipine). Although tocolytics have been shown to decrease the likelihood of birth within 24 hours of the onset of labor, they have not been found to reduce the incidence of births before 30 weeks' gestation, 32 weeks' gestation or 37 weeks' gestation (Gyetvai et al., 1999). However, delaying birth for 24 to 48 hours does have an impact on neonatal morbidity and mortality, since delaying the preterm birth allows time for maternal treatment with corticosteroids, which is associated with fetal lung maturation.

Currently ritodrine is the only agent approved by the Food and Drug Administration for tocolysis. Beta-adrenergic agonists interact with myometrial neuroreceptors, leading to an activation of cyclic adenosine monophosphate–dependent protein kinase, which reduces myometrial contractility by decreasing the effect of calcium at the cellular level. Although most of the published research studying the use of these drugs had numerous methodologic problems, review of randomized control trials indicate they may decrease delivery within 48 hours of onset of preterm labor and decrease delivery within 7 days of the acute episode of preterm labor (Gyetvai et al., 1999). Dosage for ritodrine suggested by the manufacturer is to start intravenous administration at 0.1 mg/min, with an increase of 0.05 mg every 10 minutes until contractions stop or until dosage reaches the maximum recommended rate of 0.35 mg/min. The dosage is maintained at the effective level for 12 hours after contractions cease. Dosage for terbutaline is 0.25 mg subcutaneously every 3 hours or 2.5 μg/min intravenously, with an increase of 2.5 μg/min every 20 minutes until contractions stop or until the maximum dosage of 20 μg/min is reached. Both drugs should be stopped immediately if side effects are experienced. Beta-adrenergic agonists are contraindicated in patients with cardiac disease, hyperthyroidism, and diabetes. Women with impaired renal function are at risk for increased severe side effects when treated with these drugs.

Maternal side effects and complications of parenteral beta-mimetic tocolysis include apprehension and jitteriness, tachycardia, pulmonary edema, myocardial ischemia and dysrhythmias, hypotension, hyperglycemia, hyperinsulinemia, hypocalcemia, hypokalemia, and altered thyroid function. Fetal effects include tachycardia and cardiac arrhythmias, myocardial and septal hypertrophy, myocardial ischemia, cardiac failure, hyperglycemia, hyperinsulinemia, and intrauterine fetal death.

Prostaglandin synthesis inhibitors generate their effect in preterm labor by inactivating cyclo-oxygenase, the enzyme necessary in the synthesis of prostaglandin 2 from arachidonic acid. Since this is the initial step in prostaglandin synthesis, these drugs inhibit the production of a substance essential for uterine contractility. Indomethacin decreases the gap junction formation and decreases the concentration of intracellular calcium. Dosage for indomethacin is 50 mg orally or 50 to 100 mg per rectum as a loading dose, then 25 mg orally every 6 hours. Indomethacin is usually not given for more than 2 days because of the potential fetal effects. Fetal effects include constriction of the ductus arteriosis and right-sided heart failure, oligohydramnios related to decreased urine production, and pulmonary hypertension. Maternal side effects include nausea and heartburn, gastrointestinal bleeding, alterations in coagulation, and thrombocytopenia. Women who are sensitive to aspirin may develop asthma, and women with hypertension may experience a significant rise in blood pressure. Since these drugs are antipyretic agents, fever related to infection may be masked. Maternal contraindications to indomethacin tocolysis include renal or hepatic disease, active peptic ulcers, poorly controlled hypertension, asthma, and coagulation disorders (Gabbe, Niebyl, and Simpson, 1999).

Calcium channel blockers inhibit the transport of extracellular calcium across the cell membranes, leading to decreased myometrial contractility. Recent research suggests that calcium channel blockers may prolong labor better than beta-adrenergic agonists, possibly because of the side effects associated with the latter that may lead to discontinuation of the treatment (Papatsonis et al., 1997). Dosage for nifedipine is 10 to 20 mg orally every 6 hours. An alternate loading dose regimen is 10 mg orally every 20 minutes for up to three doses. Maternal side effects include headache, flushing, dizziness, nausea, decrease in blood pressure, increase in pulse, and mild increase in serum glucose. Research suggests that neonatal effects are lessened with the use of nifedipine when compared to use of the beta-sympathomimetic tocolytic agents (Papatsonis et al., 2000).

Although magnesium sulfate is the most frequently used tocolytic in the United States and is assumed to have tocolytic effects similar to those of the beta-mimetics, a recent meta-analysis found that magnesium sulfate administration was not associated with decreases in birth 24 hours, 48 hours, and 7 days after the initial onset of PTL (Gyetvai et al., 1999). Dosage is usually a 4- to 6-g loading dose intravenously and continued intravenous infusion of 2 to 4 g/hr. Since magnesium is excreted through the renal system, women with impaired renal function need close monitoring of serum levels. Magnesium sulfate is contraindicated in patients who have myasthenia gravis. Maternal side effects include flushing, nausea, vomiting, headache, muscle weakness, shortness of breath, and pulmonary edema. There are few fetal effects, although lethargy and respiratory depression in the neonate have been reported. Magnesium sulfate is commonly the drug of choice in treatment of acute preterm labor since it has less side effects and complications than ritodrine.

Maternal contraindications to tocolysis include severe preeclampsia or chronic hypertension, antepartum hemorrhage, chorioamnionitis, advanced dilation, and cardiac disease. Fetal contraindications include gestational age greater than 37 weeks, estimated birth weight greater than 2500 g, fetal demise, lethal anomaly, or signs of fetal compromise.

Recent preterm labor prevention programs have included more aggressive treatment in the home setting. Home uterine monitoring, use of infusion pumps that allow for continuous administration of pharmacologic agents, and home visits by specially prepared nurses appear to be well accepted by patients. However, further research is necessary to determine whether this approach actually decreases the rate of preterm birth.

Once a woman has experienced an acute episode of preterm labor, she should be evaluated weekly by the provider for assessment of the cervix. Digital examination or transvaginal ultrasound can be used to determine whether there has been cervical change. Women who have been treated for preterm labor should be advised to avoid activities that increase uterine contractility (nipple stimulation, orgasm). In addition, they should be encouraged to stay well hydrated; limit heavy lifting and prolonged standing; and avoid cigarettes, drugs, and alcohol. Recent studies in France suggest that their national program that included education regarding self-identification of contractions, reduction of physical exercise, and work-leave for women with heavy or physically demanding work requirements is associated with a decrease in preterm births in singleton pregnancies (Papiernik and Grange, 1999).

POSTDATES PREGNANCY

Etiology/pathology. Term pregnancy is considered to be 37 to 42 completed weeks of pregnancy dating from the first day of the last period (assuming a 28-day cycle). Term pregnancy can also be considered to be 35 to 40 weeks from conception. Postdates pregnancy exceeds 42 weeks' gestation of menstrual age. Prolonged pregnancy exceeds 40 weeks' conception age and applies when there is relative certainty about the dating of the pregnancy. It should be noted, however, that more research has identified that the median duration of a first pregnancy in white women is 274 days, 8 days longer than that predicted using Naegle's rule. Median duration of subsequent pregnancies is 3 days longer than that assumed by Naegle's rule (Mittendorf et al., 1990). The incidence of postdates pregnancy varies by definition applied and methods used in determining gestational age. There is also evidence that length of gestation varies by race, resulting in race-dependent differences in the incidence of post-dates (Papiernik, Alexander, and Paneth, 1990). The incidence of postdates pregnancy when relying on menstrual history alone is estimated to be 10%. The incidence when combining menstrual history with early ultrasound findings is 1% to 2%.

Postmaturity can be diagnosed only after the birth when it is found that the newborn exhibits characteristics associated with dysmaturity.

Signs and symptoms. Postdates pregnancy is suspected when the gestation exceeds 42 completed weeks by menstrual dating.

Postmaturity syndrome is the delivery of the fetus after 42 weeks' gestation with the following findings:

- Oligohydramnios
- Meconium-stained fluid
- Neonatal characteristics, including loss of subcutaneous fat, long fingernails, peeling skin, absence of lanugo, absence of vernix, and wide-eyed, alert facies

Screening/diagnosis. Using early ultrasound dating to confirm dating obtained through other parameters increases the accuracy of diagnosis of postdates pregnancy. Postmaturity syndrome can only be diagnosed at delivery.

Management—community-based. It is essential that dating be done using a variety of indicators at the first prenatal visit and at each revisit. In this respect, management of postdates pregnancy begins early in pregnancy. Once an estimated due date (EDD) has been determined through the best dating parameters available, it should not be changed unless there is strong clinical evidence supporting the change. For example, when a woman reports a known last menstrual period, positive pregnancy test correlates with probable date of conception, early sizing is consistent with the EDD, and second trimester ultrasound is consistent with the original dating, it would be irrational to change the due date late in pregnancy for any reason. When conception is known (e.g., through in vitro fertilization or maintenance of a basal body temperature graph), it is not rational to change an original EDD on the basis of the findings of a second or third trimester ultrasound examination.

When postdates gestation is encountered, the clinician is faced with the decision to manage expectantly or to induce labor. In a midwifery approach to care, decisions must be made in collaboration with the woman. Her decisions about use of interventions are going to be influenced by her beliefs about pregnancy and birth, her values regarding biotechnology, and her sense of well-being. Since there are benefits and risks to each approach, the woman's decision should be respected and should guide the plan of care.

Expectant Management When the woman desires expectant management, the midwife should collaboratively develop a plan that provides fetal assessment and supports activities that foster the normal, healthy transition to active labor. The most common approach to fetal assessment in pregnancy that exceeds 40 weeks is a baseline NST and amniotic fluid index (AFI) by 41 weeks' gestation, followed by twice weekly NSTs and weekly AFIs until delivery (ACOG, 1999a). Women should also be counseled to assess fetal movement. This can be done either by using one of the common fetal kick counts approaches such as the Cardiff Count-to-Ten chart or by having the woman identify specific times of day in which she relaxes and subjectively notes her baby's movements. Many women demonstrate that they know and appreciate their baby's wake and sleep cycles.

When the cervix is not ripe, the woman may be interested in self-care interventions that foster cervical ripening and onset of labor. Sexual intercourse is associated with cervical ripening, most likely because of the prostaglandins in semen (Toth, Rehnstrom, and Fuchs, 1989). Evening primrose oil is thought to aid in ripening the cervix, and sources on use of herbs suggest one capsule three times per day for up to a week (Weed, 1986). Nipple stimulation can be used, with women instructed to roll the nipple or provide stimulation by sucking or use of a breast pump. Women should stop stimulation when contractions are 3 minutes apart or if the stimulation causes contractions that are greater than 60 seconds in length. Although hyperstimulation is a theoretic risk, research has not found that to be the case (Elliott and Flaherty, 1984). Castor oil has long been thought to stimulate labor, although there are no randomized control studies to evaluate the effectiveness. One small study exploring use of castor oil when women experience premature rupture of membranes suggests that castor oil may stimulate labor with increased effectiveness in multiparas (Davis, 1984). "Stripping the membranes" is also commonly suggested as a means of increasing prostaglandin release, but research findings conflict when evaluating effectiveness (Crane et al., 1997; Goldenberg et al., 1996) (Research Box 26-1).

Induction of Labor When gestational dating is sound and indicates completion of 41 weeks, many sources recommend induction of labor to decrease the risks of macrosomia and fetal intolerance in labor (Cunningham et al., 1997; Gabbe, Niebyl, and Simpson, 1999). The rate of induction of labor in the United States doubled between 1989 and 1997, and evidence suggests that the

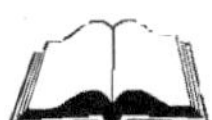

Research Box 26-1

McColgin SW et al: Stripping membranes at term: can it safely reduce the incidence of post-term pregnancies? *Obstet Gynecol* 76(4):678-680, 1990.

Background

Intentional digital separation of the chorionic membranes from the wall of the lower uterine segment ("stripping the membranes") has been believed to promote the initiation of labor. However, little research has explored the safety and efficacy of this common intervention.

Research Question

Does membrane stripping in appropriately selected patients reduce the incidence of postdates pregnancy?

Methods

Women with firmly established gestational dating were recruited at 38 weeks' gestation for participation in this randomized control trial. The experimental group received a weekly cervical examination that included membrane stripping, or, if the cervix was uneffaced and closed, the cervix was stretched digitally until membrane stripping could be accomplished. The control group received a weekly cervical examination that assessed the Bishop score. Outcome measures included time from first examination to delivery, week of gestation at delivery, mode of delivery, and maternal and neonatal complications.

Sample

One hundred and eighty women were recruited into the study from a practice that provided care for approximately 6000 childbearing women during the 16 months of data collection. No data are presented to assess whether the participants were representative of the patient population of women with term singleton pregnancies with firm gestational dating. The two groups were similar for maternal age, Bishop scores, and number of nulliparas and multiparas. However, the mean parity was significantly higher in the experimental group. There is no information given regarding the statistical power of the sample size of 90 participants per group.

Results

The most significant finding was a reduction of postterm pregnancy from 15.6% (n = 14) in the control group to 3.3% (n = 3) in the treatment group. The gestational age at delivery was significantly less in the experimental group, and the mode of delivery was not different when comparing the two groups. There were similar rates of maternal and neonatal complications.

Clinical Application

Membrane stripping is an intervention commonly used in midwifery practice, so the results of this study are compelling. The authors conclude that routine stripping of membranes for select women at term with firm dating has the potential to reduce the incidence of postdates pregnancy with a reduction in the associated fetal surveillance, the number of office visits, patient and physician anxiety about the complications associated with postdates pregnancy, and "difficult" inductions. However, clinicians need to recognize the limitations of this study, particularly the possibility that the small sample size contributed to a type I error in analysis or that other confounding variables were not identified.

rate continues to increase (Ventura et al., 1999). Induction of labor should be considered only when the benefits of the expeditious delivery outweigh the risks of continuing the pregnancy (ACOG, 1999b). When induction is indicated and the cervix is not favorable, cervical ripening should be considered. Prostaglandin $E_1$and E_2 and misoprostol have all been found to be effective in softening the cervix. Contraindications to induction of labor include complete placenta previa, vasa previa, umbilical cord prolapse, transverse fetal lie, and previous uterine surgery (excluding low transverse cesarean scar). The following situations carry increased maternal and fetal risk when induction is implemented: previous low-transverse cesarean deliveries, breech presentation, multiple pregnancy, polyhydramnios, non-reassuring fetal heart rate, and maternal cardiovascular disease.

Management—referral. When out-of-hospital birth is planned, referral for in-hospital labor and delivery may be indicated when greater than 42 weeks' gestation is experienced. This recommendation is based on the increased risk of oligohydramnios, meconium-stained fluid, and fetal intolerance of labor in prolonged pregnancy. In many sites, the midwife can collaboratively care for women experiencing prolonged pregnancy. Medical referral is indicated with findings suggestive of fetal compromise.

MULTIPLE GESTATION

Etiology/pathology. Multiple gestation occurs when a single fertilized egg divides into two individuals (monozygotic) or when two or more ova are fertilized (dizygotic) in a single ovulatory cycle. Monozygotic twins are genetically identical. Dizygotic twins are as similar as any siblings of the same parents. Dizygotic twins are commonly called fraternal twins. The incidence of monozygotic twins is 4/1000 births. The incidence of dizygotic twins varies by race and age, with less dizygotic twinning in Asian populations and young women, and more in black populations and in women who are 35 to 40 years of age. There can be a familial tendency to dizygotic twinning, most likely the result of hormonally induced multiple ovulation. Developed countries are experiencing an increase in multiple births secondary to the increased use of assisted reproductive techniques. Gestations with greater than two fetuses can be any combination of monozygotic and dizygotic twinning. With the increased use of ovulating-inducing drugs and in vitro fertilization, it is now estimated that the incidence of multiple gestation has increased in the United States to 3% of all pregnancies (Ventura et al., 1998).

Increased perinatal morbidity and mortality in multiple gestation have been well documented. Preterm labor and IUGR are more common with multiple gestation. Multiple gestation is also associated with increased rates of placenta previa, placental abruption, preeclampsia, cord accidents, malpresentation, and congenital anomalies.

Since dizygotic twins have different genetic makeup, their blastocysts always form different placentas and membranes. Even if the blastocysts implant in close proximity to each other, the placentas may fuse at their junction, but the placental vasculature and membranes remain distinct (Figure 26-3, *B*). In monozygotic twinning the development of placenta(s) and membranes depends on the timing of cleavage of the fertilized ovum (Figure 26-3, *A*). If cleavage occurs in the first 2 to 3 days following fertilization, two chorions and two amnions form. However, if cleavage occurs after 3 days, the differentiation of cells that form the chorion has occurred, and only one chorion develops. If the cleavage occurs between days 3 and 8, two amnions form, resulting in a di-

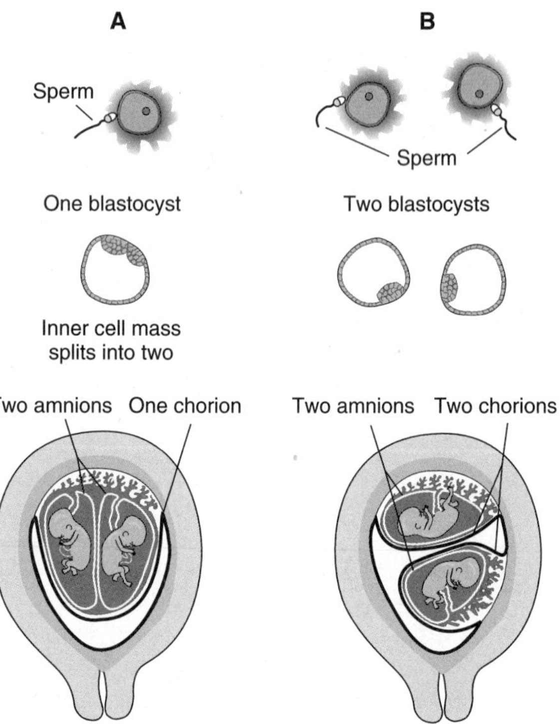

Figure 26-3 Twin pregnancy. **A,** Identical twins; **B,** fraternal twins.

amniotic, monochorial placenta. If cleavage occurs between days 8 and 13 after fertilization, only one amnion develops, resulting in a monoamniotic, monochorionic placenta. When the membranes are monoamniotic, there is a significant risk for cord accident, and it is estimated that the risk of fetal death is greater than 50% when there is only one amnion. If cleavage occurs on days 13 to 15, conjoined twins develop.

Almost all monochorionic placentas have vascular communication between the two fetuses. This can be artery-to-artery, artery-to-vein, and vein-to-vein. An arteriovenous anastomosis results in twin-to-twin transfusion in which the twin donor is smaller, with anemia, hypoglycemia, cardiac atrophy, decreased muscle mass and small, pale placenta. The twin recipient may be up to 1000 g larger than her or his sibling and often has polycythemia, hemolysis, cardiac hypertrophy, and a large placenta.

Early wastage has been identified in multiple gestation. Multiple gestational sacs and embryos may be noted on early first trimester ultrasound examinations, only to have follow-up scans identify only one fetus. One theory is that when there is a blighted ovum, there may be resorption of the sac without any effect on the other developing embryo. Commonly, first trimester vaginal spotting may indicate the regression of a blighted ovum in a multiple gestation.

Signs and symptoms. Women with multiple gestations are more likely to experience severe nausea and vomiting. Once quickening occurs, they may report fetal movements that are greater than those experienced with a singleton pregnancy. Abdominal and pelvic examination identifies a uterus larger than expected for the gestational age after 12 weeks' gestation. Two or more distinct fetal heart rates may be heard. Abnormally high hCG and alpha-fetoprotein levels suggest multiple gestation.

Screening/diagnosis. Diagnosis is made by clinical examination and confirmed by ultrasound examination.

Management—community-based. The community-based midwife may manage women experiencing multiple gestation collaboratively with an obstetrician according to practice and institutional policies. Women with multiple gestation have increased nutritional needs, and the recommended weight gain for women carrying twins is about 50% greater than that expected for a singleton pregnancy. Since women carrying multiple fetuses are at increased risk for anemia, attention should be paid to adequate iron and folic acid intake. Prenatal supplementation is recommended using a multiple vitamin preparation (Institute of Medicine, 1992). Hematocrit and hemoglobin levels should be evaluated at the first prenatal visit and in late second trimester.

Since fetal chromosome abnormalities are increased in dizygotic twins and structural abnormalities are increased in monozygotic twins, parents should be offered genetic counseling. Counseling should include a discussion regarding the ethical issues surrounding findings that one or more of the fetuses are abnormal. Ethical issues also arise when multifetal pregnancy reduction is considered. Higher-level multiple gestations (greater than three fetuses) carry increased risk of maternal and perinatal morbidity and mortality. By reducing the number of fetuses to three, the risks may be decreased. Whether reducing triplets to twins improves outcomes remains controversial.

Since women experiencing multiple gestation are at increased risk for preterm labor, instruction in identification of preterm labor symptoms is indicated. Use of risk assessment, serial cervical assessment, and home uterine monitoring has not consistently been shown to decrease preterm labor and birth in multiple gestation. Women carrying twins, triplets, or higher-order multiples should be referred to a perinatologist when preterm labor is identified.

Ultrasound examination is useful in identifying multiple gestations, screening for anomalies, and monitoring the growth of the fetuses. Although the Routine Antenatal Diagnostic Imaging with Ultrasound (RADIUS) study did note that, in women in the routine screening group, 100% of multiple gestations were identified by 24 weeks' gestation, the outcomes for those pregnancies did not differ from those of the control group who received ultrasound assessment only for medical indication (Crane et al., 1994; Ewigman et al., 1993; LeFevre et al., 1993). However, if multiple pregnancy is identified early in the pregnancy, the clinician has greater opportunity for counseling regarding behavioral changes that are associated with improved pregnancy outcome. ACOG recommends an ultrasound examination in second trimester to identify placentation, amnionicity, chorionicity, number of fetuses, amniotic fluid or placenta abnormalities, and assessment of fetal growth (ACOG, 1998b). Serial ultrasound for fetal growth identifies IUGR, growth discordance, and abnormal amniotic fluid volumes. When these problems are identified or when pregnancy-induced hypertension, fetal anomalies, and monoamnionicity are identified, fetal assessment using NSTs and/or biophysical profile is indicated. Currently, routine fetal assessment for all multiple pregnancies is not recommended (ACOG, 1998b).

Management—referral. Referral to a perinatologist or obstetrician skilled in managing multiple pregnancies is necessary for all women carrying greater than two fetuses and when practice guidelines determine that multiple gestation is a contraindication to midwifery or community-based care.

Implications for current pregnancy. Since multiple pregnancy carries the risk of preterm delivery, the woman and her family experience increased stress related to the potential problems for mother and infants. For this reason, case management by an experienced perinatal nurse may coordinate management and enhance the family's coping mechanisms. Referral to social service agencies may be indicated if the woman needs assistance for modified activity and home care.

ABNORMAL PRESENTATION AT TERM

Etiology/pathology. Factors associated with malpresentation include lax abdominal muscles, uterine anomalies, increased or decreased fetal mobility, and obstruction of the pelvic inlet. Prematurity and hydramnios are associated with increased fetal mobility and therefore are strongly associated with malpresentation.

Incidence of breech presentation at term is estimated to be 3%. Before term, estimates of incidence range from 7% to 16% at 32 weeks' gestation (Gabbe, Niebyl, and Simpson, 1999; Hughey, 1985). Spontaneous version to vertex presentation occurs in 57% of cases between 32 and 36 weeks' gestation, and 25% of the time after 36 weeks. Breech presentation is associated with fetal weight less than 2500 g, uterine anomalies, contracted pelvis, use of anticonvulsant drugs, placenta previa, cornual placenta, decreased or increased amniotic fluid volume, fetal anomalies, multiple pregnancy, and short umbilical cord. Adequate fetal movement is necessary to allow the fetus to actively orient itself, and normal fetal neuromuscular development and normal amount of fluid facilitate the fetus to assume the cephalic presentation.

Delivery of a fetus in the breech presentation is associated with increased fetal and maternal morbidity and mortality. Fetal asphyxia secondary to entrapment of the aftercoming head, extremity paralysis caused by nerve compression, and trauma from difficult delivery are recognized as potential problems. Maternal morbidity and mortality are associated with the increased rate of cesarean section.

A complete breech presentation occurs when the hips and knees are flexed. A frank breech presentation occurs when the hips are flexed and the knees are extended. An incomplete breech presentation is when one or both hips are not flexed and one or both knees or feet are located below the breech.

Oblique and transverse lies are associated with multiparity, lax abdominal tone, uterine and fetal anomalies, decreased diameters of the pelvic inlet, and pelvic masses.

Signs and symptoms. Breech presentation may be suspected when the pregnant woman notes frequent kicking in the lower abdomen, as opposed to up under her ribs. She may also note discomfort or shortness of breath secondary to the hard fetal head under her diaphragm.

A careful clinician will be able to identify probable breech presentations through abdominal examination. Suspected breech often can be confirmed by a pelvic examination when the fetal buttocks or feet are palpated through the cervix or the thin lower uterine segment.

Likewise, oblique and transverse lies may be suspected by the findings of the abdominal examination. Pelvic examination identifies either a very high presenting part, or a shoulder.

Screening/diagnosis. Screening and diagnosis are initiated with abdominal palpation in the third trimester. Suspected breech presentations can be diagnosed by definitive identification of the buttocks or feet during vaginal examination. Ultrasound examination diagnoses abnormal presentations.

Management—community-based. Because of the increased risks to the woman and her baby, it is advantageous to facilitate version of the breech to vertex presentation. Use of specific maternal positioning—that which elevates the hips above the shoulders—has been associated with increased incidence of spontaneous versions. Bung and colleagues (1987) randomly assigned women with breech presentations at term to an exercise group and a control group. The exercise group had a 70% vertex delivery rate vs. the 55% vertex rate in the control group. Midwives can suggest that women elevate the hips for 15 minutes three times per day to assist in spontaneous versions to vertex presentation (Enkin, Renfrew, and Keirse, 1995; Simkin, Whalley, and Keppler, 1991).

When women do not experience spontaneous version of the fetus, they should be given the option of assisted external version. Use of tocolytic drugs in conjunction

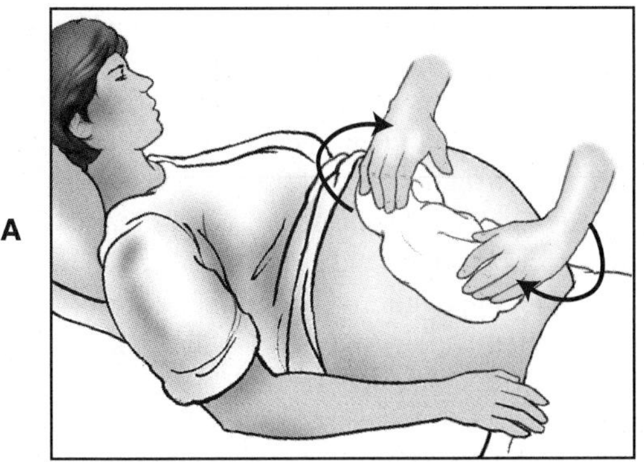

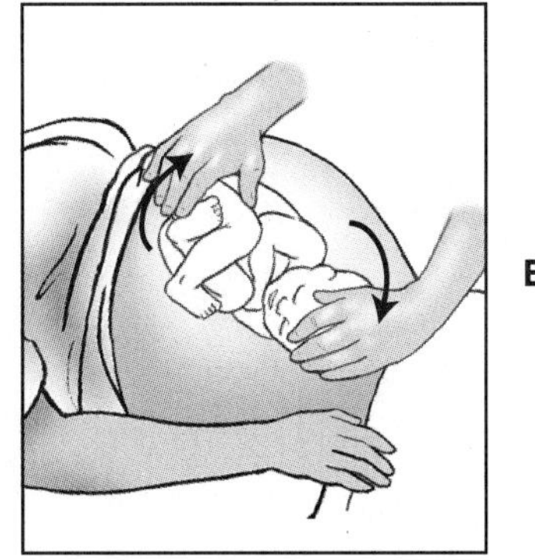

Figure 26-4 External cephalic version.

with the procedure has led to an increase in the success rate for external cephalic versions after 37 weeks (Hofmeyr, 2000). Delay of external cephalic version attempts until term allows more time for spontaneous version and provides more time for contraindications for version or indication for cesarean section to become more apparent (Chalmers, Enkin, and Keirse, 1989).

Research has suggested that external cephalic version can increase the incidence of cephalic birth after breech from 22% to 70% (Hofmeyr, 1983, 2000). More recent studies have suggested increased success in external version when tocolytics are used during the procedure (Hofmeyr, 2000; Marquette et al., 1996).

The procedure is done in a site in which ultrasound placentation, fetal position, and cord positioning can be confirmed. After tocolysis, gentle pressure is applied to the fetal head and back as a "forward roll" is attempted (Figure 26-4, *A* and *B*). When version is successful, women are often given the option to induce labor if the cervix is favorable in order to decrease the risk that the fetus will revert to a breech presentation. Factors associated with failure of version include obesity, engagement of the presenting part, oligohydramnios, and posterior positioning of the fetal back (Gabbe, Niebyl, and Simpson, 1999).

Risks of external cephalic version are primarily fetal in nature. Fetal bradycardia and decreased variability have been noted following external cephalic version, but these findings have been transitory, and perinatal outcomes have been no worse than the general population. Fetal-maternal hemorrhage and fetal spinal cord injury have been reported as rare outcomes.

Alternate approaches to external version include visualization, hypnosis, and the use of moxibustion. Further research is needed to confirm the effectiveness of these approaches. However, it can be noted that Eastern medicine has used moxibustion for generations, and one randomized control trial suggests that the success rate may be higher than medical external version (Cardini and Weixin, 1998).

Implications for current pregnancy. Interventions to increase the likelihood that the fetus will be vertex in labor decrease the morbidity and mortality associated with vaginal breech births and cesarean deliveries for breech births. The challenge in many communities is the identification of clinicians who are skilled in the procedure.

DEVIATIONS IN FETAL GROWTH—SMALL FOR GESTATIONAL AGE

Etiology/pathology. Small-for-gestational-age (SGA) infants are defined as those who have birth weights at or below the tenth percentile for gestational age. Many SGA babies are clinically normal and are small because of genetics rather than a pathologic process. IUGR, a growth pattern that is less than expected for gestational age, usually results in a baby who is SGA, although a fetus may not reach its growth potential yet be above the tenth percentile. Risk factors for IUGR are listed in Box 26-5.

Impaired placental perfusion is the most common reason for SGA in infants without anomalies. Impaired perfusion is associated with preeclampsia, placental abruption, placenta previa, and placenta mosaicism.

IUGR is associated with intrapartal and neonatal problems. Intrapartal problems include abnormal fetal

Box 26-5 *Risk Factors for Intrauterine Growth Restriction*

Maternal Medical Factors

Hypertension
Renal disease
Diabetes (with vascular compromise)
Cyanotic heart disease
Antiphospholipid syndrome
Collagen-vascular disease
Hemoglobinopathies

Maternal Social Factors

Smoking
Substance use and abuse
Severe malnutrition
Exposure to teratogens

Obstetric Factors

Multiple gestation
Primary placental disease
Perinatal infections
Previous IUGR infant

Fetal Factors

Genetic disorders

IUGR, Intrauterine growth restriction.

heart rate patterns in labor, oligohydramnios, and increased cesarean delivery rate. Neonatal problems include polycythemia, hyperbilirubinemia, hypoglycemia, hypothermia, apnea, low APGAR scores, umbilical artery pH less than 7.0, seizures, and neonatal death (ACOG, 2000).

Signs and symptoms. Signs of IUGR include fundal height less than expected in third trimester and estimated fetal weight less than expected for gestational age. Signs associated with IUGR include hypertension, poor weight gain, and signs of substance abuse.

Screening/diagnosis. Screening occurs at each prenatal visit when the clinician screens for risk factors associated with IUGR and performs a complete abdominal assessment in second and third trimesters. The assessment of size-less-than-dates must rule out other causes of the size-dates discrepancy, including inaccurate gestational dating, presenting part deep in the pelvis, transverse lie, and intrauterine fetal demise.

When IUGR is suspected, serial ultrasound examinations should be obtained to monitor the growth pattern. Measurements that usually are included in ultrasound assessment include fetal abdominal circumference, head circumference, biparietal diameter, and femur length. A less than normal abdominal circumference or estimated fetal weight suggests IUGR. Since IUGR is associated with anomalous fetuses, a careful anatomy scan should be done to detect structural defects. The woman should also be offered genetic counseling, particularly when anomalies are noted.

Because IUGR is associated with oligohydramnios, amniotic fluid volume should be assessed. Oligohydramnios is found in 77% to 83% of pregnancies with IUGR (ACOG, 2000).

In most cases the midwife can continue to manage the care of a pregnancy complicated with IUGR and normal amniotic fluid volume in consultation with an obstetrician. The midwife, obstetrician, and pregnant woman develop a plan not only to assess the fetus, but also to identify the underlying cause of the growth restriction. Counseling should address interventions that will increase uterine perfusion, including hydration, rest in the left lateral position, and no smoking or exposure to other vacoconstricting agents. Nutritional counseling should emphasize the importance of adequate caloric and protein intake.

Management—referral. When IUGR is suspected, referral to a perinatal diagnostic center that offers Doppler ultrasonography to measure umbilical artery waveforms is indicated. The measurement of waveforms has poor positive predictive value, but absent or reversed end-diastolic flow is associated with poor perinatal outcome and increased perinatal mortality (Kingdom, Burrell, and Kaufmann, 1997).

Referral to an obstetrician is indicated when IUGR is accompanied by oligohydramnios. In some settings the midwife may be able to manage these cases collaboratively with the obstetrician or perinatologist.

Implications for current pregnancy. Since IUGR is associated with increased perinatal morbidity and mortality, the woman and her family experience numerous stressors. The recommended changes in behaviors and activities may have a significant impact on the family's function. Perinatal counseling should be offered, and referrals to agencies that can provide resources, including home care assistance and financial support, may be indicated.

DEVIATIONS IN FETAL GROWTH—LARGE FOR GESTATIONAL AGE

Etiology/pathology. Macrosomia is defined as birth weight greater than 4000 or 4500 g and/or birth weight above the 90th percentile for gestational age. Large-for-gestational-age (LGA) infants are at increased risk for perinatal morbidity and mortality. Most LGA infants are normal large babies secondary to genetics and maternal nutrition. A small proportion of LGA babies are associated with diabetes in pregnancy. LGA babies of diabetic mothers develop increased fat and muscle mass across the shoulders and abdomen, resulting in chest circumference abnormally greater than head circumference. This growth pattern is termed asymmetric macrosomia. Infants of obese women with normal glucose control have excessive growth of both the head and the chest/abdomen, resulting in symmetric macrosomia.

Signs and symptoms. Signs of macrosomia include fundal height that is greater than expected for gestational age and estimated fetal weight that is greater than expected for gestational age. Increased maternal weight gain is also associated with macrosomia.

Screening/diagnosis. Screening is done at each prenatal examination in third trimester when the clinician does a complete abdominal assessment. Although numerous formulas have been developed to estimate fetal weight using ultrasound measurements, ultrasound prediction continues to have poor sensitivity and poor positive predictive value (Chauhan et al., 1998; Chauhan et al., 2000; Combs et al., 2000; Gonen, Spiegel, and Abend, 1996). Diagnosis is made when birth weight is determined.

Management—community-based. When measurement of fundal height indicates size-greater-than-dates, further data are needed to determine the underlying cause of the discrepancy. In addition to an LGA fetus, differential diagnoses for size-greater-than-dates include incorrect dating, polyhydramnios, multiple gestation, uterine myomata, or other pelvic masses that displace the uterine fundus. A review of historical data should clarify the gestation age, identify previous LGA births, and identify family history of large infants. Ultrasound examination can rule out abnormalities in amniotic fluid, multiple gestation, and masses.

When probable macrosomia is identified, glucose screening results should be reviewed. If glucose screening was done at 24 weeks and found to be normal, a repeat screen during the third trimester may be indicated, particularly when additional risk factors (e.g., obesity, Latino, or Native American ethnicity) are present. A thorough nutritional history should be obtained, and counseling provided to decrease intake of excessive calories.

Induction of labor at term when macrosomia is suspected has been suggested as an approach to decrease the risks of dysfunctional labor and fetal injury during birth. Research findings have not demonstrated a decrease in risk of maternal or neonatal morbidity when elective induction is done (Irion and Boulvain, 2000). Cesarean delivery for fetuses with estimated fetal weight greater than 4500 g or fetuses of mothers who have diabetes has also been suggested as a means to decrease maternal and neonatal morbidity (Gabbe, Niebyl, and Simpson, 1999). However, the imprecision of estimating macrosomia and the documented increase in maternal morbidity and mortality must be considered when discussing elective surgery with the mother.

Management—referral. Referral to a facility in which anesthesia and surgical availability is assured 24 hours per day may be indicated when the community-based clinician believes there is a high risk of dysfunctional labor and shoulder dystocia.

RH ALLOIMMUNIZATION

Etiology/pathology. Before the development of anti-D immunoglobulin, the incidence of fetal and neonatal hemolytic disease was 9% to 10% of pregnancies. When women are Rh D negative (Rh D−), alloimmunization is associated with mild-to-moderate hemolytic anemia in the fetus, hyperbilirubinemia, and fetal hydrops. Alloimmunization occurs when there is fetomaternal transfusion from an Rh D positive (Rh D+) infant to the Rh D− mother. Alloimmunization can occur with as little as 0.1 ml of fetal blood. The most common time for fetomaternal transfusion is at the time of delivery. Other events that increase the risk of transfusion include elective and spontaneous abortions, ectopic pregnancy, placental abruption, chorionic villi sampling, amniocentesis, and percutaneous fetal procedures.

Alloimmunization does not occur in all Rh D− women carrying an Rh D+ fetus. About 30% of these women do not have an immune response to the antigen. In addition, women who experience ABO incompatibility with their fetuses do not mount an immune response to the fetal Rh D+ antigen. However, because it is not possible to identify women who are protected from alloimmunization, prophylactic interventions are carried out with all Rh D− women when the father of the baby is Rh D+ or presumed to be Rh D+.

The use of passively administered antibody to prevent active immunization by an antigen is termed antibody-mediated immune suppression. The administration of anti-D immunoglobulin to Rh D− individuals exposed to Rh D+ cells has been shown to prevent the immune response. The original research suggested that 300 μg of Rh immune globulin would prevent immunization in individuals exposed to 10 ml of Rh D+ cells (Gabbe, Niebyl, and Simpson, 1999). It is now known that over 99% of postpartum women have less than 5 ml of fetal cells in their system and that 300 μg of anti-D immunoglobulin can prevent alloimmunization after exposure to 30 ml of Rh D+ blood or 15 ml of fetal cells. Therefore theoretically the dosage could be decreased to 100 to 150 μg to protect almost all susceptible women; however, the 300-μg dose of Rh D immunoglobulin remains the standard in the United States for administration in second and third trimesters and in the postpartum period. It is recommended that all women who deliver an Rh D+ infant have laboratory testing to determine the extent of fetomaternal hemorrhage in order to ensure that sufficient anti-D immunoglobulin is given. In most facilities this is done using the Kleihauer-Betke test. When there is risk for fetomaternal transfusion in the first trimester, the dose of anti-D immunoglobulin is 50 μg to prevent protection against sensitization for up to 2.5 ml of fetal red blood cells (ACOG, 1999c).

Signs and symptoms. Identification of Rh D antibody is the sign of alloimmunization. If the alloimmunization is not identified early and fetal effects occur, size-greater-than-dates secondary to fetal hydrops is a sign of the pathologic process.

Screening/diagnosis. All women should have their blood type and Rh determined at the first prenatal visit. When previous records are available, they can be used to validate the blood type. All Rh D− women should have an antibody screen to identify alloimmunization.

Management—community-based. All clinicians should offer Rh D− women antenatal prophylaxis at 28 weeks' gestation. When the father of the baby is known to be Rh negative, Rh D immunoglobulin may be withheld. One study has found the development of alloimmunization when delivery occurred more than 12 weeks after the administration of prophylaxis at 28 weeks (Bowman, 1985). Because of this, some sources suggest repeating the dose if more than 12 weeks has passed since the original administration. However, since the literature is so limited, there is no consensus on whether this is an appropriate approach to prophylaxis.

The American Association of Blood Banks recommends that all Rh D− postpartum women be screened for antibodies before giving the anti-D immunoglobulin at 28 weeks to identify women who have become alloimmunized (ACOG, 1999b). However, because the incidence of Rh D alloimmunization before 28 weeks is estimated to be 0.18%, ACOG recommends that rescreening should be at the discretion of the provider.

Women who are identified as Du+ or weakly D positive should be considered Rh D+ and therefore not candidates for anti-D immunoglobulin.

Management—referral. Women who have developed alloimmunization must be referred to a perinatologist for management.

Implications for current pregnancy. When women choose not to have anti-D immunoglobulin prophylaxis, the clinician should document the counseling that was done and the level of understanding of the woman and her partner. When the father of the baby is Rh+ or presumed Rh+, the Rh− woman should be followed with monthly antibody screens to identify antibody reaction. If antibody titer of greater than 1:4 is identified, she should be referred to a perinatologist for management.

ABO INCOMPATIBILITY

It is estimated that 20% to 25% of pregnancies are ABO incompatible. In these cases the mother's serum contains anti-A or anti-B antibodies, and the fetus' red blood cells contain A or B antigen (Gabbe, Niebyl, and Simpson, 1999). ABO incompatibility results in mild-to-moderate hemolytic anemia in the neonate associated with hyperbilirubinemia. Less than 1% of cases require exchange transfusion. ABO incompatibility has not been shown to lead to fetal hemolysis since the IgM anti-A or anti-B do not cross the placenta well. Because of this, screening for anti-A and anti-B antibodies is not recommended in pregnancy.

References

ACOG: *Medical management of tubal pregnancy (Practice Bulletin 3),* Washington, DC, 1998a, American College of Obstetricians and Gynecologists.

ACOG: *Special problems of multiple gestation (Educational Bulletin 253),* Washington, DC, 1998b, American College of Obstetricians and Gynecologists.

ACOG: *Antepartum fetal surveillance (Practice Bulletin 9),* Washington, DC, 1999a, American College of Obstetricians and Gynecologists.

ACOG: *Induction of labor (Practice Bulletin 10),* Washington, DC, 1999b, American College of Obstetricians and Gynecologists.

ACOG: *Prevention of Rh D alloimmunization (Practice Bulletin 4),* Washington, DC, 1999c, American College of Obstetricians and Gynecologists.

ACOG: *Intrauterine growth restriction (Practice Bulletin 12),* Washington, DC, 2000, American College of Obstetricians and Gynecologists.

Andrews WW et al: Second-trimester cervical ultrasound: associations with increased risk for recurrent early spontaneous delivery, *Obstet Gynecol* 95(2):222-226, 2000.

Ankum WM et al: Risk factors for ectopic pregnancy: a meta-analysis, *Fertil Steril* 65(6):1093-1099, 1996.

Bentley DL et al: Relationship of uterine contractility to preterm labor, *Obstet Gynecol* 76(1)(suppl):36S-38S, 1990.

Bowman JM: Controversies in Rh prophylaxis. Who needs Rh immune globulin and when should it be given? *Am J Obstet Gynecol* 151:289-294, 1985.

Brustman LE et al: Education does not improve patient perception of preterm uterine contractility, *Obstet Gynecol* 76(suppl):93S-96S, 1990.

Bung P et al: Is Indian version a successful method for decreasing the incidence of breech presentation? *Geburtshilfe Frauenheillkd* 47(3):202-205, 1987.

Cardini F, Weixin H: Moxibustion for correction of breech presentation: a randomized controlled trial, *JAMA* 280(18): 1580-1584, 1998.

Centers for Disease Control and Prevention: Ectopic pregnancy—United States, 1990-1992, *MMWR* 44:46-48, 1995.

Chalmers I, Enkin M, Keirse MJNC, editors: *Effective care in pregnancy and childbirth,* New York, 1989, Oxford University Press.

Chauhan SP et al: Limitations of clinical and sonographic estimates of birth weight: experience with 1034 parturients, *Obstet Gynecol* 91(1):72-77, 1998.

Chauhan SP et al: Sonographic measurements of fetal parts to predict pulmonary maturity among twins and singletons, *J Miss State Med Assoc* 41(3):516-520, 2000.

Combs CA et al: Sonographic EFW and macrosomia: is there an optimum formula to predict diabetic fetal macrosomia? *J Matern Fetal Med* 9(1):55-61, 2000.

Crane JP et al: A randomized trial of prenatal ultrasonographic screening: impact on the detection, management, and outcome of anomalous fetuses: RADIUS Study Group (see comments), *Am J Obstet Gynecol* 171(2):392-399, 1994.

Crane JM et al: Transvaginal ultrasound in the prediction of preterm delivery: singleton and twin gestations, *Obstet Gynecol* 90(3):357-363, 1997.

Creasy RK, Gummer BA, Liggins GC: System for predicting spontaneous preterm birth, *Obstet Gynecol* 55(6):692-695, 1980.

Cunningham FG et al: *Williams obstetrics,* ed 20, Stanford, Conn, 1997, Appleton & Lange.

Davis L: The use of castor oil to stimulate labor in patients with premature rupture of membranes, *J Nurse-Midwifery* 29(6):366-370, 1984.

Edenfield SM et al: Validity of the Creasy risk appraisal instrument for prediction of preterm labor, *Nurs Res* 44(2):76-81, 1995.

Elliott JP, Flaherty JF: The use of breast stimulation to prevent postdate pregnancy, *Am J Obstet Gynecol* 149(6):628-632, 1984.

Enkin M, Renfrew M, Keirse MJ et al: *A guide to effective care in pregnancy and childbirth,* ed 2, Oxford, 1995, Oxford University Press.

Ewigman BG et al: Effect of prenatal ultrasound screening on perinatal outcome: RADIUS Study Group (see comments), *N Engl J Med* 329(12):821-827, 1993.

Fedrick J, Anderson ABM: Factors associated with spontaneous preterm birth, *Br J Obstet Gynecol* 83:342-344, 1976.

Gabbe SG, Niebyl JR, Simpson JL: *Pocket companion to obstetrics—normal and problem pregnancies,* ed 3, New York, 1999, Churchill Livingstone.

Goldenberg M et al: Stretching of the cervix and stripping of the membranes at term: a randomised controlled study, *Eur J Obstet Gynecol Reprod Biol* 66(2):129-132, 1996.

Goldenberg RL et al: Bed rest in pregnancy, *Obstet Gynecol* 84(1):131-136, 1994.

Gonen R, Spiegel D, Abend M: Is macrosomia predictable, and are shoulder dystocia and birth trauma preventable? *Obstet Gynecol* 88(4 Pt 1):526-529, 1996.

Gyetvai K et al: Tocolytics for preterm labor: a systematic review, *Obstet Gynecol* 94(5):869-877, 1999.

Hofmeyr GJ: Effect of external cephalic version in late pregnancy on breech presentation and caesarian section rate: a controlled trial, *Br J Obstet Gynaecol* 90(5):392-399, 1983.

Hofmeyr GJ: External cephalic version facilitation for breech presentation at term. In Neilson JP et al, editors: *Pregnancy and childbirth module of the Cochrane database of systematic reviews (updated December 2, 1997).* Available in The Cochrane Library (database on disk and CD-ROM). The Cochrane Collaboration, Issue 1, Oxford, 1998, Update Software. Updated quarterly.

Hueston WJ et al: The effectiveness of preterm-birth prevention educational programs for high-risk women: a meta-analysis, *Obstet Gynecol* 86(4):705-712, 1995.

Hughey MJ: Fetal position during pregnancy, *Am J Obstet Gynecol* 153(8):885-886, 1985.

Iams JD, Johnson FF, Parker M: A prospective evaluation of the signs and symptoms of preterm labor, *Obstet Gynecol* 84(2):227-230, 1994.

Institute of Medicine: *Nutrition during pregnancy and lactation: an implementation guide,* Washington, DC, 1992, National Academy Press.

Irion O, Boulvain M: Induction of labour for suspected fetal macrosomia. In Neilson JP et al, editors: *Pregnancy and childbirth module of the Cochrane database of systematic reviews (updated December 2, 1997).* Available in The Cochrane Library (database on disk and CDROM). The Cochrane Collaboration, Issue 1, Oxford, 1998, Update Software. Updated quarterly.

Kaplan BC et al: Ectopic pregnancy: prospective study with improved diagnostic accuracy, *Ann Emerg Med* 28(1):10-17, 1996.

Khan KS et al: Misleading authors' inferences in obstetrics diagnostic test literature, *Am J Obstet Gynecol* 181(1):112-115, 1999.

Kingdom JC, Burrell SJ, Kaufmann P: Pathology and clinical implications of abnormal umbilical artery Doppler waveforms, *Ultrasound Obstet Gynecol* 9(4):271-286, 1997.

Knuppel RA, Drukker JE: *High-risk pregnancy—a team approach,* ed 2, Philadelphia, 1993, WB Saunders.

LeFevre ML et al: A randomized trial of prenatal ultrasonographic screening: impact on maternal management and outcome: RADIUS Study Group (see comments), *Am J Obstet Gynecol* 169(3):483-489, 1993.

Macones GA, Berlin M, Berlin JA: Efficacy of oral beta-agonist maintenance therapy in preterm labor: a meta-analysis, *Obstet Gynecol* 85(2):313-317, 1995.

Main DM et al: Prospective evaluation of a risk scoring system for predicting preterm delivery in black inner city women, *Obstet Gynecol* 69(1):61-66, 1987.

Marquette GP et al: Does the use of a tocolytic agent affect the success rate of external cephalic version? *Am J Obstet Gynecol* 175(4 Pt 1):859-861, 1996.

Mittendorf R et al: The length of uncomplicated human gestation, *Obstet Gynecol* 75(6):929-933, 1990.

Morrison JC: Preterm birth: a puzzle worth solving, *Obstet Gynecol* 76(suppl):1, 1990.

Owen J et al: Evaluation of a risk scoring system as a predictor of preterm birth in an indigent population, *Am J Obstet Gynecol* 163(3):873-879, 1990.

Papatsonis DN et al: Nifedipine and ritodrine in the management of preterm labor: a randomized multicenter trial (see comments), *Obstet Gynecol* 90(2):230-234, 1997.

Papatsonis DN et al: Neonatal effects of nifedipine and ritodrine for preterm labor, *Obstet Gynecol* 95(4):477-481, 2000.

Papiernik E, Grange G: Prenatal screening with evaluated high risk scores, *J Perinatal Med* 27(1):21-25, 1999.

Papiernik E, Alexander GR, Paneth N: Racial differences in pregnancy duration and its implications for perinatal care, *Med Hypotheses* 33(3):181-186, 1990.

Simkin P, Whalley J, Keppler A: *Pregnancy, childbirth and the newborn,* New York, 1991, Meadowbook Press.

Toth M, Rehnstrom J, Fuchs AR: Prostaglandins E and F in cervical mucus of pregnant women, *Am J Perinatol* 6(2):142-144, 1989.

Ventura SJ et al: Births: final data for 1997, *Natl Vital Statistics Rep* 47(18):1-96, 1999.

Ventura SJ et al: *Report of final natality statistics, 1996,* Monthly vital statistics report, vol 46, no. 11 (suppl), Hyattsville, Md, 1998, National Center for Health Statistics.

Weed S: *The woman's herbal for the childbearing year,* 1986, Ash Tree Publishers.

Williams MA et al: Adverse infant outcomes associated with first-trimester vaginal bleeding, *Obstet Gynecol* 78(1):14-18, 1991.

Yost NP et al: Pitfalls in ultrasonic cervical length measurement for predicting preterm birth, *Obstet Gynecol* 93(4):510-516, 1999.

Zaccardi R, Abbott J, Koziol-McLain J: Loss and grief reactions after spontaneous miscarriage in the emergency department (see comments), *Ann Emerg Med* 22(5):799-804, 1993.

Chapter 27

Complications of Labor and Delivery

Midwives and family practice physicians are prepared to care for women experiencing healthy pregnancies. It is essential that these clinicians practice within a health care system that ensures the availability of an obstetrician in case deviations from normal are identified. When obstetric or medical problems are encountered in labor, the midwife may continue to provide care while consulting with the obstetrician or work in collaboration with the obstetrician as care is given. In high-risk situations, transfer of care to the obstetrician is expected.

There are times when midwives and obstetricians may disagree in their interpretation of "risk" in a particular clinical situation. Open and honest discussion is necessary to objectively evaluate the state of knowledge reflected in the literature. Each provider needs to attempt to reject opinions that reflect protection of turf or politics rather than science.

Problems encountered in labor may require reconsideration of site of birth. When collaborative care or referral requires a move from home to hospital or from birth center to hospital, it is essential that a process for safe transfer has been identified. Clinicians working outside the hospital need to constantly consider the time necessary for transfer when making decisions regarding care. For example, a midwife practicing at home may discuss using artificial rupture of membranes with the woman rather than waiting until the membranes rupture spontaneously in second stage in order to identify moderate-to-thick meconium-stained fluid, a finding that would make transfer necessary.

Although most healthy women experience normal labors and deliveries, severe problems occasionally occur. For this reason, midwives and family practice physicians must maintain competency in emergency procedures in order to respond appropriately until the obstetric or neonatal specialist arrives.

COMPLICATIONS RELATED TO THE PROGRESS OF LABOR

Dysfunctional labor (dystocia) is characterized by unusually slow progress and is associated with abnormalities of the expulsive forces (power); abnormalities in presentation, position, or size of the fetus (passenger); and abnormalities of the maternal pelvis (passage). Prolongation of labor is associated with increased maternal and infant morbidity and mortality. The art of midwifery care is the ability to acknowledge and validate individual variation in labor while recognizing the labor factors that increase risk for the mother and/or baby.

Prolonged Latent Phase

Prolonged latent phase is diagnosed when the period from onset of regular, uncomfortable contractions until the onset of rapid cervical dilation exceeds 20 hours in nulliparas and 14 hours in multiparas. These time frames were originally identified by Friedman (1954) as two standard deviations from the mean of his study population and have held consistent in more recent work in different populations. More recently, prolonged latent phase has been defined as greater than 12 hours for nulliparas and greater than 6 hours for multiparas (Chelmow, Kilpatrick, and Laros, 1993). Prolonged latent phase is commonly considered a minor deviation from normal, and management decisions often are based on provider belief in conservative or aggressive management. Recent evidence suggests that prolonged latent phase is associated with increased maternal and neonatal morbidity (Chelmow, Kilpatrick, and Laros, 1993; Friedman and Neff, 1987). Even after controlling for other factors, prolonged latent phase is associated with other labor abnormalities and increased cesarean section rate, suggesting that the prolongation may reflect abnormalities in the underlying physiology of labor. Neonatal outcomes associated with prolonged latent phase include increased perinatal death rates and decreased mean APGAR scores.

Prolonged latent phase is probably a result of alterations in the myometrial function and contractile patterns. These alterations are influenced by myogenic, neurogenic, and hormonal systems (Wiznitzer, 1995). The resulting contractile patterns can be either hypotonic or hypertonic, and management should be guided by the assumed underlying problem.

Box 27-1

Historical Data

Gestational age
Onset of contractions
Frequency of contractions and trend over time
Duration of contractions and trend over time
Intensity of contractions and trend over time
Presence or absence of leaking fluid
Presence or absence of bloody show
Fetal activity
Rest in past 24 hours
Fluid and nutritional intake in past 24 hours
Use of analgesia or sedatives
Chart review for history of this pregnancy, obstetric history, medical/surgical history

Physical Examination Data

General appearance, including skin turgor
Fetal presentation, position, and estimated fetal weight
Fetal heart rate pattern
Palpation of contractions for frequency, duration, and intensity
Cervical effacement
Cervical dilation
Consistency of cervix
Station of presenting part
Application of presenting part to cervix
Status of membranes
Clinical pelvimetry

Laboratory and Other Studies

Urine specific gravity and ketones

Diagnosis of prolonged latent phase. Prolonged latent phase should be suspected when a nullipara complains of painful, regular contractions for more than 20 hours and cervical examination identifies dilation less than or equal to 3 cm with or without effacement. Prolonged latent phase should be suspected if this labor pattern without progression to active phase is greater than 14 hours in multiparas. Box 27-1 identifies the data to be collected in order to appropriately manage the labor. It is important the prolonged latent phase not be confused with false labor—irregular contractions that don't lead to cervical change.

Management of prolonged latent phase. Conservative management includes supportive measures that assist the woman in conserving energy, maintaining fluid and nutrition requirements, and providing psychologic and emotional support. Maternal and fetal status may be assessed in the outpatient setting or the obstetric triage area of the labor and delivery unit, and, once it is determined that there are no factors that would make outpatient care contraindicated, options can be discussed with the woman. The options available today are essentially the same as those recommended by Friedman almost 20 years ago—therapeutic rest or augmentation (Friedman, 1983).

The influence of time of day and the woman's own circadian rhythm should be considered in making a plan of management. If the woman is well rested and the assessment is done during her usual waking hours, ambulating at home or in the community is an option. Ambulation is associated with increasing effectiveness of contractions, most likely from the positional effect on the application of the presenting part on the cervix. Ambulation also provides distraction for the woman, which in turns increases her ability to cope with discomfort. Continued intake of fluids and light, nutritious foods is appropriate. Counseling regarding contacting the provider if the contractions become more uncomfortable or if she experiences spontaneous rupture of membranes, together with the provider's recommendation for timing of the next assessment, should be completed before the end of the visit.

If the assessment is done during the usual sleeping hours, rest may be encouraged. A warm bath or shower, as well as massage, may assist in efforts to nap between or through contractions.

If the woman is not well rested or not coping well with the labor, sedation or analgesia may be considered. Use of morphine to enhance sleep appears to be the most effective approach. Morphine, 15 to 20 mg intramuscularly or subcutaneously, can be given, and, if after 20 minutes contractions have not decreased and maternal respirations are not depressed, an additional 10 mg of morphine can be given (Hunter and Chern-Hughes, 1996). This regimen should provide 6 to 10 hours of sleep. Eighty-five percent of women treated with therapeutic rest can be expected to awaken in active phase labor. Approximately 10% of women experience cessation of regular contractions, in which case a retroactive diagnosis of false labor can be made. The remainder continue an ineffective labor pattern, and augmentation of labor may be indicated. If history or laboratory results reveal that adequate fluids have not been taken, intravenous hydration may be initiated.

If the cause of the prolonged latent phase at term is thought to be caused by a hypotonic contraction pattern, augmentation with oxytocin may be offered as an option. Oxytocin augmentation is discussed under management of protracted active phase labor. Other approaches to labor augmentation include nipple stimulation, acupressure, and use of herbs. Research suggests that nipple rolling, breast massage, application of warm compresses to the breast before nipple rolling, and use of a breast pump are effective for stimulating uterine contractions (Moenning and Hill, 1987; Salmon et al., 1986; Chayen, Tejani, and Verma, 1986; Stein et al., 1990). The association between breast stimulation and tetanic contractions resulting in decelerations in the fetal heart rate (FHR) has been noted in the literature, although research findings have been conflicting (Hill et al., 1984; Salmon et al., 1986). It appears that stimulating only one breast at a time decreases the risk of decelerations.

Acupressure to the Bladder 67 point on the outside of the little toe on both feet next to the nail has been associated with uterine stimulation (Weed, 1986).

Blue cohosh has been recommended as an herbal stimulant for labor. Blue cohosh contains the alkaloid methylcytosine that causes physiologic responses similar to those caused by nicotine, including increased pulse, blood pressure, and gastric mobility. It also contains the glycoside caulosaponin, which provides the oxytocic effect. Caulosaponin is a vasoconstrictor and particularly exerts an effect on the coronary arteries (Tyler, 1987). For these reasons, contraindications to the use of blue cohosh include cardiovascular disease, hypertension, and diabetes. One regimen for its administration is 3 to 8 drops of blue cohosh tincture in warm water or tea, repeated every 30 minutes until contractions are established. If labor is not established in 4 hours, the tincture can be put directly onto the tongue every hour for up to 9 hours or until labor is established (Hunter and Chern-Hughes, 1996). Uterine contraction pattern and FHR should be monitored closely when blue cohosh is used.

Prolonged latent phase should not be considered an indicator of dystocia, and cesarean delivery for this labor pattern alone is not appropriate (ACOG, 1995a).

Protracted Active Phase

Protracted or slow-slope active phase has been described as rate of cervical change less than 1.2 cm/hr for nulliparas and less than 1.5 cm/hr for multiparas once the cervix has reached 4 cm dilation or rapid cervical change has begun. Rate of descent is often considered in the def-inition. Protracted active phase has been associated with increased cesarean section rates and maternal exhaustion. Slow-slope active phase is often caused by a hypotonic contraction pattern, but occasionally hypertonic contraction patterns also contribute to poor progress. Protracted active phase may also be a result of fetopelvic disproportion associated with macrosomia, compromised inlet or midpelvis, or malposition contributing to increased diameters of the presenting part.

Diagnosis of protracted active phase. Diagnosis is made when progressive cervical change (1.2 cm/hr for nulliparas; 1.5 cm/hr for multiparas) is not noted by the same examiner on at least two successive vaginal exam-

Box 27-2 *Data Collection for Protracted Active Phase*

Historical Data

Gestational age
Onset of contractions
Frequency of contractions and trend over time
Duration of contractions and trend over time
Intensity of contractions and trend over time
Presence or absence of leaking amniotic fluid
Presence or absence of bloody show
Fetal activity
Rest in past 24 hours
Fluid and nutritional intake in past 24 hours
Use of analgesia or sedatives
Chart review for history of this pregnancy, obstetric history, medical/surgical history

Physical Examination Data

General appearance
Fetal presentation, position, and estimated fetal weight
Fetal heart rate pattern
Palpation of contractions for frequency, duration, and intensity
Cervical effacement
Cervical dilation
Consistency of cervix
Station of presenting part
Molding or identification of asynclitism of fetal head
Application of presenting part to cervix
Status of membranes
Clinical pelvimetry

Laboratory and Other Studies

Urine specific gravity and ketones
Ultrasound to confirm position and estimate fetal weight

inations. Data collection necessary for assessment of the problem and development of a plan of care is listed in Box 27-2.

Management of protracted active phase. If assessment confirms that the woman and her baby are healthy and coping well with the labor, conservative noninterventive support of slow active phase is appropriate. Activities that may enhance the labor pattern are change of position, ambulation, nipple stimulation, acupressure, rest, and hydration.

Augmentation of the labor through the use of amniotomy and/or oxytocin infusion is an option for active management of protracted active phase of labor. Contraindications to amniotomy include high presenting part, malpresentation or malposition, palpation of cord or vessels through the forebag, and lack of documentation of active labor. Contraindications to oxytocin infusion are summarized in Box 27-3.

Amniotomy is thought to augment labor through the release of prostaglandins and the mechanical effect of increased pressure of the presenting part on the cervix. The results of studies evaluating the use of amniotomy for augmentation have been mixed. Although some researchers have found that amniotomy decreases the length of active phase (Garite et al., 1993; Fraser et al., 1993), findings also suggest increased FHR decelerations and increased maternal infectious morbidity with use of the procedure (Garite et al., 1993; Rouse et al., 1994).

Box 27-3 *Relative Contraindications to Oxytocin Augmentation*

Known contracted pelvis
Fetal intolerance of labor
High parity
Overdistention of the uterus
Hypertonic uterine contractions

Oxytocin augmentation is most commonly used in cases of protracted active phase. The goal of oxytocin augmentation is to stimulate uterine activity to reach regular contractions every 2 to 3 minutes with pressure that is adequate to promote cervical change. There is a wide range of normal variation in the amount of oxytocin needed for individual laboring women. Research has suggested that the woman's own spontaneous contractile activity, cervical dilation, parity, and gestational age all are variables associated with the success of augmentation (ACOG, 1995a). Hyperstimulation is defined as "a persistent pattern of more than five contractions in 10 minutes, contractions lasting 2 minutes or more, or contractions of normal duration occurring within 1 minute of each other" (ACOG, 1995a, p. 5).

Oxytocin augmentation should always be administered in a dilution of a balanced salt solution using a controlled infusion pump and inserted via a secondary line to the mainline intravenously. Most institutional policies recommend a dilution of 10 U of oxytocin per 1000 ml of diluent. Ongoing assessment of the maternal and fetal response to the augmentation should be done by an experienced professional nurse and the provider. Resting tone, frequency, duration, and intensity of the contractions can be monitored with external or internal electronic monitoring or by palpation. FHR response should be monitored and documented every 15 minutes during first-stage labor and every 5 minutes during second-stage labor (ACOG, 1995a). When augmentation is initiated, a consulting physician with privileges for cesarean delivery must be readily available.

If hyperstimulation develops, immediate cessation of the oxytocin infusion is necessary. The half-life of oxytocin is 3 to 5 minutes; thus a decrease in uterine stimulation usually occurs rapidly.

As with all procedures, full explanation of augmentation, along with discussion of benefits and risks for each intervention, should take place in order for the woman to provide informed consent. If not done previously, the midwife may discuss the woman's feelings about pain relief and provide explanation of analgesia and anesthesia that may be appropriate as the contractions become more intense.

Active-Phase Arrest

Active-phase arrest has been defined as an arrest of dilation for at least 2 hours, occurring after onset of active phase (Friedman, 1954; Handa and Laros, 1993). Active-phase arrest has been associated with increased rate of cesarean section and instrumental delivery. Handa and Laros (1993) found inadequate uterine contractions in 81% of women who experienced active-phase arrest and who had documentation of intrauterine pressure catheter (IUPC) findings. Each of these women received oxytocin augmentation, but only 40% went on to deliver vaginally. Characteristics associated with active-phase arrest and subsequent cesarean delivery include estimated fetal weight of more than 4000 g and high presenting part at the time of the arrest.

Diagnosis of active-phase arrest. To diagnose active-phase arrest, it must first be determined that the woman is truly in active-phase of labor. Most sources recommend using 4 cm dilation as the minimum cervical stage to determine that latent phase of labor is complete. Diagnosis is made when no cervical change is noted by the same examiner using two vaginal examinations at least 2 hours apart. Most clinicians also include the finding of no change in descent as a requirement for diagnosis.

Management of active-phase arrest. Since most cases of active-phase arrest are associated with inadequate contractile forces, augmentation of labor is the usual approach. After discussing the benefits and risks of augmentation with the woman and obtaining her consent, administration of oxytocin using titration that leads to contractions every 2 to 3 minutes is the usual approach. There is evidence to suggest that artificial rupture of membranes may further stimulate contractions. The clinician may consider placement of an IUPC to document contractile strength. Less invasive methods to stimulate labor include encouraging rest for 1 to 2 hours, nipple stimulation, ambulation, hydrotherapy, acupressure, and intravenous hydration. Analgesia or anesthesia may be helpful in cases in which the woman is extremely tense and fearful.

The traditional recommendation regarding the length of augmentation to assess the probability of progression to vaginal delivery is to augment for 2 hours and document achieving a contractile pattern greater than 200 Montevideo units during that time. If no cervical change is made, it is assumed that there is a true active-phase arrest. Recent work suggests a trial of 4 hours of augmentation with sustained contractile pattern of 200 Montevideo units or 6 hours for women unable to sustain uterine contractile patterns of greater than 200 Montevideo units (Rouse, Owen, and Hauth, 1999). Had the researchers followed the usual practice of cesarean delivery after 2 hours of lack of progress with augmentation, the cesarean delivery rate for the cohort would have been 26% rather than the 8% achieved with more liberal time limits. There were no severe maternal or fetal complications associated with the longer augmentations.

Protracted Descent and Arrest of Descent

Protracted descent is defined as descent of the presenting part at a rate less than 1.2 cm/hr in nulliparas and less than 1.5 cm/hr in multiparas. Arrest of descent is defined as no descent in more than 1 hour in nulliparas and multiparas. The monitoring of descent is most crucial in second-stage labor. There is evidence that nulliparas who enter active-phase labor with an unengaged fetal head have an increased risk of cesarean birth. However, over 85% of these women still go on to have vaginal births, although most experience prolonged first- and second-stage labors (Roshanfeker et al., 1999).

Diagnosis of protracted descent and arrest of descent. Diagnosis is made when the same examiner finds decreased rate of descent or failure to descend on two successive vaginal examinations at least 1 hour apart. Determination of an increase in fetal head molding often accompanies true descent abnormalities.

Management of protracted descent and arrest of descent. Since descent disorders are often associated with hypotonic contractile patterns, augmentation as described in previous paragraphs is often considered. Once adequate uterine forces have been achieved and lack of descent is documented, consultation for probable cesarean section is appropriate.

Noninvasive interventions to assist with descent include maternal position changes—particularly to vertical positions—pelvic rocking, and massage, and acupressure to enhance relaxation.

Precipitate Labor

Precipitate labor is traditionally defined as labor less than or equal to 3 hours. Some authors make a distinction between short labors (<3 hours) and precipitate labor, the latter being defined as rates of cervical change or descent greater than the 95th percentile for length of labor. Precipitate labors exhibit cervical change greater than 5 cm/hour for nulliparas and 10 cm/hr for multiparas (Friedman, 1978). Although short labor theoretically has been associated with major maternal lacerations, postpartum hemorrhage, and low APGAR scores in the neonate, recent evidence disputes this (Mahan, Chazotte, and Cohen, 1994). However, precipitate labor has been associated with meconium-stained fluid, postpartum hemorrhage, and lower 1-minute APGAR scores. In Mahan's sample, women experiencing precipitate labor were more likely to have experienced placental abruption secondary to recent cocaine use.

Management of precipitate labor. Because of the association of abruption and cocaine use with precipitate labor, a thorough history to identify substance use should be taken. The actual management of the delivery does not differ significantly from normal labors and delivery. Controlled delivery of the presenting part decreases the incidence of maternal lacerations and fetal morbidity associated with expulsive birth.

MANAGEMENT OF COMPLICATIONS RELATED TO MATERNAL-FETAL STATUS

Malpresentation/Malposition: Persistent Occipitoposterior Position

Prolonged labor secondary to persistent occipitoposterior (OP) position is a commonly encountered problem. It is estimated that about 10% of fetuses are in the OP position at the beginning of labor. Most rotate spontaneously to the anterior position, often when the head is on the perineum. It has been estimated that 1% to 4.7% of births occur with the infant in the OP position (Gardberg and Tuppurainen, 1994). Women with anthropoid or android characteristics of the pelvis have an increased incidence of persistent OP position in labor. Delivery of the infant in the OP position is associated with greater incidence of severe perineal and vaginal lacerations and increased use of episiotomy, forceps, and vacuum extraction.

When the fetal head descends into the pelvis in the OP position, presenting diameters may be increased as a result of poor flexion. In addition, the fetal head may not be well applied to the cervix because of the different relationship of the fetus's head to the pelvis.

It has been reported the rupture of membranes before onset of contractions is more frequent when the fetus is in the OP position (Gardberg and Tuppurainen, 1994).

Diagnosis of persistent occipitoposterior position. Diagnosis is made through careful abdominal palpation to determine fetal position and vaginal examination to determine orientation of fetal sutures and fontanelles to the maternal pelvis. Observation of the abdomen reveals the characteristic contour of OP position—slight depression between the umbilicus and symphysis. Palpation reveals fetal back rotated toward the maternal spine, and numerous fetal small parts anteriorly. The fetal head may be nonengaged because of the poor fit in the pelvis, and the sinciput may be palpated immediately above the pubis.

Findings on vaginal examination depend on the degree of flexion of the fetal head. With adequate flexion, the anterior fontanelle is palpated in the anterior pelvis. With deflexion, the anterior fontanelle may be more mid-position Occasionally the posterior fontanelle can be reached in the posterior pelvis.

Management of persistent occipitoposterior position. Expectant management of first stage of labor is widely accepted. OP position should be suspected when the laboring woman experiences severe back pain not relieved with usual labor comfort measures during contractions. Prolonged first stage is a result of increased diameters of the fetal head and poor application of the fetal head to the cervix. Upright maternal positions and activity such as ambulation and pelvic rocking enhance descent of the presenting part. Massage, use of warm or cool compresses to the lower back, and hydrotherapy enhance coping mechanisms through the contractions.

Because of the increased incidence of prolonged labor and severe back pain, the clinician should explore feelings about pain relief with the laboring woman early in labor. Adequate pain relief can enhance coping mechanisms. Some women respond well with short-acting intravenous analgesia, particularly in late first stage. Sterile water papules have also been found to be effective in decreasing back pain. Epidural anesthesia may prove helpful in a prolonged labor, particularly by allowing the woman to rest and conserve energy for second-stage pushing. However, the relaxation of the pelvic musculature may inhibit rotation of the fetal head, leading to increased incidence of instrument-assisted deliveries.

Premature urge to push is common in late first stage. Assisting the woman into a kneeling position with the head resting on the forearms may relieve pressure on the anterior lip of the cervix. Supporting breathing patterns that prevent increased abdominal pressure may also decrease the pushing sensation.

Management of second stage is highly varied, and the use of interventions to assist the delivery remains controversial. Pushing in the upright position assists descent both because of the increased effectiveness of contractions and the better fit of the fetal head as it descends into the pelvis. Squatting increases the intraabdominal pressure with pushing and actually increases the sagittal diameter of the pelvic outlet. Kneeling may be more comfortable for some women, allows for massage and hand pressure on the lower back during pushing, and relieves pressure on the perineum, thereby decreasing perineal trauma at the time of the birth. Pearl and colleagues (1993) found that women with spontaneous OP deliveries had longer second stages of labor and higher incidence of third- and fourth-degree lacerations. Women with episiotomies had the highest incidence of severe perineal lacerations, although those with mediolateral episiotomies were less likely to have extensions into third- and fourth-degree lacerations. Perineal trauma may be increased because of the wider presenting diameters caused by incomplete flexion. Longer second stage with resultant prolonged pressure on the perineum, causing edema and friable tissue, may also be a cause of increased trauma. Increased vaginal lacerations were found when instrumental delivery was performed. Fetal morbidity (Erb's palsy, facial nerve palsy, cephalohematoma) was associated with use of instrumental delivery (Pearl et al., 1993).

Consultation with an obstetrician skilled in instrumental deliveries is warranted when a laboring woman with persistent OP position experiences a prolonged second stage of labor. Obstetric intervention is indicated when the woman is no longer tolerating the second stage or when the fetus exhibits intolerance to labor. Use of vacuum extraction may be an option for midwives and family practice physicians when state regulations and institutional policies support its use by providers who are not obstetricians.

Breech Presentation

Breech presentation is present in approximately 3% of term labors. Because of the greater amount of fluid in relationship to the mass of the fetus before term, breech presentations occur in 24% to 33% of labors in late second and early third trimesters. Many of the perinatal problems associated with breech deliveries are more related to the preterm status of the fetus rather than the breech presentation. Perinatal mortality rates at term range from 0% to 1.6% in recent published studies of breech births. By the early 1980s, cesarean section for breech presentations had become the standard of practice in North America, and in the United States about 85% of fetuses in breech presentation at the onset of labor or at term are delivered surgically (Cibils, 1995). Two randomized studies evaluating the outcomes of breech deliveries by route of delivery found no immediate perinatal benefit for the neonate delivered surgically and demonstrated increased maternal morbidity for women experiencing cesarean section (Collea, Chein, and Quilligan, 1980; Gimosky, Wallace, and Schifrin, 1983). However, the studies were completed at a time when obstetricians were being taught to attend vaginal breech births. Currently, obstetricians often complete their residencies without any experience in vaginal breech birth. Hence, there are most likely benefits to cesarean deliveries for breech when considering the lack of provider skills and practice in vaginal breech birth.

Diagnosis of breech presentation. Breech presentation can be identified by careful abdominal examination and confirmed by vaginal examination. The attitude of the breech presentation can be identified by ultrasound examination.

Box 27-4 *Important Points for Attending Emergency Breech Birth*

Keep hands off the breech until maternal expulsive efforts have delivered the infant to the level of the umbilicus.

Rotation to the sacrum anterior position is necessary for successful delivery of the fetal head.

Don't try to hasten the birth by providing traction to the trunk of the infant. This leads to deflexion of the fetal head and increases the risk of a nuchal arm.

Use a warmed towel as a sling to support the body while encouraging the mother to continue expulsive efforts to deliver the head.

Don't overextend the body as the head pivots under the symphysis pubis.

Management of breech presentation. Management of breech by the primary provider (midwife or family practice physician) depends on her or his own skills, the skills of the obstetric specialist, the practice relationship between the provider and obstetrician, and the institutional policies. When there is the opportunity for collaborative management with an obstetrician skilled in vaginal breech birth, the midwife or family practice physician may co-manage care, with the obstetrician readily available in the event that problems are encountered. More commonly the community standard is that referral to the obstetrician is expected, and management is determined by the obstetrician's beliefs and skills.

Occasionally the midwife or physician may be present at an unanticipated breech birth. Box 27-4 outlines the important points to be considered when attending an emergency breech birth. Figure 27-1 summarizes the cardinal movements of the fetus during breech birth.

Face Presentation

Face presentation occurs in approximately 1 of 250 to 500 deliveries. Hyperextension of the fetal head is associated with large infants, multiparous gestations in which there is poor abdominal tone, contracted pelvis, multiple nuchal cords, congenital anomalies, and masses in the fetal neck region as one would find with fetal goiter. Although the anteroposterior and transverse diameters of the fetal head in a face presentation are essentially the same as those of the well-flexed fetal head during dilation and descent, the actual diameter passing through the introitus is longer, thereby increasing the risk of perineal trauma. If the chin is posterior, it is impossible for the fetal head to rotate under the symphysis pubis since the bregma wedges behind the anterior pelvis. When the chin is anterior, successful vaginal delivery can usually be accomplished. The fetus/neonate usually tolerates the labor and birth but may have airway or feeding problems secondary to the edema of the face and pressure on the extended anterior neck. Although face presentation is not an absolute contraindication for out-of-hospital birth, the clinician should discuss the risk of poor labor progress and neonatal problems with parents seeking a home or birth center birth.

Diagnosis of face presentation. Diagnosis can be made by careful abdominal examination, with the examiner noting the cephalic prominence on the same side as the fetal back. Confirmation by vaginal examination can be difficult early in labor since the face can easily be confused with a breech presentation. Ultrasound examination can definitively identify face presentation and is suggested to rule out anencephaly (Wiznitzer, 1995).

Management of face presentation. Face presentations with mentum anterior can be managed expectantly, but, because of the increased risk for labor abnormalities, obstetric consultation should be obtained when the presentation is identified. When the mentum is posterior, referral to an obstetrician for cesarean delivery should be done immediately. There has been one reported series of successful reversal of face presentations under tocolysis in women who refuse cesarean delivery (Neumann et al., 1994). The option may be available when the obstetrician is skilled in the procedure and institutional policy supports it.

Unanticipated Multiple Gestation

Skilled abdominal examination and the frequency of ultrasound screening in pregnancy makes the occurrence of unanticipated multiple gestations rare. Even though the event is rare, the midwife or physician working in community-based settings must be prepared for the unexpected presentation of a laboring woman who has not had prenatal care and who is carrying twins or the rare woman who has not had an ultrasound assessment and whose body habitus precludes accurate assessment of the abdomen.

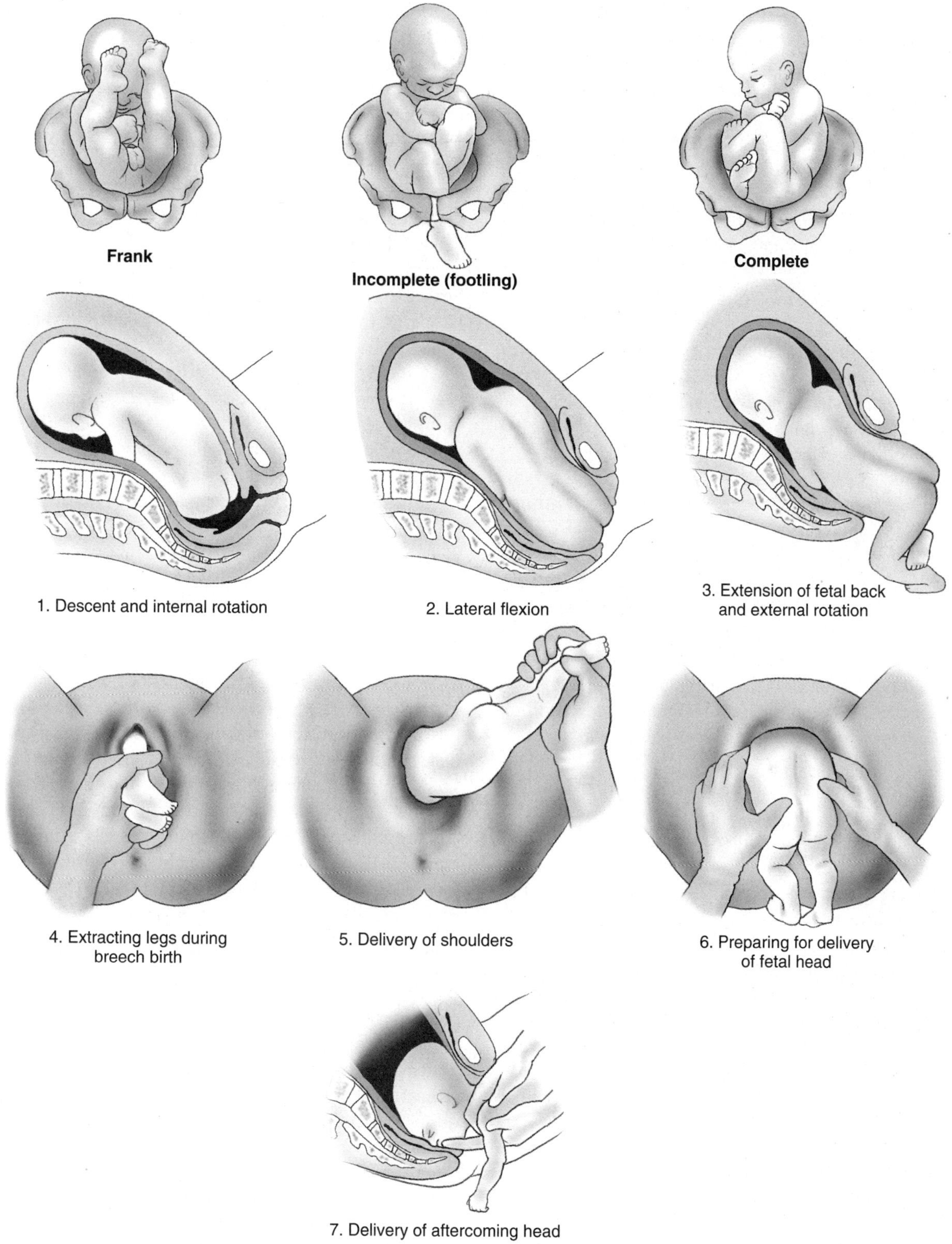

Frank

Incomplete (footling)

Complete

1. Descent and internal rotation

2. Lateral flexion

3. Extension of fetal back and external rotation

4. Extracting legs during breech birth

5. Delivery of shoulders

6. Preparing for delivery of fetal head

7. Delivery of aftercoming head

Figure 27-1 Breech birth.

Women with multiple gestation pregnancies are more likely to deliver prematurely, and their infants are more likely to experience intrauterine growth problems. Therefore, when faced with unanticipated multiple gestation, the clinician must consider the possibility of immature neonates and plan for transfer to an appropriate facility as necessary.

Diagnosis of multiple pregnancy. Careful examination of the pregnant abdomen may reveal fundal height greater than expected, palpation of two distinct fetal heads, or palpation of numerous small parts. Establishment of two or more distinct FHR patterns also indicates multiple pregnancy. Confirmation of the number of fetuses can be established using ultrasound. Multiple gestation should be suspected when an infant is delivered whose weight is clearly less than that estimated by abdominal palpation.

Management of unanticipated multiple gestation. In most communities, when a midwife or family practice physician identifies multiple gestation, the pregnant woman is referred to an obstetrician for care. In some instances, depending on the relationship between the providers and institutional policy, co-management with a midwife-obstetrician or family practice–obstetrician team is possible. This discussion addresses management of care of the woman who presents in labor with an unanticipated multiple gestation pregnancy in the community setting.

Establishment of probable gestational age is essential. When preterm birth is anticipated, the ability to transfer the woman to a hospital with at least a level II nursery before delivery needs to be addressed. If an obstetrician is immediately available, she or he should be consulted, regardless of probable gestational age. If an obstetrician is not available on site, the obstetrician covering emergencies needs to be contacted at once. Availability of a surgical team should be assessed in case cesarean section is indicated.

Determination of the position of each of the fetuses is essential. Careful abdominal examination with cervical examination to confirm position of the first fetus can be done quickly if birth is imminent. Portable ultrasound screening confirms presentation, position, and attitude of each fetus. FHR patterns for each fetus should be monitored throughout the delivery. The risk of prolapsed cord needs to be considered with small fetuses and with malpresentations.

If possible, it is helpful to have one clinician and one nurse ready for each infant's birth. In community hospital settings it is helpful to also have practitioners from the anesthesia department and the covering pediatrician available for resuscitative assistance.

Cephalic presentation of the first fetus occurs in about 75% of cases of twin gestations (Gant and Cunningham, 1993). Some authors recommend episiotomy before the delivery of the first infant in case further manipulation is necessary for the aftercoming infant. When both fetuses are vertex and there is no sign of fetal compromise, vaginal delivery is expected.

When the first fetus is in breech presentation, the birth should be managed as any emergency breech. However, the clinician needs to keep the following in mind:

- If the fetus is either unusually small or large, there may be problems with the aftercoming head.
- Prolapsed cord should be anticipated.
- If twin A is breech and twin B is vertex, there is risk for the rare but potentially lethal occurrence of locked twins.
- Because of these potential problems, cesarean delivery is recommended when the first fetus is breech (ACOG, 1998b).
- Immediate phone consultation with an obstetrician coupled with tocolysis to slow the labor may allow for preparation for surgical delivery.

Emergency delivery of the second twin demands patience and the maintenance of a calm environment. As soon as the first twin is delivered, it should be handed to the most appropriate assistant for stabilization. The size and presenting part of the second fetus is then determined. FHR pattern of the second fetus is evaluated. As long as there is no sign of fetal compromise and there is no vaginal bleeding, it is preferable to wait for the labor to resume without intervention. Labor usually resumes within 10 minutes. Gentle fundal pressure may assist the presenting part of the second fetus to descend into the pelvis if it has not entered the true pelvis. If an obstetrician is not physically present yet, phone contact for guidance as she or he is in transit is helpful. With obstetric assistance, labor can be augmented with a low-dose oxytocin infusion if labor does not resume in 10 minutes.

In summary, the role of the midwife or family practice physician when a woman presents in labor with unanticipated multiple gestation is efficient identification of the problem, immediate consultation with the covering obstetrician, maintenance of a controlled delivery if birth is imminent, and stabilization of the woman and her fetuses while awaiting the arrival of the obstetrician.

Maternal Infection—Chorioamnionitis

Chorioamnionitis is acute inflammation of the membranes. It is clinically diagnosed in 1% to 2% of all pregnancies but has been identified histologically in as many as 10% to 20%. When a woman experiences prolonged rupture of membranes, the risk of clinical infection increases to 3% to 15%. Most commonly, chorioamnionitis is caused by group B streptococcus (GBS) or *Escherichia coli,* and the mode of transmission is ascension from the vagina into the uterus. Other common pathogens include *Streptococcus faecalis, Proteus, Klebsiella,* and *Pseudomonas.* Although ascending infection tends to occur in the presence of ruptured membranes, it can also occur when the membranes are intact.

Signs of chorioamnionitis include maternal fever, maternal and fetal tachycardia, foul-smelling vaginal discharge, uterine tenderness, and leukocytosis. Fetal tachycardia usually precedes the maternal signs. Chorioamnionitis is associated with endometritis and postpartum fever. With appropriate antibiotic therapy, maternal outcome is usually good. However, chorioamnionitis may lead to septic shock, acute renal failure, and disseminated intravascular coagulation.

Neonatal infection occurs in 3% of cases in which chorioamnionitis has been identified. Infants who become infected have an increased risk of respiratory distress and intraventricular hemorrhage. The infection is usually introduced into the fetal oropharynx, leading to pulmonary and gastrointestinal effects. Occasionally the infection is introduced transplacentally, in which case the liver, brain, meninges, and heart may be affected.

Management of chorioamnionitis. Management of chorioamnionitis begins with development of a plan for delivery. Induction or augmentation of labor is preferred, since cesarean section increases the risk of systemic infection. When delivery seems remote, cesarean delivery is considered to decrease the fetus's exposure. Antibiotic therapy is initiated before delivery, and the combination of ampicillin and gentamycin is commonly used to provide broad coverage.

Suspicion of chorioamnionitis requires obstetric consultation. In cases in which the woman is stable, the fetal status is reassuring, and vaginal delivery is anticipated, co-management of the case is appropriate. In cases in which the maternal or fetal status is not reassuring, referral to the obstetric specialist is expected. The neonatal or pediatric team should be notified of the diagnosis, and a septic work-up of the neonate is usually expected.

Prelabor Rupture of Membranes at Term

The management of rupture of membranes before contractions at term remains controversial. The commonly used phrase, "premature rupture of membranes," implies that there is some "mature" time of rupture. At the time that the term "premature rupture of membranes" was coined, there had been no randomized control studies investigating the clinical options, let alone evaluating the effect of the latent time from rupture until active phase of labor (Keirse, Ottervanger, and Smit, 1996). The authors suggest the more appropriate descriptor—"prelabor rupture of membranes"—which still retains the common acronym, PROM.

Studies have found that PROM occurs in 6% to 19% of term pregnancies (Keirse, Ottervanger, and Smit, 1996). If labor is not induced, 69% of women with PROM at term will deliver within 24 hours, and 86% will deliver within 48 hours. A small proportion (2% to 5%) will not deliver until after 72 hours of rupture. Studies have suggested that, as the length of time of rupture increases, the risk of maternal and neonatal infection increases (Hannah et al., 1996). For this reason, liberal use of labor induction became popular in the 1950s to 1960s when perinatal mortality caused by infection was greater than 10%. As advances in neonatal care and development of antibiotics led to a decrease in the perinatal mortality rate, obstetricians became more concerned with the increased risk of cesarean section when early induction was used. It has only been in the last decade of the century that multicenter randomized control studies have better identified the benefits and risks of conservative or aggressive treatment. The findings of the studies, as well as those of several meta-analyses, have suggested that an active induction policy is associated with a higher rate of cesarean section, there is no difference in maternal infection when comparing active and expectant management and that an active induction policy is associated with a decrease in neonatal infection (Hannah et al., 1996; Keirse, Ottervanger, and Smit, 1996; Mozurkewich and Wolf, 1997) (Research Box 27-1).

Risk factors for chorioamnionitis and postpartum fever in PROM include more than six digital vaginal examinations and active labor longer than 12 hours. Risk factors for neonatal infection following PROM at term include chorioamnionitis, endometritis, GBS colonization, longer than 48 hours of rupture of membranes, and

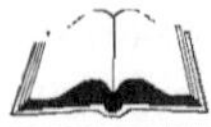

Research Box 27-1

Hannah ME et al.: Induction of labor compared with expectant management for prelabor rupture of membranes at term, *N Engl J Med* 334(16):1005-1010, 1996.

Background

Approximately 8% of pregnant women experience spontaneous rupture of membranes at term before the establishment of active labor. If labor is not induced, approximately 60% of these women begin labor spontaneously within 24 hours, and over 95% begin active labor within 72 hours. Prolonged rupture of membranes may increase the risk of infection; for this reason, many physicians recommend induction of labor if contractions don't begin shortly after rupture of membranes. However, the timing of initiation of induction is controversial; and it is strongly influenced by convenience for the physicians, nurses, and patients.

Research Questions

(1) Is the practice of inducing women with prelabor rupture of membranes at term preferable to a practice of waiting for labor to begin spontaneously if there is no evidence of fetal or maternal compromise? (2) Is there any difference in the method of induction and the outcomes of the labor?

Methods

Women who consented to participate in the study were randomly assigned to one of four groups. In one group labor was induced immediately with oxytocin infusion. In the second group labor was induced immediately using prostaglandin gel followed by oxytocin infusion as necessary. In the third and fourth groups women were managed expectantly unless there was evidence of fetal or maternal compromise or until 4 days had elapsed. Group 3 was then induced using oxytocin infusion, and group 4 was induced using prostaglandin gel followed by oxytocin infusion as necessary. The primary outcome was definite or probable neonatal sepsis. Definite sepsis was defined as presence of clinical signs of infection plus at least one of the following: positive blood, spinal fluid (CSF), urine, tracheal aspirate or lung tissue culture; positive Gram stain of CSF; positive antigen-detection tests on body fluids; or radiographic or histologic confirmation of pneumonia. Probable infection was defined as clinical signs of infection plus at least one of the following: high or low blood neutrophil count, high immature-to-total neutrophil ratio, high actual immature neutrophil count, or abnormal CSF findings. Other process variables and outcomes explored included obstetric factors (e.g., parity, previous obstetric history), reason for induction in the expectant groups, operative vaginal delivery, cesarean delivery, use of internal fetal monitoring, fetal distress, meconium-stained fluid, signs of maternal infection, administration of antibiotics, number of digital cervical examinations, time to active labor, duration of active labor, and interval from rupture to delivery. Women also were asked to evaluate their experience and the care they received.

prolonged internal fetal monitoring (Seaward et al., 1998; Yancey et al., 1996).

Management of premature rupture of membranes at term. Accurate diagnosis of PROM is the first step in management. Historical data include the woman's complaint of a sudden gush of fluid from the vagina or a constant leaking of fluid. Obvious leaking or pooling of fluid that has vernix and/or fetal hair is diagnostic. When the rupture of membranes is not obvious, sterile speculum examination can confirm the diagnosis by identification of pooling of fluid in the posterior fornix and by providing secretions that can be examined for pH and ferning.

Establishment of fetal well-being, presentation, and gestational age are necessary to determine which options are reasonable. If screening for GBS has not been done at 35 to 37 weeks, the use of the fast-acting screen for GBS should be considered. When the woman has experienced a healthy pregnancy, fetal status is reassuring, and there is a negative screen for GBS, the clinician should discuss the benefits and risks of active and conservative management. Ultimately the woman should determine which approach is in concert with her beliefs and expectations for labor. In the absence of risk factors for maternal and neonatal infection, the decision is usually influenced by her beliefs about the use of technology in an otherwise normal labor. Some women are very comfortable with the use of continuous fetal monitoring and the somewhat higher rate of epidural anesthesia that are associated with active early

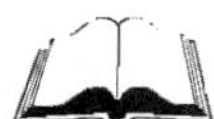

Research Box 27-1—cont'd

Sample

The study enrolled 5042 women at 72 hospitals in Canada, the United Kingdom, Australia, Israel, Sweden, and Denmark. Data were complete for all but one participant. Baseline data, including maternal age, parity, gestational age, interval from membrane rupture until delivery, and other obstetric factors were similar in the four groups. Sample size provided a power of 80% to detect a reduction of 50% or more in cases of neonatal infection (4% to 2%).

Results

Labor began spontaneously in 77% of the women in the expectant/oxytocin group and 78.5% of the expectant/prostaglandin group. Reasons for inductions in the expectant groups included obstetric complications, chorioamnionitis, rupture of membranes greater than 4 days, and request by patient or physician. The rates for cesarean delivery or instrumental vaginal delivery were similar in all groups. Women in the induction/oxytocin group experienced less chorioamnionitis, postpartum fever, administration of antibiotics, fewer digital cervical examination; they had shorter labors and shorter intervals from membrane rupture to delivery. Women in the induction/prostaglandin group had a shorter interval from membrane rupture to delivery than the expectant groups; they did experience more digital examinations than the induction/oxytocin group. There were no differences among groups in neonatal infection or morbidity. Women in the induction/oxytocin and induction/prostaglandin groups were less likely to report negative feelings about the management of care.

Clinical Implications

The overall incidence of neonatal sepsis (2.6%) was low in this sample and did not differ by management approach. Therefore there is no clear neonatal advantage to induction or expectant management when planning care for a woman who experiences prelabor rupture of membranes at term. These findings conflict with other studies that have suggested decreased neonatal sepsis rates when induction is initiated following prelabor membrane rupture. Contrary to the findings in other studies, this study did not find an increase in cesarean delivery when induction is used. The findings suggest that any of these approaches are reasonable options for women who experience term membrane rupture before labor. For this reason, the clinician should explain the benefits and risks of each option and support the woman's decision regarding induction or expectant management. Of interest is the finding that women seemed to view induction more favorably than expectant management. Further research is necessary to determine whether there are subpopulations of women who differ from this perception and to determine whether the woman's sense of control influences the evaluation of care.

induction. Others may feel very strongly about minimizing intervention as long as the labor is progressing normally.

Regardless of the decision to manage actively or conservatively, digital cervical examinations should be kept to a minimum to decrease the risk of infection. At the very least, digital cervical examination should be deferred until active labor. Active management can include the use of prostaglandin gel for cervical ripening and induction using oxytocin. Institutional policy may require that, when the primary provider is a midwife, obstetric consultation is necessary before induction.

When a woman chooses to await spontaneous labor, she and her clinician should mutually agree on a plan of care that will ensure ongoing assessment of fetal status and identification of signs of infection. Midwifery practices typically use a combination of the following screening/diagnostic procedures when managing PROM at term conservatively:

- Fetal movement counts several times per day
- Teaching the woman and/or her partner how to auscultate FHTs and identify fetal tachycardia
- Daily assessments by the midwife to evaluate fetal and maternal status
- Maternal temperature BID
- Baseline complete blood count with differential, with repeats every 24 to 48 hours

In addition, the midwife should review the following danger signs and instruct the woman to contact the midwife immediately if any are noted: fever, chills, increased maternal pulse, decreased fetal movement, meconium-stained fluid, or four-smelling fluid.

Obstetric consultation is necessary when signs of maternal infection are present and when fetal status is nonreassuring. If the practice or institution is using the risk-associated approach to neonatal GBS prevention, intrapartum antibiotic prophylaxis should be initiated at 18 hours following rupture.

Uterine Rupture

Rupture of the uterus is an obstetric emergency requiring prompt diagnosis and management to prevent or decrease maternal and fetal mortality and morbidity. Complete rupture involves all layers of the uterine wall and pelvic peritoneum with extrusion of the fetus into the peritoneal cavity. Incomplete rupture (dehiscence, silent rupture, occult rupture, creation of a uterine window) involves the separation of the myometrium, with the pelvic peritoneum remaining intact. The fetus usually remains inside the uterus in cases of incomplete rupture.

Rupture of the uterus can be spontaneous, traumatic, or rupture of a previous scar. Spontaneous rupture is a result of strong uterine contractions, often in association with obstructed labor. The rupture usually occurs in the lower uterine segment. Spontaneous rupture is associated with placental abruption and use of oxytocin. With the increase in use of "crack" cocaine in pregnancy in some communities, ruptures associated with abruption have increased. Although rare, spontaneous rupture has been documented in primigravida labors. Traumatic rupture is associated with use of instruments, intrauterine manipulation, misuse of oxytocic drugs, and severe blunt trauma to the abdomen.

Rupture of a uterine scar is more likely (estimated 2% incidence) with a classical (longitudinal) scar. The rupture may occur in late pregnancy or during labor. Rupture of a transverse scar in the lower uterine segment is most likely to occur during labor, and the incidence is estimated to be 0.82%. Although most scar ruptures involve scars from previous cesarean sections, other surgeries or procedures such as myomectomy or hysteroscopy may also increase the risk of rupture. Scar ruptures are more likely to be incomplete ruptures.

Diagnosis of ruptured uterus. Alteration of FHR patterns suggesting distress is a common early finding in cases of rupture. Complete spontaneous rupture of the uterus usually presents as severe and continuous abdominal pain, followed by cessation of rhythmic uterine contractions. Vaginal bleeding may be present. Ruptured uterus must be suspected when abdominal palpation reveals dramatic change in fetal position, distinct palpation of the fetus outside the contracting uterus, or change of station from deep in the pelvis to floating outside the pelvis.

Incomplete rupture may present with no signs or symptoms or may mimic complete rupture. Rachagan (1991) found that classic symptoms of rupture were present only in 35% of incomplete ruptures and that an increase in maternal pulse and cessation of fetal heart tones were the most common findings. Often an incomplete rupture is diagnosed only at the time of surgery or with exploration of the uterus after a birth.

Although it may seem counterintuitive, research has indicated that use of an IUPC is of little or no value in identifying rupture of the uterus (Flamm and Quilligan, 1995).

Other maternal signs and symptoms of rupture include tachycardia, syncope, vomiting, pallor, and hypotension.

Management of ruptured uterus. Management is determined by the acuity of the situation. In a complete rupture with maternal shock and fetal distress, immediate setup for surgery while calling for anesthesia and surgical support is necessary. Initiation of an intravenous line with a large-bore catheter or initiation of a second line should be accomplished immediately. Blood products should be ordered STAT. In cases in which the woman and the fetus are stable (incomplete rupture), cesarean section and repair of the site of rupture can be accomplished in a less emergent manner.

Issues surrounding vaginal birth after cesarean. Trial of labor after previous cesarean birth continues to be a controversial subject. In an effort to decrease the cesarean section rate in the United States, physicians have been encouraged to offer the option of vaginal birth after cesarean (VBAC) to women. It has been estimated that about 75% of women experiencing cesarean birth will be able to experience vaginal births in subsequent pregnancies (Flamm et al., 1988; Flamm et al., 1990; Miller, Diaz, and Paul, 1994). Many physicians are uncomfortable with the less than 1% risk of uterine rupture associated with VBAC with a low transverse uterine scar. Numerous studies have indicated that even when rupture occurs, maternal and neonatal outcomes are good. However, there has been documentation of perinatal deaths, almost always when women were attempting VBAC without close assessment during labor.

Identification of factors strongly associated with increased risk of rupture of a previous uterine scar has been difficult. However, findings in studies using different methodologies suggest that history of two or more previous cesarean deliveries, excessive use of oxytocin, and presence of dysfunctional labor may increase the risk of rupture (Leung et al., 1993; Miller et al., 1994).

A rational approach to offering VBAC as an option should include the following actions:

1. Documentation of the previous uterine scar should be attempted. Even if medical records cannot be obtained (e.g., when the delivery has occurred outside the United States), documentation of the attempt to confirm the scar is important. When documentation of the scar is not possible, it is important to gain as much information regarding the reason for the cesarean from the woman in order to identify situations in which a classical or vertical incision may have been made. Cesarean deliveries that are performed for "failure to progress," suspicious FHR patterns, breech presentation, or genital herpes almost always use low transverse uterine incisions. Transverse lie, placenta previa, or sudden severe fetal distress present situations in which there is a greater chance of the use of a vertical incision (Flamm and Quilligan, 1995).
2. The provider should present the benefits and risks of VBAC prenatally to all women for whom it appears that VBAC is an option. Written material at her level of literacy and in her language should be shared with the woman so that she makes a decision based on sound understanding of the benefits and risks.
3. Oxytocin induction or augmentation should be used with extreme care. Although use of the IUPC is not helpful in diagnosing rupture, it is warranted with oxytocin use in labor to better monitor the intensity of the contractions.
4. The FHR pattern should be monitored throughout the labor, and obstetric consultation should be obtained immediately for any sudden, moderate-to-severe variable decelerations or bradycardia. Immediate cesarean birth is warranted with these signs of fetal distress.
5. A physician credentialed to perform an emergency cesarean section should be immediately available.
6. The surgical team, including an anesthesiologist, should be immediately available in case emergency cesarean section is necessary.

It is important to consider that most of the studies that have supported the safety of VBAC have been conducted in teaching hospitals with immediate availability of obstetricians, anesthesiologists, and neonatologists. There has been little evaluation of the safety of VBAC in community hospitals when all of these specialists may not be on site. It seems reasonable to include the immediate availability of resources for emergency cesarean section in VBAC policies in community hospitals or birth centers.

Inversion of the Uterus

Inversion of the uterus is a potentially life-threatening event that occurs in approximately 1:2,500 to 15,000 births. Factors associated with inversion include multiparity, placenta accreta, uterine atony, leiomyomas, and mismanagement of the third stage of labor. Partial inversion occurs when only the fundus inverts into the uterus. Complete inversion occurs when the fundus passes through the cervix into the vagina.

Diagnosis of inversion of the uterus. Diagnosis is made when the care provider notes an abnormal decrease in fundal height or inability to palpate the fundus abdominally following the birth of the infant or when the uterus is seen in the vaginal vault or at the introitus. Inversion is usually accompanied by hemorrhage and resultant maternal shock.

Management of inversion of the uterus. The most important management is prevention of inversion. Tension of the cord to try to hasten third stage is not appropriate and may prove dangerous to the mother.

Treatment requires immediate replacement of the uterus into the pelvis. Immediate replacement of the uterus can be accomplished using a fist or several fingers on the dominant hand. Once replaced, bimanual compression can further reduce hemorrhage. Intravenous fluids should be given for stabilization, and oxytocin or methylergonovine administered to prevent atony. If immediate replacement is not accomplished, anesthesia and emergency surgical support are required.

Prolapsed Cord

Prolapsed cord describes the presence of the umbilical cord below the presenting part of the fetus. Occult cord presentation occurs when the cord is compressed above the level of the presenting part. In term pregnancy with the fetus in a vertex presentation and occipitoanterior position, the fetal head usually fills the pelvis well, decreasing the risk of prolapse. When there is a poor fit of the presenting part (e.g., in cases of malpresentation, malposition, and preterm labor), there is increased risk for prolapse. Additional risk factors for prolapsed cord include rupture of membranes with an unengaged presenting part, multiple gestation, and displacement of an engaged presenting part during cervical examination or intervention.

Diagnosis of prolapsed cord. Vaginal examination that reveals presence of cord behind fetal membranes is diagnostic. When membranes rupture, vaginal examination reveals presence of cord in the vaginal vault or even extending through the introitus. Sudden deceleration of FHR immediately with rupture of membranes, particularly with a contraction, should make the clinician suspicious of prolapse. Vaginal examination should be done immediately to confirm the diagnosis. Occasionally cord prolapse is diagnosed during ultrasound examination.

Management of cord prolapse. Management of cord prolapse is guided by the stage of labor and the condition of the fetus. If FHR is present, the clinician must prepare for delivery while attempting to keep the fetus well oxygenated. If fetal heart tones are absent, labor is allowed to continue with the eventual delivery of a stillborn infant.

When the diagnosis of prolapsed cord is made during first stage with presence of FHR, the clinician should call for immediate operative support. While staff prepare the woman for an immediate cesarean section, the midwife or labor nurse should position the woman in knee-chest position, elevate the foot of the bed, and insert two to three fingers or the entire hand into the vagina to elevate the fetal head off the cord. Care should be taken to not manipulate a prolapsed cord since stimulation may lead to cord spasm. If the cord is protruding outside the vagina, it should be protected with warm saline–soaked gauze. Fetal heart tones should be monitored throughout the preparation for surgery. The counterpressure against the presenting part should not be removed until the surgical delivery of the infant.

Fetal Intolerance of Labor

Fetal intolerance of labor is an indication for surgical delivery. It is inappropriate to use the older term, fetal distress, since that term is imprecise and nonspecific in describing the fetal status (ACOG, 1998a). When assessing FHR patterns, the terms "reassuring" and "nonreassuring" should be used, along with a further description of the interpretation of findings.

Nonreassuring patterns are nonspecific without further assessment by the physician or midwife. Associated fetal factors such as presence or absence of problems identified during the pregnancy must be considered when seeking to determine the underlying cause of the patterns. Management should reflect appropriate actions to affect the probable underlying problem.

Nonreassuring baseline patterns. FHR baseline must be assessed between contractions and between periodic changes such as accelerations and decelerations for at least a 10-minute period of time. Baseline tachycardia is associated with infection, hypoxemia, anemia, prematurity, cardiac dysrhythmias, maternal fever, maternal dehydration, and anxiety (Simpson and Creehan, 1996). Beta sympathomimetic drugs can also cause fetal and maternal tachycardia.

The management of fetal tachycardia associated with maternal infection includes monitoring maternal temperature, intravenous hydration, and consideration of administration of intravenous antibiotics. Consultation with an obstetrician is warranted, and cesarean section is appropriate if delivery is not imminent. Fetal tachycardia associated with late or variable decelerations suggests fetal hypoxemia. Maternal position change, fetal scalp stimulation to assess response, administration of intravenous fluids, and administration of oxygen via face mask to the mother may alleviate the decelerations. If the increased baseline and decelerations continue following these initial interventions, obstetric consultation is necessary.

Baseline bradycardia is associated with hypoxemia or asphyxia, vagal stimulation, cardiac anomalies, or hypothermia (Simpson and Creehan, 1996). Bradycardia requires immediate obstetric consultation. Bradycardia with normal fetal activity is associated with complete atrioventricular heart block. No intervention is necessary during labor, but the neonatal team should be alerted for assessment and possible cardioversion or pacemaker insertion following the birth. Second-stage bradycardia may occur, and, as long as the variability remains normal and the FHR does not fall below 80 to 90 beats/min, no intervention to expedite birth is usually needed. Management of bradycardia includes maternal position change, hydration, and maternal oxygen administration via face mask.

When bradycardia follows a nonreassuring pattern, immediate cesarean section is indicated. This pattern of terminal bradycardia may be a result of hypoxia and can precede intrauterine death.

Baseline variability. Variability reflects the ability of the cardiac system to maintain balance between the sympathetic and parasympathetic aspects of the autonomic nervous system. Normal variability is one of the best indicators of intact integration of the central nervous system and cardiac functioning (Gabbe, Niebyl, and Simpson, 1999). Decrease in variability is associated with administration of medications that depress the central nervous system, fetal tachycardia, prematurity, fetal sleep cycles, hypoxemia, and cardiac or central nervous system anomalies. When the fetus has had average variability and variability decreases following the administration of pharmacologic agents such as narcotics or tranquilizers, no interventions are necessary. Persistent absent or minimal variability requires obstetric consultation along with maternal position change and hydration. Marked variability may be an early sign of mild hypoxia and is usually associated with normal pH.

A sinusoidal heart rate is a smooth, undulating pattern of uniform variability with an amplitude of 5 to 20 beats/min and resembling a sine wave (Gabbe, Niebyl, and Simpson, 1999). Sinusoidal patterns are associated with fetal anemia, including the anemia secondary to the hemolysis found in Rh alloimmunization. Pseudosinusoidal patterns can be noted with narcotic analgesia. When sinusoidal patterns are identified, fetal scalp sampling can be used to assess hematocrit and pH. Identification of sinusoidal patterns requires obstetric consultation.

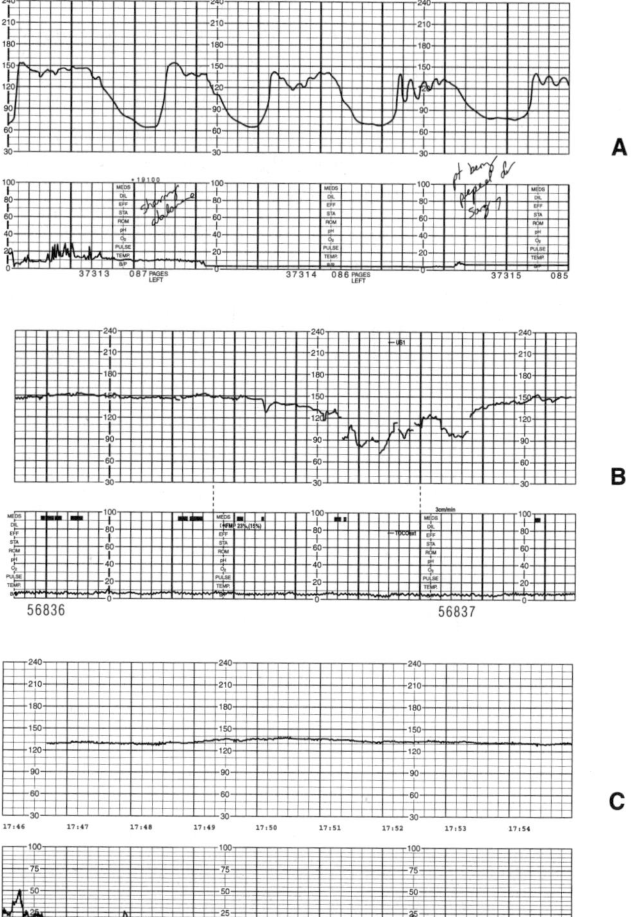

Figure 27-2 **A,** Moderate-to-severe variable decelerations with decreased variability; **B,** prolonged variable deceleration; **C,** absent variability. (**A** to **C** from Tucker SM: *Pocket guide to fetal monitoring,* ed. 4, St. Louis, 2000, Mosby.)

Periodic changes in FHR patterns

Early Decelerations Early decelerations are most commonly caused by fetal head compression with a resulting vagal response. As long as nonreassuring aspects of the FHR pattern are absent, there is no intervention necessary since early decelerations are not associated with fetal hypoxemia.

Moderate-to-Severe Variable Decelerations Variable decelerations occur in response to umbilical cord compression or vagal stimulation. Variable decelerations are reassuring when they last less than 60 seconds, when there is normal baseline and variability, and when they return rapidly to the baseline. Variable decelerations that are persistent and that progress to lower and lower FHR during their nadir are considered nonreassuring. When the FHR decreases to 60 to 70 beats/min and when a slow return to baseline occurs, there is an increased risk of hypoxia. Fetuses who are acidotic often demonstrate severe variable decelerations with slow return to baseline, accompanied by baseline tachycardia (ACOG, 1995b). Figure 27-2, *A* to *C,* illustrates nonreassuring patterns.

Management for moderate-to-severe variable decelerations includes maternal position change and administration of intravenous fluids and oxygen per face mask at 8 to10 L/min. Administration of maternal oxygen may increase the fetal PO_2 by 30% to 40% (ACOG, 1995b). When these interventions do not alleviate the problem, obstetric consultation is required. If oligohydramnios has been identified, amnioinfusion may decrease the extent of cord compression.

Moderate-to-severe variable decelerations may progress to prolonged decelerations, which may last from 2 to 10 minutes. A deceleration of greater than 10 minutes is considered a baseline change. Prolonged decelerations may be a result of a solitary episode of cord compression, maternal hypotension, hyperstimulation of the uterus, or vagal stimulation (Simpson and Creehan, 1996). Management includes the actions for variable decelerations, plus the discontinuing of any oxytocin infusion. Vaginal examination is also indicated to rule out prolapsed cord.

Late Decelerations Late decelerations are associated with transient fetal hypoxia associated with decreased placental perfusion (ACOG, 1995b). Chronic impaired perfusion can be associated with placental abnormalities and maternal medical problems, including hypertension, diabetes, and collagen disorders. Acute impaired perfusion is associated with uterine hyperstimulation, maternal hypotension, and placental abruption.

Isolated late decelerations do not require specific intervention other than ongoing assessment. Persistent late decelerations are always considered nonreassuring and require obstetric consultation. Persistent late decelerations that are a result of central nervous system reflex secondary to hypoxia become deeper as the hypoxia becomes more severe. When persistent late decelerations are associated with metabolic acidosis from tissue hypoxia, the depth of the deceleration is not correlated with severity of hypoxia (ACOG, 1995b). Management of persistent late decelerations includes all of the interventions noted previously to increase perfusion to the fetus (i.e., maternal position change, administration of intravenous fluids, discontinuation of oxytocin infusion, and oxygen by face mask).

In all cases of apparent fetal intolerance to labor, the decision to intervene surgically or with instrumental delivery depends on the likelihood of hypoxia and metabolic acidosis and the estimated time to vaginal delivery. Even in the face of nonreassuring decelerations, when there is normal variability and no tachycardia, the risk of acidosis is very low (ACOG, 1995b). Management of fetal intolerance to labor requires, at the minimum, ongoing obstetric consultation. When the fetus appears to be relatively stable, co-management with the obstetric specialist is appropriate. When the fetus is not stable, referral for full obstetric management is necessary.

Shoulder Dystocia

True shoulder dystocia occurs when the anterior shoulder becomes impacted behind the symphysis pubis. "Tight" shoulders, in which there is soft tissue resistance to delivery, is a condition often misdiagnosed as shoulder dystocia. Shoulder dystocia occurs in 0.2% to 0.6% of vaginal deliveries (Baskett and Allen, 1995). Shoulder dystocia is suspected when the fetal head delivers and there is delay in rotation of the shoulders to the anteroposterior diameter and/or inability to deliver the shoulders with usual hand maneuvers. Dystocia should also be suspected when the fetal head is immediately pulled back against the vulva following delivery ("turtle sign"). One consistent finding in studies of shoulder dystocia is that, although there are factors associated with increased risk of shoulder dystocia, most cases occur with no risk factors at all.

The following associated factors have been identified:

- *Uncontrolled diabetes.* The association of uncontrolled diabetes and macrosomia is well-established. The important factor to keep in mind is the fact that these babies develop shoulder and body diameters greater than head diameters secondary to increased body fat (Nocon et al., 1993).
- *Birth weight greater than 4000 g.* Increased birth weight in and of itself is not a factor, but rather the occurrence of true macrosomia in which there is an increase in body size in relation to the diameters of the fetal head. Because true macrosomia is difficult to diagnose, many authorities use birth weight greater than 4000 or 4500 g as a proxy indicator (McFarland et al., 1995; Nocon et al., 1993; Spong et al., 1995).
- *Prolonged second stage of labor.* Prolonged second stage has long been considered a factor in shoulder dystocia, but more recent studies stress that prolonged second stage in the presence of a large fetus is more predictive. Other investigators have found no association between length of second stage and shoulder dystocia (McFarland et al., 1995).
- *Midpelvis instrumental deliveries.* The use of midpelvis instrumental deliveries continues to be a consistent factor associated with shoulder dystocia (McFarland et al., 1995). The use of forceps or vacuum assistance may lead to delivery of the large fetal head, but the following large shoulders may become impinged above the symphysis.
- *Oxytocin induction or augmentation used when macrosomia is suspected.* Since there is an increased risk of dysfunctional labors with large infants, oxytocin is frequently used to facilitate

delivery. The multiple factors of large infant, dysfunctional labor, and induction or augmentation increase the risk of shoulder dystocia.

Shoulder dystocia is associated with increased maternal and neonatal morbidity. Because of the association among increased birth weight, use of instruments, and prolonged second stage labor, maternal complications include increased perineal and vaginal trauma and blood loss. Neonatal complications associated with shoulder dystocia include brachial plexus nerve damage and paralysis, fractured clavicles, cerebral hemorrhage, and asphyxia. However, recent research suggests that brachial plexus may be related to other factors, including malpresentation (Gherman, Ouzounian, and Goodwin, 1999; Gilbert, Nesbitt, and Danielsen, 1999). Asphyxia and cerebral hemorrhage may lead to perinatal death.

Diagnosis of shoulder dystocia. Shoulder dystocia may be diagnosed when maneuvers in addition to gentle downward traction of the fetal head are necessary to deliver the shoulders. Spong and colleagues (1995) suggest use of more objective criteria to more accurately identify all cases of shoulder dystocia, and propose that consideration be given to use of total head-to-body delivery time be used to define shoulder dystocia. In their sample, head-to-body delivery times greater than 60 seconds appeared to be related to true shoulder dystocia.

Management of shoulder dystocia. As soon as shoulder dystocia is suspected, the clinician should call for help and ask an assistant to note the time. Response from obstetrics, anesthesia, and pediatrics should be expected. It is helpful to keep in mind that, during the first 5 minutes, maneuvers are chosen to decrease risk of injury to mother and baby. During the second 5 minutes, knowing that further delay could lead to death, more dramatic measures can be taken, balancing potential injury to the mother and/or baby with the more severe harm that is done by not delivering the body within 10 minutes.

- Apply firm yet gentle downward traction to the fetal head for 1 minute. During this time it may be helpful to hyperflex the mother's thighs onto her abdomen (McRobert's maneuver) to increase pelvic outlet diameters (Figure 27-3).
- During the second minute, have an assistant provide firm suprapubic pressure while again providing firm downward traction of the head.
- During the third minute, attempt to deliver the posterior shoulder, followed by the anterior shoulder.
- During the fourth minute, attempt to rotate the fetal shoulders into the oblique diameter using two to three fingers on the dominant hand, and repeat firm downward pressure.
- During the fifth minute, attempt the Screw maneuver (Figure 27-4).

Throughout the management of the shoulder dystocia, it is helpful to have the assistant call out the time elapsed each minute. With the sense of urgency to complete delivery of the infant's body, the clinician may think that more time has elapsed than truly has. This sense of urgency may lead to more vigorous attempts of extraction than necessary during these first 5 minutes. The most important process is the consistent firm downward pressure on the fetal head. Excessive pressure and lateral flexion of the fetal head are associated with increased risk of brachial palsy injuries.

If these steps are not successful, reposition the mother and start again. There is evidence that moving the mother onto all-fours may facilitate delivery of the shoulders (the Gaskin maneuver) (Bruner et al., 1998). In most cases the repositioning alone accompanied by renewed efforts to deliver the shoulders will be successful. If the new efforts fail, intentional fracturing of the clavicle is recommended. This is accomplished by the clinician putting the thumb on the anterior fetal clavicle and the second and third fingers on the posterior aspect of the clavicle. The clavicle is then snapped, much like a matchstick can be snapped between thumb and fingers. The maneuver is difficult because of the tight presentation of the shoulders.

Older texts and articles suggest fundal pressure to assist with delivery. Fundal pressure should be avoided since it further impinges the anterior shoulder against the symphysis pubis. Excessive fundal pressure is also a factor in premature separation of the placenta.

Many authorities recommend cutting a large episiotomy as soon as shoulder dystocia is suspected. An episiotomy does not alter the bony dystocia, but gives the clinician more room to maneuver her or his hands in attempting to free the impacted shoulder.

Early Postpartum Hemorrhage

Postpartum hemorrhage remains a significant contributor to maternal morbidity and mortality. It can occur without warning, and the clinician must be ready to provide prompt, effective intervention to limit blood loss and ultimately to prevent death.

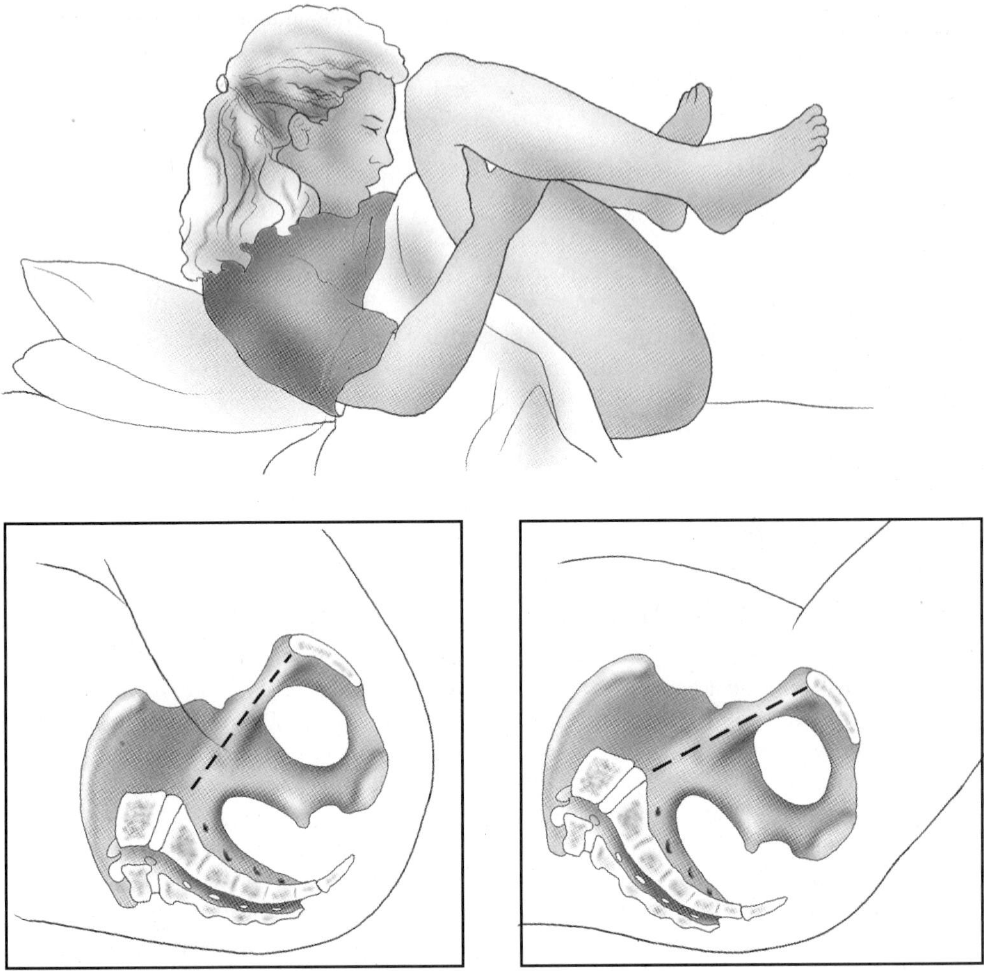

Figure 27-3 McRobert's maneuver.

Traditionally postpartum hemorrhage has been defined as blood loss of greater than 500 ml after the birth, although some sources now suggest using 1000 ml as the cut-off. Pregnancy hypervolemia normally increases blood volume by about 1000 to 2000 ml, so that blood loss during delivery is usually tolerated without significant decrease in hematocrit. Hemorrhage can be defined as a decrease in hematocrit of at least 10%. A decrease in hemoglobin of 1 to 1.5 g/dl or hematocrit of 3% corresponds with blood loss of 450 to 500 ml. Hemorrhage can occur because of bleeding from the placental site, bleeding from sites of trauma, or dysfunctional coagulation mechanisms. Eighty to ninety percent of early postpartum hemorrhage occurs during the first hour after delivery. Hemorrhage occurring after 24 hours following delivery is usually referred to as late or delayed postpartum hemorrhage. Conditions that increase the risk of postpartum hemorrhage are listed in Box 27-5.

The most common cause of postpartum hemorrhage is uterine atony. Often the atony is caused by mismanagement of the third stage of labor. Attempting to deliver the placenta before full separation can result in adherent pieces of placenta and membranes that inhibit the contractibility of the myometrium, resulting in continued patency of uterine vessels at the site. Atony can also be related to the use of certain drugs (oxytocin, magnesium sulfate, beta-adrenergic tocolytic agents, diazoxide, calcium channel blockers, and halothane) (Simpson and Creehan, 1996).

Management of postpartum hemorrhage. Anticipation of postpartum hemorrhage is the first management strategy. Women with increased risk of hemorrhage should have an intravenous line placed during labor and should have blood drawn for typing and screening in case of need for transfusion. Immediately after the de-

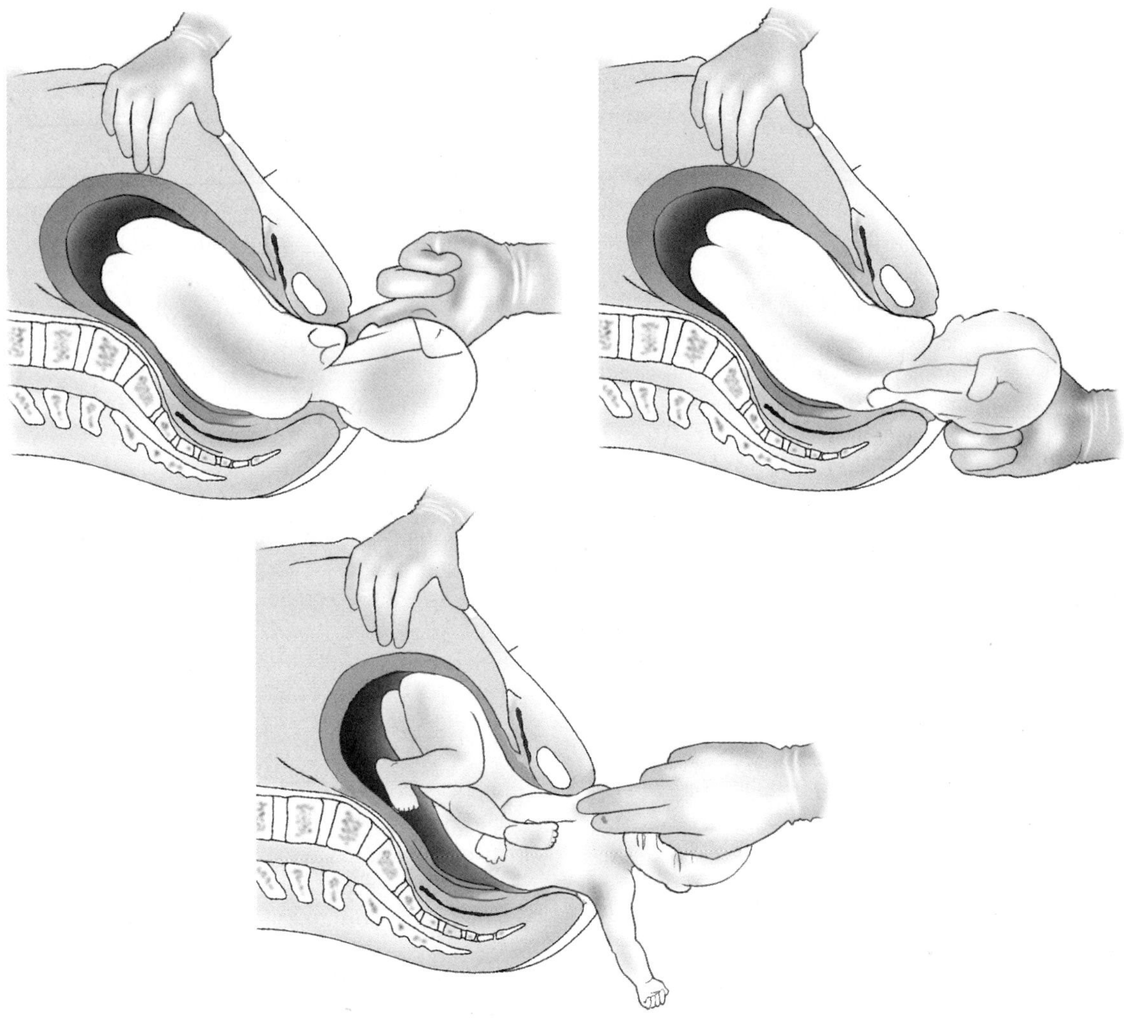

Figure 27-4 Screw maneuver.

Box 27-5 *Conditions Associated with Postpartum Hemorrhage*

Uterine Atony

Overdistended uterus
Anesthesia or analgesia
Rapid labor
Prolonged labor
Induction or augmentation of labor
History of postpartum hemorrhage
Grand multiparity

Tissue Trauma

Perineal or vulvar lacerations
Episiotomy
Cervical or vaginal lacerations
Uterine rupture

Placental Conditions

Low-lying placenta
Placenta accreta

Other

Large fibroids
Chorioamnionitis

livery of the placenta, a birth assistant should assess the fundus to determine whether it is firm or boggy. If the uterus is not contracting well, massage should be administered until there is sustained contractile activity. When women have risk factors for postpartum hemorrhage, it is reasonable to give oxytocin or methylergonovine prophylactically.

Early postpartum hemorrhage usually presents as excessive vaginal bleeding, often with clots. At times the hemorrhage may present as a constant "trickle" of bleeding. Blood pressure alone is not accurate in assessing the degree of hypovolemia since vasoconstriction shunts blood to the vital organs early in the process of hypovolemic shock. A decrease in mean arterial pressure to 30 mm Hg or less is suggestive of hypovolemia (Simpson and Creehan, 1996). When hemorrhage is diagnosed, it is advisable to begin administration of 20 U of oxytocin in 1000 ml of lactated Ringer's intravenous solution at a rate of 10 ml/min. If necessary, prostaglandin F_{2a}, 0.25 mg intramuscularly, can be given and repeated at 15- to 90-minute intervals.

If initial fundal massage and administration of medication to contract the uterus do not control the bleeding, the clinician should call for help and initiate bimanual compression (Figure 27-5). If bimanual compression is not effective within moments, blood should be ordered for transfusion, and uterine exploration for retained fragments should be done. Preparation for transfer to an operating room for surgical intervention should be completed while awaiting the surgical team.

If bleeding continues and the fundus remains firm, the clinician must consider that the source is soft tissue trauma. The perineum, vagina, and cervix should be inspected closely to identify previously overlooked lacerations. Inspection requires excellent visualization, which may require using stirrups and additional light sources. Any lacerations that are actively bleeding must be repaired immediately. Consultation and co-management are warranted when severe lacerations are identified.

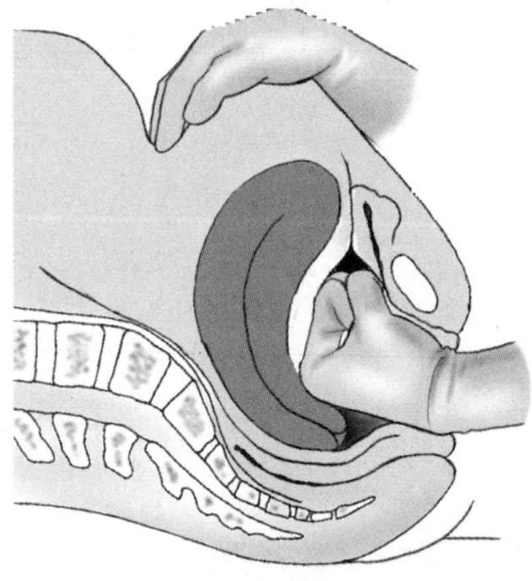

Figure 27-5 Bimanual compression of the uterus.

The clinician should note whether the blood is clotting and whether the clot is firm or friable. Unstable clot formation is a sign of coagulopathy, and immediate consultation with a perinatologist is in order.

Following control of hemorrhage, frequent fundal assessments should be done to ensure adequate contractile activity. Continuing the intravenous oxytocin infusion for several hours should be considered. Administration of oral methylergonovine, 0.2 mg every 4 to 6 hours for six doses can be considered, particularly for women with a history of postpartum hemorrhage in previous pregnancies and for those who are not breastfeeding. Follow-up determination of hemoglobin and hematocrit should be obtained 24 hours after the hemorrhage to estimate total blood loss and evaluate postpartum hemodynamics.

Amniotic Fluid Embolism

Amniotic fluid embolism occurs when there is passage of fluid from the uterus into the maternal vascular system. Ruptured or leaking membranes, opened uterine or cervical veins, and a pressure gradient sufficient to force the amniotic fluid into the veins are necessary for this emergency condition. Unrecognized and untreated, amniotic fluid embolism can be rapidly fatal.

Labor in which there is hyperstimulation of the uterus can be instrumental in providing the pressure necessary to force the fluid into the maternal system. Partial or full separation of the placenta, either as abruption or during third-stage labor, provides the vascular entry. Lacerations of the cervix or uterus can also open the maternal vascular system. Passage of meconium by the fetus creates a more irritating fluid, should it enter the maternal system.

Diagnosis of amniotic fluid embolism. Signs of amniotic fluid embolism include respiratory distress and circulatory collapse. Occasionally the woman experiences seizures. Often fetal distress is the initial sign. The following sequence is usually noted:

- Respiratory distress
- Cyanosis
- Cardiovascular collapse
- Hemorrhage
- Coma (Gabbe, Niebyl, and Simpson, 1999)

If the condition is not immediately fatal, disseminated intravascular coagulation develops, and bleeding is noted from the vagina and sites of intravenous insertions. Severe hemorrhage can lead to death.

Management of amniotic fluid embolism. Immediate referral to a perinatologist and intensive care team is essential. While awaiting their response, mechanical ventilation or resuscitation should be initiated as necessary. Blood replacement can be initiated in preparation for possible bleeding disorders. When the amniotic fluid contains thick meconium and other particulate matter (lanugo, vernix), the chance of full recovery is diminished.

References

ACOG: *Dystocia and the augmentation of labor (Technical Bulletin),* Washington, DC, 1995a, American College of Obstetricians and Gynecologists.

ACOG: *Fetal heart rate patterns: monitoring, interpretation and management (Technical Bulletin 207),* Washington, DC, 1995b, American College of Obstetricians and Gynecologists.

ACOG: *Inappropriate use of the terms fetal distress and birth asphyxia (Committee Opinion 197),* Washington, DC, 1998a, American College of Obstetricians and Gynecologists.

ACOG: *Special problems of multiple gestation (Educational Bulletin 253),* Washington, DC, 1998b, American College of Obstetricians and Gynecologists.

Baskett TF, Allen AC: Perinatal implications of shoulder dystocia, *Obstet Gynecol* 86(1):14-17, 1995.

Bruner JP et al: All-fours maneuver for reducing shoulder dystocia during labor, *J Reprod Med* 43:439-443, 1998.

Chayen B, Tejani N, Verma U: Induction of labor with an electric breast pump, *J Reprod Med* 31:116-118, 1986.

Chelmow D, Kilpatrick SJ, Laros RK: Maternal and neonatal outcomes after prolonged latent phase, *Obstet Gynecol* 81: 486-491, 1993.

Cibils LA: Breech presentation. In Flamm BL, Quilligan E J, editors, *Cesarean section: guidelines for appropriate utilization,* New York, 1995, Springer-Verlag.

Collea JV, Chein C, Quilligan EJ: The randomized management of term frank breech presentation, *Am J Obstet Gynecol* 137:235-244, 1980.

Flamm BL, Quilligan EJ, editors: *Cesarean section: guidelines for appropriate utilization,* New York, 1995, Springer-Verlag.

Flamm B et al: Vaginal birth after cesarean section: results of a multicenter study, *Am J Obstet Gynecol* 158:1079-1084, 1988.

Flamm B et al: Vaginal birth after cesarean section: results of a five-year multicenter study, *Obstet Gynecol* 76:750-754, 1990.

Fraser WD et al: The Canadian Early Amniotomy Study Group—effect of early amniotomy on the risk of dystocia in nulliparous women, *N Engl J Med* 328:1145-1149, 1993.

Friedman EA: The graphic analysis of labor, *Am J Obstet Gynecol* 68:1568-1575, 1954.

Friedman EA: *Clinical evaluation and management,* New York, 1978, Appleton-Century-Crofts.

Friedman EA: Dysfunctional labor. In Cohen WR, Friedman EA, editors: *Management of labor,* Baltimore, 1983, University Press.

Friedman EA, Neff RK: *Labor and delivery: impact on offspring,* Littleton, Mass, 1987, PSG Publishing.

Gabbe SG, Niebyl JR, Simpson JL: *Pocket companion to obstetrics—normal and problem pregnancies,* ed 3, New York, 1999, Churchill Livingstone.

Gant NF, Cunningham FG, editors: *Basic gynecology and obstetrics,* Norwalk, Conn, 1993, Appleton & Lange.

Gardberg M, Tuppurainen M: Persistent occiput posterior presentation—a clinical problem, *Acta Obstet Gynecol Scand* 73: 45-47, 1994.

Garite TJ et al: The influence of elective amniotomy on fetal heart rate patterns and the course of labor in term patients: a randomized study, *Am J Obstet Gynecol* 168:1827-1832, 1993.

Gherman RB, Ouzounian JG, Goodwin TM: Brachial plexus palsy: an in utero injury? *Am J Obstet Gynecol* 180:1303-1307, 1999.

Gilbert WM, Nesbitt TS, Danielsen B: Associated factors in 1611 cases of brachial plexus injury, *Obstet Gynecol* 93:536-540, 1999.

Gimosky MI, Wallace RL, Schifrin BS: Randomized management of the nonfrank breech presentation at term: a preliminary report, *Am J Obstet Gynecol* 146:34-40, 1983.

Handa VL, Laros RK: Active-phase arrest in labor: predictors of cesarean delivery in a nulliparous population, *Obstet Gynecol* 81:758-763, 1993.

Hannah ME et al: Induction of labor compared with expectant management for prelabor rupture of membranes at term, *N Engl J Med* 334(16):1005-1010, 1996.

Hill WC et al: Characteristics of uterine activity during breast stimulation stress test, *Obstet Gynecol* 64:489-492, 1984.

Hunter LP, Chern-Hughes B: Management of prolonged latent phase labor, *J Nurse-Midwifery* 41:383-388, 1996.

Keirse MJNC, Ottervanger HP, Smit W: Controversies: prelabor rupture of membranes at term: the case for expectant management, *J Perinatal Med* 24:563-572, 1996.

Leung AS et al: Risk factors associated with uterine rupture during trial of labor after cesarean delivery: a case-control study, *Am J Obstet Gynecol* 168(5):1358-1363, 1993.

Mahan TR, Chazotte C, Cohen WR: Short labor: characteristics and outcome, *Obstet Gynecol* 84:47-51, 1994.

McFarland M et al: Are labor abnormalities more common in shoulder dystocia? *Am J Obstet Gynecol* 173(4):1211-1214, 1995.

Miller DA, Diaz FG, Paul RH: Vaginal birth after cesarean: a 10-year experience, *Obstet Gynecol* 84(2):255-258, 1994.

Moenning RK, Hill WC: A randomized study comparing two methods of performing the breast stimulation stress test, *J Obstet Gynecol Neonatal Nursing* 16:253-257, 1987.

Mozurkewich EL, Wolf FM: Premature rupture of membranes at term: a meta-analysis of three management schemes, *Obstet Gynecol* 89(6):1035-1043, 1997.

Neumann M et al: Intrapartum bimanual tocolytic-assisted reversal of face presentation: preliminary report, *Obstet Gynecol* 84(1):146-148, 1994.

Nocon JJ et al: Shoulder dystocia: an analysis of risks and obstetric maneuvers, *Am J Obstet Gynecol* 168(6):1732-1737, 1993.

Pearl ML et al: Vaginal delivery from the persistent occiput posterior position—influence on maternal and neonatal morbidity, *J Reprod Med* 38(12):958-961, 1993.

Rachagan SP et al: Rupture of pregnant uterus—a 21-year review, *Aust NZ J Obstet Gynaecol* 31(1):37-40, 1991.

Roshanfeker D et al: Station at onset of active labor in nulliparous patients and risk of cesarean delivery, *Obstet Gynecol* 93:329-331, 1999.

Rouse DJ, Owen J, Hauth JC: Active-phase arrest: oxytocin augmentation for at least 4 hours, *Obstet Gynecol* 93:323-328, 1999.

Rouse DJ et al: Active-phase labor arrest: a randomized trial of chorioamnion management, *Obstet Gynecol* 83(6):937-940, 1994.

Salmon YM et al: Cervical ripening by breast stimulation, *Obstet Gynecol* 67:21-24, 1986.

Seaward PG et al: International multicenter term PROM study: evaluation of predictors of neonatal infection in infants born to patients with premature rupture of membranes at term, *Am J Obstet Gynecol* 179(3 Pt 1):635-639, 1998.

Simpson KR, Creehan PA: *Perinatal nursing*, Philadelphia, 1996, JB Lippincott.

Spong CY et al: An objective definition of shoulder dystocia: prolonged head-to-body delivery intervals and/or the use of ancillary obstetric maneuvers, *Obstet Gynecol* 86(3):433-436, 1995.

Stein JL et al: Nipple stimulation for labor augmentation, *J Reprod Med* 35:710-714, 1990.

Tyler VE: *The new honest herbal—a sensible guide to herbs and related remedies,* Philadelphia, 1987, George F Stickley.

Weed S: *Wise woman herbal for the childbearing year,* Woodstock, NY, 1986, Ash Tree Publishing.

Wiznitzer A: Obstructed labor and shoulder dystocia, *Curr Opin Obstet Gynecol* 7:486-491, 1995.

Yancey MK et al: Risk factors for neonatal sepsis, *Obstet Gynecol* 87(2):188-194, 1996.

Chapter 28

Complications of the Postpartum Period

As discussed in Chapters 22 and 24, the postpartum period involves physical and emotional transitions for women. Physically the woman's body goes through significant changes as it returns to the nonpregnant state. Emotionally the processes of attachment and realignment of relationships among family members progress on a continuum as the woman and her significant others incorporate the new infant into their lives. Although this is usually a healthy time for families, complications may occur requiring intervention and possible referral to other professionals. This chapter presents selected complications that typically occur after the first 4 hours after delivery. When the birth has occurred in a hospital or birth center, the woman and her family may have returned to their home, and the problems or potential problems are identified through maternal contact of the provider or during a scheduled office/clinic visit.

DELAYED (LATE) POSTPARTUM HEMORRHAGE

Delayed postpartum hemorrhage is blood loss greater than 500 ml after the first 24 hours after delivery. Suggested causes of delayed hemorrhage include sloughing of the placental scar, retained fragments of placenta or membranes, and subinvolution of undetermined etiology. Delayed hemorrhage occurs most frequently between 8 and 14 days after delivery.

Diagnosis. Delayed hemorrhage is suspected when the client reports increased vaginal bleeding or lochia that becomes rubra following a normal transition to serosa or alba. Interval history may identify an increase in physical activity, although often there are no associated factors.

Physical examination includes general assessment for signs of acute or chronic blood loss, abdominal palpation of the fundus, and assessment of the amount and color of bleeding on the peripad. Vital signs may indicate hypotension and increased pulse. A complete blood count or hemoglobin and hematocrit should be obtained for comparison with previous studies. Ultrasound may be used to identify retained tissue, although it may be difficult to differentiate between tissue and blood clots.

Management—community-based. Management depends on the degree of bleeding and the amount of maternal compromise secondary to the blood loss. Mild cases in which the woman is not symptomatic can be managed with oral administration of methylergonovine (0.2 mg PO every 4 hours for 6 doses), increased frequency of breast-feeding, and rest. Education regarding fundal massage and assessment of the amount of bleeding should be offered.

Increased bleeding in association with a firm fundus suggests bleeding from a laceration or hematoma and requires close inspection of the perineum, vagina, and cervix. Risk factors for hematoma formation include instrument delivery and ineffective hemostasis with laceration or episiotomy repair. Occasionally bleeding can be secondary to inadvertent damage to a vessel during administration of local or pudendal anesthesia. The classic sign for hematoma is severe pain out of proportion to the expected level of pain following birth. Inspection of the perineal area reveals swelling, often with discoloration of the overlying tissue if there is a vulvar or vaginal hematoma. The tissue overlying the hematoma may become necrotic and break down, resulting in profound hemorrhage. Signs of broad ligament hematoma include pain lateral to the uterus, with extension of pain into the flank and abdominal distention. Broad ligament hematomas are associated with cervical or deep vaginal lacerations and ruptured uterus. Identification of hematoma or unrepaired laceration necessitates obstetric consultation and probable referral for medical intervention.

Management—referral. When the blood loss is associated with signs of shock, hematocrit less than 20%, or uterine atony not responsive to methylergonovine, immediate medical referral is indicated. Hospitalization for intravenous hydration, blood replacement, and suction curettage may be necessary.

INFECTIONS

Before the advent of antibiotics in the 1930s, infection was one of the primary causes of maternal mortality. Pharmacologic intervention has contributed to a dramatic decrease in puerperal infection, but there is now a danger of increasing resistant strains of organisms. It is imperative that the clinician practice in a way that decreases risk of infection, provide early diagnosis when infection occurs, and treat appropriately to foster rapid recovery.

Endometritis

Postpartum febrile morbidity is defined as a temperature of 38° C or higher on any 2 of the first 10 days after delivery, excluding the first 24 hours (Bowes, 1996). It is estimated that 2% of patients experiencing vaginal birth and 10% to 15% of those experiencing cesarean birth develop endometritis, usually caused by an ascending infection from the lower genital tract. Risk factors for endometritis include prolonged rupture of membranes, prolonged labor, multiple vaginal examinations, instrumental/surgical delivery, preeclampsia, retention of placental fragments, postpartum hemorrhage, and anemia.

Endometritis usually involves invasion of the decidua by the infecting organisms. The invasion most commonly occurs at the placental site, although it can also occur in the vascular tissue of the remaining decidua or at the site of cervical lacerations. Infections presenting in the first 1 to 2 days after delivery are usually caused by group A streptococcus. Those occurring 3 to 4 days after delivery are more likely to be caused by enteric pathogens *(Escherichia coli)* or anaerobes. Endometritis that presents more than 1 week after the birth is most likely caused by *Chlamydia trachomatis.* Endometritis is commonly a polymicrobial infection.

Diagnosis. Symptoms of endometritis include fever and chills, malaise, and lower abdominal discomfort. Signs include fever, uterine tenderness, mucopurulent vaginal discharge, and heavy lochia rubra. When anaerobic or coliform organisms are present, foul-smelling lochia is noted. When beta-hemolytic streptococcus is present, lochia may be scant and odorless. Subinvolution is almost always associated with endometritis.

Management—community-based. Because of the virulence of some organisms, it is prudent to initiate antibiotics before the availability of culture results based on a probability of specific infective organisms. Cervical cultures or cultures of a wound site may be helpful in confirming the infecting organism and its antibiotic sensitivities. Blood cultures are indicated when systemic infection is suspected. Table 28-1 identifies commonly used antibiotics for infections in the reproductive tract. Hospitalization or out-patient therapy is decided on the basis of the severity of the disease process.

Patients with mild-to-moderate infections, particularly if they have had a normal vaginal delivery, can be treated with a short-course of single-agent intravenous antibiotic followed by oral antibiotics once there has been no fever for 24 hours. A broad-spectrum cephalosporin or penicillin is the drug of choice. In most settings this regimen can be followed in an ambulatory care unit or through the use of a home care nurse. In addition to antimicrobial therapy, bed rest, hydration, and

Table 28-1 *Antibiotics for Infections of the Reproductive Tract*

Drug	Dosage	Infection
Ampicillin	1-2 g IV q6h	Streptococci, *Escherichia coli, Proteus mirabilis, Neisseria gonorrhea,* enterococci (when used in conjunction with cefotaxime, ceftriaxone, or gentamycin), pneumococci
Cefotaxime	1-2 g IV q8h	*Streptococcus pneumoniae, Streptococcus viridans, Staphylococcus aureus, Staphylococcus epidermidis, E. coli, P. mirabilis, Klebsiella pneumoniae, Haemophilus influenzae* (ampicillin sensitive and resistant), *N. gonorrhoeae*
Cefotetan	1-2 g IV q12h	*S. pneumoniae, S. viridans, S. aureus, S. epidermidis, E. coli, P. mirabilis, K. pneumoniae, H. influenzae* (ampicillin sensitive and resistant), *N. gonorrhoeae,* anaerobes below the diaphragm *(Bacteroides fragilis)*
Cefoxitin	1-2 g IV q6h	See Cefotetan
Ceftizoxime	1-2 g q8h	See Cefotetan; has greater activity against certain strains of bacteroides and lesser activity against enteric bacilli
Clindamycin	600-900 mg IV q6h; 300 mg PO q6h for moderate infections	*S. pneumoniae, S. viridans, S. aureus, S. epidermidis,* anaerobes below the diaphragm *(Bacteroides fragilis);* drug of choice in combination with an aminoglycoside when patient is penicillin allergic
Doxycycline	100-200 mg IV q12-24h; 100 mg PO q12h	*Chlamydia trachomatis, S. pneumoniae, S. viridans,* anaerobes below the diaphragm *(Bacteroides fragilis)*
Gentamycin	1-2 mg/kg IV q8h	Effective against *Streptococcus* and *Staphylococcus* when used in conjunction with ampicillin, *E. coli, P. mirabilis, H. influenza, Pseudomonas aeruginosa;* used with metronidazole or clindamycin for anaerobic coverage
Metronidazole	500 mg IV q8h; 500 mg PO q8h	Anaerobes below the diaphragm *(Bacteroides fragilis)*

Adapted from McCormack J et al.: *Drug therapy decision-making guide,* Philadelphia, 1996, WB Saunders.

analgesia are recommended to support the healing process. If outpatient therapy is planned, it is important to assess the woman's home environment to determine whether she has the support necessary for her care and that of her baby. A plan should be formulated to ensure that recommended rest and supportive care will be carried out. Occasionally hospitalization may be necessary for adequate treatment and rest. In many settings endometritis can be managed using consultation with the obstetrician; in others referral for inpatient care may be required.

When hospitalization is necessary, continued care of the infant, including breast-feeding, depends on the woman's condition. Once she is stable, it is preferable to allow the infant to "room-in" with the mother to maintain the process of maternal-infant attachment. Additional rooming-in by the partner, relative, or friend facilitates the ongoing care of the mother and infant.

Management—referral. Referral to an obstetrician is indicated if there is no response to antibiotic therapy within 48 hours or if pelvic abscess or pelvic thrombophlebitis is suspected.

Septic Shock

Septic shock is a rare but life-threatening condition that may be a complication of reproductive tract infections in the postpartum period. The organisms most commonly responsible for septic shock include *Escherichia coli, Klebsiella pneumoniae,* and *Proteus* spp. The aerobic gram-negative organisms release endotoxins into the circulatory system, causing immunologic, hematologic, neurohormonal, and hemodynamic changes that lead to multiorgan compromise.

Diagnosis. Patients initially exhibit fever, restlessness, disorientation, hypotension, and tachycardia. Early in the process the skin is warm secondary to vasodilation, but, as the disease progresses, vasoconstriction leads to coolness, particularly in the extremities. Cardiac arrhythmias, jaundice, and anuria develop. Disseminated intravascular coagulation and adult respiratory distress syndrome are common.

Differential diagnoses include hypovolemic and cardiogenic shock, diabetic ketoacidosis, anaphylactic shock, anesthetic complications, and amniotic fluid or venous embolism (Duff, 1996). Elevated white blood count with a large percentage of bands; decreased hematocrit; abnormal coagulation studies; and increased transaminase enzyme, bilirubin, blood urea nitrogen and creatinine levels support the diagnosis. Computed tomographic scan, magnetic resonance imaging, or ultrasound studies are helpful in identifying an abscess contributing to the process.

Management—referral. Septic shock requires intensive care to monitor the hemodynamic status. Immediate referral to a perinatologist and a critical care team is expected. Vasoactive drugs and oxygen support are usually necessary. Aggressive use of intravenous broad-spectrum antibiotics and intravenous therapy to maintain fluid balance are the usual processes of care during the acute stage of the disease.

Wound Infections

Wound infections can occur in perineal/vaginal lacerations, the episiotomy site, or cesarean delivery incisions. Women with cesarean wound infections also are likely to have endometritis. Risk factors for wound infections include poor suturing technique, prolonged labor, prolonged rupture of membranes, preexisting infection (e.g., chorioamnionitis, symptomatic vaginitis), obesity, insulin-dependent diabetes, immunodeficiency disorders, immunosuppressive therapy, corticosteroid therapy, and low socioeconomic status. The most common organisms identified in wound infections are *S. aureus,* aerobic streptococci, and aerobic and anaerobic bacilli (Gibbs, Blanco, and St. Clair, 1983).

Diagnosis. Symptoms of wound infection include complaint of pain at the site, seropurulent discharge from the site, foul odor at the site, and fever. Inspection identifies erythema, induration, and tenderness. Seropurulent discharge may or may not be present. Diagnosis is made primarily by clinical examination.

Management—community-based. In many cases of wound infection, the repair will have already begun to break down. When purulent discharge is present, the entire wound must be opened for drainage. Medical referral or collaboration is necessary for this treatment. Antibiotic therapy using agents specific for staphylococcal infections is recommended. Nafcillin, 2 g IV q6h, or vancomycin, 1 g IV q12h, are acceptable regimes (Duff, 1996).

In mild-to-moderate cases of wound infection, continued outpatient treatment with medical consultation can be considered. Oral antibiotic therapy should be initiated and continued for at least 1 week. Warm soaks or sitz baths will keep the area clean and foster healing. Hydration and rest should be encouraged. The importance of good handwashing before and after contact with the wound should be emphasized. The woman should be instructed to contact the provider if fever continues, if the wound does not seem to improve over 48 hours, or if signs of systemic infection occur.

Management—referral. Necrotizing fasciitis is an extremely serious complication that may develop in both cesarean delivery incisions and episiotomies. The condition should be suspected when the wound edges are cyanotic and devoid of sensation. Since it is a life-threatening condition, necrotizing fasciitis must be aggressively managed with antibiotics, and all necrotic tissue must be debrided. Immediate referral to a perinatologist is indicated if this diagnosis is suspected.

Urinary Tract Infection

In addition to the gestational changes that increase the risk of urinary tract infection (UTI) during pregnancy, the birth process and management of the labor contribute further risk factors for infection. Trauma to the bladder and urethra and urinary catheterization during labor or immediately after delivery increase the risk of development of infection during the puerperium. When evaluating puerperal fever, UTI must be considered in the differential diagnoses.

Diagnosis. The usual symptoms of burning and urgency are also associated to trauma to the structures surrounding the vaginal introitus. Thus the woman may initially make the assumption that the pain is caused by lacerations or bruising. Lower tract infection should be suspected when fever and risk factors such as catheterization or bladder trauma are present. A true "clean-catch urine" is difficult to obtain because of the lochia. Therefore a catheterized specimen should be obtained for diagnosis. Upper tract infection presents with fever, back pain, and general malaise. Urine colony counts of greater than 10^2 colonies/ml of urine obtained by catheterization confirm the diagnosis of infection (Duff, 1996).

Management—community-based. When UTI is suspected, antibiotic therapy is usually initiated before obtaining the results of urine cultures. Lower tract infections can be treated with oral antibiotics that are effective against gram-negative organisms. Since 20% to 30% of strains of *E. coli* are resistant to ampicillin, amoxicillin (250 mg TID), or nitrofurantoin (100 mg BID) are preferred. Upper tract infection requires parenteral treatment. Ceftriaxone, 2 g intramuscularly or intravenously daily is commonly used. The decision to treat in hospital or through a home health agency depends on the severity of the infection. Upper tract infection or lower tract infection that is unresponsive to therapy requires consultation, collaboration, or referral to the obstetric consultant.

When recurrent UTIs have been a problem during the perinatal period, an evaluation by a urologist after the 6-week postpartum examination is indicated.

Mastitis

Lactation mastitis is any inflammation of breast tissue in a lactating woman, although the term is frequently used to describe only infection. Lactation mastitis is associated with maternal discomfort, cessation of breast-feeding, and development of breast abscess. Infective mastitis occurs when organisms are introduced into breast tissue, usually through a crack in the nipple. *S. aureus* is the most common organism implicated in mastitis, and the organism is passed from the infant's oropharynx during breast-feeding. When infective mastitis is left untreated, it will progress to a breast abscess.

Mastitis can also occur when a blocked duct with its overdistended alveoli forces milk substances into surrounding tissue, activating the immune system. This noninfective form of lactation mastitis is characterized by breast tissue inflammation and, left untreated, may progress to infective mastitis. Since it can be extremely difficult to differentiate between infective and noninfective mastitis, most clinicians usually assume an infective process and treat accordingly.

The usual time of onset of mastitis is within 2 weeks of the birth, although it can occur anytime during the period of lactation and nursing. Some studies suggest an increase in incidence at 5 to 6 weeks after delivery. Incidence has been estimated at 4% to 33% of nursing mothers, with a recurrence rate of 6.5% (Fetherston, 1998).

Risk factors for mastitis for women nursing for the first time include blocked ducts, attachment difficulties, and nipple pain. Risk factors for experienced nursing mothers include past history of mastitis, blocked ducts, and stress. Frequent feeding has been identified as the most significant protective factor for both new and experienced mothers. In addition, in first-time nursing mothers use of nipple creams has been identified as protective (Fetherston, 1998).

Diagnosis. Symptoms of mastitis include fever, malaise, unilateral breast pain, and tenderness over the affected area. Signs include fever, erythema, and/or a firm lesion at the affected site. Swelling under the affected area and pitting edema of the skin suggest breast abscess.

Management—community-based. When the signs and symptoms of mastitis are present, most clinicians treat with antibiotics before receiving the results of any cultures since mastitis can progress rapidly. Most infections are caused by *Staphylococcus;* thus antibiotics that commonly cover the organism are the first line of treatment. Dicloxacillin (250 to 500 mg q6h for 10 days) is commonly used. Studies suggest that, when antibiotics are initiated within 48 hours of the onset of the infection, the risk of developing an abscess is reduced.

Continuation of breast-feeding is to be encouraged. If the woman feels too ill to nurse her infant, the breasts should be pumped to prevent stasis and further inflammation. Analgesia, rest, and hydration should be encouraged to enhance healing.

Management—referral. Recurrent infections and infections associated with resistant organisms may lead to abscess formation. Suspicion of a breast abscess requires referral to a physician, and diagnosis usually requires hospitalization and intravenous antibiotic therapy.

THROMBOEMBOLYTIC DISORDERS

Venous thromboembolism is estimated to occur in 1 in 1000 to 2000 pregnancies. Deep vein thrombosis (DVT) is estimated to affect 0.71 in every 1000 pregnancies, with an incidence of 0.51/1000 deliveries occurring antenatally and 0.21/1000 deliveries occurring during the puerperium (McColl et al., 1997). The risk of DVT after cesarean delivery is about three to five times greater than following vaginal birth (Gabbe, Niebyl, and Simpson, 1999). About 15% to 25% of individuals who develop DVT experience pulmonary embolus when treatment is not adequate. Septic pelvic vein thrombophlebitis is rare, occurring in less than 1% of women with endometritis. Pathogens from intrauterine infection spread into the venous circulation, where they damage the vascular endothelium, thereby initiating thrombus formation.

The major predisposing factors for common venous thromboembolism are the venous stasis in the lower extremities caused by the weakening of the vessel walls and the compression on the major veins by the enlarging uterus. The increase in factors I, II, VII, VIII, IX, X, and XII; increase in fibrinogen; decrease in protein S; and inhibition of the fibrinolytic system contribute to the fivefold increase in thrombus formation during the perinatal period. It is estimated that about 50% of thromboses occur in the postpartum period (Ray and Chan, 1999). Even though the clotting system returns to normal nonpregnant levels by 3 weeks after delivery, the risk of thrombosis continues until 4 to 6 weeks after delivery.

Superficial thrombophlebitis is characterized by swelling, redness, and tenderness over the affected vessel, usually the saphenous vein. The thrombus formation occurs primarily in varicose veins and does not usually lead to pulmonary embolism. DVT, conversely, may predispose to pulmonary embolism. DVT should be suspected if there is pain with walking or pain with pressure over the affected veins. DVT is more common in the left leg (McColl et al., 1997; Ray and Chan, 1999). If the clot does not obstruct the vessel, the woman may not experience pain. Postpartum DVT usually occurs within the first 2 weeks after delivery.

Diagnosis. The most common symptom of superficial thrombophlebitis is tenderness over the affected vein. Inspection of the affected limb may reveal redness and swelling. Symptoms of DVT include pain with walking and swelling. Signs of DVT include demonstrated swelling and positive Homans' sign (dorsiflexion of the foot). Impedance plethysmography, real-time ultrasonography and Doppler ultrasonography can accurately identify proximal vein thrombosis but may miss some calf vein thromboses. Venography remains the standard for making the diagnosis but may miss pelvic vein DVT, a common location in the puerperium. Computed tomography is considered superior in identifying abdominal and pelvic DVT when compared to other modalities.

Symptoms of septic pelvic vein thrombophlebitis include lower abdominal pain in the first 96 hours after delivery, fever, nausea, vomiting, and complaint of abdominal bloating. Signs include tachycardia; abdominal tenderness, including guarding; and decreased or absent bowel sounds. More than half of affected women have a tender, ropelike mass originating near one cornua and extending toward the upper abdomen (Duff, 1996). Tachypnea, stridor, and dyspnea will be present if pulmonary embolism is present. Septic pelvis vein thrombophlebitis can also present with temperature instability. Differential diagnoses include pyelonephritis, appendicitis, broad ligament hematoma, adnexal torsion, pelvic abscess, nephrolithiasis, drug fever, and viral syndrome.

Management—referral. Treatment of superficial thrombophlebitis includes use of compression stockings, analgesia, and bed rest. Although the condition is usually benign, the clinician must rule out DVT. Physician consultation and collaboration are indicated.

Diagnosis of probable DVT requires immediate referral to a physician for treatment. Compression stockings, anticoagulant therapy of intravenous heparin up to 40,000 U daily, analgesics, and bed rest are usually included in the treatment plan.

Diagnosis of septic pelvic vein thrombophlebitis requires immediate referral to a physician for treatment. Management usually includes heparin administration, antibiotic therapy, analgesia, and rest. At times surgery may be indicated for ligation of the affected vessel or embolectomy.

Pulmonary Thromboembolism

Incidence of pulmonary thromboembolism (PTE) is 0.07/1000 deliveries (McColl et al., 1997). PTE is usually a result of emboli associated with DVT and is more common in the postpartum period than during pregnancy.

Diagnosis. Symptoms of PTE include the complaints of sudden-onset chest pain and difficulty breathing. Signs include dyspnea, tachypnea, tachycardia, cough, and anxiety. Arterial blood gases verify hypoxemia and hypocapnia. Chest x-ray film confirms atelectasis, and an electrocardiogram usually identifies tachycardia with right-sided cardiac strain. Ventilation-perfusion scanning identifies the probability of the presence of PTE. Pulmonary angiography confirms the diagnosis.

Management—referral. When PTE is suspected, immediate referral to a physician skilled in intensive care for hematologic and pulmonary pathology is necessary. While awaiting medical intervention, the woman should be positioned in a sitting position and given oxygen via mask. Vital signs should be taken at least every 15 minutes, and preparation for cardiopulmonary resuscitation should be made. Intravenous heparin therapy is usually initiated immediately with the suspicion of PTE to prevent further compromise. Intravenous heparin is usually used for 5 to 10 days. When the activated partial thromboplastin time is stable at 1.5 to 2.5 times normal, heparin administration can be shifted to subcutaneous or oral antiembolic agents.

POSTPARTUM PSYCHOLOGIC DISORDERS

Postpartum psychologic disorders are usually divided into three categories: postpartum "blues," nonpsychotic postpartum depression, and postpartum psychosis. About 30% to 75% of women experience mild and transient "blues." Determination of the prevalence of postpartum depression is difficult because of the use of a variety of definitions of the disorder in the literature. Onset from 4 weeks to 6 months after delivery has been cited in definitions. When a more narrow definition—onset within 6 to 9 weeks of the birth—is used, incidence of depressive symptomatology is estimated to be 12% to 16% of childbearing women. When a more liberal definition—onset in the first 6 months after delivery—is used, it is estimated that up to 22% of women may experience postpartum depression (Hendrick and Altshuler, 1998). It is further estimated that 0.1% to 0.2% of women experience postpartum psychosis. Women hospitalized for psychologic disorders during the postpartum period most commonly are diagnosed with an affective illness, either unipolar depression or bipolar disorder (Nonacs and Cohen, 1998).

Women at increased risk for postpartum psychologic disorders appear to include those with family and personal history of major depressive symptomatology during or following pregnancy, marital discord, and stressful child care events (Hendrick and Altshuler, 1998). It is estimated that women with a history of postpartum depression have a 50% to 62% risk of recurrence in subsequent pregnancies (Altshuler, Hendrick, and Cohen, 1998). Beck (1996), in a meta-analysis of 44 studies to determine the magnitude of the relationship between postpartum depression and predictor variables, identified moderate effect size for history of previous depression, poor social support, increased life stress, child care stress, presence of postpartum "blues," and decreased marital satisfaction. A large effect size was found for prenatal depression as a predictor variable.

The etiology of postpartum psychologic disturbances remains unclear. Hormonal changes have been implicated in the development of psychologic changes during the puerperium. However, research findings have been conflicting and limited by numerous methodologic problems. The dramatic decrease in estradiol after delivery may be associated with increased breakdown of serotonin, leading to depressive symptomatology, but research findings failed to discover a difference in magnitude of change of total estradiol or free estriol in depressed and nondepressed women (Hendrick and Altshuler, 1998). Studies of the effectiveness of estrogen supplements in the postpartum period have been limited by numerous confounding variables. The decline of progesterone following birth has also been implicated in the development of depressive symptomatology, but studies have failed to find an association between depressive symptoms and levels of total or free progesterone. No controlled studies have explored the effect of progesterone supplementation for prevention of treatment of depressive symptoms. Studies have failed to find an association between oxytocin, vasopressin, prolactin, and cortisol levels and the development of depression. Women with thyroid antibodies may be at increased risk for developing postpartum depression (Harris, Othman, and Davies, 1989), and thyroid dysfunction has been shown to contribute to postpartum mood disturbances.

Lower levels of tryptophan have been associated with depressive symptoms. Altered neurotransmission function, hyperactivity of the hypothalamic-pituitary-adrenal axis, and decreased responsiveness of the hypothalamic-pituitary-adrenal axis have all been suggested as possible physiologic explanations for the occurrence of the blues and postpartum depression (Bowes, 1996).

Untreated maternal psychologic disorders have been shown to be associated with development of cognitive, emotional, and social problems in children (Nonacs and Cohen, 1998). Untreated depression may lead to development of chronic and refractory mood disorders over time.

Diagnosis. Symptoms of the "blues" include tearfulness, depression, restlessness, mood lability, confusion, forgetfulness, and irritability, as well as sleep and appetite disturbances. Some women may express negative feelings about their infants. Symptoms usually develop within a few days of the birth, peaking on the fourth or fifth day and disappearing by the tenth day after delivery. By definition, postpartum "blues" are time limited and benign.

Postpartum depression usually begins within the first month after delivery, although there may be signs of depression in late pregnancy. The signs and symptoms are similar to those seen in depressive disorders in nonpregnant women—depressed mood, inability to experience happiness, low energy, and guilt. Fossey, Papiernak, and Bydlowski (1997) offer the following description of postpartum depressive state:

> The mother is stricken by a malaise she has never felt before, one that gives her a feeling of slowness and heaviness. She cries, feels sad, and is unable to face daily events. She feels incapable of and overwhelmed by child care. She has feelings of guilt and of shame about her lack of love and inadequacy toward her child (Fossey, Papiernak, and Bydlowski, 1997, p. 17).

Women experiencing postpartum depression may also entertain suicidal ideation. Because the symptoms (excluding thoughts of suicide) are usually seen as normal feelings and behaviors following birth, less severe presentations of postpartum depression may be missed.

Postpartum psychosis usually has a dramatic onset within the first 2 weeks following delivery. Early symptoms include restlessness, irritability, and sleep disturbance. The disorder progresses rapidly to include depressed or elated mood, disorganized behavior, mood lability, and delusions and hallucinations (Nonacs and Cohen, 1998).

Most scales to identify or rate depression have not been validated in the postpartum period. The Edinburgh Postnatal Depression Scale (EPDS) has been shown to have satisfactory sensitivity and specificity in diagnosing postpartum depression. Some sources recommend using the EPDS as a screening tool in routine care to childbearing women. Postpartum obstetric visits and well-baby examinations are excellent times for screening for psychologic disorders.

Management—community-based. Since postpartum "blues" are self-limiting, treatment includes support and education regarding the normal nature of the feelings. Women can be reassured that the symptoms usually recede by 10 to 14 days after delivery, but that, if they continue beyond that period, the provider should be notified. When symptoms persist, evaluation for identification of more severe affective illness is warranted.

Lavender and Walkinshaw (1998) found that providing women the chance to discuss their birth experiences with a midwife during the first few days after the birth decreased depression and anxiety scores after delivery. This opportunity for discussion and counseling can easily be integrated into postpartum teaching and counseling, regardless of site of care. During this time, assessment for signs of depression can be made, with plans for additional assessments for women with risk factors for postpartum depression. Medical consultation is indicated when postpartum depression is suspected. Moderate-to-severe depression should be treated with the same course of treatment as nonpuerperal depression (Nonacs and Cohen, 1998). Although studies on the effectiveness of pharmacologic and nonpharmacologic treatment have been limited, findings suggest that the use of antidepressants is appropriate in the postpartum period. Breast-feeding women need to be informed that all psychotropic medications are passed into breast milk, and although there aren't any apparent direct side effects to infants, the effects of trace amounts of drugs on the development of the neonate's neurologic system are not known. Interpersonal psychotherapy has also been found to be useful in treating acute episodes of depression (Nonacs and Cohen, 1998). Hospitalization may be indicated in cases of severe depression, particularly when there is a risk of suicide.

Management—referral. Postpartum psychosis includes schizophrenia and manic-depressive reactions and should be considered a medical emergency. Immediate referral to a facility with resources for prompt treatment is necessary. Treatment typically includes antipsychotic medications and mood stabilizers, and electroconvulsive therapy may be used. Untreated postpartum psychosis has been associated with infanticide, and it is estimated that infanticide may occur in up to 4% of cases (Nonacs and Cohen, 1998).

Women who are identified at increased risk for postpartum depression and psychosis should be offered consultation prenatally with a physician skilled in treatment of psychologic disorders for consideration of prophylactic therapy to prevent relapse. Studies suggest that women with history of bipolar disorder or postpartum psychosis may benefit from initiation of lithium late in third trimester or within 48 hours of delivery. When breast-feeding is highly desired by these women, valproic acid or carbamazepine may be a safer choice for the neonate.

INCONTINENCE OF URINE, STOOL, AND FLATUS

Urinary stress incontinence affects up to 40% of women, and it is estimated that over 75% of all female urinary stress incontinence is associated with childbearing. Although most women report onset during pregnancy, some may not experience problems until after delivery (Dumoulin et al., 1995). The prevalence of urinary incontinence increases as parity and maternal age increase. Some studies have suggested a relationship between episiotomy, lacerations, forceps and suturing with the prevalence of incontinence, but it has been suggested that these variables may have been proxy indicators for the vaginal birth itself (Foldspang, Mommsen, and Djurhuus, 1999).

Fecal incontinence occurs following childbirth in 4% of women, and it is estimated that many more women experience incontinence of flatus (McArthur, Bick, and Keighley, 1997). Anorectal incontinence is associated with use of forceps and vacuum extraction.

Research suggests that trauma to the pelvic musculature and anal sphincter and injury to the pudendal and sacral nerves contribute to both urinary and fecal incontinence (Wynne et al., 1996). Changes in the anal sphincter occur most dramatically in first vaginal births, and long-term lower resting pressures of the internal and external sphincters have been documented.

Perhaps most troubling is the fact that few women report signs and symptoms of urinary and fecal incontinence to their health care providers (McArthur, Bick, and Keighley, 1997). Embarrassment and the belief that incontinence is an annoyance that is to be expected with childbearing are the most likely reasons for underreporting.

Diagnosis. Urinary incontinence is diagnosed through patient report of urgency and leakage of urine, with or without associated physical activity. Fecal incontinence is also diagnosed through patient report of urgency, soiling, and frank incontinence of stool.

Management—community-based. Signs and symptoms of urinary or fecal incontinence should be assessed during prenatal visits, during the first week after delivery, and at the 6-week postpartum examination. Anticipatory counseling that includes instruction on perineal strengthening exercises (Kegel's exercises) may decrease the degree of incontinence experienced by the woman. Pelvic floor muscle exercises do not appear to be useful in cases of neurologic damage during childbirth. Most neurologic injury recovers spontaneously within 3 months of delivery (Sweet, 1997).

Management—referral. If incontinence continues beyond 6 weeks after delivery, referral to a physician for further evaluation is warranted.

THYROIDITIS

Postpartum thyroiditis (PPT) is a syndrome involving transient hyperthyroidism or hypothyroidism occurring in the first postpartum year. Incidence varies by race and geography and has been reported to be 1.9% to 16.7%. The number of cases may be underreported since the condition involves nonspecific symptoms and women typically may not associate the symptoms with childbearing since they may not occur for 6 to 9 months after the birth. PTT is considered an autoimmune disorder, perhaps precipitated by the postpartum immunologic changes when antibody titers and numbers of T-cell helper cells increase (Terry and Hague, 1998). The presence of thyroid autoantibodies in maternal serum is strongly associated with the development of PPT. The syndrome tends to follow three phases. Transient thyrotoxicosis occurs 1 to 3 months after delivery and about 1 to 2 months before the development of hypothyroidism. Transient hypothyroidism develops 3 to 8 months after delivery, followed by a return to euthyroidism (Terry and Hague, 1998).

Diagnosis. Many women remain asymptomatic during the transient hyperthyroid period. Others may complain of lack of energy, nervousness, or irritability. The hypothyroid period is associated with more symptoms, including dry skin, lack of energy, fatigue, aches and pains, poor memory, and cold intolerance. An increase in the size of the thyroid gland is usually noted. Laboratory tests useful in assessing thyroid status include thyroid-stimulating hormone (TSH), free triiodothyronine, and free thyroxine (T4). During the hyperthyroid phase, elevated T4 and depressed TSH are noted, microsomal antibodies may be present, and there is low ^{131}I uptake. The hypothyroid phase is characterized by elevated TSH, decreased free T4, and elevated antimicrosomal and antithyroglobulin antibody titers.

Management—community-based. Symptoms usually are not dramatic enough to require treatment, and the course of PPT is self-limiting. For this reason, education and reassurance are often all that is necessary.

When the symptoms of the thyrotoxic phase interfere with quality of life, use of beta blockers may be helpful. Physician consultation is indicated for treatment of PPT.

Because of the association with other autoimmune diseases, some authors suggest screening women with documented autoimmune disorders for antibodies either prenatally or at the time of delivery (Terry and Hague, 1998). Such an approach will detect most women affected with the disorder.

VIOLENCE AGAINST WOMEN IN THE POSTPARTUM PERIOD

Injuries are the leading cause of death in the postpartum period, but these deaths are usually not included in maternal mortality statistics (Dietz et al., 1998; Fildes et al., 1992). Stresses inherent in the care of the woman and her infant during the first 6 weeks after delivery may precipitate domestic abuse. Homicide is the leading cause of injury deaths in postpartum women, and data suggest that women in the 15- to 19-year age group may be at increased risk when compared to older women (Dietz et al., 1998). For this reason, screening for abuse should continue in the postpartum period. When women are at increased risk for abuse, they should be screened before their return to the home.

GRIEF AND BEREAVEMENT

Childbirth is expected to be a happy experience in a woman's life. She and her partner usually have fantasized about what their child will look like, the personality of the child, and their anticipated life as a family. Unexpected outcomes, including the death of an infant or the birth of an infant with abnormalities or medical problems requiring ongoing intervention, come as a shock, and grief and bereavement follow. Even when perinatal death, anomalies, or medical problems have been anticipated, coping with the reality of the actual problems at the time of the birth is still difficult for parents. The midwife and other professional care providers are often the primary facilitators as the parents cope with the many issues surrounding the birth and death of their child. Understanding the phases of bereavement will assist the provider in providing supportive, compassionate care during this extremely stressful time.

Bereavement refers to the "state of being bereaved or deprived of something" (Corr, Nabe, and Corr, 1996, p. 220). Conceptually, bereavement is the individual's reaction to the loss of anything strongly valued. In this context, bereavement can occur not only when a parent experiences the death of an infant, but also when labor complications deprive the woman of an anticipated normal birth experience or when the infant doesn't fit the fantasy of the "perfect baby."

Grief is the individual's response to a loss (Corr, Nabe, and Corr, 1996). Grief is manifest in the following ways:

- Feelings—sadness, anger, guilt, self-reproach, anxiety, loneliness, fatigue, helplessness, shock, yearning, numbness
- Physical sensations—emptiness in the gut, tightness in the throat or chest, oversensitivity to noise, shortness of breath, lack of energy, muscle weakness, dry mouth, loss of coordination
- Cognitive changes—disbelief, confusion, preoccupation, sense of presence of the deceased, paranormal experiences
- Behavioral changes—sleep or appetite disturbances, absentmindedness, social withdrawal, loss of interest in activities that previously were enjoyable, dreams of the deceased, crying, avoiding reminders of the deceased, sighing, restlessness
- Social difficulties—problems in relationships or in functioning in social roles
- Spiritual searching—looking for sense of meaning, anger at God (Worden, 1991, as quoted in Corr, Nabe, and Corr, 1996)

Bereavement is commonly seen as a two-staged process summarized in Table 28-2. The acute stage begins with shock at the death, even when it has been anticipated. Shock may include denial or a sense of "This can't be happening." The bereaved individual progresses into a phase of searching for the reasoning or cause of the death. Looking for blame is common; and the parent may place blame on himself, herself, or the health care provider. The searching produces grief reactions that are influenced by the parent's personality, relationship experiences, and cultural beliefs. Depression, sadness, loneliness, and disorientation are common grief reactions. Acceptance of the separation leads to the chronic stage of reintegration and acceptance of the finality of the death. Individuals vary in the time frames necessary to complete the process.

Some theorists propose that maternal bereavement has somewhat different dimensions (Table 28-3). Edelstein argues that maternal grieving differs in two distinct ways from bereavement experienced with other relationship losses (Edelstein, 1984). First, the fact that many perinatal deaths are unexpected intensifies the dis-

Table 28-2 *Stages in the Mourning Process*

Stage	Phase	Associated Effect
Acute	Shock	Numbness, disbelief, shrieking, motor retardation
	Grief reactions	Yearning for the lost object; weeping
	Separation reactions	Despair, sadness, depression, fatigue, helplessness, anger, anxiety
Chronic	Reintegration	Acceptance of loss

Edelstein L: *Maternal bereavement—coping with the unexpected death of a child,* New York, 1984, Praeger Publishers.

Table 28-3 *Stages in Maternal Bereavement*

Stage	Major Dynamics
Disorganization	Disruption in the equilibrium
Holding-on/ Letting go	Struggle to relinquish the child as living; retaining memories and identifications
Reorganization	Loss is integrated into life

Edelstein L: *Maternal bereavement—coping with the unexpected death of a child,* New York, 1984, Praeger Publishers.

organization phase, making it a distinct stage. Second, death of a child appears to intensify and lengthen the mourning period. Investigators have found that women may exhibit grief behaviors for years following the death of a child (Edelstein, 1984; Finkbeiner, 1996; Schaap et al., 1997). As one mother reported, "An infant's death haunts the parents daily from the time it happens. The hurt comes out in many different ways and to different degrees and at all different times" (Covington and Theut, 1993, p. 218). A woman's previous experience with relationships and loss and her perinatal attachment to the infant influence her transition through the emotionally difficult period of bereavement.

Bereavement is mediated by cultural beliefs and values. Beliefs about good or evil spirits, healing practices, life after death, and death-related rituals influence an individual's reaction to death. It is helpful for health care providers to familiarize themselves with common grieving behaviors in cultural groups, while recognizing that there will be variants in sanctioned behaviors across communities. Table 28-4 presents common variants in mourning behaviors in cultural groups.

Research and evaluation of the impact of perinatal grief support programs have demonstrated that guided interaction with the infant, along with creation of mementos, including photographs, locks of hair, and hospital name tags, validate the life of the infant and the loss for the parents. Validation of the infant's being facilitates the parents' movement through the mourning period. Use of supportive groups and short-term therapy have been suggested to help parents through bereavement. Occasionally a parent exhibits unresolved grief, refusal to grieve, or inability to grieve (Leon, 1990). In these cases, referral to a mental health specialist is warranted, with consideration for long-term therapy. Inability to process the death may be associated with previous experiences with loss or underlying psychologic problems.

Grieving and Perinatal Death

Care of parents experiencing perinatal death has moved from "protecting" them from the stress of mourning to the actively supporting them as they move through the grieving process. Most hospitals have policies that allow parents to see and hold their baby, encourage naming the baby, produce photographs that can be kept on file in case the parents decide at a future date that they would like them, assist with funeral arrangements, and refer family members to support groups and other supportive resources. Studies have found that most parents want to see and hold their infant, regardless of the circumstances of the death and the gestational age. Contact with the stillborn infant has been associated with less anxiety and depression in mothers 3 to 4 years after the death (Rand et al., 1998).

Lemmer (1991) found that parents' perceptions of caring behaviors could be described as "taking care of" and "caring for or about." "Taking care of" behav-

Table 28-4 *Death-Related Behaviors in Six Cultural Groups*

Religious Attitudes	Grief Expressions	Death Rituals	Resources for Support
Asian—Chinese			
Believe in reincarnation Believe it is best to die with bodies intact; may refuse surgical procedures	Not publicly expressed	Chanting ceremony at bedside after death Accepting clothing of deceased may not be considered appropriate	Families
Asian—Indochinese			
After death, soul lives in land of "tian" Deceased baby returns in body of another child Stillborns are "marked" on the soles of the feet May assign a number rather than name for first few days of life to hide baby from "evil spirits"	May weep/ wail aloud	May cover baby's head after the death as a sign of respect for the soul Mourning attire consists of a white outfit worn by women and black armband worn by men	Families
Asian—Japanese			
Shinto belief—illness caused by evil spirits Illness caused by contact with polluting agents (blood, corpses)	Tend to suppress emotions	Hindu—priest ties thread around neck or wrist to signify blessing (should not be removed); family washes body of the deceased	Family
Mexican Americans			
Illness/death is God's will	Very expressive	Dependent on religious beliefs Roman Catholic—infant baptism mandatory; anointing of the sick by a priest Religious medals should not be removed from body	Family
Native Americans			
No life after death—return to ancestors Believe in spirits and need to be in harmony with nature	May or may not be publicly expressive	Chanting, singing over dead to appeal to spirits	Families, shaman, tribal group
Arabs			
Anticipatory grief work not acceptable; always hold out hope for a cure Islam—family washes and prepares body; only friends and relatives may touch body	Express grief openly	Much touching of the dead infant's body Remain with body until transported to funeral home	Family
African Americans			
Believe in heaven/hell Serious illness may be sent as punishment by God	Very expressive	Funeral rite is a gathering including prayers, scripture readings, songs, public crying, wailing	Minister, family friends; strong, family kinship

iors exhibited by nurses and physicians include providing expert care to meet physiologic and safety needs for mother and infant and providing information in a way that parents can understand and process. "Caring for or about" behaviors include providing direct emotional support, providing individualized family-centered care, facilitating the creation of memories, and respecting the rights of parents. Noncaring behaviors include the failure of health providers to acknowledge the parents' loss, express emotional support, and recognize individual needs of the family members. Parents also express dissatisfaction with care when they believe that they have not been given accurate or complete information about the circumstances surrounding their child's death (Crowther, 1995). Because of the shock of perinatal death and the resulting disorganization in thinking, it is helpful to provide explanations not only at the time of the death, but also at postpartum visits.

Because of the disorganization, parents also usually need help in making basic decisions surrounding care. States require appropriate disposal of remains for infants more than 20 weeks' gestational age or larger than 500 g. Parents need to make a decision regarding private burial arrangements or hospital-generated arrangements. When appropriate, clergy or another spiritual leader may be helpful in guiding the parents in this decision making. Depending on the circumstances surrounding the death, consent for an autopsy may be desired. Many parents seek autopsy to better understand the cause of death. For others, autopsy may represent desecration of the body, leading them to refuse consent.

The Compassionate Friends,* a national support group for parents who have experienced the death of a child, offers the following suggestions to medical and nursing personnel when caring for a family who has experienced death of a child:

- Allow parents as much time as they need to be with their child (alone if they wish) after the death.
- Take pictures of newborns who die and put them in the infants' charts in case parents want them in future weeks or months.
- Don't hold back if you want to put your hand on a parent's arm or your arm around a parent's shoulder. Touching is our most basic form of comfort and communication.
- Understand that parents do not wish to hear rationalizations about their child's death. Never tell a parent such things as: "Your child would have been a burden to you as he was," or "She just would have suffered if she had lived."
- Be available to listen, knowing it will take years to adjust to what many people consider the worst loss of all.
- Don't be in a big hurry to offer medication. Drugs can interfere with the normal expression of grief.

Either before hospital or birth center discharge or during a postpartum home visit following home birth, it is helpful to prepare parents for the reality of returning to home and community without the anticipated infant. Stating that "Many parents [mothers] find it difficult to tell friends about their baby's death. How do you think you will tell friends and neighbors that your baby died?" often creates the opportunity for discussing possible conversation and role playing. Postpartum teaching should emphasize the usual behaviors to facilitate postpartum involution and return to the nonpregnant state. The importance of a well-balanced diet, rest, exercise, and avoidance of alcohol and mind-altering drugs during bereavement should be emphasized. If grieving behaviors affect care of self, further counseling and assessment should be recommended.

In addition to the usual 2- and 6-week postpartum examinations, it is helpful to suggest a provider visit at 4 months after the death. At this point in time, the provider can assess whether there are signs of profound grief requiring mental health intervention. Anniversaries of the baby's birth and death dates are particularly stressful, and the woman can be encouraged to make an appointment for an "annual" examination at that time. Families should also be given written information about bereavement support resources in the community.

Discussion about the differences between mothers' and fathers' grieving patterns may be helpful for couples. Women may show higher levels of anxiety and depression than their partners, especially if there has been a stillbirth (Schwab, 1996; Vance et al., 1995a; Vance et al., 1995b). Males may also exhibit anxiety and depression and demonstrate heavier alcohol use compared to men who have not experienced perinatal loss. The stressors associated with perinatal death may contribute to anger or hostility directed at the partner. Couples should be encouraged to be patient with one another and to recognize that individuals have unique ways of coping with tragedy. In American society the father may feel pressured to be the "strong" partner. Discussion regarding

*Adapted from "Suggestions for Medical Personnel," The Compassionate Friends, Inc, Oak Brook, Ill.

strategies to allow him to grieve fully is helpful in allowing him to cope with his loss.

Most midwives and physicians recommend waiting at least 1 year following the death before attempting another pregnancy. This is in recognition that the progress from acute grieving to chronic grief and reintegration can take up to 1 year. When grieving has not progressed, it is difficult for a parent to appreciate a new baby as a separate individual. Before planning another pregnancy, parents should be encouraged to discuss risk factors for future pregnancies with the midwife or physician to address medical concerns or make lifestyle changes before pregnancy.

There is a myth that midwives and physicians should not become "emotionally" involved in their patients' loss experiences. However, when a provider has developed a healthy, positive relationship with the woman and her family, there are naturally resulting "emotional" bonds. Increasingly, studies have identified that parents appreciate the provider sharing their feelings about the loss, and parents retain negative feelings about providers who are perceived as distant and uncaring. Although it can be difficult to discuss an infant's death with parents, simple sentences such as, "I'm sorry for your loss," or "I'm sorry that you and your baby had to go through this experience," will be remembered with appreciation (Chez, 1995). When a funeral or memorial service is held for an infant, the provider's presence is almost always seen as a validation of the reality of the infant and the loss experienced by the parents.

Grieving and the Birth of an Infant With Abnormalities

With the routine use of ultrasound technology, many anomalies are identified before the birth. However, even with preparation for neonatal problems, parents experience stress and grieving at the birth. Factors that influence the degree of bereavement parents experience when an infant is diagnosed with medical problems include:

- The characteristics of the anomaly or medical problem, including any apparent disfigurement
- The potential for long-term physical or mental impairment
- The extent of the infant's acute care needs, as well as the costs involved
- Previous experience with similar problems
- The impact of the condition on family functioning and alteration of maternal and paternal roles
- The support from family and friends, and the anticipated ongoing assistance that is available from loved ones

When the infant has been admitted to a Neonatal Intensive Care Unit (NICU), numerous factors contribute to stress for the mother and father. The physical separation from the mother at a time when she is recovering from childbirth puts physical and emotional strain on her. The infant's condition may prohibit extended contact with either parent, and parents may feel tremendous loss of control as expert physicians and nurses provide the ongoing care of the infant. Culture clashes may be experienced when interventions that are not consistent with the family's beliefs and values are proposed or carried out.

The woman's health care provider continues to be a primary supportive resource when the infant is experiencing problems. Sharing information and continuing a caring presence as the woman recovers from the birth are important aspects of care. The obstetric provider often becomes the source for information about possible causes of the problem, and parents may want to discuss aspects of the pregnancy as they seek understanding of the event. As with perinatal death, postpartum visits and continued assessments through the year following the birth provide support for the woman and her family and provide the opportunity for referrals that may be necessary when grieving is not progressing in a healthy way.

Grieving and the Midwife/Physician

Very little has been written about the emotions experienced by midwives and physicians who face perinatal death. The impact of death-related stress has been explored in NICU nurses (Downey et al., 1995), but articles about obstetric provider experience express opinions rather than scientific findings.

Midwives and physicians commonly go through a period of searching and disorganization following a perinatal death or other perinatal loss. Providers ponder whether anything they did or didn't do contributed to the outcome. There is very real concern for the feelings and recovery of the mother and for the fact that the grieving process will be a difficult time for family and friends. In addition, providers are faced with the possibility of a liability charge arising out of the case—a threat that has the potential for years of stress and possible ramifications for practice.

Chez (1995) offers several observations about things he has learned over years of obstetric practice:

- Most losses don't make sense.
- I am not an advocate of hospital grief teams that

take over my role. I want to have the primary therapeutic relationship if the patient also wants it.

- Much of what happens around the time of delivery is remembered.
- Too often I am confronted with the fact that there is no explanation for the death despite an autopsy.
- I do burn out at intervals. I get tired, frustrated, and withdrawn and have an intense personal sense of loss. This occurs whether I do or do not hold myself responsible for the outcome.
- Some women speak about their pain in exceptionally poignant and poetic ways . . . Sitting down with a patient, purposeful silence, and the expenditure of time allows this to happen. I have to step back and let the patient set the pace. Some patients do not want me to help, and I have to withdraw without always knowing why.

Psychologic stress in the face of perinatal grieving is an expected part of caring for childbearing families. Providers who deny stress are not being honest with themselves or have isolated themselves from the human element of practice. Midwives and physicians need to develop ways to have "safe" space to work through the emotions of attending the birth of a stillborn, delivery of an infant with major anomalies, or facing a neonatal death after an otherwise normal pregnancy. One practice in Northern California brings in a facilitator several times each year so that staff within the practice can discuss feelings and emotions arising out of difficult cases. Staff report that this process not only helps individuals cope but assists staff members in retaining a cooperative, supportive group identity that fosters growth and satisfaction in all participants.

Midwives and physicians need to nurture themselves as individuals in times of stress. Stress-associated problems with sleep may contribute to fatigue and restlessness. Changes in appetite may contribute to further decrease in well-being. Providers should identify interventions that may help in regaining balance. For some it may be going away for several days, attending a retreat, participating in spiritual community activities, or spending time with loved ones. For others, it may be spending time with colleagues in activities that validate one's expertise and skill in providing perinatal care. All professionals caring for families who face crises need to recognize signs of unhealthy coping. Deterioration of professional relationship with colleagues and patients, dysfunctional family relationships, and chronic somatic complaints associated with stress are indications that referral for professional counseling is indicated.

References

Altshuler LL, Hendrick V, Cohen LS: Course of mood and anxiety disorders during pregnancy and the postpartum period, *J Clin Psychiatry* 59(suppl 2):29-33, 1998.

Beck CT: A meta-analysis of predictors of postpartum depression, *Nurs Res* 45(5):297-303, 1996.

Bowes WA: Postpartum care. In Gabbe SG, Niebyl JR, Simpson JL, editors: *Obstetrics—normal and problem pregnancies,* ed 3, New York, 1996, Churchill Livingstone.

Chez RA: Acute grief and mourning: one obstetrician's experience, *Obstet Gynecol* 85(6):1059-1061, 1995.

Corr CA, Nabe CM, Corr DM: *Death and dying, life and living,* Pacific Grove, Calif, 1996, Brooks/Cole Publishing.

Covington SN, Theut SK: Reactions to perinatal loss: a qualitative analysis of the National Maternal and Infant Health Survey, *Am J Orthopsychiatry* 63(2):215-222, 1993.

Crowther ME: Communication following a stillbirth or neonatal death: room for improvement, *Br J Obstet Gynaecol* 102(12):952-956, 1995.

Dietz PM et al: Differences in the risk of homicide and other fatal injuries between postpartum women and other women of childbearing age: implications for prevention, *Am J Public Health* 88(4):641-643, 1998.

Downey V et al: Dying babies and associated stress in NICU nurses, *Neonatal Network* 14(1):41-46, 1995.

Duff P: Maternal and perinatal infections. In Gabbe SG, Niebyl JR, Simpson JL, editors: *Obstetrics—normal and problem pregnancies,* ed 3, New York, 1996, Churchill Livingstone.

Dumoulin C et al: Pelvic-floor rehabilitation. Part 2. Pelvic-floor reeducation with interferential currents and exercise in the treatment of genuine stress incontinence in postpartum women—a cohort study, *Phys Ther* 75(12):1075-1081, 1995.

Edelstein L: *Maternal bereavement—coping with the unexpected death of a child,* New York, 1984, Praeger Publishers.

Fetherston C: Risk factors for lactation mastitis, *J Hum Lactation* 14(2):101-109, 1998.

Fildes J et al: Trauma: the leading cause of maternal death, *J Trauma* 332:643-645, 1992.

Finkbeiner AK: *After the death of a child—living with loss through the years,* New York, 1996, The Free Press.

Foldspang A, Mommsen S, Djurhuus JC: Prevalent urinary incontinence as a correlate of pregnancy, vaginal childbirth, and obstetric techniques, *Am J Public Health* 89(2):209-212, 1999.

Fossey L, Papiernak E, Bydlowski M: Postpartum blues: a clinical syndrome and predictor of postnatal depression? *J Psychosom Obstet Gynaecol* 18(1):17-21, 1997.

Gabbe SG, Niebyl JR, Simpson JL: *Pocket companion to obstetrics—normal and problem pregnancies,* ed 3, New York, 1999, Churchill Livingstone.

Gibbs RS, Blanco JD, St Clair PJ: A case-control study of wound abscesses after cesarean delivery, *Obstet Gynecol* 62:498-502, 1983.

Harris B, Othman S, Davies JA: Association between postpartum thyroid dysfunction and thyroid antibodies and depression, *Br Med J* 305:152-156, 1989.

Hendrick V, Altshuler LL: Hormonal changes in the postpartum and implications for postpartum depression, *Psychosomatics* 39(2):93-101, 1998.

Lavender T, Walkinshaw SA: Can midwives reduce postpartum psychological morbidity? a randomized trial, *Birth* 25(4):215-219, 1998.

Lemmer CM: Parental perceptions of caring following perinatal bereavement, *West J Nurs Res* 13(4):475-493, 1991.

Leon I: *When a baby dies—psychotherapy for pregnancy and newborn loss,* New Haven, 1990, Yale University Press.

McArthur C, Bick DE, Keighley MRB: Faecal incontinence after childbirth, *Br J Obstet Gynaecol* 104:46-50, 1997.

McColl MD et al: Risk factors for pregnancy associated venous thromboembolism, *Thromb Haemost* 78:1183-1188, 1997.

Nonacs R, Cohen LS: Postpartum mood disorders: diagnosis and treatment guidelines, *J Clin Psychiatry* 59 (suppl 2): 34-40, 1998.

Rand CSW et al: Parental behavior after perinatal death: twelve years of observations, *J Psychosom Obstet Gynecol* 19(1):44-48, 1998.

Ray JG, Chan WS: Deep vein thrombosis during pregnancy and the puerperium: a meta-analysis of the period of risk and the leg of presentation, *Obstet Gynecol Surv* 54(4):265-271, 1999.

Schaap AHP et al: Long-term impact of perinatal bereavement—Comparison of grief reactions after intrauterine versus neonatal death, *Eur J Obstet Gynecol* 75:161-167, 1997.

Schwab R: Gender differences in parental grief, *Death Studies* 20(2):103-113, 1996.

Sweet BR: *Mayes' midwifery—a textbook for midwives,* ed 12, London, 1997, Baillière Tindall.

Terry AJ, Hague WM: Postpartum thyroiditis, *Semin Perinatol* 22(6):497-502, 1998.

Vance JC et al: Gender differences in parental psychological distress following perinatal death or sudden infant death syndrome, *Br J Psychiatry* 167(6):806-811, 1995a.

Vance JC et al: Psychological changes in parents eight months after the loss of an infant from stillbirth, neonatal death, or sudden infant death syndrome—a longitudinal study, *Pediatrics* 96(5):933-938, 1995b.

Wynne JM et al: Disturbed anal sphincter function following vaginal delivery, *Gut* 39:120-124, 1996.

Unit

V

Maintaining Quality Maternal-Infant Health Care

Chapter 29

Ethical Aspects of Care

Joyce E. Thompson, CNM, DrPH, FAAN, FACNM,
and Henry O. Thompson, MDiv., PhD (In memoria)

When women and their state of health, especially when they choose to carry out their reproductive role, are the primary foci of health care services, ethics and ethical concerns are many and complex. Ethics is a major concern for all health professionals, and the ethics of caring with and for women is but one important subset of this concern. As noted in the highly acclaimed document on women's reproductive health from the World Health Organization, *Mother-Baby Package: Implementing Safe Motherhood in Countries* (1996), all efforts to support, maintain, and enhance the health of women during childbearing are built on the basic foundation of equity for women—a key philosophic, moral, and theologic concept.

Equity for Women

Building on the outcomes of the Fourth World Conference on Women in Beijing 1995, the *Platform for Action* and *Beijing Declaration* (United Nations, 1996, p. 56) reinforced the notion of equity when they stated, "women have the right to the enjoyment of the highest attainable standard of physical and mental health." The IPPF *Charter on Sexual and Reproductive Rights* (1996) embodies many of the actions affirmed by United Nations Conventions and global meetings, beginning with the 1948 Charter of the United Nations and World Health Organization affirming equal rights for men and women, through the 1979 *Convention on the Elimination of All Forms of Discrimination Against Women,* the Cairo population conference in 1994, and the Beijing Fourth World Conference on Women in August 1995. The deliberations and outcomes of each of these international conferences and declarations with, for, and about women are essential background for any student in the health profession who plans to work with women and provide health care services.

Health as a Basic Human Right for All

This chapter follows the "health as a basic human right" line of reasoning and highlights some of the key ethical issues, including equity, that women, childbearing families, and health professionals who provide services during the childbearing year must recognize and face on a daily basis (Cook, 1997). The emphasis is on the ethical concerns in the promotion and maintenance of health and the prevention of disease and disability for women and their newborns during the childbearing year, from before conception through the postpartum period. The chapter concludes with an exploration of how women and health professionals can reason morally and make ethical decisions that promote the health of women and their families.

MAJOR ETHICAL CONCERNS DURING THE CHILDBEARING YEAR

Ethical concerns during the childbearing year begin for most women when they are born female. Many societies value women primarily for their reproductive roles, and such cultural conditioning for motherhood begins at a very young age. When a person's self-esteem and self-worth is tied to such a strong culturally defined reproductive role, is it any wonder that massive technologic efforts to produce a pregnancy (and the resultant child) have far outstripped the human capacity to fully understand the ethical issues raised by new reproductive technologies such as in vitro fertilization, gamete intrafallopian transfer, and zygote intrafallopian transfer, as well as the centuries-old technology of artificial insemination (Corea, 1985; Singer and Wells, 1985; Stanworth, 1987)? In fact, one of the key ethical issues within health and illness care in general, including reproductive health care, is the extremely high "value" placed on technology and technologic solutions to poor health or the results of unhealthy lifestyles—often viewed at the expense of the concern for the person on whom such technology is used (Thompson and Thompson, 1985; Verny, 1985). And yet, technology was developed as an adjunct to clinical decision-making, not as a replacement. Midwives and others need not only to understand the technology available to them as clinicians, but how to apply that technology in an ethical manner.

Ethical Use of Technology

The ethical use of technology during reproduction is a hotly debated topic in many areas of society, within health facilities and within families. Consider the basic push to have all women birth in a hospital for "safety's" sake, which is often a thinly veiled cover-up for having women placed in a strange environment that allows others to control their birth experience (Freda, 1994; Rothman, 1996; Stauning, 1994; Thompson and Thompson, 1980; Verny, 1985). This control includes close proximity to technology (electronic fetal monitoring, ultrasound imaging, cesarean section), which cannot be "used" if women choose to birth at home or in most free-standing birth centers.

The overuse of technology during labor and birth often leads to unnecessary intervention or a cascade of events that result in more technology being required to "treat" the effects of the initial use of unwarranted technology (e.g., epidural, oxytocin augmentation, failure to progress in labor that leads to a cesarean section). However, it must be noted that this comment refers to situations in which such technologic interventions are begun for the convenience of the staff or family, not situations that require such intervention to save the life of mother or infant. Technology in and of itself is neither good nor bad; how it is used by human beings determines that. What is your value related to the use of reproductive technology as a health professional? What do your patients want? Will you agree to the newest "baby picture" from ultrasound imaging when there is no indication to perform an ultrasound? Will you agree to elective induction of labor or cesarean section for a woman who is tired of being pregnant or wants no labor? These and other questions raise important ethical concerns on a daily basis for health workers who care for women and childbearing families. How will you respond as a primary care provider?

The *technologic imperative* to use technology just because it is available is not an ethical approach to the use of technology. Technology should be used (1) when indicated, (2) when the benefits of its use far outweigh the potential harm it might cause, (3) when there is no other way to accomplish the needed task (i.e., get the information), and (4) when the woman on whom the technology will be used has been given full, understandable information about the proposed technology and comprehends what it will or will not do and then is allowed to make the needed decision without coercion or threat of loss of care. The ethical use of technology is based on the ethical principles of respect for human dignity (self-determination, autonomy); doing good (beneficence) and, above all, not harming anyone (nonmaleficence); honesty and integrity (being able to say "I don't know" or that the potential harm is unknown at this time); and scientific evidence, not wishful thinking. The ethical decision-making process is described in more detail later in this chapter.

Ethics and Genetics

Ethical issues raised by the expanding knowledge of genetics and the human genome project that has nearly completed the mapping of our body's genetic material give rise to even more complex ethical questions and concerns. Less than 30 years ago, amniocentesis raised very emotional questions about whether a pregnancy might be terminated if it was found that a fetus was genetically imperfect. This technology was originally introduced in the 1950s to test for Rh-hemolytic disease in the third trimester of pregnancy (Walker, 1957; Verny, 1985) but quickly opened the door to genetic information as science forged ahead to understand genetic disease and disability. Will the newest genetic information lead to societal limits on who will be "allowed" to reproduce? Will cloning in animals be allowed to proceed to cloning human beings? And should our society allow experimentation on "left-over" fertilized zygotes from assisted reproductive events? These are the questions that are filling the popular press, and the health professionals caring for today's women and their families need to be aware of the issues or, at best, know to whom the couple can be referred to for further information. These issues are important, but they are not the essence of the focus on ethical aspects of childbearing care as addressed in this chapter for the beginning clinician.

Daily Ethical Concerns in Childbearing

Contraception, genetics, and abortion. The ethical aspects of childbearing care of note in this chapter include the daily interactions and decisions needed during the care of women and childbearing families who are anticipating a healthy pregnancy and birth. These ethical concerns begin before conception with selection of a method of contraception and planned choice of pregnancy. However, it is foolish to assume that our society is close to full choice for pregnancy and parenting and that only those who are ready, willing, and able to raise a child are the ones who are pregnant. This is false. It is a known fact that nearly half of all pregnancies are unwanted at the time of conception (e.g., wrong time, wrong situation, wrong partner). It is also known that many women choose abortion to terminate unwanted pregnancies and this "choice" may be morally offensive to some clinicians who are deeply, morally opposed to abortion (Thompson and Thompson, 1988). We suggest that producing an unwanted infant who is later abused, ignored, or allowed to die is even more tragic—a moral offense, we suggest, against an unsuspecting newborn who has neither the power nor the ability to fight back. And what will you, the health professional, do when a 12-year-old girl asks you for contraception? Do you, the clinician, know what your moral stance and value position is on these issues you will face in practice?

The prenatal period. If we move on to the prenatal period, ethical decisions surrounding genetic testing, use of the results, and whether abortion should be an option when a genetic disease is discovered in the fetus frequently surface for the clinician. And what is a thoughtful response to parents who request a selective termination of pregnancy because the sex of the fetus is not what is wanted? Will you enter into dialogue with such potential parents or simply refer to a provider who will support their choice of abortion for sex selection?

It is incumbent on each health care professional to understand her or his own values and moral positions on the issues raised by sexual behavior, reproductive choices, and the provision of prenatal care to minors. How will you respond when a 14-year-old appears in your office with her second pregnancy well advanced? How will your personal values and moral attitudes influence your ability to give quality care to this young girl? How will you respond when a woman asks for an ultrasound image of her fetus for the baby book? What will you say when your competency as a midwife is challenged by families who think they should have the "best" care—that of a doctor? What will you do? These and other questions form the essence of need for understanding the ethical dimensions of childbearing care that begins well before the pregnancy itself.

Choice of provider and site of birth. Because the choice of health care provider and site of birth are such common events, the ethical concerns surrounding them are even more difficult at times. The issue of "competent" health professionals should be the ethical basis for such choices, but are women/families given full information about each type of midwife, each type of doctor, each type of medical assistant or nurse practitioner who offers prenatal and birth care? What should the consumer look for in selecting a health professional to guide them through pregnancy, birth, and the postpartum/parenting periods (ACNM and Jacobs, 1993)? Are some professional groups deliberately falsifying information about other groups that they wish would go away? Why are these professional "turf wars" so prevalent in today's health care market? Do some groups of women's health providers fear loss of patients or loss of income? Do we really believe that all persons who call themselves midwives are equally competent? And what is the basis for competency comparison between physicians and midwives? These are just a few of the questions that surface when health professionals discuss the ethical concept of "competence"; confusion abounds. This confusion transfers to the consumer.

There is general agreement that, for the 5% to 7% of women who are ill or severely debilitated by pregnancy, hospitals and specialist physicians are "best." However, as one of the authors (J.E.T.) questioned some years ago, why should the pattern of childbearing care established for the 5% to 7% of women who are ill during pregnancy be forced on the 92% to 95% of women who are healthy during pregnancy and birth? How would you respond to client questions about safety, competence, and choices during pregnancy and birth? What resources would you offer for information and understanding of the basis for choice of health care provider and site of birth? Do you support freedom of choice for women and childbearing families, especially when they wish care from someone else? (Brown, 1996)

Established medicine often uses the "safety" and "qualified" provider issues to lobby against free choice of nonmedical practitioners such as midwives. The irony of such discussions is that obstetricians who work with midwives and the American College of Obstetricians and Gynecologists support the inclusion of professional midwives on the team caring for women's health and childbearing needs within a joint statement on practice relationships. It is both interesting and unfortunate that other types of physicians, generalists, and specialists are the ones who argue against midwives and advanced practice nurses. It would seem that legitimate concern for the quality of care during pregnancy and birth is less the issue for these medical organizations than maintaining their dominance over women, control of female health professionals, and control of the birth process itself (Rothman, 1996; Thompson and Thompson, 1980; Verny, 1985).

VALUE PERSPECTIVES IN MIDWIFERY CARE

Values are often used interchangeably with ethics (Steele and Harmon, 1983; Thompson and Thompson, 1985), but we choose another approach explained as follows. Values underlie decisions and actions in daily life in that they determine what information we will gather/use or ignore in decision-making. Unexamined values can lead to the unconscious imposition of the midwife's personal and professional values on an unsuspecting public. Values give direction to our choices, but they do not necessarily lead to ethical actions or decisions (Thompson and Thompson, 1990; Thompson and Thompson, 1995). Some of our values are inherently wrong for others when put to public scrutiny. For example, holding a strong work ethic and acting on that in one's daily life may lead to a bias against the vulnerable populations of women who do not have access to gainful employment or wages and who then fall onto the welfare rolls of this country. Or maybe you, the reader, were on welfare at some time in your own life and "made it" off by hard work, and thus you think that everyone should be able to do the same. To then conclude that women on welfare are less than human and less than deserving of public support and/or quality health services does not fit the ethical reasoning of caring for the less fortunate, the vulnerable, the poor, or those who have suffered many societal injustices that result in poor health—mandates inherent in the concept of equity (Cook, 1997).

Because values are so important to understanding who we are as people and what influences the decisions we make in our lives, we think it is important for the reader to understand the dominant values within this chapter on ethics, many of which have already been highlighted in the previous discussion. We believe that in knowing and understanding one's values and how those values might bias or influence decision making during the care of women, the midwife is better prepared to make decisions that reflect ethical health care for each woman and childbearing family (Thompson and Thompson, 1985).

Women Are Persons

We hold three basic values that inform the approach to ethics and the application of ethics to clinical practice in the care of women and childbearing families. The first is that *women are persons,* not objects. This also relates to Immanuel Kant's dictum that persons are ends in themselves and never to be used as a means to accomplish another's goals (Thompson and Thompson, 1985). Women who choose to carry out their reproductive role need to be viewed as whole, as human, as competent persons who will become competent and trustworthy mothers. The personhood of women begins with the understanding that human rights are women's rights and women's rights are human rights (Clinton, 1995; United Nations, 1979; IPPF, 1996). Some of the sexual and reproductive rights of particular concern for women are the right to information and education, the right to be treated with respect, the right to understand what is happening to their own bodies, the right to privacy, the right to liberty and security, the right to choose whether or not to carry and to found and plan a family, and the right to participate actively in decisions about their own health care (IPPF, 1996). And along with these human rights comes the need to act responsibly in making choices and the willingness to accept the consequences of these choices. Thus midwives and women need to understand the inherent *responsibilities* that go along with having rights.

Childbearing Is Normal

The second value is that childbearing is a normal biopsychosocial and cultural event in the lives of most women. It is a healthy life event with many cultural traditions and beliefs that influence how women, families, and health professionals interact during the childbearing year. The approach to midwifery care (ACNM, 1990; ICM, 1993) viewing pregnancy as "normal" is quite distinct from a traditional medical view of pregnancy as disease and pregnant women as a potential disaster waiting to happen. The midwife's decision to value health and health promotion leads to a very different approach to providing childbearing services than the disease orientation of other health professionals. Rothman (1996) wrote that "childbirth in America is dominated by a management perspective that emphasizes the efficient removal of a fetus from a woman's body, thus leaving the woman with little power or control—or worse, little trust in her own body." Valuing the woman as a capable human being with unique needs and wants during childbearing leads to a partnership model of health service delivery (Brown, 1996; Freda, 1994; Thompson and Thompson, 1985; Verny, 1985) rather than a paternalistic model (Scully, 1980).

Childbearing Care Is a Partnership

Our third basic value position is that women and families are willing and able to participate actively in decisions about their health care, given comprehensive and comprehensible information that informs those decisions. As noted previously, this value leads to a *partnership model of health service delivery* that is central to the discussion of ethics and ethical issues during the childbearing year. Contrary to popular myth in our society today, pregnancy and birth do not alter the woman's ability to think and act. However, how information is given, when such knowledge is shared, and the level of comprehension of shared information are important components of a partnership model of health service delivery. If the health worker believes that the woman and her family will not understand the "complexity" of the situation or proposed technology, the health worker has already made an unethical decision to not share information based on a lack of respect for the humanness of the woman. Health professionals do not automatically know "what is best" for those who seek professional health services, and such strong parentalism does not fit into an ethical approach to childbearing care for women as persons, childbearing as normal, and shared decision making.

Women who want someone else to "take care of them" during pregnancy and birth are challenging to health professionals who prefer to work on a shared model of decision making. This challenge begins with respecting the woman's right "not to know" and therefore not to participate in decision making while working to help the woman understand the crucial role and responsibility she carries for her own health and the health of her developing fetus. Health care workers know they cannot eat, sleep, or exercise for pregnant women nor can they avoid hazardous work environments or illicit drugs. The woman must be strengthened and supported in her efforts to adopt healthy behaviors, beginning with understanding that her health is important because *she* is important, of value, worthy. The midwife's commitment to and effective sharing of information about one's body and the process of pregnancy and birth, together with support and encouragement for the woman as she begins to take responsibility for her own health, including decisions that will keep her healthy, begin an important path to empowerment and enhanced self-esteem. As a new mother said when asked to reflect on her childbearing experience at the Childbearing Center of Morris Heights, "I did it! I gave birth! If I can give birth, I can do anything!" She went on to say that birth empowers women who can then empower their families and their communities (Maternity Center Association, 1994). What a powerful lesson in self-esteem and empowerment for all health professionals who work with women during childbearing.

INFORMED DECISION MAKING AND CONSENT

The three elements of information sharing that provide the basis for shared decision making (i.e., how, when, and what is understood) are all grounded in the ethical concept of *informed consent.* The ethical concept of informed consent is grounded in respect for persons—autonomy and self-determination (Bandman and Bandman, 1995; Davis et al., 1997; Thompson and Thompson, 1981). When a woman decides a course of action based on necessary and clear information, she can be said to be acting autonomously. As stated in the ACNM *Code of Ethics* (1990), "nurse-midwives share professional information with their clients that leads to informed participation and consent. This sharing is done without coercion or deception." Except in emergency and selected complex situations, health professionals are obligated to support the informed decision of the woman, even when it disagrees with the choice of the professional (Brown, 1996; Freda, 1994; Thompson and Thompson, 1988). The promotion of "good" and avoidance of "harm" are other key ethical principles that provide the basis for the doctrine of informed consent.

It is not easy to implement the doctrine of informed consent, however. Much of the information shared with pregnant women and families is "filtered" by and through the values of the teacher, whether it be midwife, childbirth educator, or physician. How much can this woman understand, how should one present this information, how much information is reasonable for the time the health professional has available with the client, and what level of language will lead to understanding are several of the questions that filter the sharing of information. If the woman has not read widely about pregnancy and birth, she may have personal/family experiences that inform her understanding of this life event. Some of these are positive, others negative. The same happens with those who read about an experience they have yet to have themselves; some writings enhance understanding, and others enhance fear. The important thing for health professionals is to begin where the woman is and proceed from there. This takes time and genuine interest in learning about the woman and her life experiences, time that too often is cut short because of competing demands of health systems, financial expediency, or conflicting loyalties of the midwife. Time and caring go together, and the midwife is a critical force in making sure both are available to each woman.

The ethical doctrine of informed consent contains the mandate to explain, to offer alternatives, to discuss risks and benefits of a particular choice of action, to make sure the information is understood by the client, and then to encourage the client to choose the action best for her (Thompson and Thompson, 1981). If the midwife decides "not to tell" or withholds some crucial details about a needed decision, the midwife ends up coercing the woman to choose what the midwife wants done rather than what the woman may have chosen. Such coercion is unethical, especially when done intentionally. Informed participation in decisions for health care is the ethical ideal, but it is very difficult to achieve at times. Sometimes the woman does not want to make the needed decision, sometimes the provider is not aware of her or his own value biases, and sometimes the emergency nature of the situation does not allow time for fully shared decisions. The ideal is important, however, for we are working with essentially healthy women who are participating in a normal life event. We are working with human beings deserving of respect and who have a right to information, a right to "know," and a right to choose what is best for themselves and their developing fetus, after careful reflection and due consideration of alternatives.

WHY BE CONCERNED WITH ETHICS

Some might ask, "Why we should be concerned with ethics in a text on community-based childbearing care for women and families. After spending many years learning to be a midwife or nurse or physician, don't we already know what to do and how to care for women? Don't we *know* what is 'right' or appropriate in a given situation?" Others might view a discussion of ethics as simply a mini course in religion and then ask, "What about those who read this text who espouse no religion?" Still others suggest that a discussion of ethics does not necessarily lead to ethical practice (we often *know* how to be better practitioners than we are) or demand, as a physician colleague challenged, "Tell me how studying ethics will make me a better doctor!" Although there is an element of "truth" in each of these perspectives, none reflect a full understanding of the nature of health care ethics and why this understanding can lead to better midwives, nurses, and doctors and to ethical practice as professionals.

Goal of Ethical Practice

The goal of ethical midwifery practice (as with all other health professionals) is to *do the right thing for the right reason* (Veatch and Fry, 1987). So how do we know what is "right" action or reason? Understanding the nature of ethics, how one develops morally, and how to apply moral reasoning to clinical decision making are the rationale for including ethics content in this text. For many, it should be Chapter 1 in any health care text as the content pervades everything we learn about and do as health care professionals. The nature of being a professional is to be ethical in everything we say and do. The moral standards of behavior espoused by the profession must be known and adopted if we truly care about the women and families we purport to serve. These standards are often embodied in a series of statements called an "ethics code."

Codes of Ethical Conduct

At minimum, each health professional who works with women needs to know and understand their own profession's code of ethics. For midwives, such codes include the ACNM *Code of Ethics for Certified Nurse-Midwives* (1990), the MANA *Statement of Values and Ethics* (1991), or the ICM *International Code of Ethics for Midwives* (1993). For nurses the ANA *Code of Ethics for*

Nursing (1998) is an excellent resource for understanding the values, duties, and obligations of the nurse. For physicians the AMA *Principles of Medical Ethics* (1968) is a helpful reference. For a more global perspective on women's reproductive health, the reader is referred to the IPPF *Charter on Sexual and Reproductive Rights* (1996) or the Commonwealth Medical Association's *The Guiding Principles* (1993) on medical ethics and human rights and *1997 Declaration* from an interdisciplinary consultation on "Ethics and a Woman's Right to Health." Statement 1 of this Declaration reinforces the interrelationship of ethics and human rights in the health care of women. It reads, in part, "The health status, including sexual and reproductive health, of women is adversely affected by a wide range of human rights violations. Health professionals are well placed to detect many such violations. . . . " It is also suggested that every health professional working with women and their reproductive health concerns be informed about human rights as discussed in such documents as the 1979 *United Nations Convention on the Elimination of All Forms of Discrimination Against Women (CEDAW)* and the 1996 *Platform for Action and the Beijing Declaration* following the Fourth World Conference on Women.

The essential precepts of ethical codes for midwives include respect for women as persons, shared decision making, maintenance of confidentiality and privacy, informed participation and consent for care, nondiscrimination in caregiving, protection of clients from harm, and maintenance of competence in one's practice. Other moral duties include participating in the education of future midwives, promotion of health policies that support quality care for childbearing families and women, participation in advancing the knowledge of the profession, and respectful interaction with other health workers. The ACNM code begins with, "Nurse-midwifery exists for the good of women and their families . . ." (ACNM, 1990). This value perspective of a professional dedicated to the service of others is an important facet of midwifery practice as it is for all health professionals.

Ethical codes define the moral behaviors expected of the professional and thus socialize the individual to the values of that particular professional group. Yet it is important for each individual health worker to begin with herself or himself—to understand the gut-level and other personal values that she or he has adopted throughout the teen and adult years to date. And health professionals need to begin with self-respect and self-esteem as a basis for enhancing the self-respect and self-esteem in others. They must also go beyond the self—beyond values to know, understand, and apply ethics as the core of being a professional. They must do good and avoid harming those who come to us for health care. Health professionals must always be responsible in their caring and accountable for the decisions and actions they take (Thompson and Thompson, 1996). Women deserve our best! We must help them continue their education in ethics.

Ethical Practice Is Learned

The inclusion of ethics in any basic text for health care professionals gives credence to our view that ethical practice is learned behavior; it is not automatic. Just as noted earlier concerning the often unconscious nature of values, "intuitive ethics" is rarely sufficient for health care practice in today's complex world of technology and choices in childbearing, reflected by such questions as when, how, with whom, and where? Simply knowing the "good" or "right" action to take in a given situation does not guarantee that the action will be taken. It is also important to note that, because we live and work in a society that supports ethical pluralism, sensitive, caring, and intelligent human beings can select different reasons and actions in the same situation (Thompson and Thompson, 1988). Does this imply that "anything goes?" Absolutely not! What it implies is that moral reasoning and ethical decision making require critical thinking, reflection, an awareness of personal and professional values, an understanding of how we develop morally, and the use of moral philosophy to support one's choices. Once these choices are made, ethics requires that we accept responsibility for the outcomes of our choices. This is what it means to be a moral agent (Thompson and Thompson, 1996).

THE "WHAT" OF ETHICS

Definitions

To answer the "what" of ethics, we begin with some definitions and concepts. Over the years we have found it helpful to distinguish "ethics" from "morals," although they are often used interchangeably. If one considers "morals" to be the complex *shoulds* and *oughts* of professional practice (i.e., what one should do in a given situation, what one ought to say to a grieving parent), then "ethics" is the reason for doing or saying (i.e., the "why" of action). When health professionals take the time to ask, "Why?" or when they explain the "why" of their actions, they are being ethical. Moral behavior is extremely important for the safety of all concerned, and there must be an understanding of why it is important to always strive to *be* good, as well as *do* good (Thompson and Thompson, 1995).

Virtue and Normative Ethics

Fowler and others (Davis et al., 1997) distinguish between virtue and normative ethics—the difference between what kind of person (virtue) you should be as a midwife (or health care professional) and what kind of actions (norms) you should take in the care of others. Some of the notable virtues of midwives include integrity, honesty, caring, and respect for self and others. On the other hand, codes of ethics for midwives prescribe moral behavior (i.e., what the midwife *should* or *ought* to do in providing care for women and childbearing families). But the precepts of a code of ethics are ideals and will not provide "answers" to the myriad types of situations that arise on a daily, if not hourly, basis during care of childbearing women and families. The midwife must think critically, reflect, and reason through the situation; the midwife must be a moral agent.

The Midwife As a Moral Agent

The newest draft of the ANA *Code of Ethics for Nursing* (1998) includes for the first time a provision that addresses the moral agency of the health professional. Provision 4 reads, "The nurse has responsibilities to her or himself as a person of moral worth, including duties of moral self-respect, competence, continuing professional growth and the preservation of integrity." The authors believe that any person in the health professions should be a moral agent first and foremost. Being a moral agent requires that midwives be both responsible and accountable not only for the choices/actions they take but for the results or outcomes of those choices or actions. One cannot be accountable when following the "orders" or directions of others without thinking for oneself whether the "order" is correct, right, or appropriate, regardless of whether the "other" is a physician, a supervisor, or the woman who comes to us for pregnancy care. The partnership model of woman- or family-centered care is based on respect, equity, accountability, knowledge-sharing, and joint discussion of possible actions. As noted in Statement 3 of the ACNM *Code of Ethics for Certified Nurse-Midwives* (1990), "Decisions regarding nurse-midwifery care require client participation in an ongoing negotiation process in order to develop a safe plan of care. This process considers cultural diversity, individual autonomy and legal responsibilities." It should be clear to the midwife that letting someone else dictate how to practice midwifery violates the very nature of being a moral agent. In the end, whoever makes the choice and carries out the decision is responsible for the results of that choice. A moral agent needs to understand how both the mind (rational, cognitive being) and the heart (feeling, affective) work together for good. Therefore moral agency combined with a willingness to be ethical in practice provides the framework for ethical childbearing care. Now let us explore some of the components of how to reason morally.

Components of Moral Philosophy

In the western world the "ethical why" of moral action often comes from moral philosophy. In other words, we use various ethical theories within moral philosophy to justify our choices in ethics. Moral philosophy includes utilitarianism, deontology, and natural law approaches to justifying actions. *Utilitarianism* reasons that the correct choice/action would be the one that promotes the greatest good for the greatest number of people or, alternately, the end result justifies what we had to do to get there (e.g., a cesarean section certainly causes bodily harm to the woman, but if this "means" is required to ensure a healthy infant, the outcome is considered good for all concerned [a "good" or acceptable end justifies the means]). *Deontology* reasons that certain principles or "rules" support action in a given situation. Such principles include respect for human dignity (autonomy), doing good (beneficence) and, when you can't do good, at least do no harm (nonmaleficence). Another umbrella principle is justice as being "fair" (Beauchamp, 1982). Telling the truth, maintaining confidentiality, and protecting clients from unethical practice are other ethical principles embodied within codes of ethics for nurses, midwives, and physicians, as noted earlier. *Natural Law* is primarily concerned with what is "natural" or what exists in nature as a justification for moral action. Others view natural law as a combination of concerns for both ends and means, both utilitarianism and deontology (Thompson and Thompson, 1985). As might be expected, each of these ethical theories engenders a variety of definitions. The reader is urged to consult a basic ethics theory text for an expanded discussion of them.

MORAL REASONING AND ETHICAL DECISION-MAKING

The Process of Moral Reasoning and Decision Making

This chapter has repeatedly asked, "What will you do in a given situation? What should be done? What do you value and how will that influence how you care for women?" Let us examine *how* we make decisions as health professionals and the ethical dimensions of those decisions that require moral reasoning and a knowledge of ethical theory as well as understanding the nature of persons as moral beings. Moral reasoning is very similar to the midwifery care process, the nursing process, and the medical decision process (scientific method). Moral reasoning includes steps of analysis, weighing, justifying, choosing, and evaluating (Harron, Burnside, and Beauchamp, 1983). The primary difference is that moral reasoning is applied to the moral dimensions of the clinical situation as well as the scientific dimensions (e.g., what is known, data-based). The process of making ethical decisions in clinical practice is based on knowledge of self (values, biases), knowledge of ethics and moral reasoning, knowledge of the science and the art of caring, time to critically reflect on possible choices and the potential outcomes of each of those choices, and a willingness to commit oneself to thinking and caring at all times.

Knowing one's values and value-biases begins with a process of values clarification—a reasoned, reflective process of looking at who we are, what we believe, what we value, and the biases inherent in those values that affect our ability to provide health care services with and for women. Morris Massey (1981), a value theorist, suggests that 90% of our basic or gut-level values were programmed into us by the age of 10 from such sources as family, peers, geography, economics, religion, education, and media (e.g., television, books, music). The processes include imprinting, modeling, and intense socialization. Therefore our first notion of what it means to be a boy or girl comes from this period of intense imprinting and socialization. What were your parents' views of women and men, of their roles, and how one was to interact with another on a gender basis? If you wish to understand your most deeply held personal values, begin by asking, "Where were you . . . when you were ten?" This reflection may help you understand some of the current values you hold. Adult values are added as we experience life events and include such dimensions as being freely chosen from among alternatives after thoughtful consideration of outcomes, continuing to be prized and cherished, being made known to others, and being integrated into daily decision and actions (Raths, Harmin, and Simon, 1978). Professional values from nursing, midwifery, or medicine are learned through socialization into the profession, as well as direct education and moral discourse. It is important to note that values will be "caught" if they are not taught; just by watching and listening to teachers, other midwives, clinicians, and students of the health professionals "catch" what is important to value. Values can be changed, but most value theorists suggest that you first have to know what your values are and recognize and admit you have them before you will be able to change them if they do not fit the present situation. Morris Massey (1981) suggests that values can be highlighted and changed in response to a "significant emotional event" (e.g., reading a book, a near-death experience, or discussion with someone whose value perspective is quite different from your own [affective dissonance]). Values will not change, however, unless you are willing to admit that a change is needed, put in the time and effort to understand why current values you hold are wrong for your chosen career (e.g., bigot, view of women as less than human), and then put in the time and effort to change.

Knowledge of ethics and moral reasoning comes from reading, moral discussion, and exposure to others willing to take the time to share their approach to ethical analysis and moral reasoning. Ethics texts abound, and the brief introduction earlier in this chapter speaks to the western philosophic view of ethics theory. Eastern thought includes more psychology and religion (Thompson and Thompson, 1985).

Factors that contribute to ethical decision making include such things as time, a commitment to reason and reflection, knowledge of self and others, and competence in one's chosen profession. The process requires effort, and the end result may not always be the right action or decision, but the time and effort are well worth the outcomes of better health professionals and better health care for women.

Thompson and Thompson Bioethical Decision Model

Since 1980, we have been using a framework for moral reasoning and ethical decision making (Box 29-1). It is pluralistic in nature, allowing for differences in personal and professional values and for change over time in one's view of what constitutes ethical practice in health care.

Box 29-1 *Thompson and Thompson Bioethical Decision Model (1998)*

Step One

Review the situation to determine:

1. The health problems and scientific data available
2. Decision(s) or action(s) needed first while noting further decisions needed after the initial decision
3. Key individuals (participants or players) involved in or affected by decision

Step Two

Gather additional information to clarify the situation and:

1. Understand why that information is needed (values)
2. Understand legal constraints, if any
3. Understand potential impact of information not obtainable in the situation
4. Identify other constraints (e.g., lack of time, lack of decision capacity of key individual)

Step Three

Identify the ethical issues or concerns raised in the situation:

1. Explore the historical roots of each issue
2. Explore current philosophic/religious positions on the issue
3. Explore current societal views/taboos on each issue

Step Four

Define personal and professional moral positions on the issues/concerns identified in Step Three, including:

1. Review of personal constraints raised by the issues
2. Review of professional code(s) for guidance (e.g., ACNM, ICM, ANA, AMA)
3. Identification of conflicting loyalties/obligations of health professionals
4. Identification of levels of moral development operant in self

Step Five

Identify the moral positions of key individuals involved as well as level of moral development where possible

Step Six

Identify value conflicts, if any, and:

1. Attempt to understand basis for conflict
2. Attempt possible resolution of conflict
3. Determine if outside help is needed for resolution

Step Seven

Determine who should make the needed decision(s) and your specific role in the situation

Step Eight

Identify the range of possible actions/decision and:

1. Describe the anticipated outcome for each alternative
2. Include moral justification for each (which ethical principles are upheld, which are not; utilitarian reasoning or natural law)
3. Decide which action/decision fits the criteria for decision making in this situation (may be best among good alternatives or least harmful among equally bad alternatives)

Step Nine

Decide on a course of action and carry it out:

1. Know the reasons for the choice of action/decision
2. Be able to explain the reasons to others
3. Establish a time frame for review of outcomes

Step Ten

Evaluate the results of decision/action taken, including:

1. Did the expected outcomes occur? If not, why not?
2. Is a new decision needed? If so, return to steps of the model and make a new selection based on new information now available.
3. Was the decision process complete?

Adapted from Thompson JE, Thompson HO: *Bioethical decision making for nurses,* Norwalk, 1985, Appleton-Century-Crofts.

The model has been used successfully by a range of health care professionals and in a variety of clinical and health policy situations. It acknowledges some of the common constraints on ethical decision making that health professionals encounter, including conflicting loyalties (patient, family, other midwives, physicians, employer), legal rules, cultural taboos, and the potential impact on decision making that failure to obtain certain information might have (e.g., neonates cannot tell us preferences, untested technology risks). The model also asks the user to consider the historical basis for the ethical issue that might inform current judgments (understanding).

The theoretic basis of the decision model is moral reasoning—a critical inquiry into the ethical dimensions of health care with awareness that one may agree or disagree with others during the process, noting that the important characteristics of the user are the willingness to try to understand other points of moral discourse and reasoning, to respect the differences, and to be willing to put forth one's own reasoning on the issue for examination by others. It is vital to also note that the 10-step decision model for decision making represents a *process* rather than a fail-safe formula for choosing the right or best alternative for action (Thompson and Thompson, 1985).

The best use of this model is with others that are willing to be honest, to respect one another, and to hold their own moral point of view out for others. You, the health professional, have to be willing to think, care, and act in a professional manner because the success of the model depends on the user, it depends on you as a moral agent. The model can be used during ethics rounds, during classroom discussion of actual case studies (protecting the confidentiality of the client, of course), during ethics consultations, or as a framework for daily practice in interaction with others, including the women who come for health care. It is our hope that the reader of this text is stimulated to understand herself or himself and her or his values and personal perspective on providing community-based childbearing care for women and families. We also hope that ethics will be such an integral part of women's health care that questions of gender bias, role discrimination, and freedom of choice will be openly examined and freely discussed and previously conceived prejudices overcome in the interest of providing the "best" of health care for women—health care rooted in the value of women as persons with full rights as human beings and based on a partnership model of service delivery. Women and childbearing families have a right to receive and deserve ethical care from caring professionals.

References

American College of Nurse-Midwives: *Code of ethics for certified nurse-midwives,* Washington, DC, 1990, ACNM.

American College of Nurse-Midwives, Jacobs S: *Having your baby with a nurse-midwife,* New York, 1993, Hyperion.

American Medical Association: *Principles of medical ethics,* 1968, The Association.

American Nurses Association: *Code of ethics for nursing: provisions,* Washington, DC, 1998, ANA (draft version).

Bandman EL, Bandman B: *Nursing ethics through the life span,* ed 3, Stamford, Conn, 1995, Appleton & Lange.

Beauchamp TL: "Ethical theory and bioethics." In Beauchamp TL, Walters L, editors: *Contemporary issues in bioethics,* ed 2, Belmont, Calif, 1982, Wadsworth.

Brown C: Freedom of choice: an expression of emerging power relationships between a childbearing woman and her caregiver, *Int J Childbirth Ed* 11(3):12-16, 1996.

Clinton H: Women's rights as human rights. Paper presented at 4th World Conference on Women, 1995, Beijing, China.

Commonwealth Medical Association: *Guiding principles of medical ethics and human rights,* London, 1993, CMA.

Commonwealth Medical Association: *Declaration on ethics and a woman's right to health,* London, 1997, CMA.

Cook RJ: Advancing safe motherhood through human rights. Paper presented at WHO technical consultation on Safe Motherhood, 1997, Colombo, Sri Lanka.

Corea G: *The mother machine,* New York, 1985, Harper & Row.

Davis AJ et al: *Ethical dilemmas and nursing practice,* ed 4, Stamford, Conn, 1997, Appleton & Lange.

Freda MC: Childbearing, reproductive control, aging women, and health care: the projected ethical debates, *JOGNN* 23(2):144-152, 1994.

Harron F, Burnside J, Beauchamp T: *Health and human values: a guide to making your own decisions,* New Haven, 1983, Yale University Press.

International Confederation of Midwives: *International code of ethics for midwives,* London, 1993, ICM.

International Planned Parenthood Federation: *IPPF Charter on sexual and reproductive rights: vision 2000,* London, 1996, The Federation.

Massey M: *What you are is,* Series of three videotapes on values, 1981, CBS Fox Video.

Maternity Center Association: *Hope reborn: empowering families in the south Bronx* (video), New York, 1994, MCA.

Midwives Alliance of North America: Statement of values and ethics, *MANA News Special Supplement,* Summer, 1991.

Raths LE, Harmin M, Simon SB: *Values and teaching: working with values in the classroom,* ed 2, Columbus, 1978, CE Merrill Publishing.

Rothman BK: Women, providers and control, *JOGNN* 25:253-256, 1996.

Scully D: *Men who control women's health,* Boston, 1980, Houghton-Mifflin.

Singer P, Wells D: *Making babies: the new science and ethics of conception,* New York, 1985, Charles Scribner's Sons.

Stanworth M, editor: *Reproductive technologies: gender, motherhood and medicine,* Minneapolis, 1987, University of Minnesota Press.

Stauning I: Women, health, and medical technology, *Int J Technol Assess Health Care* 10(2):273-281, 1994.

Steele SM, Harmon VM: *Values clarification in nursing,* ed 2, Norwalk, 1983, Appleton-Century-Crofts.

Thompson HO, Thompson JE: The ethics of being a female patient and a female care provider in a male dominated health-illness system, *Issues Health Care Women* 2(3-4):25-54, 1980.

Thompson JB, Thompson HO: *Ethics in nursing,* New York, 1981, Macmillan.

Thompson JE, Thompson HO: *Bioethical decision making for nurses,* Norwalk, 1985, Appleton-Century-Crofts.

Thompson JE, Thompson HO: Living with ethical decisions with which you disagree, *MCN* 13(July/August):245-250, 1988.

Thompson JE, Thompson HO: Values: directional signals for life choices, *Neonatal Network* 8:4, 1990.

Thompson JE, Thompson HO: Handbook of Ethics for Midwives University of Pennsylvania Graduate Program in Nurse-Midwifery, Philadelphia, 1995.

Thompson JE, Thompson HO: Why should midwives be concerned with ethics? *Midwifery Today,* Winter 1996, pp 36-40.

Thompson JE, Thompson HO: Thompson and Thompson Bioethical Decision Model, revised 1998.

United Nations: *Convention on the elimination of all forms of discrimination against women,* New York, 1979, United Nations.

United Nations: *Beijing declaration and platform for action,* New York, 1996, United Nations.

Veatch R, Fry S: *Case studies in nursing ethics,* Philadelphia, 1987, JB Lippincott.

Verny TR: The psycho-technology of pregnancy and labor, *Neonatal Network* 3(5):12-22, 1985.

Walker AHC: Liquor amnii studies in the prediction of haemolytic disease of the newborn, *Br Med J* 2:376, 1957.

World Health Organization Division of Family Health: *Mother-baby package: implementing safe motherhood in countries,* Geneva, 1996, WHO.

Chapter 30

Continuous Quality Improvement in Maternal-Infant Care

Anne Scupholme, CNM, MPH, FACNM

The focus of this chapter is the evolving role of continuous quality improvement (CQI) programs in the field of maternal-infant care, with particular emphasis on the roles of the clinical practitioners—midwife, nurse practitioner, physician, physician assistant—in an interdisciplinary health care team. Systems for evaluating quality of care are established for three reasons:

1. To improve the quality of health care delivery to patients
2. To reassure institutions, regulators, and the public that the care provided is both monitored and, when necessary, modified
3. To reduce liability

It is a professional standard of responsibility for practitioners to monitor the quality of care that they provide because of their commitment to provide patients the best care possible, wherever that care is given, and regardless of the population served. The American College of Nurse-Midwives (ACNM) Position Statement entitled *Quality Management in Midwifery Care* notes:

> Promotion and evaluation of high quality care are a priority for the midwifery profession, and ACNM strongly recommends that practicing midwives participate in all aspects of quality management: quality assurance (QA), peer review, and quality improvement (ACNM, 1997).

In addition, the ACNM Standards for Practice specifically notes that "Nurse-midwifery care is evaluated according to an established program for quality assessment that includes a plan to identify and resolve problems," and "The nurse-midwife participates in a program of QA/improvement for the evaluation of nurse-midwifery practice within the setting in which it occurs and within legal requirements" (ACNM, 1993).

RATIONALE FOR CONTINUOUS QUALITY IMPROVEMENT STRATEGIES

Historically the quality of patient care was measured by the outcome statistics of the care given by a provider. Although this focused on the performance of the practitioner, it was insufficient to improve the quality of care. There are increasing expectations among patients, their families, and third-party payers concerning the scope of services provided, including the convenience factors of access, availability, and comfort amenities, and the quality of care. Determining the definition of high-quality care is difficult. The philosophy of quality management and the process of quality improvement seek to identify measurable characteristics of high-quality care by redesigning corporate culture and preparing employees for assessment, measurement, and evaluation of client care (Wendt and Vale, 1999). Health care practitioners are an integral part of this community system that evaluates individual and system performance.

Box 30-1 *Definitions of Terms Commonly Used When Evaluating Health Services*

Quality assurance: A system that evaluates the outcomes of clinical performance and includes measures to improve those outcomes.

Quality management: A philosophy that defines a corporate culture emphasizing customer satisfaction, innovation, and employee involvement.

Quality improvement: An ongoing process of innovation, prevention of error, and staff development used by institutions who adopt a quality management philosophy.

Continuous quality improvement: A philosophy applied to the organization-wide system to improve the structure, process, and outcome of its mission to provide high-quality health care.

Risk management: A process that analyzes problems and minimizes losses after a patient care error occurs.

Peer review: An evaluation of performance of a colleague by professionals with similar education and professional preparation.

Standard: A criterion to measure the appropriateness of a response to a specific event or stimulus. A standard of care may be established at the national level through professional organizations; at the state level through licensing bodies; or at the community level through guidelines for practice, protocols, and credentialing procedures in institutions and agencies.

Clinical indicator: A measurable dimension (e.g., a medical event, procedure, diagnosis, or outcome) that is a reflection of some aspect of clinical care. Clinical indicators are used as part of a screening process to make a preliminary determination about the quality of care given by a practitioner or an agency/institution.

Sentinel event: An occurrence of significant importance that requires in-depth evaluation. Examples of this in maternal-infant care are maternal or neonatal death, perinatal asphyxia, and severe birth trauma.

Threshold level: The rate or minimal acceptable level at which care can be perceived to be safe.

Outliers: Cases that do not fit the established criteria and require further investigation before quality of care can be measured.

Traditional QA activities focused heavily on the clinical care provided by individual practitioners. However, models from industry have demonstrated that no performance can be measured without evaluating the systems in which the care was provided. Quality management and CQI provide the broad system processes that assess the practitioner's clinical care in the context of the work culture (Box 30-1).

Benefits of quality management include development of more efficient mechanisms for providing services in the face of limited resources, the adoption of the assumption that there is a correct way to provide specific services, and increased job satisfaction related to participants' belief that their input is valued by the institution or agency (Yoder-Wise, 1999). The participatory process inherent in quality management requires a democratic rather than hierarchic or bureaucratic structure. Many health care institutions have moved to using this model to foster employee innovation and cross-training for greater flexibility in responding to organizational needs.

EVOLUTION OF QUALITY MANAGEMENT PROCESSES

During the post-World War II era, the manufacturing industry began looking at ways to improve quality of production. The link between development of a high-quality product and cost control was identified early in the development of models of quality control. Philip Crosby recognized the link between quality and cost and broadened the approach to include conformance to standards to ensure adequate quality at reasonable cost. His work emphasized the expectation that the work involved in production will be done right the first time and stressed the use of standards or specifications to determine to level of quality. W. Edwards Deming developed strategies to help Japanese businesses rebuild after the war, and his approach also stressed doing the job right the first time. His work differed from that of Crosby in that he emphasized the importance of meeting both corporate and customer expectations. Joseph Juran developed the model of quality planning, quality control, and quality improvement. Quality planning determines who the customers are and identifies the customers' needs. Quality control is the evaluation of performance to identify discrepancies between performance and goals. Quality improvement provides the system-wide infrastructure to carry out process improvement (Katz and Green, 1997).

Aspects of each of these early approaches to quality production have become integrated into the assessment of health care delivery. The relationships between quality of care and cost have been explored by institutional administrators, third-party payers, health care providers, and consumers. Numerous proposals have been made to decrease costs while maintaining high quality. Managed care has evolved out of this effort to control health care spending. Standards have been promulgated to identify criteria that characterize high or acceptable quality of care. Process standards identify how a health service is to be delivered. Process standards include practice guidelines and approved procedures against which the activities in provision of care can be measured and can be authorized by institutional or agency bodies, state regulatory bodies, and national accrediting bodies.

Federal and state governments play multiple roles in promoting quality health care. Governments are purchasers of care (e.g., Title XVIII and Title XIX), regulators of the processes of care, and funders for evaluation of care delivery models. Federal regulations for Title XVIII (Medicare) and Title XIX (Medical Assistance) provide standards that health care providers and institutions must meet in order to participate in the programs. Included in these regulations are requirements to collect data and disclose performance measurements (Katz and Green, 1997). The National Association of Health Data Organizations promotes the development of publicly accessible data bases at the state level. Hospital discharge data are an example of the type of data collected to assess care delivery.

Numerous models of data collection have been developed to compare the quality of health care delivery among organizations. Perhaps the most commonly used are the Health Plan Employer Data and Information Set (HEDIS) developed by the National Committee for Quality Assurance (NCQA) and the IMSystem developed by the Joint Commission on Accreditation of Healthcare Organizations (JCAHO).

Performance measures in HEDIS cover the areas of prevention, acute illness, chronic illness, mental health, and substance abuse. Examples of measures used to compare maternal-infant services are listed in Box 30-2. HEDIS indicators are used by public payers (Medicaid, Medicare), private managed-care organizations, and state departments that monitor health care delivery. Results of the data collection allow for assessing trends in care over time and comparing health delivery systems. Many states have developed "report card systems" that allow consumers to review data to make decisions about their sources of health care. For example, the Harvard Community Health Plan in Massachusetts uses HEDIS indicators to publish reports on the care delivery of multiple health plans covering over 3 million enrollees (Katz and Green, 1997).

The IMSystem is a measurement tool that attempts to integrate standards and performance measures into an

Box 30-2 *Health Plan Employer Data and Information Set (HEDIS) Indicators Reflecting Quality of Maternal-Infant Health Care*

Effectiveness of Care

Prenatal care in the first trimester
Check-ups after delivery
Cervical cancer screening
Breast cancer screening
Chlamydia screening in women
Advising smokers to quit
Childhood immunization status

Access/Availability of Care

Initiation of prenatal care
Availability of language interpretation services

Use of Services

Frequency of ongoing prenatal care
Well-child visits in the first 15 months of life
Discharge and average length of stay—maternity care
Cesarean section
Vaginal births after cesarean section rate
Births and average length of stay, newborns

Adapted from NCQA: HEDIS 2000 List of Measures, Web page, 2000, http://www.ncqa.org/pages/policy/hedis/h00meas.htm.

evaluation process (Katz and Green, 1997). IMSystem includes indicators developed by both JCAHO and other organizations, and examples of its obstetric indicators are noted in Box 30-3.

The federal government works closely with private nonprofit organizations to evaluate health care delivery in the United States. In 1965 when Titles XVIII and XIX were established, the Health Care Financing Administration (HCFA) approved Joint Commission for Accreditation of Hospitals (JCAH) standards as the benchmark of quality in the auditing of programs covered by Medicare and Medicaid. JCAH was established in 1948 as an independent organization whose mission was voluntary accreditation of health care organizations. The original composition of JCAH included representatives from the American Hospital Association, the American Medical Association, the American Dental Association, the American College of Practitioners and Surgeons, and two consumers (Koch and Fairly, 1993). If a hospital was accredited by JCAH, it was considered to be in compliance with Medicare and Medicaid regulations. So, although the accreditation process was technically voluntary, hospitals could not afford to be out of compliance for federal reimbursement for services. It wasn't until the 1980s that JCAH moved from minimal standards to standards that reflected optimal or expected standards that addressed the quality of care more completely. In 1987 the organization expanded its mission, becoming the Joint Commission on Accreditation of Healthcare Organizations (JCAHO), to assess quality of care in all sites in which health care was offered. This change moved the organization from accreditation of only hospitals to accreditation of outpatient facilities and managed-care organizations.

QA began in the early 1900s when the American College of Surgeons (ACS) approved minimum standards for their members. The standards allowed for a review of the quality of care of hospitalized patients, and early reviews were informal and subjective. By the 1970s JCAH folded much of the ACS work into its medical audit methodology, and by 1980 JCAHO published its first standard on QA.

Box 30-3 *Selected IMSystem Obstetric Indicators*

Focus: Prenatal patient evaluation, education and treatment selection
Numerator: Patients delivered by cesarean section
Denominator: All deliveries

Focus: Prenatal patient evaluation, education and treatment selection
Numerator: Patients with vaginal births after cesarean section
Denominator: Patients delivered with a previous cesarean section

Focus: Prenatal patient evaluation, intrapartum monitoring, and clinical intervention
Numerator: Live-born infants with a birth weight less than 2500 g
Denominator: All live births

Focus: Prenatal patient evaluation, intrapartum monitoring, neonatal patient evaluation, and clinical intervention
Numerator: Live-born infants with a birth weight greater than or equal to 2500 g who have at least one of the following: APGAR score of less than 4 at 5 minutes, a requirement for admission to the neonatal intensive care unit within 1 day of delivery for greater than 24 hours, a clinically apparent seizure, or significant birth trauma
Denominator: All live-born infants with a birth weight of greater than 2500 g

Additional Indicators (Data May Not Be As Easy to Consistently Collect)

Maternal readmissions within 14 days of delivery
Intrahospital maternal deaths occurring within 42 days after delivery
Infants with a birth weight of less than 1800 g delivered in a hospital without neonatal intensive care unit
Patients with excessive maternal blood loss

Adapted from JCAHO: *1996 Comprehensive accreditation manual for hospitals,* Oakbrook Terrace, Ill, 1995, Joint Commission on Accreditation of Healthcare Organizations, pp. 579-587.

INTRODUCING CONTINUING QUALITY IMPROVEMENT INTO MIDWIFERY CARE

Because the commitment of midwifery to delivery of high-quality care to women and their infants, it is imperative that midwives develop a process of CQI in their practices. Many midwives practice in institutions that have incorporated a CQI program into their culture. In these cases the midwives can use the data collected to closely monitor practice activities and effectiveness. However, when institutional CQI programs are in place, midwives may want to develop additional indicators that address unique aspects of midwifery practice in order to address practice effectiveness in greater depth using a midwifery perspective.

To understand the relationship between QA and CQI, a comparison of the two systems is shown, based on the JCAHO 10-step model (Table 30-1).

Measuring Care—What You Will Need to Identify

Scope of practice. The scope of care provided by the organization or practice is delineated by the services that are provided, the clients served, the demographic characteristics of the clients, the diagnostic and treatment modalities commonly used, the referrals made to other practi-

Table 30-1 *Comparison of Quality Assurance/Improvement Systems*

JCAHO 10-step model	Quality assurance approach	Continuous quality improvement
Assign responsibility	Director of QA responsible; the focus is the practitioner level	Responsibility starts with the chief executive/administrator; the focus is organizational, office-wide or practice-wide
Delineate scope of care	Each specialty delineates its mission	The organization, office, or practice asks—What services do we provide? Do we meet the needs of the clients? Can we do it better?
Identify important aspects of care	Look for high-risk, problem-oriented areas	Identification of the most important clinical, administrative, and support services
Identify indicators	Indicators are determined by specialty	Teams or individuals use data to set priorities and opportunities for the organization or practice
Establish thresholds	Each specialty determines the level of tolerance	The nature of the opportunity is determined by a team for overall improvement
Collect and organize data	Each specialty monitors its own indicators	Data from many sources are used to analyze the care processes of the organization, practice, or site
Evaluate care	Unsatisfactory threshold levels trigger intensive review	Group identifies problems based on data analysis and initiate plan(s) to address the problems
Take action by improvement	Focus of action plan is change of behavior of outliers, with feedback, education, or sanctions	The action plan implemented includes who, what, when, where, and how
Assess effectiveness and document improvement	Continue to monitor indicators for return to norm	Continue to monitor to verify and maintain gains and institute change as needed.
Communicate results	Provide feedback to practitioners	Report to all parties and integrate findings

tioners or facilities, and the accessibility of services. As businesses have learned, perhaps the first question that needs to be addressed is, "Who is the customer?" Although it is easy to identify the client as the customer, further analysis identifies a variety of customers involved in the delivery of health care. Other customers of midwifery care, in the broad sense of the term, include the third-party payers, the employers in the community who contract with the insurers, physicians with whom the midwives consult and collaborate, nurses with whom the midwives work in the clinical units, support staff in the units, and administrators in the institution/agency. The relationships with all of these individuals and groups influences the delivery of midwifery care in any particular site.

The actual recipients of care obviously have a strong influence on the scope of services provided. For example, a practice that provides prenatal and intrapartum care to primarily unmarried pregnant adolescents has different service demands than one that provides care primarily to married, well-educated career women. Likewise, providing care in a community whose cultural beliefs include birth as a normal process best managed with ongoing female support is different than providing care in a community in which there is great belief in the use of technology during the birthing process.

Employers and third-party payers also will influence the climate in which care is given. When providing care at the cheapest rate possible is seen as more valued than offering a variety of approaches or options in order to meet cultural expectations, options become limited.

Aspects of care. Services provided by the practice need to be analyzed to further define the scope of practice. Three categories are used when addressing scope of practice:

1. *High volume.* This category addresses the activities that occur most often and affect the greatest number of patients.
2. *High risk.* This category addresses cases that are significant enough to be reviewed after every occurrence. These are termed sentinel events. Examples include maternal or fetal death, rupture of the uterus, and placenta abruption.
3. *Problem prone.* This category addresses activities that tend to produce or be associated with problems with patients or staff. Patient-related problems include birth injuries related to interventions at birth. Staff-related problems include clashes that occur when there are strong differences of opinion regarding management of particular cases.

Identification of Indicators

A clinical indicator is a measurable dimension that is considered to be an important aspect of care and for which the data can easily be collected. The number of the total population of individuals or events and the identification of the number of occurrences of the indicator both are necessary for meaningful measurement. For example, identifying the number of uterine ruptures during attempted vaginal birth after cesarean delivery without knowing the number of women laboring with a prior history of cesarean delivery does not give sufficient information to track trends or compare practices. Table 30-2 provides some examples of indicators for use by practitioners in a variety of institutions or agencies. Some indicators are sentinel events in which every case needs review using both peer review and systems improvement review. Other indicators can be reported as a rate, and review is only triggered if the established threshold is exceeded.

Establishment of Thresholds

The literature provides many acceptable rates of occurrence using recommendations promulgated by professional organizations, panels of experts (e.g., the USPHS Expert Panel on the Content of Prenatal Care), managed-care organizations, and governmental regulators. Thresholds must reflect the population characteristics of the practice.

When there are differing thresholds identified by different credible groups, the one that is most in concert with the community's norms should be used. For example, one guideline may set a threshold for birth weight less than 2500 g at 10% of live births; another may set it at 6%. In a setting in which care is provided to primarily healthy, well-educated women who do not experience barriers to prenatal care, the threshold for low birth weight should be set at the lower level of 6%.

Development of Criteria Sets

Criteria sets are developed to provide tools for the evaluation of the quality and appropriateness of care. The purpose of a criteria set is to identify a level of care activities below which most providers would agree that the care is inadequate or unacceptable. Criteria sets are typically written in clear, concise language that allows non-providers to audit patient care records to assess compliance with the accepted level of services. Criteria sets are usually developed by authoritative sources using na-

Table 30-2 *Clinical Indicators in Maternal-Infant Care*

Perinatal care	Well woman gynecology	Neonatal/infant care
Birth at <37 weeks gestation	Abnormal Pap smear	Birth injury
Birth weight <2500 g	Abnormal breast lump	Incomplete immunization schedule
Hgb <10 g/dl postpartum	Telephone triage documented and plan implemented appropriately	Neonatal death
Abnormal glucose screen in pregnancy	Oral contraceptive use monitored per protocol	Admission of a term infant to the neonatal intensive care unit
Eclampsia	Medical problems identified and referred as appropriate	
Cesarean delivery	Recommended screening(s) documented with follow-up consistent with protocol	
Estimated blood loss >500 ml after vaginal birth; >1000 ml after cesarean section		
Maternal death		
Administration of antibiotics following a term vaginal delivery		
Referral to a higher level of care (e.g., level 1 hospital to level 3 hospital)		
Lost to follow-up		

tional standards for practice. Once accepted for use in a practice or institution, criteria sets should be circulated among all staff so that all individuals involved in the delivery of services understand the expectations. Currently, criteria sets addressing obstetric care are approved and published by ACOG; ACNM has not yet published criteria sets based on expected midwifery standards. An example of one of ACOG's criteria sets is illustrated in Box 30-4.

MODEL FOR ESTABLISHING A COMPLETE QUALITY IMPROVEMENT PROGRAM IN A MATERNAL-INFANT COMMUNITY-BASED PRACTICE

Step 1. Assign responsibility. A clinical practitioner (e.g., Director of the Midwifery Practice) should oversee the organizing, managing ,and reporting of CQI activities for the practice. In some settings the coordinator may delegate many of the administrative responsibilities to a nonclinician. A plan for communication of identified problems and opportunities for improvement should be developed, and a forum such as a CQI committee for discussing findings with representatives of all areas of staff should be identified.

Step 2. Delineate scope of care. The scope of care and service to be monitored should be agreed on by committee members. Patient characteristics, including demographic information and payment source, should be identified. Provider characteristics, including credentialing and the ability to provide special services, should be delineated. Any special procedures or treatments unique to the practice setting should be noted and should reflect the specialties represented by the practice. In a midwifery practice these will most likely include prenatal, intrapartum, and postpartum care. Additional services that will depend on the training and credentialing of personnel may include antepartum fetal testing, ultrasound examinations, and colposcopy services.

Box 30-4 *ACOG CRITERIA SET: Quality Evaluation and Improvement in Practice*

Diagnosis:

Postterm pregnancy

Definition:

A pregnancy lasting more than 2 weeks beyond the confirmed expected date of delivery (EDD)

Confirmation of Diagnosis: (any of the following)

1. Estimate length of gestation from an initial clinical examination early in pregnancy (uterine size should be compatible with dates).
2. Determine the EDD by ultrasonography performed before 24 weeks of gestation.
3. Document conception associated with infertility treatment.

Antepartum Management:

1. Request patient to observe and record fetal movement.
2. Perform antepartum fetal surveillance by 42 weeks using standard protocols (e.g., nonstress test [NST], contraction stress test, biophysical profile, modified biophysical profile [amniotic fluid volume and NST]).
3. Effect delivery for nonreassuring antepartum testing results
4. Assess the appropriateness of induction of labor:
   a. If patient has a favorable cervix at or after 42 weeks of gestation, induction of labor is recommended unless contraindicated.
   b. If patient has an unfavorable cervix at or after 42 weeks of gestation, use of cervical ripening agents and induction of labor should be considered.
5. Expectant management is appropriate for the patient after 42 weeks with an unfavorable cervix and reassuring antepartum fetal tests.
6. Consider cesarean delivery for sonographically estimated macrosomia (greater than 4500 g).
7. Counsel patient regarding the importance of notifying her obstetrician when any of the following occurs:
   a. Reduction in fetal movement
   b. Onset of uterine contractions
   c. Rupture of membranes

Intrapartum Management:

1. Initiate fetal monitoring.
2. Document progress in labor.
3. Perform amniotomy unless inappropriate.
4. Document presence or absence of meconium when membranes rupture.
5. In the presence of meconium, document appropriate suctioning of the upper airway before the body of the fetus is delivered.

Unless otherwise stated, each numbered and lettered item must be present.

Bibliography

American College of Obstetricians and Gynecologists: *Diagnosis and management of postterm pregnancy (ACOG Technical Bulletin 130),* Washington, DC, 1989, ACOG.

American College of Obstetricians and Gynecologists: *Antepartum fetal surveillance (ACOG Technical Bulletin 188),* Washington, DC, 1994, ACOG.

Cunningham FG, MacDonald PC, Gant NF, Leveno KJ, Gilstrap LC III: Postterm pregnancy. In *Williams obstetrics,* ed 19, Norwalk, Conn, Appleton & Lange, 871-875, 1993.

The American College of Obstetricians and Gynecologists (ACOG), through its Committee on Quality Assessment, develops criteria sets intended to assist in the evaluation of the quality and appropriateness of care. Using criteria sets, nonphysician reviewers should be able to identify problematic trends or patterns in chart review. The purpose of this criteria set is to identify a threshold below which most physicians would agree that the care may be inappropriate. Other clinical approaches, also considered acceptable by a significant portion of physicians, are not all recognized in each criteria set. Therefore, peer review must make the final determination as to whether variations in care are deemed appropriate. Criteria sets are intended for quality review and are not designed to be used primarily as utilization review criteria. Use of criteria sets alone as utilization review criteria or to deny payment may represent an inappropriate use of these documents.

Step 3. Identify important aspects of care. Patient-related aspects of care may include access, continuity of care, compliance, satisfaction, and risk minimization. Access to care measures the ability of patients to obtain needed health services and the potential barriers that exist. A common measurable indicator used in prenatal services is the ability for a patient to be scheduled for an initial prenatal visit within 2 weeks of her initial contact with the practice. Potential barriers to timely scheduling of the initial prenatal visit include inadequate number of providers, inadequate number of clinical hours, and clinical hours that conflict with the community's usual employment hours.

Continuity of care is demonstrated when the care plan is implemented in a timely manner and continues smoothly without interruption. Interruptions of care include missed appointments, lost or omitted laboratory tests, and omitted screening studies. Problems may be identified when patients have difficulty rescheduling appointments or when appointments for special studies (e.g., ultrasound examinations) cannot be made in a reasonable period of time. Compliance is closely associated with continuity of care and represents the degree to which patients assume responsibility for their activities to complete the care plan. An example of compliance is the patient's ability to keep an appointment for special studies once that appointment has been made.

Patient satisfaction represents the degree to which the health care delivery meets the usual patient's reasonable needs, wants, and expectations. Survey data are commonly collected to establish patient satisfaction with the appointment process, waiting time, financial arrangements, perceived communication with practice staff, and availability of providers. Conflicts occur when either the provider or the patient perceives that the other is being unreasonable. A common area of conflict occurs in group practices when the patient desires to see only one provider and have the assurance that the provider will be available for the labor and delivery. The patient perceives this as a reasonable expectation. Providers, on the other hand, recognize their need to have established personal time off—time that is not available if the provider is "on-call" for a patient 24 hours per day, 7 days per week.

Patient risk minimization involves methods to reduce medical risk to patient and includes processes such as allergy documentation on patient records, infection control measures, and maintenance of drug profile.

Provider-Related Aspects of Care

Provider-related aspects of care include provider and support staff performance and the appropriateness of services that are offered. Provider staff performance covers the practitioner's ability to use knowledge, skills, and judgment to obtain optimum health outcomes. Peer review is a mechanism that assesses the provider's performance. Support staff performance includes the certification, training, experience, and competency of the support staff in providing both quality care and quality service to the patient. Indicators may include specific communication skills (e.g., introduces self to patient), appropriate data collection and assessment of patients, documentation, ability to assist the provider, preparation for procedures, and postprocedural patient care. Appropriateness of services measures whether a particular service that was provided was actually indicated. It also identifies when a service was indicated but not given. Diagnostic procedures, prescription of medication, and therapeutic regimens are often included in the indicators for assessing appropriateness of care.

Organizational and System Aspects of Care

Organizational and system aspects of care include the medical record system, the environment, quality control of equipment and supplies, policies and procedures, and cost of services provided in the practice. There are numerous tools to measure the degree to which the practitioner implements a medical record system that provides a timely and accurate record of all appropriate clinical information. Environmental aspects of care include hazardous waste management, infection control measures, standard precautions, fire and emergency preparedness, electrical safety, and provision of privacy. Environmental aspects that address patient comfort include the ambiance of the office, cleanliness, comfort, and the appropriateness of the furnishings for the patient population. Quality control of equipment and supplies should be designed to measure their functioning, preventive maintenance and service, and cleaning and testing.

It should be possible to review the operational systems of an office or clinic based on the written policies and procedures. For example, the mechanisms for the follow-up on abnormal laboratory studies should be evaluated. Policies to ensure compliance with federal, state, and local regulations should be in place and reviewed periodically. Cost of services analyzes several aspects of the relationship between coast and quality of care.

Step 4. Identify indicators. Indicators are described as objective and measurable variables related to the structure, process, or outcome of care.

Structure indicators are designed to answer the question, "Can this office/clinic site provide quality care?"

Examples of structural measures include the number and preparation of staff, the presence of equipment necessary for the provision of services, and other physical resources. An example of a structure indicator is the presence of an up-to-date log for monitoring the appropriate storage of laboratory specimens.

Process indicators are designed to monitor the standard of care that the practice provides and are designed to answer the question, "How does this setting provide quality care?" An example of a process indicator is the determination of whether there is an established protocol for evaluating blood glucose results, including documentation, intervention, and communication with the patient.

Outcome indicators are designed to answer the question, "Does this practice provide quality care?" Outcomes are observable and measurable results attributable to the antecedent structures and processes. An example of an outcome indicator is a formula that identifies adequate prenatal care using entry into care and number of visits for gestational age.

Clinical indicators are activities that occur that are associated with potential deficiencies in ambulatory management of care. An example of a clinical indicator is the rate of inpatient admissions for pregnant women with pyelonephritis, a diagnosis associated with lack of recognition of and treatment for lower urinary tract disease.

Step 5. Establish thresholds. Thresholds are established to provide a trigger for the evaluation of care. They can be based on the literature or on the experience of the practice setting. It is important that populations be matched to similar populations receiving care from similar practitioners. For example, it may be possible for one practice to establish a threshold for macrosomia as 5%, whereas this might be too low a threshold where women traditionally have vaginal deliveries of large babies without any evidence of abnormal blood glucose levels during pregnancy. Thresholds should reflect the cultural beliefs held in the community. Thresholds for genetic testing may not apply in communities in which there are strong beliefs against taking tissue or fluid from the body.

Step 6. Collect and organize data. Trained staff members should collect data pertaining to the indicators and organize it for comparison with established thresholds.

Step 7. Evaluate care. Cumulative data should be evaluated using the established thresholds, and the outcomes should be analyzed by providers and staff members skilled in identifying factors associated with specific outcomes. An adverse patient outcome may not result from provider performance but from system or patient failure to complete the treatment plan. Patterns or trends that relate to specific staff, skills, procedures, or patient populations may reveal opportunities for interventions that will improve care.

Step 8. Take action for improvement. All key individuals involved in the provision of care should work collaboratively to establish action plans. These actions should identify *who* is responsible for doing *what* and *when.* Action should be appropriate to the issue and may include providing education, training, or mentoring; making changes in policies and procedures; altering staff assignments; and counseling or discipline.

Step 9. Assess effectiveness and document improvement. The effectiveness of actions taken are assessed and documented through further data collection. If the findings are similar to the previous findings, other action plans must be considered to remedy the cause of the undesirable outcome. It is inappropriate to continue to use the same plans if they are shown to be ineffective.

Step 10. Communicate results. Findings and conclusions are shared with all of the ambulatory care staff. It is particularly important to recognize the successes or achievements to engender a sense of pride and accomplishment in delivering quality care. Too often staff may believe that programs to evaluate quality target the negative aspects of practice and not the positive.

SUMMARY

A growing number of practitioners and health care organizations are promoting the use of continuing quality management as a means of improving the delivery of health care. Inherent in the pure model of CQI is the active participation of the customer of service; in the case of maternal-infant care, the customer is the mother-infant dyad. The midwifery model of care assumes active participation of the women; yet we continue to see ineffective integration of patient expectations and feedback into the ongoing evaluation of care in the health care system. However, one needs to recognize that the patient role as "customer" of care differs from the customer role in industry. The patient not only is a consumer of health care but also is a direct object of those very health care processes. The psychologic and emotional component inherent in the reason for seeking treatment may influence the patient's ability to assertively make informed decisions about the processes of care and the evaluation of the quality of care (Lehr and Strosberg, 1991).

In addition to patient surveys that collect data regarding satisfaction with the quality of care following pregnancy and birth, some practices are encouraging patient input through their inclusion on community advisory boards or Boards of Directors for practices or agencies. This model provides the community participation to truly evaluate the degree to which the practice is meeting the needs and expectations of women and their families.

References

ACNM: *Standards for the practice of nurse-midwifery 1993,* Washington, DC, 1993, American College of Nurse-Midwives.

ACNM: *Quality management in midwifery care* (Position Statement), Washington, DC, 1997, American College of Nurse-Midwives.

Katz JM, Green E: *Managing quality—a guide to system-wide performance management in health care,* ed 2, St Louis, 1997, Mosby.

Koch MW, Fairly TM: *Integrated quality management,* St Louis, 1993, Mosby.

Lehr H, Strosberg M: Quality improvement in health care: is the patient still left out? *QRB Qual Rev Bull* 17(10):326-329, 1991.

Wendt D, Vale D: Managing quality and risk. In Yoder-Wise PS, editor: *Leading and managing in nursing,* ed 2, St Louis, 1999, Mosby.

Yoder-Wise. PS: *Leading and managing in nursing,* ed 2, St Louis, 1999, Mosby.

Chapter 31

Maintaining Midwifery in a Rapidly Changing Health Care Environment

During the last decade, the United States has seen a dramatic swing from a medical care system dominated by fee-for-service plans to one dominated by managed care organizations. By mid-1998 it was estimated that more than 85% of those insured through medium and large employers, 40% of those insured by Title XIX (Medicaid), and 15% of those insured by Title XVIII (Medicare) were enrolled in some type of managed care organization (Paine, Dower, and O'Neill, 1999). The debate continues regarding whether these changes in payment mechanisms will facilitate the growth of the midwifery model of care or strengthen the medical model of care, thereby reversing the growth in midwifery that has occurred in the past decade. If the health care delivery system had been a rational one in which policy decisions were based on evidence provided by clinical research and program evaluation research, we could predict that the midwifery model of care for childbearing would become the gold standard against which other models would be measured. Research has demonstrated that the midwifery approach is associated with decreased infant and maternal morbidity and mortality, due, in part, to the emphasis on patient education and counseling, the development of strong patient-provider relationships, the decreased use of surgical interventions during birth, and the emphasis on developing positive mothering behaviors in the postpartum period (e.g., the strong emphasis on breast-feeding). However, the American medical system is highly influenced by professional rivalries, for-profit development of pharmaceutic and biotechnologic agents, and the activities of highly paid lobbyists on the federal and state levels.

If we are truly committed to the development of a system that is effective in maintaining the health status of the majority of pregnant women, we must shift emphasis from the current pathology-oriented obstetric system to a wellness-oriented system of care. Although a small proportion of women with medical and obstetric problems will continue to need the expertise of perinatal specialists, the majority of pregnant women in this country would benefit from the midwifery model of care.

The midwifery model of care can be summarized by the following characteristics:

- Monitoring the physical, psychologic, and social well-being of the woman throughout the childbearing cycle
- Providing the woman with individualized education, counseling, and prenatal care
- Continuous hands-on assistance during labor and delivery

- Postpartum support
- Minimal use of technologic intervention
- Identification of obstetric problems, with referral to appropriate providers for care (Pew Health Professions Commission and UCSF Center for Health Professions, 1999)

KEEPING WOMEN CENTRAL IN THE HEALTH CARE EXPERIENCE

As indicated throughout this text, the foundation of midwifery care is that the woman must be the central figure in the care process. The midwifery philosophy supports the woman as the expert in determining her health care needs, and it is the woman who, after being given sound information about options in care, makes the determination of the best approach for her needs. The health care professional with her or his unique knowledge and skills assists the woman in the decision-making process and respects the woman's choices. This approach assumes that the woman is developmentally, emotionally, psychologically, and cognitively able to reason.

One way to assess what women desire in health care is to review the literature exploring satisfaction with care. Factors that have been found to be associated with obstetric patient satisfaction include communication, control, participation in decision making, continuity of care, presence of a support person, information (e.g., prenatal and parenting classes), nursing care services, and physical environment. Providers using a midwifery model of care have been found to practice in a way that is consistent with these expectations.

The communication style used by midwives encourages active participation by the woman and her partner. Information is given in a way that promotes understanding, and the woman is given authority to make decisions based on that information. Communication is enhanced through the relationship that develops between the midwife and the woman. The care process can be described as a partnership in which the participants work together to meet goals. This is in contrast to the traditional obstetric model in which physicians are more likely to see themselves as the key decision makers (Rooks, 1999). The results of one research project found that women preferred providers who demonstrated the ability to empower the woman, to enable her to feel special, and to help her relax and be in control, and to be her advocate (Fraser, 1999). Use of the midwifery model of care fosters this preferred style of communication.

Midwives and other practitioners who practice in the midwifery model have traditionally provided the personal service that women seek. Comments noted in Fraser's study included:

"The midwife has time for you, the doctor checks you and you're out."

"I feel more comfortable with the midwife . . . she knows me . . . the doctor doesn't . . . He doesn't listen or talk to me . . ."

"You can talk to the midwife and can't so much to doctors."

"The doctors discussed around me, not with me" (Fraser, 1999).

Communication conveys the values and beliefs held by the individual. In general, the language used by obstetricians tends to be mechanistic and controlling (Davis-Floyd, 1992; Fraser, 1999; Kitzinger, 1999; Martin, 1987). Terminology reflects concepts found in science and architecture (the pubic arch, pelvic floor, abdominal wall, birth canal) as well as judgments about the production ability of the machine (inadequate labor forces, incompetent cervix, failure to progress) (Kitzinger, 1999). In this context the caregiver becomes a manager who controls the production, as in "active management of labor." This controlling approach is in sharp contrast with the midwifery approach in which the woman and her perceived needs are the center of decision making. Although the expert knowledge of the midwife is important in supporting the woman and responding to emergency situations, the woman's lived experience and expectations should guide the experience of pregnancy and birth.

Women expect expert, or at least competent, clinical skills in their providers. Other factors, including the quality of the relationship perceived, the open sharing of information, the empathy shown toward the woman's life experience, and the feeling that each pregnant woman is treated as an individual with unique needs affect the overall evaluation of the woman's experience in the health care system. Ultimately satisfaction with care is associated with outcomes of care. Individuals who are satisfied with their care continue with the practice, thereby maintaining continuity of care. Individuals who are satisfied tend to follow through with treatment regimens and follow-up care. It stands to reason, then, that by creating a system that enhances satisfaction with care, we will provide an environment that has the potential to improve the health status of women and their children.

EVIDENCED-BASED PRACTICE

It is important for health care professionals to assess women's expectations and desires for their childbearing experiences in the context of the evidence provided by clinical and systems research. As noted in Chapter 2, the design of a study directly affects the strength of the findings. The U. S. Preventive Services Task Force identifies several levels of evidence (findings) ranked here as strongest to weakest:

1. Experimental. randomized control trials, considered the gold standard, with well-designed control trials without randomization considered acceptable but limited because of greater chance of bias
2. Well-designed cohort studies or case-controlled studies, preferably using a multi-site approach
3. Multiple time series
4. Dramatic results from uncontrolled experiments
5. Opinions of respected authorities, observational studies, case studies, and expert committee reports—considered the least compelling when evaluating the findings and recommendations

Research findings traditionally published in obstetric journals tend to reflect knowledge obtained from the lower levels of evidence. One recent review of a 12 issues of *Obstetrics and Gynecology* found that 76% of published studies were observational, 14% were experimental, and 10% were "other" (Funai, 1997). Likewise, midwifery research findings have historically been limited by observational studies, many with small sample sizes. Partially in response to the move toward creating a new paradigm of evidence-based practice, The American College of Obstetricians and Gynecologists (ACOG) now uses a process for developing their clinical practice guidelines that relies on analyzing and grading the strength of findings based on the research methodology used. Leaders in both ACOG and the American College of Nurse-Midwives (ACNM) have increasingly called for greater attention to evidence-based practice.

The Cochrane Collaboration was established in 1993 to develop an electronic database of readily available information on the effectiveness of care practices across medical specialties. Using meta-analyses and a critique of the study design, reviewers produce summaries of the strength of the evidence supporting or not supporting specific interventions or approaches to care. The Cochrane pregnancy care database uses the following categories in classifying the potential benefit or harm from practices:

1. Clearly beneficial
2. Likely to be beneficial
3. Trade-off between beneficial and adverse effects
4. Unknown effectiveness
5. Unlikely to be beneficial
6. Likely to be ineffective or harmful

In a similar process, the World Health Organization (WHO) has published *Care in Normal Birth: a Practical Guide,* a compilation of reviews by the WHO technical working group. The WHO group summarized the strength of evidence for selected interventions and care practices using four categories:

1. Demonstrably safe and useful; should be encouraged
2. Clearly harmful or ineffective; should be eliminated
3. Insufficient evidence to support a clear recommendation; use with caution while further research clarifies the issue
4. May be necessary for some women but used too often; frequently used inappropriately

Taken together, these two resources provide strong support to the midwifery model of care. Examples of care practices identified as "Clearly beneficial"/"Demonstrably safe and useful" that are typically found in the midwifery model include:

- Emotional and psychologic support during labor and birth
- Maternal mobility and choice of position during labor
- Consistent support for breast-feeding mothers
- Unrestricted breast-feeding

Care practices "likely to be beneficial" that are consistently found in midwifery practice include:

- Respecting women's choice of companions during labor and birth
- Maternal movement and position changes to relieve pain in labor
- Encouraging early mother-infant contact

Conversely, practices considered "clearly harmful or ineffective" that have been rejected in the midwifery model include routine enemas in early labor, routine perineal shaving, and routine use of episiotomies.

It is less clear whether the practices that "have tradeoffs between beneficial and adverse effects" or "are frequently used inappropriately" are typically used by midwives. Examples of care practices that had been determined to fall into these categories include:

- Use of continuous electronic fetal monitoring
- Use of oxytocin to increase the strength and frequency of labor contractions
- Use of epidural analgesia for pain control in labor

Recent analysis of birth certificate data suggests that midwives are as likely as physicians to use electronic fetal monitoring and oxytocin for stimulation of labor (Curtin, 1999). However, limitations to the birth certificate data include the fact that one cannot determine whether the use of electronic fetal monitoring was continuous or intermittent. In addition, one needs to consider that nurse-midwives working in hospitals are often expected to follow obstetric protocols that reflect the medical rather than the midwifery model of care. The consumer demand for interventions that may be used too frequently or inappropriately also contributes to the use of these practices. Over 60% of women surveyed at a large teaching hospital indicated that they planned to definitely or probably request epidural analgesia (Lieberman, 1999). Both consumers and providers often opt for induction of labor once the estimated date of delivery has passed, and consumers expect at least one ultrasound scan during the pregnancy.

To provide the greatest benefits of the midwifery model of care for healthy women, midwives must be recognized and authorized to practice as autonomous health professionals. Requiring physician supervision or approval of practice guidelines used by a midwifery practice is akin to having dentists supervise physical therapists. The disciplines, while sharing some scientific knowledge, are distinct and unique in their approaches to meeting the health care needs of individuals and populations. The paradigm of medicine is centered around pathology and the interventions that are effective in curing disease. The paradigm of midwifery is centered on health and interventions to promote health and prevent disease. When considered in this way, it is clear that obstetricians are as prepared to provide care for women experiencing healthy pregnancies as midwives are to surgically intervene in complicated pregnancies.

INTEGRATING MIDWIFERY MODEL INTO MANAGED CARE

Health care analysts suggest that the emerging managed-care system is built on three values—lowering costs, enhancing patient/consumer satisfaction, and improving the overall quality of care (Pew Health Professions Commission and UCSF Center for Health Professions, 1999). The current system has emphasized three components: (1) accessibility to the primary care provider, (2) coordination of referrals, and (3) understanding of the family and community context of health. Both the for-profit and not-for-profit managed-care organizations have done well in performing the first two tasks. However, most health care systems have not developed approaches that maximize the third (Grumbach et al., 1999).

Most patients recognize the benefit of having a designated primary care provider. The primary care provider is more than a "gatekeeper." In theory, the primary care provider manages common health problems, screens for and diagnoses health problems, and coordinates consultations and referrals. There continues to be a debate regarding whether obstetricians-gynecologists are prepared to address all of the responsibilities inherent in being a primary care provider since until recently obstetrics and gynecology has developed primarily as a surgical specialty. Even though residency programs have now added more primary care experience to their rotations, the physicians being prepared will not be out in practice for several years.

In addition, debate continues regarding whether non-physicians can assume the role of primary care provider. Research suggests that nurse practitioners and midwives are comparable to physicians in screening for disease, and may be more effective in creating an atmosphere in which patients follow through with treatment recommendations (Brown and Grimes, 1995). Midwives are prepared to meet the usual health care needs of most healthy women both during pregnancy and during the non-pregnant periods of their lives. Midwives have demonstrated the ability to increase access to care, not just by increasing the numbers of providers available, but also by providing care that is community-based and culturally sensitive. Numerous studies have found that nurse-midwives provide a disproportionate amount of care to those populations most vulnerable to poor pregnancy outcomes with outcomes similar to or better than national statistics. With the discipline's roots in public health and with its emphasis on the psychosocial aspects of health, midwives are unique in their preparation to provide care in the context of family and community health.

Several developments in the evolution of managed care have already had or have the potential to have an impact on midwives and the midwifery model of care. First, the move to consolidate care through mergers of hospitals, agencies, and medical care groups may threaten the survival of the midwifery model of care in several ways. The consolidation of large institutions may increase the power held by a small group of people (e.g., physicians and administrators). Without pressure from external forces, there will be an inherent protection of the status quo, which is the obstetric model of care. With many midwives working as employees of institutions or physicians, they will be further removed from levels of decision making. Second, consolidation is leading to organizational changes that integrate formerly disparate services to lower cost, increase satisfaction, and improve the quality of care. Because of their history of high patient satisfaction and quality of care, midwives may face an opportunity to increase their practice if they are assertive in convincing managed-care groups of their successes. Finally, analysts suggest that the integrated systems may lead to opportunities for innovative, creative, and nontraditional approaches to delivering high-quality health care. To this end, midwives have the opportunity to develop creative service systems using the midwifery model of care as the core, with referral to obstetric care only when obstetric problems are identified (Pew Health Profession Commission and UCSF Center for Health Professions, 1999).

COLLABORATIVE CARE MODEL

As creative new approaches are being proposed for the delivery of health care services, many policy makers and health professionals are calling for increased use of collaborative care models. Collaborative care has been described as "professionals working within their scopes of practice to meet patient needs, without duplication of services" (Hankins et al., 1996). This configuration of working relationships is not new. Following the development of a few isolated demonstration projects, federal maternal-child health funding in the 1960s stimulated the creation of interdisciplinary teams that functioned very much like the "newer" collaborative teams. The concept behind the collaborative model is that each discipline has its own unique strengths and talents, and patients should receive care from the most appropriate professional for the perceived health care needs. Benefits of interdisciplinary models of care have been increased patient satisfaction, improved outcomes, cost-effectiveness, and increased use of nonphysician providers (Singleton and Green-Hernandez, 1998). The greatest limitation to the full development of this model has been the medical profession's control of the medical marketplace. Federal, state, and local regulations and policies have supported physicians as the ultimate authority in health care, even though the education and culture of medicine are based on a paradigm appropriate for a relatively small proportion of pregnant women. Examples of the barriers faced by nonphysician health care professionals include limitations on full hospital admitting privileges, exclusion as primary providers in health maintenance organizations (HMOs) and other managed-care organizations, requirements for physician supervision in practice, and limitations on direct third-party reimbursement for care practices provided by nonphysicians. Until policies that allow for the full independent practice of nonphysician providers are enforced, these providers will lack the autonomy required for provision of services. And, as long as midwives are not accepted as autonomous providers, their ability to function as full partners in a collaborative model is threatened.

Policy and position papers issued by ACNM and ACOG further illustrate the differing interpretations of collaborative relationships. The ACNM supports that concept that the midwife is an autonomous provider who works "within a health care system that provides for consultation, collaborative management, or referral as indicated by the health status of the client" (American College of Nurse-Midwives, 1997). The Statement on Independent Nurse-Midwifery Practice adds, "The goal of collaboration is to share authority while providing quality care within each individual's professional scope of practice. Successful collaboration is a way of thinking and relating that requires knowledge, open communication, mutual respect, a commitment to providing quality care, trust and the ability to share responsibility" (American College of Nurse-Midwives, 1997). The ACNM clearly sees health care professionals in an interdisciplinary team functioning as equals to best serve client needs. In contrast, ACOG clearly sees a continued hierarchic model when using an interdisciplinary model of care:

> The team consists of obstetrician-gynecologists and other health care professionals who function within their educational preparation and scope of practice. These team members work together utilizing mutually agreed upon guidelines and policies that define the individual and shared responsibilities of each member. Although the responsibility of the obstetrician-gynecologists places them in a role of ultimate authority because of their education and training, the contributions of each member are valued and important to the quality of patient outcome. The concept of a team guided by one of its own members and the acceptance of shared responsibility for outcomes promote shared accountability (American College of Obstetricians and Gynecologists, 1994).

Until physicians are willing to recognize other health professionals as true equals, true collaborative or integrated practices will not be institutionalized in the American health care system. Individual practice models may function successfully, but they will be the product of the beliefs and values of the individual partners, not those of the disciplines or professional cultures represented. Furthermore, as roles blur in collaborative practices, the distinct qualities of the midwifery profession may be overshadowed by the dominant medical model. This decreased visibility of midwifery as a distinct profession may foster the continued view of midwives as physician extenders. It will take assertive, politically sophisticated midwives to ensure the continued recognition of midwives as the experts in the care of healthy women.

Collaborative relationships are strongly influenced by the financial structure and employment relationships among health providers, institutions, and payers. Physicians and midwives who are employed by a managed-care agency (e.g., staff-model HMO) by necessity collaborate in clinical decision making but may not have any input regarding financial decisions made by the agency. When a midwife is an employee of a physician group, clinical collaboration may be present, but she or he most likely has no input regarding financial aspects of the practice. True partnerships, or integrated practices, allow midwives and physicians to share in administrative, financial, and clinical decisions. Although there have been a few successful models that demonstrate the full integration of physicians, midwives, and other professionals, they are clearly still the exception to the rule.

The clinical role assumed by midwives in collaborative practice is influenced by the underlying beliefs about the most effective and efficient use of each professional. Midwives in collaborative practices typically serve a substitute function for physician care or serve on an interdisciplinary team in which clients receive care from all members of the group. When the midwife or group of midwives are serving as a substitute for physician services, they have a designated caseload for which they provide all services available under the sanctioned scope of practice. Physicians provide services through availability for consultation, collaboration, or referral. Advantages of the substitute function model are that clients receive the continuity of care from providers with whom they can form stronger relationships, there may be a greater emphasis on the unique midwifery model of care, and midwifery is more visible as a unique profession. In an integrated model, patients are seen by any or all members of the team, depending on the scheduling patterns agreed on by the practitioners. For example, women may receive prenatal care from midwives in the practice and physician care at the time of the birth. Or women may see midwives and physicians for prenatal visits and whichever professional is staffing the labor and delivery unit for her birth. Advantages of the integrated model include the potential increase efficiency of staffing and the broader influence the midwifery approach can have on medical practice. Disadvantages of the integrated model include the lack of continuity of care and the blurring of midwifery and obstetric approaches to care (King and Shah, 1998).

Those who support the promotion of collaborative practice note that practitioners are more likely to value the collaborative model when their educational experiences and preparation for practice are integrated. The integration can occur by having students in multiple disciplines enroll in core courses whose content crosses disciplines (e.g., core science courses), by having a multidisciplinary team of faculty teach management courses, and by having students in one discipline (e.g., medicine) taught specific course content by faculty representing another discipline (e.g., midwifery). However, experience suggests that faculty attitudes and control over the integration of interdisciplinary learning into curricula introduce many barriers to collaborative education. Professional rivalries and protection of turf need to be overcome before there is universal institutional support for collaborative learning experiences.

COST EFFECTIVENESS

The research exploring the cost effectiveness of the midwifery model of care has been limited by the problems inherent in identifying the actual costs of care, the use of indicators that do not represent many of the services provided by midwives, and the lack of analysis of long-term effects of care. Even with these methodologic problems, though, findings consistently suggest cost advantages to the midwifery model. Several studies have identified the fact that midwives, even when working within a medically dominated hospital-based system, use fewer resources than physicians (Oakley et al., 1996; Rosenblatt et al., 1997). Blue Cross of Washington data demonstrated that obstetricians used 12.2% more resources than CNMs, with most of the increase being associated with anesthesia use during labor and the increased hospital stay associated with cesarean deliveries. Analysis of midwifery care in birth centers has also demonstrated cost savings that reflect both the impact of type of provider and site of birth (Research Box 31-1). One recent study using birth certificate and hospital discharge data suggested that, if 40% of women were cared for by providers using the "noninterventive" approach (as an indicator for the midwifery model of care), the an-

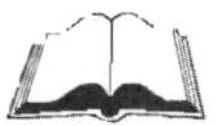

Research Box 31-1

Rosenblatt RA et al: Interspecialty differences in the obstetrics care of low-risk women, *Am J Public Health* 87(3): 344-351, 1997.

Background

Obstetric care accounts for over 10% of hospital charges, and most obstetric care in the United States is provided by obstetricians, family physicians, and certified nurse-midwives (CNMs). Intraspecialty differences between these providers have been documented; and the differences may influence the quality of care, patient satisfaction, accessibility of care, and the process and cost of care.

Research Question

Are there systematic differences in the style and resource intensity of care provided to similar groups of women by certified nurse-midwives, family physicians, and obstetricians?

Methods

Retrospective chart abstraction was used to identify number of prenatal visits, screening laboratory tests, diagnostic tests (e.g., amniocentesis), intrapartum procedures (e.g., induction, augmentation, use of epidural anesthesia, episiotomy), operative delivery, birth weight, and APGAR scores. Sociodemographic data, including payment source, ethnicity, parity, and relationship status, were gathered from the charts. An "intend to treat" protocol was used. Pair-wise comparisons and multiple regression were used to analyze the data. Total costs of prenatal and intrapartum care were estimated using the Blue Cross of Washington fee schedule.

Sample

The sampling frame was derived from lists of family physicians, obstetricians, and CNMs maintained by the relevant professional organizations in the state of Washington. All CNMs and a randomly selected sample of obstetricians and family physicians were recruited to participate in the study. The medical records for all patients initiating care with an index provider and meeting the study criteria for low-risk pregnancies were abstracted by trained abstractors.

Results

Prenatal practice was similar among groups. The only differences in interventions were that (1) obstetricians were more likely to order/perform amniocentesis than CNMs and family physicians, and (2) CNMs were more likely to obtain nonstress tests than physicians, most likely for postdates assessment rather than routine induction for postdates. Major differences were found in management during the intrapartum period. CNMs were less likely to induce or augment labor, use epidural anesthesia, use continuous electronic fetal monitoring, and perform episiotomies. The differences between obstetricians and family physicians were less marked. The average cesarean section rate for CNMs was 8.8% vs. 13.6% for obstetricians and 15.1% for family physicians. The increased use of intervention by obstetricians was associated with a use of 12.2% increase in resources. Analysis of subgroups, including nulliparous women and women with parity of one, two, and greater than two, found that patients initiating care with CNMs were less likely to be induced, continuously electronically monitored, use epidural anesthesia, receive episiotomies, or experience instrumental or operative deliveries. Multiple regression analysis found no provider characteristics (e.g., age, gender) and no patient variables statistically significant in the model.

Clinical Application

Results from this study can be used to educate policy makers about the economic benefits of CNM care. Strengths of the study include the control of biologic and sociodemographic factors that influence the process and outcome of care and the use of a random urban sample of obstetric providers in an entire state. Limitations include the use of retrospective data without random assignment to treatment groups and the probable effect of self-selection of provider. The possibility that results cannot be generalized to other states must also be considered.

Box 31-1 *Expected Outcomes in a System that Promotes the Midwifery Model of Care for the Majority of Childbearing Women*

Decreased maternal mortality rate
Decreased perinatal mortality rate
Decreased low birth weight rate
Decreased cesarean delivery rate
Increased screening and intervention for women who smoke in pregnancy
Increased screening and intervention for women who experience domestic abuse
Decreased use of induction and augmentation of labor in healthy women
Decreased use of continuous electronic fetal monitoring in healthy women
Decreased use of epidural analgesia for pain relief in labor
Decreased rate of episiotomies
Decreased rate of operative vaginal births
Decreased rate of third- or fourth-degree lacerations during birth
Increased rate of breast-feeding during the first 6 weeks postpartum
Increased mean length of breast-feeding
Decreased length of stay for postpartum women
Decreased length of stay for neonates
Decreased admissions to Neonatal Intensive Care Units

Summarized from Rooks JP: *Midwifery and childbirth in America,* Philadelphia, 1997, Temple University Press.

nual U.S. cost savings would exceed $13 billion (Schlenzka, 1999).

Opponents of the midwifery model of care point to the perception that midwifery is labor intensive, and, as such, not as cost effective as believed when looking at resource usage. Managed-care models have pushed providers to increase productivity. Those who do not are faced with termination of contracts or other punitive measures. Clinicians are forced to shorten prenatal visits and care for several women at a time on Labor and Delivery Units. Midwifery, with its focus on relationship-building, education, counseling, and ongoing support, cannot fit in a mold that limits the time of contact with clients. Efforts should be made to design research that explores the effect of the time commitment to clients. In theory, the empowerment of the woman during the prenatal care should not only have a positive effect on her experience in labor, but may also have an impact on her experience in mothering her child.

SUMMARY

If the midwifery model of care is to thrive in this era of managed care, those making policies and administrative decisions need to recognize the potential benefits of shifting from an obstetric paradigm to a midwifery paradigm. Midwifery offers distinct benefits for the three goals of managed care noted earlier.

1. Lowering costs. The midwifery model of care has demonstrated decreased costs related to decreased use of resources, particularly technologies that have been determined to be "frequently used inappropriately."
2. Enhancing patient/consumer satisfaction. The midwifery model of care consistently has been evaluated as generating high levels of consumer satisfaction.
3. Improving the overall quality of care. The midwifery model of care has consistently been found to demonstrate high levels of quality of care.

Proponents of the midwifery model of care need to act proactively in educating leaders in managed-care organizations and in regulatory arenas regarding these three points. It is essential that midwives do not do this work alone; to do so would be construed to be self-serving. Numerous consumer groups, including childbirth educators, parents, and health care advocates, can be encouraged to become activists to promote this healthy model of care. Without this grassroots activity, we are likely to face continuation of the status quo—the obstetric model of care for all childbearing women.

Establishment of a national commitment to ensure that the midwifery model of care becomes the standard for healthy childbearing women has the potential to radically change the way care is given to childbearing women. Outcomes that can be predicated from this shift in care are summarized in Box 31-1. These potential outcomes reflect findings in published biomedical literature.

Improvement in the usual indices used to assess maternal and infant health ultimately leads to improved health status of society (Research Box 31-2). The midwifery model of care has demonstrated superior outcomes for

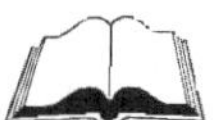

Research Box 31-2

MacDorman MF, Singh GK: Midwifery care, social and medical risk factors, and birth outcomes in the USA, *J Epidemiol Commun Health* 52(5):310-317, 1998.

Background

In spite of skyrocketing health care expenditures for obstetric and neonatal care, numerous barriers to prenatal and perinatal care continue to exist in the United States. One of the recommendations to reduce the infant mortality rate while controlling costs, expanding coverage, and improving the quality of prenatal and perinatal care is to increase the use of certified nurse-midwives (CNMs) in U.S. maternity care. Although the proportion of births attended by CNMs has increased over the past two decades, CNMs attended only 5.5% of births in 1994. Nurse-midwives provide care to a higher proportion of women in certain sociodemographic risk categories, including adolescents, women living in poverty, women with less than a high school education, and ethnic minorities.

Research Question

Are there significant differences in birth outcomes for infants delivered by CNMs compared to those delivered by physicians? Do these differences remain after controlling for sociodemographic and medical risk factors?

Methods

Data were collected from the national linked birth/infant death data set for the 1991 cohort. All U.S. births and a subset of singleton infants between 34 and 43 weeks' gestation delivered vaginally were examined using logistic and ordinary least squares regression. A sample of 100% of the CNM-attended births and a 25% random sample of physician-attended births was created for multivariate analysis. Dependent variables were infant, neonatal, and post-neonatal mortality; low birth weight; and mean birth weight. Sociodemographic and health risk factors (independent variables) included birth attendant, maternal age, race education, marital status, birth order, month pregnancy prenatal care began, gestational age, and medical risk factors.

Sample

Birth/death records for all CNM-attended births and 25% of physician births were used for analysis.

Results

Results confirmed that a greater proportion of certified nurse-midwife than physician deliveries involved mothers at increased risk for poor pregnancy outcome. When sociodemographic variables were controlled, the risk of infant mortality was 20% lower for CNM-attended births. When medical risk factors were controlled, the risk of infant mortality was 19% lower for CNM-attended births. The risk of neonatal mortality was 34% lower for CNM-attended births and the risk of low birth weight was 29% lower for CNMs when sociodemographic and medical risk factors were controlled.

Clinical Application

Findings from this study can be used to educate policy makers about the benefits of CNM care, particularly in vulnerable populations. Strengths of the study include the use of a population-based data set and the many sociodemographic and medical risk factors used in the analysis. Limitations include the cross-sectional nature of the data collection, identifying the birth attendant but not the provider of prenatal care.

healthy women experiencing normal pregnancies when compared to the traditional obstetric model of care. Yet, the obstetric model continues to be the dominant model in the United States. Change is not going to come from within the current medical system for a variety of professional and financial reasons. Forces from without hold the only hope for supporting the substitution of the medical paradigm with the midwifery paradigm of care. And, whereas the midwifery model is clearly the superior model for healthy women, it also holds the potential for increasing the health status for women at increased risk for perinatal problems (Declercq, 1993; Declercq, 1995). Collaborative care using a perinatologist-midwife team offers the perinatologist's expertise in medical/obstetric problems in pregnancy and the midwife's expertise in the normal aspects of pregnancy, including the psychosocial aspects that greatly influence the perinatal outcome.

By shifting the paradigm of care of the childbearing women to a midwifery model of care, we have the potential to bring more balance to the use of health care resources. We currently have a system that provides highly specialized care (i.e., care created for the care of women with obstetric or medical problems during pregnancy) to all women, even though greater than 90% of pregnant women will experience either no problems or minor problems during pregnancy and birth. A large proportion of pregnant women are receiving care from providers trained as surgical specialists rather than from providers prepared to support normal pregnancy and birth.

Numerous professional organizations and expert panels have called for an increased role of midwives in the health care delivery system for childbearing women. Barriers to the full incorporation of these professionals have continued for decades. Dramatic changes in societal expectations and professional power structures often accompany revolutionary change in long-standing systems and cultures. The last decade of the twentieth century has seen the shift in power in health care from physicians to financial officers, and increasingly the public sees the many problems in the current system of care. A crystal ball cannot predict what the outcome will be and what the care to childbearing women will look like in another decade. The current turbulence in the health care system has the potential to set the stage for a dramatic shift in care processes during the childbearing year, and midwives need to continue to work for change to best meet the health care needs of women and their families. The midwifery model that places the woman's needs as central in the care process is a strength that has supported previous policy successes. As long as we—providers, consumers, policy makers—work to ensure decision making based on solid evidence of effectiveness and client satisfaction, we have a greater chance of creating a system in which midwifery is the central model of care for healthy women. Midwives, obstetrician-gynecologists, family physicians, nurse practitioners, and physician assistants, working together on behalf of women and infants, have the potential to create a system that emphasizes risk appropriate levels of care that best meet the needs of society.

References

American College of Nurse-Midwives: *Statement on independent nurse-midwifery practice,* Washington, DC, 1997, ACNM.

American College of Obstetricians and Gynecologists: *Guidelines for implementing collaborative practice,* Washington, DC, 1994, ACOG.

Brown SA, Grimes DE: A meta-analysis of nurse practitioners and nurse midwives in primary care, *Nurs Res* 44(6):332-339, 1995.

Curtin SC: Recent changes in birth attendant, place of birth, and the use of obstetric interventions, United States, 1989-1997, *J Nurse-Midwifery* 44(4):349-354, 1999.

Davis-Floyd R: *Birth as an American rite of passage,* Berkeley, 1992, University of California Press.

Declercq ER: Where babies are born and who attends their births: findings from the revised 1989 United States certificate of live birth, *Obstet Gynecol* 81:997-1004, 1993.

Declercq ER: Midwifery care and medical complications: the role of risk screening, *Birth* 22:68-73, 1995.

Fraser DM: Women's perceptions of midwifery care—a longitudinal study to shape curriculum development, *Birth* 26(2):99-107, 1999.

Funai EF: Obstetrics and gynecology in 1996: marking progress toward evidence-based medicine by classifying studies based on methodology, *Obstet Gynecol* 90(6a):1020-1022, 1997.

Grumbach KJ et al: Resolving the gatekeeper conundrum—what patients value in primary care and referrals to specialists, *JAMA* 282(3):261-266, 1999.

Hankins GD et al: Patient satisfaction with collaborative practice, *Obstet Gynecol* 88(6):1011-1015, 1996.

King T, Shah MA: Integrated midwife-physician practice: obstetric Darwinism? *J Nurse-Midwifery* 43(1):55-60, 1998.

Kitzinger S: Sheila Kitzinger's letter from Europe: obstetric metaphors and marketing, *Birth* 26(1):55-57, 1999.

Lieberman E: No free lunch on Labor Day: the risks and benefits of epidural analgesia during labor, *J Nurse-Midwifery* 44(4):394-398, 1999.

Martin E: *The woman in the body: a cultural analysis of reproduction,* Boston, 1987, Beacon Press.

Oakley D et al: Comparisons of outcomes of maternity care by obstetricians and certified nurse-midwives, *Obstet Gynecol* 88:823-829, 1996.

Paine LL, Dower CM, O'Neill EH: Midwifery in the 21st century—recommendations from the Pew Health Professions Commission/UCSF Center for Health Professions 1998 Task Force on Midwifery, *J Nurse-Midwifery* 44(4):341-348, 1999.

Pew Health Professions Commission and University of California, San Francisco Center for Health Professions: *The future of midwifery,* San Francisco, 1999, UCSF Center for Health Professions.

Rooks JP: The midwifery model of care, *J Nurse-Midwifery* 44(4):370-374, 1999.

Rosenblatt RA et al: Interspecialty differences in the obstetrics care of low-risk women, *Am J Public Health* 87:344-351, 1997.

Schlenzka P: *Safety of alternative approaches to childbirth,* PhD dissertation, Palo Alto, Calif, 1999, Stanford University.

Singleton JK, Green-Hernandez C: Interdisciplinary education and practice—has its time come? *J Nurse-Midwifery* 43(1):3-7, 1998.

Appendix A

Repairing Lacerations and Episiotomies

WOUND HEALING

When tissue has been traumatized, healing occurs in three phases:

Phase 1: Immediately after injury, an inflammatory response causes increased blood flow to the area, an increase in fluid in the tissues, and an accumulation of leukocytes and fibrocysts. The leukocytes produce proteolytic enzymes that dissolve and remove injured tissue.

Phase 2: After the first several days following the injury, the fibroblasts form collagen fibers at the site of the injury.

Phase 3: Ultimately enough collagen is laid down in the damaged tissue to produce a closed, healed would.

The healing process is influenced by age, weight, nutritional status, dehydration, adequacy of blood supply to the affected area, and the individual's own immune status (Ethicon, 1994, No. 1). Some general principles to remember are:

1. Maintenance of sterile aseptic technique is essential in decreasing the risk for infection.
2. Establishment of hemostasis before repairing the laceration/epiosiotomy is essential for good visualization and prevention of hematoma formation.
3. Minimal handling of the injured tissue prevents further damage that may inhibit healing.
4. Wound edges must be well approximated to prevent dead space that would promote the growth of anaerobic bacteria.
5. Sutures should have enough tension to approximate tissue but not be so tight that they "pull" when the natural inflammatory response causes tissue edema.

Suture material used in laceration/episiotomy repair holds the wound edges together temporarily until sufficient collagen formation has occurred. Natural absorbable sutures are digested by proteolytic enzymes. Synthetic absorbable sutures are broken down by absorption of water that weakens the suture's polymer chain. It is thought that the hydrolyzation produces less inflammatory response that the enzyme-mediated response (Ethicon, 1994, No. 1).

The most commonly used natural absorbable suture is chromic gut, which retains its strength for 10 to 14 days before enzyme activity begins breaking it down. Complete absorption usually occurs by 90 days after suturing. The most commonly used synthetic absorbable suture is polyglatin 910 (Vicryl) which retains about 65% of its initial strength by 14 days after suturing and is usually completely absorbed by 70 days after the procedure.

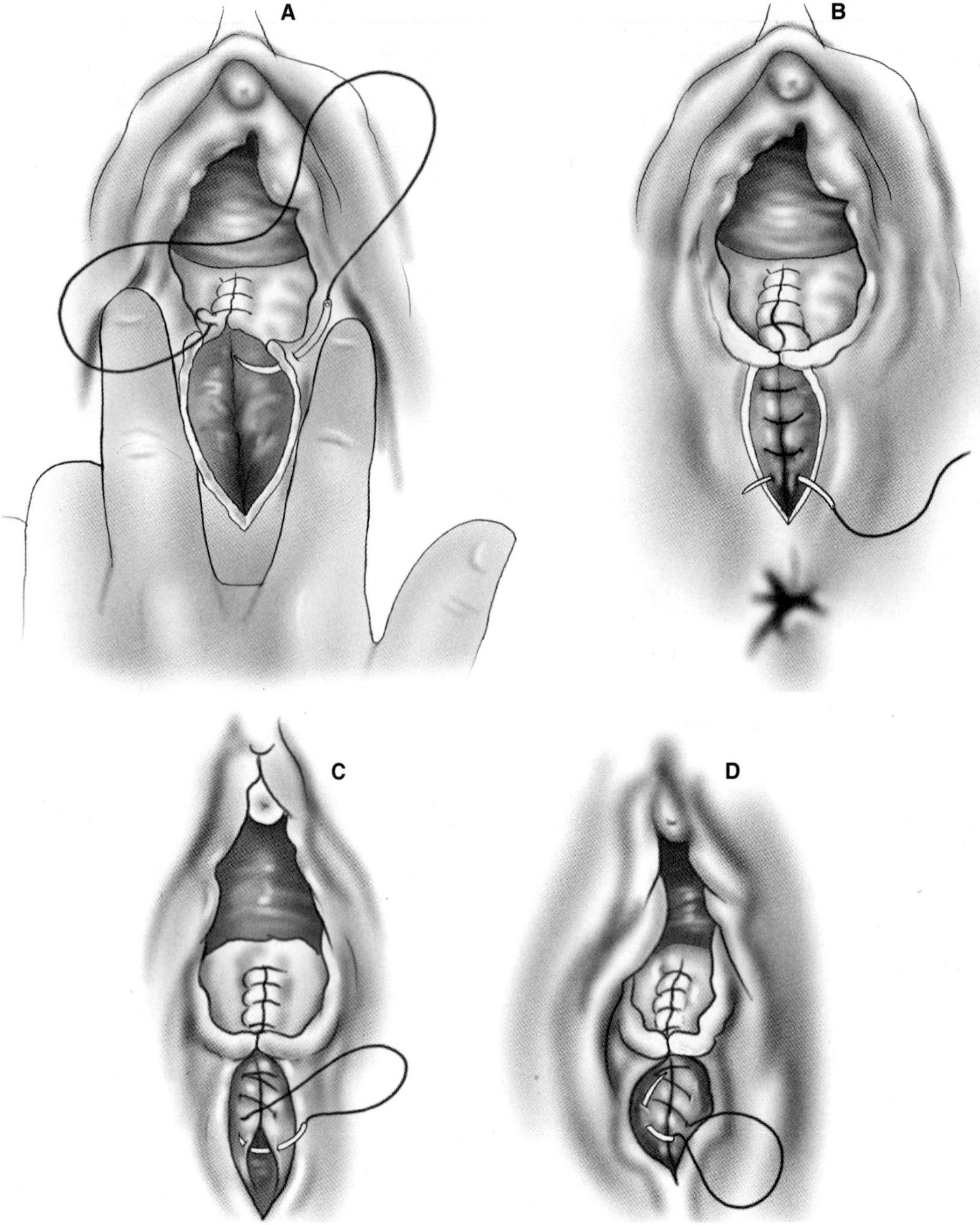

Figure A-1 Repair of median epi¶¶siotomy. **A,** Chromic 2-0 or 3-0 suture is used as a continuous suture to close the vaginal mucosa and submucosa. **B,** After closing the vaginal incision and reapproximating the cut margins of the hymenal ring, the suture is tied and cut. Next, three or four interrupted sutures of 2-0 or 3-0 chromic are placed in the fascia and muscle of the incised perineum, **C,** As continuous suture is carried downward to unite the superficial fascia. **D,** Completion of repair. The continuous suture is carried upward as a subcuticular stitch.

The diameter of the suture used in perineal repair is described using 0s. As the number of 0s increases, the diameter of the suture decreases. The most common sizes used in repairing trauma from birth are 2-0, 3-0 and 4-0, with 4-0 being the thinnest. The suture used in obstetric repair is swaged onto a needle, and almost all repairs will use a ½ circle taper point needle. Taper points pierce tissue without cutting it.

Repair of First-Degree Lacerations

First-degree lacerations involve only the skin and mucosa. They can be small superficial injuries that look more like abrations ("skid marks") or longer superficial tears. When they are less than 1 cm and are not bleeding, they usually do not need to be repaired. Essentially all first-degree lacerations heal spontaneously, usually with well-approximated edges. However, because first-degree lacerations on the vulvar may be quite painful during voiding, clinicians offer women the option of suturing to decrease discomfort.

Small labial and periurethral tears can be repaired using a 4-0 suture placed either as interrupted stitches or in a running subcuticular stitch (see below). If only one or two stitches are placed, they can usually be done without injecting local anesthesia. Spraying a local anesthetic agent over the area (using a syringe without the needle) provide adequate anesthesia for minimal repairs.

Repair of Second-Degree Lacerations and Episiotomies

Second-degree lacerations and episiotomies involve the skin, mucosa, and underlying muscle. To maintain a clear field, many clinicians place a moistened gauze pack into the vagina before beginning the repair. After ensuring adequate anesthesia, a 3-0 suture is first anchored using a square knot approximately 1 cm above the apex of the wound. This initial knot not only "anchors" the suture to healthy tissue but also compresses retracted ends of blood vessels, thereby decreasing bleeding. A continuous interlocking stitch ("locked blanket stitch") is used to close the vaginal mucosa (Figure A-1, *A*). When the mucocutaneous junction is reached, a small, downward stitch is placed, exiting the subcutaneous plane of the perineal aspect of the laceration/episiotomy. Care should be taken not to place the suture in the hymenal tags. When the laceration/episiotomy is deep, several deep interrupted stitches are placed to ensure that there is no dead space in the wound (Figure A-1, *B*). A 2-0 or 3-0 suture can be used for interrupted sutures. The 3-0 suture used to close the vaginal mucosa can then be used to continue closing the subcutaneous perineal layer, using a continuous running (noninterlocking) stitch (Figure A-1, *C*). At the apex of the perineal laceration the last stitch brings the needle to the subcuticular layer. A continuous running stitch is then used to approximate the subcuticular layer, ending at the mucocutaneous junction (Figure A-1, *D*). A final stitch is taken to create the knot to complete the repair. Once complete, the vaginal packing is removed, and the area is inspected to confirm adequate repair and hemostasis. A gentle rectal examination should be done to ensure that no stitches have penetrated the rectal wall.

Repair of Third and Fourth-Degree Lacerations

Third-degree lacerations involve anal and sphincter damage, and fourth-degree lacerations involve injury to the rectal wall. Although fourth-degree lacerations are almost always associated with sphincter damage, occasionally rectal wall injury can occur with an intact sphincter. Third- and fourth-degree lacerations require meticulous repair to preserve continence and prevent rectovaginal fistulas. In most settings, third- and fourth-degree lacerations must be repaired by a physician. However, when state regulations and practice guidelines allow midwives to do these repairs, the following should be kept in mind:

1. The torn edges of the sphincter are usually retracted and difficult to see. Once they are identified, an Allis clamp can be used to hold the torn ends. The ends are brought together using several interrupted 0-suture stitches. The capsule is then closed with three to four interrupted stitches.
2. Rectal mucosa is repaired using a 3-0 suture placed as interrupted stitches in the submucosa, approximately 0.5 cm apart. A second layer of interrupted sutures is then placed in the layer of the superficial fascia.
3. Once the rectal and sphincter tissue are repaired, the gloves should be changed to prevent contamination of the perineal repair.

Reference

Wound closure manual, Ethicon, 1994, Johnson & Johnson.

Index

t, tables; *f*, figures; *b*, boxes

M

Q

R

S